NURSING
Solved Question Papers for General Nursing and Midwifery—3rd Year (2019–2010)

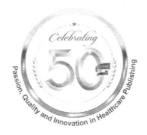

NURSING
Solved Question Papers for General Nursing and Midwifery—3rd Year (2019–2010)

(As per INC Revised Syllabus)

Fourth Edition

I Clement
Doctor of Philosophy in Nursing (PhD)
MSc Nursing (Medical Surgical Nursing)
MA (Sociology) MA (Child Care and Education)
Postgraduate Diploma in Hospital Administration

Professor and Principal
Head, Department of Medical Surgical Nursing
Columbia College of Nursing
Bengaluru, Karnataka, India

JAYPEE BROTHERS MEDICAL PUBLISHERS
The Health Sciences Publisher
New Delhi | London | Panama

Jaypee Brothers Medical Publishers (P) Ltd

Headquarters
Jaypee Brothers Medical Publishers (P) Ltd
4838/24, Ansari Road, Daryaganj
New Delhi 110 002, India
Phone: +91-11-43574357
Fax: +91-11-43574314
Email: jaypee@jaypeebrothers.com

Overseas Offices

J.P. Medical Ltd
83 Victoria Street, London
SW1H 0HW (UK)
Phone: +44 20 3170 8910
Fax: +44 (0)20 3008 6180
Email: info@jpmedpub.com

Jaypee-Highlights Medical Publishers Inc
City of Knowledge, Bld. 235, 2nd Floor
Clayton, Panama City, Panama
Phone: +1 507-301-0496
Fax: +1 507-301-0499
Email: cservice@jphmedical.com

Jaypee Brothers Medical Publishers (P) Ltd
Bhotahity, Kathmandu, Nepal
Phone: +977-9741283608
Email: kathmandu@jaypeebrothers.com

Website: www.jaypeebrothers.com
Website: www.jaypeedigital.com

© 2019, Jaypee Brothers Medical Publishers

The views and opinions expressed in this book are solely those of the original contributor(s)/author(s) and do not necessarily represent those of editor(s) of the book.

All rights reserved. No part of this publication may be reproduced, stored or transmitted in any form or by any means, electronic, mechanical, photocopying, recording or otherwise, without the prior permission in writing of the publishers.

All brand names and product names used in this book are trade names, service marks, trademarks or registered trademarks of their respective owners. The publisher is not associated with any product or vendor mentioned in this book.

Medical knowledge and practice change constantly. This book is designed to provide accurate, authoritative information about the subject matter in question. However, readers are advised to check the most current information available on procedures included and check information from the manufacturer of each product to be administered, to verify the recommended dose, formula, method and duration of administration, adverse effects and contraindications. It is the responsibility of the practitioner to take all appropriate safety precautions. Neither the publisher nor the author(s)/editor(s) assume any liability for any injury and/or damage to persons or property arising from or related to use of material in this book.

This book is sold on the understanding that the publisher is not engaged in providing professional medical services. If such advice or services are required, the services of a competent medical professional should be sought.

Every effort has been made where necessary to contact holders of copyright to obtain permission to reproduce copyright material. If any have been inadvertently overlooked, the publisher will be pleased to make the necessary arrangements at the first opportunity. The **CD/DVD-ROM** (if any) provided in the sealed envelope with this book is complimentary and free of cost. **Not meant for sale**.

Inquiries for bulk sales may be solicited at: jaypee@jaypeebrothers.com

Nursing: Solved Question Papers for General Nursing and Midwifery—3rd Year (2019–2010)

First Edition: 2010
Second Edition: 2015
Third Edition: 2017
Fourth Edition: **2019**

ISBN: 978-93-88958-80-6

Printed at Nutech Print Services - India

Preface to the Fourth Edition

It gives me immense pleasure to draft *Nursing Solved Question Papers for General Nursing and Midwifery Third Year (2019–2010)*, fourth edition. This solved question paper includes three sections—Section-1: Midwifery and Gynecological Nursing, Section-2: Pediatric Nursing, Section-3: Community Health Nursing. It has 10 years solved question papers from 2010–2019, entire contents are based on the syllabus recommended by Indian Nursing Council (INC). All the subjects in third year are covered, each questions are framed carefully with appropriate answer with needed diagrams. The entire contents are revised and reframed with recent answers. This solved question papers will help the students to prepare and present well in examination.

I Clement

Preface to the First Edition

Nursing practices and education have become challenging for today's nursing students. They need to keep pace with the fastly developed and developing technological advancement applied in provision of health care. The requirements imposed in the latest curriculum are highly standard and need more hard work from students part. Examination is the platform that determines the fate and the destiny for any student, marks that they obtain talks on behalf of them whatever they practice nurse. The first impression, they give during the interview during the requirement, acquiring good marks becomes essential, and it is an important responsibility for each student. So, keeping this in mind, twelve years solved question papers and answer book for general nursing and midwifery is prepared.

This book is student-friendly; each question paper is thoroughly examined, answers are solved quite intelligently, depicted in easy languages. This 3rd year solved question papers and answer book will definitely help the student not only to score pass marks but with high scores. Each student will gain the idea of how to present the paper during the examination; guidelines for how to write the examinations are given in this book. All the GNM students can go through and get prepared for these examinations and score good marks.

I wish all the best for the succes in your examination.

I Clement

Contents

Section 1: Midwifery and Gynecological Nursing

1. Paper-2019 (February) 1
2. Paper-2018 13
3. Paper-2017 29
4. Paper-2016 44
5. Paper-2015 69
6. Paper-2014 90
7. Paper-2013 105
8. Paper-2012 128
9. Paper-2011 145
10. Paper-2010 162

Section 2: Pediatric Nursing

1. Paper-2019 183
2. Paper-2018 194
3. Paper-2017 212
4. Paper-2016 227
5. Paper-2015 250
6. Paper-2014 267
7. Paper-2013 286
8. Paper-2012 302
9. Paper-2011 318
10. Paper-2010 (August) 330
11. Paper-2010 (February) 349

Section 3: Community Health Nursing

1. Paper-2019 369
2. Paper-2018 377
3. Paper-2017 391
4. Paper-2016 406
5. Paper-2015 423
6. Paper-2014 448

7. Paper-2013 470
8. Paper-2012 490
9. Paper-2011 506
10. Paper-2010 520

General Nursing and Midwifery Third Year

Hours of instruction

Sl. No.	Subjects	Theory (hours)	Practical (hours)
1	Midwifery and Gynecological Nursing	120	756
2	Community Health Nursing-II	100	216
3	Pediatric Nursing	70	288
	Total	290	1260

Examination scheme

Sl. No.	Subjects	Total marks	Internal assessment	Board examination	Duration of examination
1.	Midwifery and Gynecological Nursing	100	25	75	3
2.	Pediatric Nursing	100	25	75	3
3.	Community Health Nursing-II	100	25	75	3
	Practical				
1.	Pediatric Nursing	100	25	75	
2.	Midwifery and Gynecological Nursing	100	25	75	
3.	Community Health Nursing-II	100	25	75	

Community Health Nursing

Hours: **100**

Course Description

This course is designed to help the students gain in-depth knowledge of community health and community health nursing services. On completion of this course, the students will be able to function at the first level in various community health settings both in urban and rural areas.

General Objectives

Upon completion of this course, the students will be able to:
1. Describe health system and healthcare services in India.
2. Identify major health problems, national health program and specialized community health services.
3. Explain the concept of health team and describe the nurse's role at various levels of healthcare settings.
4. Describe the demographic concept and family welfare program.
    - Explain and motivate use of birth control methods to the community.
5. State the importance of health statistics.
6. Maintain records and reports required in community health nursing services.
7. Demonstrate skills in rendering effective nursing care in all community health settings.

Course Content

Unit-I: Health System in India (Organizational set-up)
1. Central level
2. State level
3. District level
4. Block and local level.

Unit-II: Healthcare Services in India
1. Healthcare concept and trends
2. Healthcare delivery system
3. Public sector: Rural areas, urban areas, health insurance, scheme, other agencies (defense, railways, etc.)
4. Voluntary health agencies
5. Indigenous system of medicine
6. Nurse's role in healthcare services.

Unit-III: Health Planning in India
1. National Health Policy
2. National Health Planning

3. Five Year Plan
4. Health Committees and Reports.

Unit-IV: Specialized Community Health Services and Nurse's Role
1. Maternal and child health (MCH): Reproductive health and child care
2. School health services
3. Industrial nursing
4. Geriatric nursing
5. Care of the handicapped: Physically and mentally challenged
6. Rehabilitation nursing.

Unit-V: Nurse's Role in National Health Program
1. Major health problems in India
2. National control and development program
3. National eradication program
4. Nurse's role in national health program.

Unit-VI: Demography and Family Welfare Demography
1. Concept of demography and family welfare
2. Trends in India and its implications
3. Concept of fertility and infertility
4. Small family norms
5. Concept of family welfare
6. Importance of family welfare
7. Aims and objectives
8. Family planning methods
9. Family welfare policy
10. National program
11. Nurse's role in family welfare program.

Unit-VII: Health Team
1. Concept
2. Composition
3. Functions.

Role of nursing personnel at various levels
1. Multipurpose health worker: Male and female
2. Lady health visitor/health supervisor
3. Public health nurse
4. Public health nurse supervisor
5. District public health nursing officer.

Unit-VIII: Vital Health Statistics
1. Concept
2. Uses
3. Sources
4. Important rates and indices
5. Vital health records and their utility.

Pediatric Nursing

Hours: **70**

Course Description

This course is designed to help the students develop and understanding of the concept of child health, the trends in child care and the health problems of children. This will enable the students to meet the needs of the children in health and sickness.

General Objectives

Upon completion of this course, the students will be able to:
1. Explain the concept of child health, the principles underlying child care and trends in pediatric nursing.
2. Describe normal growth and development of children, so as to recognize deviation(s) from normal health.
3. Demonstrate skill in meeting the needs of the sick as well as healthy children.

Course Content

Unit-I: Introduction

1. Concept in childhealth care
2. Trends in pediatric nursing
3. Role of pediatric nurse in child care
4. Child care in India
5. Emerging challenges, nursing process related to pediatric nursing
6. Concept of preventive pediatrics
7. Vital statistics.

Unit-II: The Newborn

A. Characteristics of newborn and physiological status of the newborn:
    1. Assessment of the newborn: Head to toe assessment (physical assessment), neurological assessment.
    2. Nursing care of the normal/healthy newborn including home care.
    3. Breastfeeding concept of baby-friendly hospital initiative.
B. Common health problems—medical and nursing management of:
    1. Hyperbilirubinemia, hemolytic disorder, neonatal hypoglycemia, sepsis, oral thrush, impetigo, erythema, toxemia, hypothermia, neonatal conclusions.
    2. Birth injuries: Injuries of muscles and peripheral nerves, injuries of bone, soft tissue injury and injury of nervous system.
C. High-risk newborn:
    1. Definition: Small for dates, low-birth weight.
    2. Common health problems of pre-term, post-term and low-birth weight infants and their nursing management.

3. High risk to newborn of HIV-positive mother, diabetic mother, its medical and nursing care.

Unit-III: The Healthy Child

Growth and development: Definition, principles, factors affecting growth and development, techniques of assessment of growth and development, importance of learning about growth and development.

a. **The infant:** Growth and development during infancy.
b. **Health promotion during infant**
   - Nutrition counseling and weaning, immunization
   - Safety and security including prevention of accidents, play and toys.
c. **The toddler**
   - Growth and development of toddler
   - Health promotion during toddlerhood, nutrition counseling, toilet training, immunization, safety and prevention of accidents, guidance to parent on toddler's care, play and toys.
d. **The pre-schooler**
   - Growth and development during pre-school years
   - Health promotion during pre-school years, nutritional guidance, safety and security, day care centers/nursery school, play, role of parents in sex education of child.
e. **The school age**
   - Physical, psychological and moral development during school age years
   - Health promotion during school years, nutritional guidance, sleep and rest, physical exercise and activity, dental health, sex education, play, role of parents in reproductive child health.
f. **The adolescent**
   - Physical changes, physiological and reproductive changes, reaction of adolescents to puberty
   - Health promotion during adolescence
   - Nutritional guidance, personal care, reproductive health/sex education, role of parents in health promotion of adolescents.

Unit-IV: Care of Sick Child

1. Child's reaction to hospitalization
2. Effects of hospitalization on the family of the child
3. Role of nurse in helping child and family in coping with stress of hospitalization and illness.

Nursing interventions and adaptations in nursing care of sick child

1. Examination, principles of safety observed in pediatric techniques
2. Preparation of child for diagnostic tests, collection of specimens
3. Calculation and administration of oral and parenteral medications
4. Procedures related to feeding: formula preparation, gavage, gastrostomy feeding
5. Procedures related to elimination: Enema, colostomy irrigation
6. Use of play as nursing intervention
7. Care of child in incubator
8. Administration and analysis of oxygen concentration
9. Surgical dressing
10. Steam tent inhalation
11. Immobilized child
12. Phototherapy.

Unit-V: Behavioral Disorders and Common Health Problems during Childhood, their Prevention, Medical and Nursing Management

a. **Infancy:** Nutritional disturbances, allergies, dermatitis, vomiting, diarrhea, failure to thrive, resistance to feeding, colic, anxiety.
b. **Early childhood:** Communicable diseases, poisoning, tonsillitis, otitis media, urinary tract infections, diarrhea, child abuse, breath holding spells, bed wetting, thumb sucking, nail biting, temper tantrums, masturbation.
c. **Middle childhood:** Helminthic infestations, common skin infections, animal and insect bites, stuttering, pica, tics, antisocial behavior, enuresis.
d. **Later childhood:** Problems of pubertal development: precocious puberty, tall stature, gynecomastia, acne, amenorrhea, dysmenorrhea, sexually transmitted diseases, accidents, sports injuries, juvenile delinquency, anorexia nervosa, obesity.

Unit-VI: Children with Congenital Defects/Malformations

Etiology, signs, symptoms, complications, medical, surgical and nursing management of:
1. Malformations of the central nervous system—cranial deformities, defects of spina bifida, meningocele, hydrocephalus, cerebral palsy, neural tube closure. Skeletal defects—cleft lip and palate.
2. Defects of gastrointestinal tract—esophageal atresia and fistula, anorectal malformations, hernia, congenital hypertrophied pyloric stenosis.
3. Defects of genitourinary tract—hypospadias, epispadias, exstrophy of bladder, phimosis, cryptorchidism, polycystic kidney.
4. Sexual abnormalities—ambiguous genitalia, hermaphroditism.
5. Defects of cardiovascular system—congenital heart diseases, major acyanotic and cyanotic defects.
6. Orthopedic abnormalities—clubfoot, developmental abnormalities of extremities.

Unit-VII: Children with Various Disorders and Diseases

Etiology, signs, symptoms, complications, prevention, medical, surgical and nursing management of:
1. Disturbances of fluid and electrolyte balance: Imbalance, burns, disturbance of renal function, acute and chronic glomerulonephritis, acute and chronic renal failure.
2. Disturbed respiratory functions: Acute infections of upper and lower respiratory tract, acute inflammation of lungs.
3. Gastrointestinal disorders: Malabsorption syndromes (celiac diseases) and obstructive disorders (intestinal obstruction, Hirschsprung's disease) inflammatory conditions (appendicitis, Meckel's diverticulum, ulcerative colitis), worm infestations.
4. Problems related to production and circulation of blood: Acquired heart diseases, congestive cardiac failure, infective endicarditis, and rheumatic fever.
5. Problems related to the elements of blood: Anemia's, sickle cell anemia, and thalassemia, defects of hemostasis, hemophilia, immune deficiency diseases, HIV infection (AIDS), leukemias, thrombocytopenia, and purpura.
6. Disturbances of regulatory mechanism: Disturbances of cerebral functions—altered state of consciousness, craniocerebral trauma.
7. Intracranial infections: Meningitis, encephalitis, convulsive disorders.
8. Endocrine dysfunctions: Disorder of pituitary functions, of thyroid and parathyroid function, disorders of adrenal cortex, disorders of pancreatic hormone secretion.

9. Problems that interfere with locomotion: Poliomyelitis, osteomyelitis, kyphosis, lordosis and scoliosis, rheumatoid arthritis.
10. Children with developmental problems: Handicapped children, multiple handicapped children, mental retardation.
11. Communication disorders—Hearing, vision impairment deaf and blind children.

Unit-VIII: Welfare of Children
1. Child welfare services, agencies Balwadi, Anganwadi Daycare Centers, Midday Meal Program
2. Welfare of delinquent and destitute children
3. Program and policies for welfare of working children
4. National Child Labor Policy
5. Child Act, Juvenile Justice Act
6. Internationally accepted rights of the child.

Midwifery and Gynecological Nursing

Midwifery: **100**
Gynecology: **20**

Course Description

This course is designed to help students acquire knowledge and gain skills to meet the health needs of women during the period of pregnancy, labor and puerperium. The students will be able to identify different gynecological disorders and diseases and gain skills in proving nursing care to women suffering from these disorders and diseases.

General Objectives

Upon completion of this course the students will be able to:
1. Describe the health needs of women in pregnancy, labor and puerperium.
2. Identify deviation(s) from normal pregnancy and take appropriate action.
3. Demonstrate skills in providing antepartum, intrapartum and postpartum care to the mother as well as care to the newborn.
4. List different gynecological problems and demonstrate skills in providing nursing care to women suffering form these disorders and diseases.

Course Content

Unit-I: Introduction
1. Definition: Midwifery, obstetrical nursing
2. Scope
3. Historical review
4. Development of maternity services in India.

Unit-II: Reproductive System
1. Review of genitourinary system of male and female organs structure, physiology
2. Menstrual cycle
3. Internal and external organs of reproduction
4. Female pelvis: Structure, diameters and type.

Unit-III: Embryology and Fetal Development
1. Ovum, sperm, maturation, fertilization and implantation
2. Development of fertilized ovum, morula, blastocyst, embryo
3. Development of placenta: Structure of full-term placenta, functions and abnormalities, anatomical variations
4. Formation of fetal sac, membranes. Amnion and chorion and their functions

5. Formation of liquor amni, its functions and abnormalities
6. Development of umbilical cord: Structure, functions and abnormalities
7. Fetal skull: Diameters, fontanelles, sutures and their importance
8. Fetal circulation.

Unit-IV: Nursing Management of Pregnant Women

1. Reproductive health
2. Genetic counseling
3. Physiological changes in pregnancy
4. Diagnosis of pregnancy: History, signs and symptoms and investigations
5. Influence of hormones
6. Prenatal care: Objectives, history taking, calculation of expected date of delivery, routine examinations
7. Health education: Breast care, diet in pregnancy and antenatal exercises
8. Preparation for hospital/home delivery
9. Immunization: Minor disorders of pregnancy and its management.

Unit-V: Nursing Management of Women in Labor

1. Definition, stage and duration
2. Causes of onset of labor
3. True and false labor
   a. **First Stage of Labor**
      1. Signs of onset of labor
      2. Physiological changes in first stage of labor
      3. Management: Preparation of labor room
      4. Preparation of women in labor: Physical and psychological
      5. Equipments for normal delivery
      6. Care: Physical, psychological, monitoring of maternal and fetal condition
      7. Vaginal examination: Indications, articles, technique.
   b. **Second Stage of Labor**
      1. Signs of second stage
      2. Mechanism of labor
      3. Monitoring of maternal and fetal condition
      4. Physical and psychological care
      5. Procedure for conduct of normal delivery
      6. Prevention of perineal tear
      7. Episiotomy, suturing and care.
   c. **Third Stage of Labor**
      1. Signs, physiological changes
      2. Management: Immediate baby care, technique of placental expulsion, monitoring maternal condition examination of placements and its membranes, blood loss
      3. Immediate postnatal care/fourth stage of labor.
   d. **Conduct of Home Delivery**

Unit-VI: Nursing Management of Baby at Birth

1. Assessment
2. Review of physiology of newborn
3. Apgar scoring, examination for defects (head to foot examination)
4. Infant feeding: Breastfeeding, artificial feeding
5. Care of skin, eyes, cord, buttocks
6. Psychology and perception of newborn
7. Minor disorders of newborn: Birthmarks, rashes, skin infections, sore buttocks, infections of eyes
8. Jaundice of newborn
9. Major disorders: Birth asphyxia, resuscitation measures, hemolytic disease (RH factor)
10. Infections and birth injuries.

Unit-VII: Nursing Management of Mother during Puerperium

1. Definition, objectives of care
2. Immediate postnatal care (care during IV-stage of labor)
3. Physiological changes during puerperium
4. Psychosocial aspects of care
5. Diet during puerperium
6. Establishment of lactation and breast care
7. Perineal care
8. Postnatal exercises
9. Postnatal examination, follow-up, family welfare
10. Minor ailments and its management.

Unit-VIII: Complications of Pregnancy and its Management

1. Bleeding in early pregnancy
2. Bleeding in late pregnancy
3. Pregnancy-induced hypertension, pre-eclampsia, eclampsia
4. Hydramnios, oligohydramnios
5. Hydatidiform mole
6. Pelvic inflammatory diseases
7. Intrauterine growth retardation, intrauterine death
8. Postmaturity.

Unit-IX: High-risk Pregnancy and its Management

1. Concept, factors
2. Anemia, jaundice, viral infections
3. Urinary tract infections, heart diseases, diabetes mellitus, osteomalacia, sexually transmitted diseases, AIDS
4. Teenage pregnancy, elderly primigravida, multipara, multiple pregnancy.

Unit-X: High-risk Labor and its Management

1. Malpositions, malpresentations: Occipitoposterior position face, brow, shoulder and breech presentation
2. Contracted pelvis: Definition, causes, diagnosis, management and trial of labor

3. Abnormal uterine action: Hypotonic and hypertonic action, Bandl's ring contraction, precipitates labor
4. Cervical dystocia
5. Early rupture of membranes, prolonged labor, induction of labor
6. Obstructed labor rupture of uterus
7. Obstetrical emergencies: Cord presentation, cord prolapse, amniotic fluid embolism, obstetric shock
8. Complications of third stage: Postpartum hemorrhage, atonic uterus, retained placenta and membranes, inversion of uterus.

Unit-XI: Complications of Puerperium and its Management

Puerperal pyrexia, puerperal sepsis, thrombophlebitis, embolism, puerperal psychosis.
1. Mastitis, breast abscess.

Unit-XII: Obstetric Operations

2. Manual removal of placenta
3. Version: Internal, external
4. Forceps delivery
5. Vacuum extraction
6. Cesarean section
7. Medical termination of pregnancy
8. Laparoscopic sterilization
9. Embryotomy.

Unit-XIII: Drugs Used in Obstetrics

Unit-XIV: Ethical and Legal Aspects Related to Midwifery and Gynecological Nursing

Gynecological Nursing

Hours: **20**

Course Content

Unit-I: Introduction
1. Definition related to gynecological nursing
2. Sexuality
3. Gynecological history taking, examination and investigations.

Unit-II: Puberty
1. Definition development of sex organs in females
2. Menstrual cycle
3. Disorders of menstruation: Amenorrhea, dysmenorrhea, cryptomenorrhea.

Unit-III: Fertility and Infertility
Definition, causes, investigation and management—both in male and female.

Unit-IV: Pelvic Infections
1. Vulva: Vulvitis, bartholinitis
2. Vagina: Vaginitis, trichomonas vaginalis, moniliasis
3. Metritis, salpingitis, oophoritis, pelvic abscess
4. Chronic infections, cervical erosion.

Unit-V: Uterine Displacement and Descent
1. Retroversion, retroflexion
2. Descent of the uterus: First degree, second degree, completes procidentia.

Unit-VI: Sexually Transmitted Diseases and their Prevention
1. Syphilis, gonorrhea, warts
2. Acquired immunodeficiency syndrome (AIDS)/HIV.

Unit-VII: Breast Disorders
1. Mastitis
2. Breast abscess
3. Tumors
4. Malignancy.

Unit-VIII: Benign and Malignant Neoplasms of Reproductive Organs
1. Uterine polyps, uterine fibroids
2. Cancer: Cervix, uterus
3. Ovarian cyst: Benign, malignant
4. Cancer: Chemotherapy, radiotherapy
5. Palliative care.

MIDWIFERY AND GYNECOLOGICAL NURSING

2019 (February)

Midwifery and Gynecology

SECTION-I

I. Give the meaning for the following:
   a. Menarche.
   b. Meconium.
   c. Puerperium.
   d. Amnion.

II. Fill up the blanks:
   a. Male gonad is _____
   b. Weight of a non-pregnant uterus is _____
   c. _____ suture run between the two parietal bones.
   d. Posterior fontanelle is otherwise known as _____

III. Write short notes on any *four* of the following:
   a. Episiotomy.
   b. Oligohydraminios.
   c. Placenta.
   d. Breast changes during pregnancy.
   e. Phases of lactation.

IV. a. Write about the minor disorders of pregnancy and its management.

V. a. What is Apgar score?
   b. Write the immediate care of full term healthy newborn baby.

SECTION-II

VI. State whether the following statements are *true* or *false*:
   a. One mL of oxytocin ampoule contains 10 units of oxytocin.
   b. Pseudomenstruation is seen in infants.
   c. Mastitis is the inflammatin of the breasts.
   d. Perineal tear occur due to large baby.

VII. Choose the correct answer from the following:
   a. Prophylactic methergine is administered after the delivery of:
      i. Baby   ii. Anterior shoulder   iii. Posterior shoulder
   b. The type of forceps which is applied when the fetal head is at pelvic outlet:
      i. Long curved   ii. Wrigleys   iii. Keilland

c. Painful menstruation is:
   i. Menorrhagia   ii. Dysmenorrhea   iii. Metrorrhagia

VIII. Write short notes on any *three* of the following:
   a. Cord prolapse.
   b. Causes of male infertility.
   c. Puberty.
   d. Syphilis.
   e. Breast engorgement.

IX. a. Defne placenta previa.
   b. List the types of placenta previa.
   c. Explain the management of placenta previa.

X. a. Define puerperal sepsis.
   b. List out the causes and clinical manifestation of puerperal sepsis.
   c. Explain the management of mother with puerperal sepsis.

OR

   a. Define fibroid uterus.
   b. Write the clinical features of fibroid uterus.
   c. Explain the management of fibroid uterus.

SECTION-I

I. Give the meaning for the following:

a. Menarche.

Menarche defined as the time in a girl's life when mensturation first begins. During the menarche period, menstruation may be irregular and unpredictable.

b. Meconium.

Meconium defined as dark, sticky material that is normally present in the intestine at birth and passed in the feces after birth, after trypsin and other enzymes from the pancreas have acted on it. The passage of meconium before birth can be a sign of fetal 'distress.

c. Puerperium.

Puerperium defined as the time immediately after the delivery of a baby. (In Latin a "puerpera" is a woman in childbirth since "puer" means child and "parere" means to give birth.) Puerperal fever is childbirth (or childbed) fever due to an infection usually of the placental site within the uterus. If that infection involves the bloodstream, it constitutes puerperal sepsis.

d. Amnion.

A thin, membranous sac filled with a watery fluid (called the amniotic fluid) in which the embryo or fetus of a reptile, bird, or mammal is suspended during prenatal development. Also called amniotic sac.

II. Fill up the blanks:

a. Male gonad is **Testes**.
b. Weight of a non-pregnant uterus is **60 g**.
c. **Sagittal** suture run between the two parietal bones.
d. Posterior fontanelle is otherwise known as **Lambdoid**.

III. Write short notes on any *four* of the following:

a. Episiotomy. (2016-III.a)

b. Oligohydramnios.

Oligohydramnios refers to a low level of amniotic fluid during pregnancy. It is defined by an amniotic fluid index that is below the 5th centile for the gestational age, and is thought to affect approximately 4.5% of term pregnancies.

Causes of oligohydramnios include the following:
The main causes of oligohydramnios are:
1. Preterm prelabor rupture of membranes.
2. Placental insufficiency – resulting in the blood flow being redistributed to the fetal brain rather than the abdomen and kidneys. This causes poor urine output.
3. Renal agenesis (known as Potter's syndrome).
4. Non-functioning fetal kidneys, e.g. bilateral multicystic dysplastic kidneys.
5. Obstructive uropathy.

6. Genetic/chromosomal anomalies.
7. Viral infections (although may also cause polyhydramnios).

Signs and symptoms: The common clinical features are smaller symphysio-fundal height, fetal malpresentation, undue prominence of fetal parts and reduced amount of amniotic fluid.

Treatment: The goal of treatment is to keep you pregnant for as long as it's safe. Treatment may also make you more comfortable. Treatment will depend on the symptoms, pregnancy, and general health.

c. Placenta. (2014-IV.c)
d. Breast changes during pregnancy.

Breast changes are a normal part of pregnancy and occur as a result of hormonal fluctuations. Changes to the breasts can occur as early as 1 week after conception, and they can continue right up until the birth of the baby and beyond.

First trimester breast changes: During weeks 0 to 13 of pregnancy, women may experience:
- **Tenderness and discomfort:** These changes occur because of rising hormone levels in the body and increased blood flow to the breast tissue. Breast discomfort often subsides after a few weeks, although it may return in the later stages of pregnancy.
- **Enlargement:** Going up a cup size or two when pregnant is normal for many women, especially if it is their first pregnancy.
- **Blue veins:** Prominent blue veins usually appear on several areas of the skin, including the breasts and stomach.

Second trimester: From weeks 14 to 27, the second trimester of pregnancy may bring about the following breast changes:
- **Darker areolas:** The areolas are the colored circles around the nipples. Over the course of the second and third trimesters, the areolas often become larger and darker.
- **Areola bumps:** Pregnancy causes small, painless bumps to appear on the areolas. These are oil-producing glands called Montgomery's tubercles, and they lubricate the breasts and promote easier breastfeeding.
- **Nipple discharge:** Some women may notice nipple discharge during their second trimester. For others, this may not occur until the third trimester or after labor. Discharge can occur at any time, but it is more likely when the breasts become stimulated.

Third trimester: Weeks 28 to 40 of pregnancy can lead to the following breast changes:
- **Continuing growth and other changes:** Many of the breast changes that occur in the first and second trimesters will continue throughout the final months of pregnancy.
- **Stretch marks:** Rapid tissue growth causes the skin to stretch, which may lead to striae gravidarum, or stretch marks.

e. Phases of lactation.

Stages of lactogenesis, phases of lactogenesis, breast changes that occur during the phase:

Lactogenesis I: This phase begins around week 16 in pregnancy and is the stage in which colostrum begins to be created.

Lactogenesis II: In this phase the secretion of copious milk follows the hormonal shift triggered by birth and the placenta delivery and typically occurs around day 4 postpartum.

Lactogenesis III: This phase is when the milk supply is maintained via autocrine control from around day 10 postpartum until weaning begins.

Lactogenesis IV: This phase marks breast involution, the process of decreased milk production by apoptosis of the milk-making epithelial cells.

IV. a. Write about the minor disorders of pregnancy and its management. (2014-III.e)

V. a. What is Apgar score? (2015-III.a)
   b. Write the immediate care of full term healthy newborn baby.

Immediate care: Directly after birth there should be attention to the condition of the newborn.
1. Drying the baby with warm towels or cloths, while being placed on the mother's abdomen or in her arms. This mother-child skin-to-skin contact is important to maintain the baby's temperature, encourage bonding and expose the baby to the mother's skin bacteria.
2. Ensuring that the airway is clear, removing mucus and other material from the mouth, nose and throat with a suction pump.
3. Taking measures to maintain body temperature, to ensure no metabolic problems associated with exposure to the cold arise.
4. Clamping and cutting the umbilical cord with sterile instruments, thoroughly decontaminated by sterilization. This is of utmost importance for the prevention of infections.
5. A few drops of silver nitrate solution or an antibiotic is usually placed into the eyes to prevent infection from any harmful organisms that the baby may have had contact with during delivery (e.g. maternal STDs).
6. Vitamin K is also administered to prevent hemorrhagic disease of the newborn.
7. The baby's overall condition is recorded at 1 minute and at 5 minutes after birth using the Apgar Scale.
8. Putting the baby to the breast as early as possible. Early suckling/breastfeeding should be encouraged within the first hour after birth and of nipple stimulation by the baby may influence uterine contractions and postpartum blood loss but according to the WHO, this should be investigated.
9. About 6 hours or so after birth, the baby is bathed, but the vernix caseosa (whitish greasy material that covers most of the newborn's skin) is tried to be preserved, as it helps protect against infection.

Late care:
Skin-to-skin contact: After a normal vaginal birth, your newborn baby will be put on your chest for skin-to-skin contact. The baby needs sleep and food, and they need to feel secure and warm, so they need to feel skin.

Doing this simple thing:
1. Reduces newborn crying
2. Helps start and sustain breastfeeding
3. Helps maintain your baby's body temperature
   After this first contact, they will be weighed, measured and observed to make sure they are healthy.

Weighing and measuring: After skin-to-skin contact and the first breastfeed, the midwife might offer to weigh the baby, and measure the baby's length and head circumference. The baby doesn't need to be washed for at least 24 hours.

Vitamin K: At the time of weighing, your midwife will also offer to give the baby a vitamin K injection to prevent bleeding from vitamin K deficiency.

Cord blood collection if you are Rh-negative: If the blood group is Rh-negative, some blood will be taken from the umbilical cord to determine whether your baby's blood group is compatible.

Feeding: Babies start to show signs of wanting to feed soon after birth and usually attach and suck at the breast about 50 minutes after birth. They may then breastfeed for an hour or more. Put your baby against your chest, and they will probably find your breast and start feeding. If that doesn't happen, you can ask your midwife or a lactation consultant for help. The first milk you make is called 'colostrum'. It is thick and often yellowish, rather than pure white. It is the ideal milk for your baby. Normally a small amount is produced—your baby's tummy is just the size of a marble.

Sleeping: The baby will stay with you so you can bond and respond easily to their needs. They will probably sleep soon after their first feed, and that might last 6 hours or so. They will probably sleep for more than half of their first day in the world.

Apgar scores: One of the main observations made after birth is called an Apgar score. It assesses your baby's adjustment to life outside the womb. The Apgar score is measured at 1 minute and 5 minutes after birth while the baby is on your chest. Sometimes it is measured again at 10 minutes after birth.

It records your baby's heart rate, breathing, color, muscle tone and reflexes. The maximum score is 10. A score of 7 or above usually means your baby is doing well. It is not an ability or intelligence test, and it does not predict your baby's health later in life.

Urine and meconium: Within the first 24 hours your baby will probably pass urine and meconium (newborn faeces) at least once. Meconium is black and sticky.

SECTION-II

VI. State whether the following statements are *true* or *false*:
a. One mL of oxytocin ampoule contains 10 units of oxytocin: **TRUE**
b. Pseudomenstruation is seen in infants: **FALSE**
c. Mastitis is the inflammatin of the breasts: **TRUE**
d. Perineal tear occur due to large baby: **TRUE**

VII. Choose the correct answer from the following:
a. Prophylactic methergine is administered after the delivery of:
   i. Baby   ii. Anterior shoulder   iii. Posterior shoulder
   Ans: i. Baby
b. The type of forceps which is applied when the fetal head is at pelvic outlet:
   i. Long curved   ii. Wrigleys   iii. Keilland
   Ans: ii. Wrigleys
c. Painful menstruation is:
   i. Menorrhagia   ii. Dysmenorrhea   iii. Metrorrhagia
   Ans: ii. Dysmenorrhea

VIII. Write short notes on any *three* of the following:
a. Cord prolapse.
Umbilical cord prolapse is where the umbilical cord descends through the cervix, with (or before) the presenting part of the fetus. It affects 0.1–0.6% of births.

Cord prolapse occurs in the presence of ruptured membranes, and is either occult or overt:
1. **Occult (incomplete) cord prolapse**—the umbilical cord descends alongside the presenting part, but not beyond it.
2. **Overt (complete) cord prolapse**—the umbilical cord descends past the presenting part and is lower than the presenting part in the pelvis.
3. **Cord presentation**—the presence of the umbilical cord between the presenting part and the cervix. This can occur with or without intact membranes.
   Although the incidence is relatively low, the mortality rate for such babies is high (~91 per 1000). This is largely because cord prolapse occurs more frequently in preterm babies, who are often breech, and who may also have other congenital defects.

Pathophysiology: Umbilical cord prolapse is where the umbilical cord descends through the cervix, with (or before) the presenting part of the fetus. Subsequently, **fetal hypoxia** occurs via two main mechanisms:
1. **Occlusion:** The presenting part of the fetus presses onto the umbilical cord, occluding blood flow to the fetus.
2. **Arterial vasospasm:** The exposure of the umbilical cord to the cold atmosphere results in umbilical arterial vasospasm, reducing blood flow to the fetus.

Management

Firstly, call for help—umbilical cord prolapse is an **obstetric emergency**. It should be managed as follows:
1. **Avoid handling the cord** to reduce vasospasm.
2. **Manually elevate the presenting part** by lifting the presenting part of the cord by vaginal digital examination. Alternatively, if in the community, fill the maternal bladder with 500 mL of normal saline (warmed if possible) via a urinary catheter and arrange immediate hospital transfer.

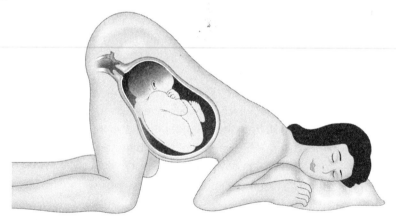

3. **Encourage into left lateral position** with head down and pillow placed under left hip OR knee-chest position. This will relieve pressure off the cord from the presenting part.
4. **Consider tocolysis (e.g. terbutaline):** If delivery is not imminently available this will relax the uterus and stop contractions, relieving pressure off the cord. It may be sufficient to allow enough time for transfer to a location where delivery is feasible (e.g. an operating theater for a cesarean section). This is a particularly useful strategy if there are fetal heart rate abnormalities while preparing for a C-section.

5. **Delivery is usually via emergency cesarean section:**
   a. If fully dilated and vaginal delivery appears imminent, encourage pushing or consider instrumental delivery.
   b. If at threshold for viability (23 + 0 weeks – 24 + 6 weeks) and extreme prematurity, expectant management may be discussed due to significant maternal morbidity with cesarean at this gestation and poor fetal outcomes.

b. Causes of male infertility.

1. **Abnormal sperm production or function:** Due to undescended testicles, genetic defects, health problems such as diabetes or infections, such as chlamydia, gonorrhea, mumps or HIV. Enlarged veins in the testes (varicocele) can also affect the quality of sperm.
2. **Problems with the delivery of sperm:** Due to sexual problems, such as premature ejaculation; certain genetic diseases, such as cystic fibrosis; structural problems, such as a blockage in the testicle; or damage or injury to the reproductive organs.
3. **Overexposure to certain environmental factors:** Cigarette smoking, alcohol, marijuana or taking certain medications, such as select antibiotics, antihypertensive, anabolic steroids or others, can also affect fertility. Frequent exposure to heat, such as in saunas or hot tubs, can raise the core body temperature and may affect sperm production.
4. **Damage related to cancer and its treatment:** Treatment for cancer can impair sperm production, sometimes severely.

c. Puberty.

Puberty is the term used to describe the developmental changes a child undergoes to become sexually mature and physiologically ready for reproduction. It normally begins between the ages of 8 to 14 in females and between the ages of 10 to 16 in males. In this article, we will discuss the hormonal and physical changes that occur during puberty in boys and girls and its clinical relevance.

Hormonal changes: Puberty and the reproductive system are controlled by the hormones of the Hypothalamic-pituitary-gonadal (HPG) axis. The hypothalamus releases gonadotrophin releasing hormone (GnRH) in a pulsatile manner, which stimulates the release of follicle stimulating hormone (FSH) and luteinizing hormone (LH) from the anterior pituitary gland.

Precocious puberty is defined as the appearance of secondary sexual characteristics before the age of 8 in girls or before the age of 9 in boys. There are a variety of causes/types:

1. **Iatrogenic:** This occurs as a result of exposure to exogenous estrogens, e.g. via creams or lotions, etc.
2. **True/complete:** Due to early maturation of the HPG axis resulting in high levels of GnRH, FSH and LH. This may be due to CNS lesions near or in the posterior hypothalamus, CNS neoplasms, hamartomas, primary hypothyroidism.
3. **Incomplete:** Due to increased levels of estrogens in girls and androgens in boys that are independent of GnRH.

Precocious puberty may either be isosexual (early sexual development consistent with the genetic and gonadal sex of the child) or contrasexual (early sexual development associated with feminisation of a male or virilisation of a female).

d. Syphilis.

Syphilis is a sexually transmitted infection caused by the spirochete gram-negative bacterium *Treponema pallidum* subspecies *pallidum*. Other subspecies of Treponemes are responsible for non-sexually transmitted diseases, such as Bejel, a chronic skin and tissue disease, Yaws, a disease of the bones and joints, and Pinta, a skin disease. Unlike syphilis, these diseases are transmitted by any close contact (sexual or not) and do not pass from mother to fetus.

Risk factors
1. Engaging in unprotected sex—especially with high risk partners.
2. Multiple sexual partners.
3. Men who have sex with men (MSM).
4. HIV infection.

Clinical features: Syphilis is divided into congenital and acquired. Acquired syphilis is further divided into early (2 years since infection). Acquired syphilis can be asymptomatic (latent) or symptomatic, which can be primary, secondary or tertiary (cardiovascular, neurological or gummatous).

Management: Penicillin is the treatment of choice. Patients with penicillin allergy should be considered for desensitisation. As *Treponema pallidum* subspecies *pallidum* replicates slowly, prolonged courses of antibiotics are required for late disease.

e. Breast engorgement.

Breast engorgement means your breasts are painfully overfull of milk. This usually occurs when a mother makes more milk than her baby uses. Your breasts may become firm and swollen, which can make it hard for your baby to breastfeed. Engorged breasts can be treated at home.

Symptoms of engorged breasts include:
1. Swollen, firm, and painful breasts. If the breasts are severely engorged, they are very swollen, hard, shiny, warm, and slightly lumpy to the touch.
2. Flattened nipples. The dark area around the nipple, the areola, may be very firm. This makes it hard for your baby to latch on.
3. A slight fever of around 100.4°F (38°C).
4. Slightly swollen and tender lymph nodes in your armpits.

IX. a. Defne placenta previa.

Placenta previa is where the placenta is fully or partially attached to the lower uterine segment. It is an important cause of antepartum hemorrhage—vaginal bleeding from week 24 of gestation until delivery.

Placenta previa is a problem of pregnancy in which the placenta grows in the lowest part of the womb (uterus) and covers all or part of the opening to the cervix. The placenta grows during pregnancy and feeds the developing baby. The cervix is the opening to the birth canal.

b. List the types of placenta previa.

The types of placenta previa include:
1. Complete placenta previa occurs when the placenta completely covers the opening from the womb to the cervix.
2. Partial placenta previa occurs when the placenta partially covers the cervical opening

3. Marginal placenta previa occurs when the placenta is located adjacent to, but not covering, the cervical opening.

c. Explain the management of placenta previa.

Any woman presenting with a significant antepartum hemorrhage should be resuscitated using an ABCDE approach. Do not delay maternal resuscitation in order to determine fetal viability.

Placenta previa may be identified in an asymptomatic patient at their 20-week ultrasound scan:
1. Placenta previa minor—a repeat scan at 36 weeks is recommended, as the placenta is likely to have moved superiorly.
2. Placenta previa major—a repeat scan at 32 weeks is recommended, and a plan for delivery should be made at this time.

    In cases of confirmed placenta previa, Cesarean section is the safest mode of delivery. Placenta previa major usually warrants an elective Cesarean section at 38 weeks.

    In all cases of antepartum hemorrhage, give anti-D within 72 hours of the onset of bleeding if the woman is rhesus D negative.

X. a. Define puerperal sepsis.

Puerperal sepsis was defined as infection of the genital tract occurring at any time between the onset of rupture of membranes or labor, and the 42nd day postpartum in which two or more of the following are present:
1. Pelvic pain.
2. Fever, i.e. oral temperature 38.5°C/101.3°F or higher on any occasion.
3. Abnormal vaginal discharge, e.g. presence of pus.
4. Abnormal smell/foul odor of discharge.
5. Delay in the rate of reduction of the size of the uterus (involution).

b. List out the causes and clinical manifestation of puerperal sepsis.

Causes:
1. Postpartum infections are less common since the introduction of antiseptics and penicillin. However, skin flora, such as *Streptococcus* or *Staphylococcus* and other bacteria still cause infections. These thrive in moist and warm environments.
2. Postpartum infections often start in the uterus after delivery. The uterus can become infected if the amniotic sac becomes infected. The amniotic sac the membranes that contain the fetus.

Symptoms and signs may include:
1. Fever
2. Pain in the lower abdomen or pelvis caused by a swollen uterus
3. Foul-smelling vaginal discharge
4. Pale skin, which can be a sign of large volume blood loss
5. Chills
6. Feelings of discomfort or illness
7. Headache
8. Loss of appetite
9. Increased heart rate.

c. Explain the mangement of mother with puerperal sepsis.

Antibiotics have been used to prevent and treat these infections however the misuse of antibiotics is a serious problem for global health. It is recommended that guidelines be followed which outline when it is appropriate to give antibiotics and which antibiotics are most effective.

The operations employed were colpotomy, abdominal drainage and removal of diseased structures and hysterectomy, each operation being employed in certain pathological states. Vein ligation has been done so rarely in this hospital and the mortality in these people so low that the tendency is entirely towards conservative management with repeated blood transfusions.

Cesarean sections: Sepsis can develop after any type of surgery. Cesarean sections are major abdominal surgeries with all the associated risks.

Choosing the right hospital is critical: Women should make sure they choose a facility with excellent cleanliness. Family members should also emphasize that doctors follow proper sanitation guidelines when treating the mother. There should be no untrained medical professional touching the pelvic or any other region on the body of the mother.

Proper hygienic practices: Apart from ensuring complete sanctity of the health facility, the professionals should be extremely careful during the delivery. All equipment should be properly sterilized and all hands must wear medical gloves. Midwifes and other professionals must have full training on taking a high vaginal swab, maintaining optimum vulva hygiene, and best practices to obtain a blood culture. Above everything, healthcare professionals must not give in to a sense of callousness stemming from handling numerous deliveries. Every woman is special and unique, deserving of maximum attention.

Timely postpartum checkups: Do not skip postpartum appointments thinking you are too busy and all the discomfort is normal.

OR

a. Define fibriod uterus.

Uterine fibroids (leiomyomas) are benign smooth muscle tumors of the uterus. They are the most common benign tumors in women, with an estimated incidence of 20-40%. The risk of a fibroid becoming malignant is 0.1%.

b. Write the clinical features of fibroid uterus.

Many women who have fibroids don't have any symptoms. In those that do, symptoms can be influenced by the location, size and number of fibroids. In women who have symptoms, the most common symptoms of uterine fibroids include:

1. Heavy menstrual bleeding
2. Menstrual periods lasting more than a week
3. Pelvic pressure or pain
4. Frequent urination
5. Difficulty emptying the bladder
6. Constipation
7. Backache or leg pains.

Rarely, a fibroid can cause acute pain when it outgrows its blood supply, and begins to die.

c. Explain the management of fibroid uterus.

There are both medical and surgical options for the management of uterine fibroids. Asymptomatic patients with small fibroids often do not need treatment.

Medical
1. Tranexamic or mefanamic acid.
2. Hormonal contraceptives.
    a. Useful to control menorrhagia.
    b. Includes the COCP, POP and Mirena IUS.
3. GnRH analogues (Zolidex):
    a. Suppresses ovulation, inducing a temporary menopausal state.
    b. Useful pre-operatively to reduce fibroid size and lower complications.
    c. Can be used for 6 months only, due to the risk of osteoporosis.
4. Selective progesterone receptor modulators (Ulipristal/Esmya):
    a. Reduces size of fibroid and menorrhagia.
    b. Useful preoperatively or as an alternative to surgery.

Surgical
1. Hysteroscopy and transcervical resection of fibroid (TCRF):
   Useful for submucosal fibroids
2. Myomectomy: Option in women wanting to preserve their uterus.
3. Uterine artery embolization (UAE):
    a. Performed by a radiologist via the femoral artery.
    b. Commonly causes pain and fever postoperatively.
4. Hysterectomy.

2018
Midwifery and Gynecology

SECTION-I

I. **Give the meaning of the following:**
   a. Bregma.
   b. Leukorrhea.
   c. False pelvis.
   d. Dystocia.

II. **Fill in the blanks:**
   a. The bony canal through which the fetus pass through during birth is _____
   b. The graphical record of cervical dilatation against duration of labor is _____
   c. The term placenta weighs about _____ g
   d. The name given to the lochia between 1 and 4 days is called _____

III. **Write short notes on any *four* of the following:**
   a. Minor disorders during pregnancy.
   b. Temporary family planning methods.
   c. Causes of onset of labor.
   d. Fetal circulation.
   e. Genetic counseling.
   f. Immediate care of the newborn.

IV. **Define the following:**
   a. Define pelvis.
   b. List the types of pelvis.
   c. Explain in detail about female pelvis.

V. a. Define postnatal care.
   b. List the objectives of postnatal care.
   c. Explain in detail about the care of postnatal mother.

SECTION-II

VI. **State whether the following statements are *true* or *false*:**
   a. Methergin is used to decrease the uterine contraction.
   b. Hydrops fetalis is the most serious form of Rh hemolytic disease.
   c. Oligohydraminos is a state where liquor amni exceeds more than 2,000 mL.
   d. Episiotomy is surgically planned incision on the abdomen.

VII. **Choose the correct answer from the following:**
   a. The condition where the presentation of the fetus is constantly changing even beyond 36 weeks is:
      i. Longitudinal   ii. Unstable lie   iii. Transverse lie   iv. Oblique lie

b. Inability to conceive the child after regular unprotected intercourse is:
   i. Sterility   ii. Infertility   iii. Subfertility lie   iv. Fertility
c. Impaired involution of the uterus is called as:
   i. Subinvolution   ii. Anteversion   iii. Retroversion   iv. Extroversion

VIII. Write short notes on any *four* of the following:
   a. Manual removal of placenta.
   b. Levels of care in NICU.
   c. Tocolytic agents.
   d. Cryptomenorrhea.
   e. Breast abscess.
   f. Bishops score.

IX. Answer the following:
   a. Define breech presentation.
   b. Explain the types of breech presentation.
   c. Describe the obstetrical and nursing management of breech presentation.
   OR
   a. Define cesarean section.
   b. List the indications of cesarean section.
   c. Explain the management of mother underwent cesarean section.

X. a. What is sexually transmitted diseases (STDs).
   b. List down sexually transmitted diseases.
   c. Discuss the diagnosis and management of the mother with HIV infection.
   OR
   a. Define menopause.
   b. List the physiological and psychological changes of menopause.
   c. Explain hormonal replacement therapy for menopause.

Midwifery and Gynecological Nursing: 2018   15

SECTION-I

I. **Give the meaning of the following:**

a. **Bregma.**

The bregma is the anatomical point on the skull at which the coronal suture is intersected perpendicularly by the sagittal suture.

b. **Leukorrhea**

Leukorrhea is a white, yellowish, or greenish white viscid discharge from the vagina resulting from inflammation or congestion of the uterine or vaginal mucous membrane.

c. **False pelvis.**

The false (or greater) pelvis is bounded on either side by the ilium. In front it is incomplete, presenting a wide interval between the anterior borders of the ilia; behind is a deep notch on either side between the ilium and the base of the sacrum.

d. **Dystocia.**

Obstructed labour, also known as labour **dystocia**, is when, even though the uterus is contracting normally, the baby does not exit the pelvis during childbirth due to being physically blocked.

II. **Fill in the blanks:**

a. The bony canal through which the fetus pass through during birth is **Vaginal canal**.
b. The graphical record of cervical dilatation against duration of labor is **Partograph**.
c. The term placenta weighs about **600 g**.
d. The name given to the lochia between 1 and 4 days is called **Lochia Rubra**.

III. **Write short notes on any four of the following:**

a. Minor disorders during pregnancy. (2014-III-e)

b. Temporary family planning methods. (2015-x-C)

c. Causes of onset of labor.

1. **Oxytocin:** There is oxytocin receptor in the uterus. Oxytocin receptors are increased in the uterus with the onset of labor. And then oxytocin promotes the release of prostaglandins from the decidua. Oxytocin synthesis is increased in the decidua and in the placenta. Oxytocin level reaches the maximum at the moment of birth.

2. **Progesterone:** A decrease in progesterone production may stimulate prostaglandins (PG) synthesis and enhance the effect of estrogen which has a stimulating effect on uterine muscle.

3. **Estrogen:** The probable mechanisms are:
   a. Increases the release of oxytocin from maternal pituitary.
   b. Promotes the synthesis of receptors for oxytocin in the myometrium and decidua.

4. **Prostaglandins:** Prostaglandins are the important factors which initiate and maintain labor. Prostaglandins stimulate smooth muscle to contract. The major sites of synthesis of prostaglandins are amnion, chorion, decidual cells and myometrium.

d. Fetal circulation. (2013-III-b)
e. Genetic counseling. (2013-III-b)
f. Immediate care of the newborn. (2016-III-c)

IV. Define the following:

a. Define pelvis.

The pelvis is a hard ring of bone, which supports and protects the pelvic organs and the contents of the abdominal cavity. The muscles of the legs, back and abdomen are attached to the pelvis, and their strength and power keep the body upright and enable it to bend and twist at the waist, and to walk and run.

b. List the types of pelvis.

S.No.	Features	Gynecoid	Android	Anthropoid	Platypelloid
1.	Brim	Rounded	Heart-shaped	Long-oval	Kidney-shaped
2.	Fore pelvis	Generous	Narrow	Narrowed	Wide
3.	Sidewalls	Straight	Convergent	Divergent	Divergent
3.	Ischial spines	Blunt	Prominent	Blunt	Blunt
4.	Sciatic notch	Rounded	Narrow	Wide	Wide
5.	Sub-pubic angle	90°	<90°	>90°	>90°
6.	Incidence	50%	20%	25%	5%

c. Explain in detail about female pelvis.

1. The cross-sectional anatomy of the female pelvis shows five bones—two hip bones, sacrum, coccyx and two femurs.
2. Each hip bone is formed by the fusion of three bones—the ilium, pubis and ischium.
3. The sacrum and coccyx are also comprised of smaller bones. The first is formed by the fusion of the five sacral vertebrae (S1-S5), and the latter by the fusion of the four coccygeal vertebrae.
4. The femur is the strong thigh bone. It articulates with the hip, forming the ball-and-socket hip joint.
5. There is a numerous variety of muscles that can be seen in the female pelvis, depending on the level of the cross section.
6. The abdominal region includes the external oblique, internal oblique, transversus abdominis, rectus abdominis and pyramidalis muscles.
7. The muscles of the back region include the quadratus lumborum, latissimus dorsi, serratus posterior inferior, erector spinae, interspinales and transversospinalis muscles.
8. The muscles present in the thigh region can be split into three sections, anterior, medial and posterior. The anterior compartment is comprised of the iliopsoas, quadratus femoris, sartorius, and pectineus.
9. The medial compartment is comprised of the adductor magnus, adductor longus, adductor brevis, obturator externus, and gracilis.

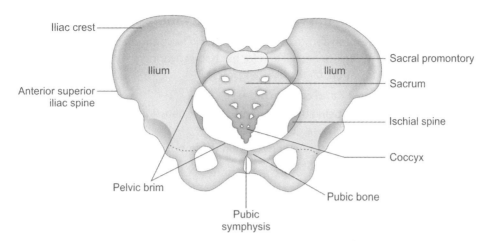

10. The posterior compartment is comprised of the biceps femoris, semitendinosus and semimembranosus muscles.
11. In the gluteal region, the muscles seen there are the gluteus maximus, gluteus medius, gluteus minimus and tensor fascia latae, as well as the deeper piriformis, gemellus superior, gemellus inferior and obturator internus muscles.
    The pelvic floor includes the levator ani, bulbospongiosus and the deep transverse perineal muscles.
12. The major organs present in a female pelvis cross section are those of the digestive, urinary and reproductive systems.
13. Organs of the digestive tract include the ascending and sigmoid colon, ileum of the small intestine, rectum and anal canal. Organs of the urinary system include the urethra, bladder and the two ureters.
14. Organs of the female reproductive system present in the pelvis are subdivided into internal and external genitalia. The internal genitalia consist of the uterus, two uterine tubes, two ovaries and the vagina.

V. a. Define postnatal care.

Postnatal care (PNC) is the care given to the mother and her newborn baby immediately after the birth and for the first 6 weeks of life.

b. List the objectives of postnatal care.

1. Support of the mother and her family in the transition to a new family constellation, and response to their needs
2. Prevention, early diagnosis and treatment of complications of mother and infant, including the prevention of vertical transmission of diseases from mother to infant
3. Referral of mother and infant for specialist care when necessary
4. Counseling on baby care
5. Support of breastfeeding
6. Counseling on maternal nutrition, and supplementation if necessary
7. Counseling and service provision for contraception and the resumption of sexual activity
8. Immunization of the infant.

c. Explain in detail about the care of postnatal mother.

An important aspect of the midwife/nurse works whether in hospital or at home is her educational role. Advice the mother to care for herself and for her baby covering a wide range of subjects like hygiene nutrition, immunization, family planning, etc.

The basic principles of post natal care include:
1. Promotion of physical well-being by good nutrition, adequate fluid intake, comfort, cleanliness, and sufficient exercises to ensure good muscle tone.
2. Early ambulation is insisted to prevent deep vein thrombosis.
3. Establishment of emotional well-being.
4. Promotion of breastfeeding.
5. Prevention of complications.

Admission to postnatal ward: The mother and baby are usually transferred to the postnatal ward within an hour or 2 after delivery. The midwife/nurse should well come the mother and help her to settle in the ward. She will observe her general condition, palpate the uterus to note whether it is contracted or not and observe the lochia.

Sleep and rest: The mother should have sufficient sleep and rest. Keep a quiet comfortable atmosphere without disturbance. Inability to sleep must be regarded with concern and Doctor should be consulted. Hypnotics may be needed and it is given without hesitation. Undue anxiety, sleeplessness and loss of appetite should be rewarded as serious. Rest is usually encouraged during the day preferably in prone position as this aids drainage from the uterus and vagina.

Ambulation: Mothers benefit a feeling of well being from this early activity and this reduces the incidence of thrombi embolic disorders.

Diet: A good balanced diet should be taken as advised in pregnancy. The woman's appetite usually returns very quickly after labor is ended and has had some sleep. Protein foods are important particularly if she is breastfeeding. Excess fruit should be avoided as substances from this will pass to the baby in the milk and may cause diarrhea. The daily fluid intake should be from 2.5 to 3 liters of which at least 600 mL should be milk.

Postnatal exercises – Advantages
1. Gives the women a sense of wellbeingness
2. Maintains good circulation, lessens possibility of venous thrombosis.
3. Restores muscle tone of the abdominal wall and pelvic floor.
4. Promotes for normal drainage of lochia
5. Prevents hypostatic pneumonia
6. Helps in emptying the bladder, bowels and uterus
7. Permits her to enjoy a daily bath
8. Enables her to take early care of her baby.
9. Restores her body figure

Pelvic floor exercises (Kegel exercise): The pelvic floor muscles have been under strain during pregnancy and stretched during delivery and it may be both difficult and painful to contract these muscles postnatally. Mothers should be encouraged to do the exercise (as explained in the antenatal section) as often as possible in order to regain full bladder control, prevent uterine prolapsed and ensure normal sexual satisfaction in future.

SECTION-II

VI. State whether the following statements are *true* or *false*
a. Methergin is used to decrease the uterine contraction: **FALSE**
b. Hydrops fetalis is the most serious form of Rh hemolytic disease: **TRUE**
c. Oligohydraminos is a state where liquor amni exceeds more than 2,000 mL: **FALSE**
d. Episiotomy is surgically planned incision on the abdomen: **FALSE**

VII. Choose the correct answer from the following:
a. The condition where the presentation of the fetus is constantly changing even beyond 36 weeks is:
   i. Longitudinal   ii. Unstable lie   iii. Transverse lie   iv. Oblique lie
   Ans: ii. Unstable lie
b. Inability to conceive the child after regular unprotected intercourse is:
   i. Sterility ii. Infertility   iii. Subfertility lie   iv. Fertility
   Ans: ii. Infertility
c. Impaired involution of the uterus is called as:
   i. Subinvolution   ii Anteversion   iii. Retroversion iv. Extroversion
   Ans: i. Subinvolution

VIII. Write short notes on any *four* of the following:
a. Manual removal of placenta.

Manual placenta removal is the evacuation of the placenta from the uterus by hand. It is usually carried out under anesthesia or more rarely, under sedation and analgesia.

Indications
1. Placenta not yet expelled 30 to 45 minutes after delivery.
2. Hemorrhage prior to spontaneous expulsion of the placenta.

Technique
1. Follow precautions common to all intrauterine procedures and specific precautions for manual procedures.
2. Cup the fundus with one hand and hold it down.

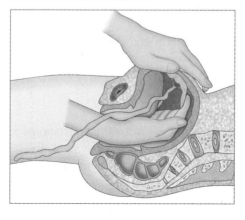

3. Advance the other hand, fully pronated, directly to the fundus and locate the cleavage plane between the uterine wall and the placenta with the fingertips. This hand is inserted all the way up to the forearm in the genital tract.
4. Once the cleavage plane has been located, use the side of the pronated hand like a spoon to detach the placenta and bring it out.
5. Immediately reinsert the hand to perform uterine exploration.

Manual Removal of the Placenta = TIA FATS R2O2

T: Try Syntocinon 20 units into the umbilical vein
I: Get IV access
A: Anesthesia or Analgesia is required
F: Follow the cord to find the cervix
A: Abdominal hand on the fundus to fix the uterus
T: Tent the fingers to dilate the cervix and enter the uterus
S: Separate the placenta working between the two hands
R2 Remove the placenta and Recheck the cavity
O2 Oxytocin by infusion to contract the uterus. Antibiotics Optional.

b. Levels of care in NICU.

The American Academy of Pediatrics categorizes hospitals into four levels based on the care a facility can provide to newborns. These levels of care correspond to the therapies and services provided. Facilities offering neonatal intensive care must meet health care standards through federal/state licensing or certification. The four categories are:

Level I: Well newborn nursery: Level I units are typically referred to as the well baby nursery. These facilities have the capability to provide neonatal resuscitation at every delivery; evaluate and provide postnatal care to healthy newborn infants; stabilize and provide care for infants born at 35 to 37 weeks' gestation who remain physiologically stable.

Level II: Special care nursery
1. Provide care for infants born at 32 weeks gestation or older and weighing more than or equal to 1500 g who have physiologic immaturity or who are moderately ill with problems that are expected to resolve rapidly and are not anticipated to need subspecialty services on an urgent basis
2. Provide care for infants who are feeding and growing stronger or recovering after intensive care
3. Provide mechanical ventilation for a brief duration or continuous positive airway pressure
4. Stabilize infants born before 32-weeks gestation and weighing less than 1500 g until transfer to a neonatal intensive care facility

Level III: Neonatal intensive care unit (NICU)
1. Provide sustained life support
2. Provide comprehensive care for infants born at all gestational ages and birth weights with critical illness
3. Offer prompt access to a full range of pediatric medical subspecialists, pediatric surgical specialists, pediatric anesthesiologists and pediatric ophthalmologists

4. Provide a full range of respiratory support that may include conventional and/or high-frequency ventilation and inhaled nitric oxide
5. Perform advanced imaging, with interpretation on an urgent basis, including computed tomography, MRI and echocardiography.

Level IV: Regional neonatal intensive-care unit (regional NICU): Regional NICUs have all of the capabilities of level I, II and III units. In addition to providing the highest level of care, Level IV NICUs:
1. Are located within an institution that has the capability to provide surgical repair of complex congenital or acquired conditions
2. Maintain a full range of pediatric medical subspecialists, pediatric surgical subspecialists and pediatric anesthesiologists at the site
3. Facilitate transport and provide outreach education
4. Provide extracoporeal membrane oxygenation (ECMO).

c. Tocolytic agents.

Drugs that prevent preterm labor and immature birth by suppressing uterine contractions. Agents used to delay premature uterine activity include magnesium sulfate, beta-mimetics, oxytocin antagonists, calcium channel inhibitors, and adrenergic beta-receptor agonists.

Beta-sympathomimetics

Action: Relaxation of the smooth muscle fibers by stimulating the beta receptors present on the cell membrane.
Examples: Ritodrine (Yutopar):

Calcium Antagonists

Action: Antagonise the action of calcium within the myometrial cells so reduce its contractility, e.g. Nifedipine 10 mg oral tablet.

TABLE 1 Common tocolytic agents

Agent	Common dosage	Comments
Magnesium sulfate	4-6 g IV bolus followed by 2-3 g/h IV infusion	May cause maternal flushing, lethargy, headache, weakness, dry mouth, pulmonary edema, cardiac arrest; may cause neonatal lethargy, hypotonia respiratory depression; recommended by ACOG to reduce cerebral palsy risk
Terbutaline	0.25 mg SC every 20 min-3 h or 2.5-10 mcg/min continuous infusion, gradually increased to 17.5-30 mcg/min	May cause maternal cardiac arrhythmias, pulmonary edema, myocardal ischemia, hypotension, tachycardia, metabolic abnormalities, nausea, vomiting, fever, hallucinations; may cause neonatal tachycardia, hypoglycemia, hypocalcemia, hyperbilirubinemia, hypotension, intraventricular hemorrhage
Nifedipine	30 mg po followed by 10-20 mg q4-6h	May cause maternal flushing, headache, dizziness, nausea, transient hypotension; no fetal or neonatal effects reported
Indomethacin	50 mg rectally or 50-100 mg po followed by 20-50 mg po q4-6h for 48 h	May cause maternal nausea, heartburn; may cause neonatal constriction of ductus arteriosus, pulmonary hypertension, decreased renal function, intraventricular hemorrhage, hyperbilirubinemia, necrotizing enterocolitis
Ketorolac	60 mg IM followed by 30 mg IM q6h for 48 h	No maternal, fetal, or neonatal effects reported
Sulindac	200 mg po q12h for 48 h	No maternal, fetal, or neonatal effects reported

Magnesium Sulfate

Action: The intracellular calcium is displaced by magnesium ion leading to inhibition of the uterine activity.

Dosage: The initial dose is 40 cc of 10% solution given slowly IV. The subsequent doses depend upon the response and the development of $MgSO_4$ toxicity so reflexes and respiratory rate should be observed.

Prostaglandin Inhibiting Agents

Action: Inhibition of uterine contractions by inhibiting prostaglandin synthesis.

Dosage: For example, indomethacin 100 mg suppository initially, followed by 25 mg orally every 6 hours for up to 24 hours after contractions ceased.

Ethyl Alcohol

Action

1. Inhibits the release of oxytocin from the posterior pituitary gland.
2. Suppresses the myometrial activity directly.
3. Inhibits prostaglandin F2 a synthesis.

d. Cryptomenorrhea.

Cryptomenorrhea or cryptomenorrhoea, also known as hematocolpos, is a condition where menstruation occurs but is not visible due to an obstruction of the outflow tract.

Specifically the endometrium is shed, but a congenital obstruction such as a vaginal septum or on part of the hymen retains the menstrual flow. A patient with cryptomenorrhea will appear to have amenorrhea but will experience cyclic menstrual pain. The condition is surgically correctable.

Signs:
1. Abdominal examination: Swelling is felt on palpation.
2. On vulval inspection: A tense, bulging, bluish membrane is seen, this finding varies according to the thickness of the obstructing membrane. It may be absent in patients with complete or partial vaginal agenesis.
3. On rectal examination: A large bulging mass is felt.

Treatment: A simple cruciate incision followed by excision of tags of hymen allows drainage of the retained menstrual blood. A thicker transverse vaginal septum can be treated with Z-plasty. A blind vagina will require a partial or complete vaginoplasty. Hematosalpinx may require laparotomy or laparoscopy for removal and reconstruction of affected tube. Infertility may require assisted reproductive techniques.

e. Breast abscess.

A breast abscess is a localized collection of pus in the breast tissue. It is usually caused by a bacterial infection. Breast infections, including mastitis and breast abscesses, are most often seen in women aged 15 to 45 years.

Symptoms: The signs and symptoms of breast abscesses are:
1. A tender swelling or lump in an area of the breast;
2. Pain in the affected breast;
3. Redness, warmth, swelling, and tenderness in an area of the breast;

4. Fever;
5. Muscles aches; and
6. Feeling generally unwell.

Treatment: Treatment for breast abscesses includes antibiotics, surgical removal of pus and self-care measures.

Antibiotics: Antibiotics are usually needed to treat the infection that caused the breast abscess. The most common type of bacteria causing breast abscesses is *Staphylococcus aureus*.

Surgery

1. The pus in the breast abscess usually needs to be drained.
2. Most breast abscesses can be drained using a needle.
3. Local anesthetic is used to numb the skin before the needle is inserted.
4. Drainage with a needle may be done with the help of an ultrasound scan, to locate the position of the abscess and guide the needle to the right area.
5. Large abscesses may need to be treated with a small surgical cut (incision) and drainage.

Self-care

1. In addition to resting as much as possible and drinking plenty of fluids, there are several other self-care measures that can help.
2. Take simple painkillers such as paracetamol or a non-steroidal anti-inflammatory medicine (NSAID). If you are breastfeeding, check with your doctor before taking any medicines.
3. Cold compresses can also be used to help reduce pain.

f. Bishops score.

1. The Bishop score (also known as pelvic score) is the most commonly used method to rate the readiness of the cervix for induction of labor.
2. The Bishop score gives points to 5 measurements of the pelvic examination dilation, effacement of the cervix, station of the fetus, consistency of the cervix, and position of the cervix. The calculator below will calculate a Bishop score.
3. The Bishop's score was originally developed to predict the likelihood of a woman entering labor naturally in the near future.
4. A woman with a low score of 1 would not be expected to go into labor for about 3 weeks. A woman with a higher score score of 10 could be expected to go into labor within a few days.

Score	0	1	2
Cervical dilatation (cm)	<1	1-2	3-4
Length of cervix (cm)	>2	1-2	<1
Station of presenting part (cm)	Spines-3	Spines-2	Spines-1
Consistency	Firm	Medium	Soft
Position	Posterior	Central	Anterior

Dilatation (Dilation): The most important element of the Bishop score is dilatation. Dilatation is the distance the cervix is opened measured in centimeters (cm). For reference a penny is about 2 cm across. Points are given from 0 to a maximum of 3 points for a cervix dilated to 6 cm or greater.

Effacement: Effacement (also called shortening or thinning) is reported as a percentage from zero percent (normal length cervix) to 100% or complete (paper thin cervix). Points are given from 0 to a maximum of 3 points for a cervix effaced to 80 % or greater.

Station: Station is the position of the baby's head relative to the bony projections of the lower pelvis called the ischial spines. When the baby's head is at 0 station its head is even with the ischial spines. Stations divide the pelvis above and below the ischial spines into 3rds Negative numbers indicate that the head is above the ischial spines. Positive numbers indicate its head is below the ischial spines.

Position: The position of the cervix relative to the fetal head and maternal pelvis.

IX. Answer the following:

a. Define breech presentation. (2016-X-a)
b. Explain the types of breech presentation. (2016-X-b)
c. Describe the obstetrical and nursing management of breech presentation. (2011-X-a)

1. Mother was kept in the comfortable position.
2. Assessment of physical and mental status: A complete physical examination was done to find out any abnormalities including general condition of the patient, vital signs, FHS.
3. Psychological preparation: Emotional support was given to the patient and explained about the procedure.
4. Ordered investigations were sent like RBS, CBC and urine R/E and reports were also collected.
5. Half hourly monitoring of fetal heart sound and correct recording and reporting was done.
6. Augmentation with injection oxitocin was started according to doctor's order.
7. Partograph was filled to monitor the progress of labour.
8. Intake and output was monitored.
9. Mother was encouraged for adequate fluid intake like black tea, hot soups etc. to prevent dehydration

Management in the second stage of labor:
1. Mother was shifted to the second stage (delivery room) and kept comfortably on the delivery bed with the head elevated 45°.
2. Mother's vital signs and fetal heart sound was also monitored and recorded.
3. She was encouraged to push during strong contraction.
4. Strict aseptic technique was maintained during delivery.
5. She delivered a live female baby at 08:00 pm weighing 2,250 g.
6. Kangaroo mother care was provided to the baby.
7. Baby's sex was shown to the mother.

Management of the third stage of labor:
1. As soon as the baby was delivered injection Syntocin 10 units IM was given.
2. Post delivery vital signs were taken and recorded.
3. Placenta was delivered using control cord traction and placenta was observed; which was complete and normal.
4. Vagina was carefully observed and cleaned.
5. Wet dress of the mother was changed.

6. She was encouraged to massage the uterus every 15 minutes for 5 minutes.
7. Teaching about breast feeding, perineal hygine, cord care was given.
8. Mother was transferred to the postnatal ward.

OR

a. Define cesarean section.

Cesarean section is the delivery of a baby through a surgical incision in the abdomen and uterus.

b. List the indications of cesarean section.

A planned or 'elective' Cesarean section is performed for a variety of indications. The following are the most common, but this is not an exhaustive list:

1. **Breech presentation** (at term)—planned cesarean sections for breech presentation at term have increased significantly since the 'Term Breech Trial'.
2. **Other malpresentations**, e.g. unstable lie (a presentation that fluctuates from oblique, cephalic, transverse etc.), transverse lie or oblique lie.
3. **Twin pregnancy**—when the first twin is not a cephalic presentation.
4. **Maternal medical conditions** (e.g. cardiomyopathy)—where labor would be dangerous for the mother.
5. **Fetal compromise** (such as early onset growth restriction and/or abnormal fetal Dopplers) – where it is thought the fetus would not cope with labor.
6. **Transmissible disease** (e.g. poorly controlled HIV).
7. **Primary genital herpes** (herpes simplex virus) in the third trimester—as there has been no time for the development and transmission of maternal antibodies to HSV to cross the placenta and protect the baby.
8. **Placenta previa**—'low-lying placenta' where the placenta covers, or reaches the internal os of the cervix.
9. **Maternal diabetes** with a baby estimated to have a fetal weight >4.5 kg.
10. **Previous major shoulder dystocia**.
11. **Previous 3rd/4th perineal tear where the patient is symptomatic**—after discussion with the patient and appropriate assessment.
12. **Maternal request**—this covers a variety of reasons from previous traumatic birth to 'maternal choice'. This decision is after a multidisciplinary approach including counseling by a specialist midwife.

c. Explain the management of mother underwent cesarean section. (2011-VIII-a)

X. a. What is sexually transmitted diseases. (2011-VIII-b)
   b. List down sexually transmitted diseases.

1. Chlamydia
2. Gonorrhea otherwise known as "the clap," is another common bacterial sexually transmitted diseases (STD)
3. Syphilis
4. *Mycoplasma genitalium*
5. Trichomoniasis

6. Human papilloma virus (HPV)
7. HIV/AIDS
8. Crabs/Pubic Lice.

c. Discuss the diagnosis and management of the mother with HIV infection.

Human immunodeficiency virus (HIV) is a retrovirus that causes HIV infection by infecting CD4 T cells and can lead to acquired immunodeficiency syndrome (AIDS). Pregnancy in women living with HIV is complicated not only by HIV infection itself but also by the medical and psychosocial comorbidities associated with HIV. HIV infection in pregnancy poses a threat to maternal immune health and can lead to perinatal transmission of HIV in utero, intrapartum, or through breastfeeding postnatal.

Diagnosis

1. HIV-1 western blot
2. HIV-1 indirect immunofluorescence assay (IFA)
3. HIV-1 nucleic acid test (NAT)
4. CD4 count
5. Maternal HIV-1/HIV-2 antigen/antibody enzyme-linked immunosorbent assay (ELISA)
6. Maternal HIV-1/HIV-2 antibody differentiation immunoassay
7. Neonatal HIV DNA or RNA polymerase chain reaction (PCR)

General Guidance

1. Pregnant women with HIV should receive at least the minimum package of recommended antenatal visits and pregnancy care, and additional interventions such as screening for sexually transmitted infections, nutritional support and infant feeding and family planning counseling should be considered.
2. There is a high risk of HIV transmission during labor and delivery. This risk can be minimized by following several key principles and practices, including reinforcing recommended antenatal clinic visits, especially high-risk management in the late third trimester; promoting facility-based delivery by trained skilled birth attendants; avoiding unnecessary instrumentation and premature rupture of membranes by using a partograph to monitor stages of labor; and non-invasive suction of nasogastric secretions and washing away blood in the newborn.

Treatment

The goals in the use of antiretroviral drugs during pregnancy are twofold:
1. Treatment of maternal infection and
2. Reduction of the risk of perinatal transmission.

Antiretroviral Therapy:

1. The primary treatment for HIV is antiretroviral therapy (ART), which has been shown to improve survival rates and immune system function, decrease the risk of complications, and reduce the likelihood of HIV transmission.
2. Therapy typically consists of a regimen of 3 or more antiretroviral (ARV) drugs.

OR

a. Define menopause.

Menopause is nothing but a hormonal deficiency. The absence of estrogen production is one of the main causes of the physical changes in menopause suffered by women during this period.

b. List the physiological and psychological changes of menopause.

1. Psychological symptoms are frequently reported around the time of menopause. Symptoms include depression, loss of memory, irritability, poor concentration, tiredness and loss of confidence.
2. Women also experience sleep disturbances and insomnia, which could partly be due to night sweats and hot flushes.
3. Menopause can be a difficult time for a woman as it not only marks the end of her reproductive capacity, but can also be associated with changes in domestic arrangements and feelings of loss of youth and femininity. Therefore, the symptoms experienced may not be entirely due to a lack of estrogen.
4. A combination of physical and psychological influences can result in a complete loss of libido, decreased sexual satisfaction and avoidance of intercourse.

Effects of menopause: Changing hormone levels can cause severe discomfort and some health risks.

1. Vaginal dryness
2. Bone thinning, or osteoporosis
3. Urinary problems
4. Thinning hair
5. Sleep problems
6. Hot flashes and night sweats
7. Moodiness
8. Lower fertility
9. Irregular periods
10. Concentration and memory difficulties
11. Smaller breasts and an accumulation of fat in the abdomen.

c. Explain hormonal replacement therapy for menopause.

Hormone therapy (HT) is one of the treatments for relief of menopausal symptoms. These symptoms, caused by lower levels of estrogen at menopause, include hot flashes, sleep disturbances, and vaginal dryness.

There are two basic types of HT:
1. ET means estrogen-only therapy. Estrogen is the hormone that provides the most menopausal symptom relief. ET is prescribed for women without a uterus due to a hysterectomy.
2. EPT means combined estrogen plus progestogen therapy. Progestogen is added to ET to protect women with a uterus against uterine (endometrial) cancer from estrogen alone.

There are two general ways to take HT:
1. Systemic products circulate throughout the bloodstream and to all parts of the body. They are available as an oral tablet, patch, gel, emulsion, spray, or injection and can be used for hot flashes and night sweats, vaginal symptoms, and osteoporosis.
2. Local (nonsystemic) products affect only a specific or localized area of the body. They are available as a cream, ring, or tablet and can be used for vaginal symptoms.

Benefits of HRT
1. HRT remains the most effective treatment for the relief of menopausal vasomotor symptoms (e.g. hot flushes and night sweats), psychological symptoms (e.g. mood swings and irritability) and genitourinary symptoms (e.g. vaginal dryness and urinary frequency).
2. In symptomatic women, HRT results in a considerable improvement in quality of life.
3. HRT has also been used for the prevention and treatment of osteoporosis, one of the long-term consequences of the menopause.
4. HRT prevents and, to some extent, reverses post-menopausal bone loss, reduces bone turnover – primarily by reducing bone resorption – and, thus, maintains the micro-architecture of bone.
5. These actions result in a reduced risk of osteoporotic fractures, including those of the vertebrae, distal forearm and proximal femur.

2017

Midwifery and Gynecology

SECTION-I

I. **Write the meaning of the following:**
   a. Polarity.
   b. Oral thrush.
   c. Lie.
   d. Amnion.

II. **Fill in the blanks:**
   a. _____ is the name given to the endometrium during pregnancy.
   b. First milk secreted from the mother is called _____
   c. _____ is the graphic representation to assess the progress of labor
   d. A dark line running from symphysis pubis to umbilicus during pregnancy is called _____

III. **Write short notes on any *four* of the following:**
   a. Internal and external organs of female reproductive system.
   b. Prevention of birth injuries.
   c. Methods of placental expulsion in 3rd stage of labor.
   d. Signs and symptoms of pregnancy.
   e. Vaginal examination in labor.

IV. **Answer the following:**
   a. Define reproductive health.
   b. Explain physiological changes of reproductive system during pregnancy in detail.

V. a. **Define puerperium.**
   b. Enumerate physiological changes during puerperium.
   c. Explain role of midwife in postnatal care.

SECTION-II

VI. **State whether the following is *true* or *false*:**
   a. Implantation and development of fertilized ovum outside the normal uterine cavity is called Hydatidiform mole.
   b. In breech presentation denominator is occiput.
   c. Leg exercise and early ambulation are encouraged to prevent deep vein thrombosis in puerperium.
   d. Tocolytic drugs are used to produce uterine contractions.

VII. Choose the correct answer from the following:
   a. During abdominal palpation midwife can suspect polyhydramnios by feeling:
      i. Fluid thrill   ii. Position of fetus   iii Breech
   b. Brandt Andrews maneuver means:
      i. Bimanual contractions   ii. Delivering the placenta by cord traction iii. Expel the fetus
   c. Tenderness of calf muscle on deep pressure in deep vein thrombosis is:
      i. Hegars signs   ii. Osianders sign   iii. Homans sign

VIII. Write the short notes on any *four* of the following:
   a. Forceps delivery.
   b. Management of obstetrical shock.
   c. Indications of prostaglandins and role of midwife in drug administration.
   d. Teenage pregnancy.
   e. Contracted pelvis.
   f. Hydatidiform mole.

IX. Answer the following:
   a. Define uterine prolapse.
   b. Enumerate causes, signs and symptoms of uterine prolapse.
   c. Explain the management of uterine prolapse.

   OR

   a. **Define obstructed labor.**
   b. List out the causes and clinical features of obstructed labor.
   c. Explain role of midwife in management of obstructed labor.

X. a. **Define post-term pregnancy.**
   b. Enumerate the causes and clinical features and management of women in post-term pregnancy.

   OR

   a. Define puerperal sepsis.
   b. Explain predisposing factors and management of woman with puerperal sepsis.

SECTION-I

I. Write the meaning of the following:

a. **Polarity.**

The condition of having poles. The condition of a body or system in which it has opposing physical properties at different points, esp magnetic poles or electric charge. The particular state of a part of a body or system that has polarity an electrode with positive polarity.

b. **Oral thrush.**

Oral thrush occurs when a yeast infection develops on the inside of your mouth and on your tongue. This condition is also known as oral candidiasis, oropharyngeal candidiasis, or, simply, thrush. The *Candida albicans* (C. albicans) fungus causes oral thrush.

c. **Lie. (2016-I-d)**

d. **Amnion.**

Amnion: A thin membrane that surrounds the fetus during pregnancy. The amnion is the inner of the two fetal membranes (the chorion is the outer one), and it contains the amniotic fluid.

II. Fill in the blanks:
   a. **Gravida** is the name given to the endometrium during pregnancy.
   b. First milk secreted from the mother is called **Colostrum**
   c. **Partograph** is the graphic representation to assess the progress of labor.
   d. A dark line running from symphysis pubis to umbilicus during pregnancy is called **Linea Nigra.**

III. Write short notes on any *four* of the following:

a. Internal and external organs of female reproductive system.

External Genital Organs

The **vulva** is the external portion of the female genital organs. It includes:
1. **Labia majora**—two large, fleshy lips, or folds of skin.
2. **Labia minora**—small lips that lie inside the labia majora and surround the openings to the urethra and vagina.
3. **Vestibule**—space where the vagina opens.
4. **Glands of Bartholin**. The glands of Bartholin are two tiny ducts located on each side of the opening of the vagina. It is here that the mucus, which serves as the lubrication for intercourse, is produced upon stimulation.
5. **Prepuce**—a fold of skin formed by the labia minora.
6. **Clitoris**—a small protrusion sensitive to stimulation.
7. **Fourchette**—area beneath the vaginal opening where the labia minora meet.
8. **Perineum**—area between the vagina and the anus.

9. **Anus**—opening at the end of the anal canal.
10. **Urethra**—connecting tube to the bladder.

Internal reproductive organs: The main internal female genital organs and their functions are explained briefly below:
1. The **vagina** is the passageway through which fluid passes out of the body during menstural periods. It is also called the **birth canal**. The vagina connects the cervix (the opening of the womb, or **uterus**) and the vulva (the external genitalia).
2. The **uterus**, also called the **womb**, is a hollow, pear-shaped organ located in a woman's lower abdomen, between the bladder and the rectum. The main parts of the uterus are:
   a. **Cervix:** The narrow, lower portion of the uterus.
   b. **Corpus:** The broader, upper part of the uterus.
   c. **Myometrium:** The outer layer of the corpus; the muscle that expands during pregnancy to hold the growing fetus.
   d. **Endometrium:** The inner lining of the uterus.
3. The **ovaries** are female reproductive organs located in the pelvis. There are two of them, one on each side of the uterus. The ovaries produce eggs and the female hormones estrogen and progesterone.
4. The **fallopian tubes** are 2 extensions from the upper left and right hand sides of the uterus to each of the 2 ovaries.

b. Prevention of birth injuries.

A birth injury is a health problem that an infant is born with that is, in most cases, completely preventable. The most common types of preventable birth injuries are caused by:
1. Pulling and/or twisting the infant improperly during the delivery period.
2. Improper handling and use of birth-assisting tools, such as forceps or a vacuum extraction tool.
3. Administering the wrong amount or the wrong type of medication to the mother during pregnancy and during labor.
4. Failure to monitor the infant properly for distress, including failure to regularly monitor fetal heartbeat.
5. Failure to schedule and perform an emergency cesarean surgery (C-section).

c. Methods of placental expulsion in 3rd stage of labor. (2013-IV-b)

d. Signs and symptoms of pregnancy.

Nausea and vomiting: Nausea and vomiting may come as early as a week into the pregnancy. Many women experience illness in the morning (morning sickness), some in the afternoon or evening, others feel nausea throughout the entire day.

Breast tenderness: Breasts may be very tender, swollen and start to enlarge. Many times the veins within the breast will become more visible.

Frequent urination: Pregnancy causes the uterus to swell and it will start to enlarge for the growing fetus immediately. The uterus puts pressure on bladder making to feel the need for more frequent urination.

Feeling tired/sluggish: This one is pretty obvious. When pregnant your body is going through some major hormonal changes. HCG levels alone go from 0 – 250,000 mIU/mL in just twelve weeks.

Missed period/Light bleeding: Light bleeding (spotting) may occur approximately 8–10 days from ovulation. It usually happens around the same time you would have gotten your menstrual period.

Dizziness and/or fainting: When standing in one place you may feel dizzy or even faint. The growing uterus compresses major arteries in your legs which causes your blood pressure to drop making you extremely light headed.

Constipation: Pregnancy hormones will slow down bowel functions to give maximum absorption time of vitamins and nutrients.

Irritability: Raging hormones are the cause of this…along with having to put up with all the other symptoms. This symptom should decrease soon into the second trimester but until then, a healthy diet, moderate exercise and plenty of sleep should help the crabbiness somewhat.

Heartburn: The uterus is very swollen and starts to push upward as it grows. The increasing levels of HCG will also slow down digestion making your stomach not empty as fast which increases the stomach acid.

e. Vaginal examination in labor.

A vaginal examination is an intimate procedure that should only be performed when it is absolutely necessary and will provide information that will aid in the decision-making process. The examination should always be approached in a sensitive manner that maintains the dignity of the client at all times. The midwife should ensure that the woman is in a comfortable position, she has emptied her bladder and that the examination is explained in full. Informed consent must be obtained before the procedure is carried out.

Indications for vaginal examination are to:
1. Confirm the onset of labor
2. Identify the presentation and position of the fetus
3. Assess progress or delay in labor
4. Ascertain the presence of forewaters (carry out rupture of membranes if indicated)
5. Assess prior to administering analgesia
6. Apply a fetal scalp electrode

The procedure
1. Communicate with the woman, while undertaking the examination
2. Ensure that she is in a comfortable position and her dignity is maintained at all times
3. Wash hands
4. Set up the trolley and open the vaginal examination pack
5. Put on gloves
6. Swab vulva from front to back
7. Use individual sterile lubricating gel
8. Use 'dirty' hand to hold labia apart
9. Then gently insert 'clean' fingers downwards and backwards into the vagina.

Findings

Inspect external genitalia for signs of:
1. Varicosities
2. Edema
3. Warts
4. Previous scarring
5. Mutilation and type
6. Discharge or bleeding

IV. Answer the following:

a. Define reproductive health.

Reproductive health refers to the diseases, disorders and conditions that affect the functioning of the male and female reproductive systems during all stages of life.

1. Disorders of reproduction include birth defects, developmental disorders, low birth weight, preterm birth, reduced fertility, impotence, and menstrual disorders.
2. Research has shown that exposure to environmental pollutants may pose the greatest threat to reproductive health.
3. Exposure to lead is associated with reduced fertility in both men and women, while mercury exposure has been linked to birth defects and neurological disorders.
4. A growing body of evidence suggests that exposure to endocrine disruptors, chemicals that appear to disrupt hormonal activity in humans and animals, may contribute to problems with fertility, pregnancy, and other aspects of reproduction.

b. Explain physiological changes of reproductive system during pregnancy in detail. (2015-V-b)

V. a. Define puerperium. (2014-V-a)
b. Enumerate physiological changes during puerperium.

Pueriperium defined as the period from delivery of the placenta to the end of 6th postnatal week.

Uterus change:
1. Change from a cavity capable containing 4–5 L of fluid, to a cavity barely capable of containing an adult finger
2. The uterus changes it mass over the 4 weeks from 1,000 g to 50–100 g, with discharges changing from red to brown/pink and finally yellowish/white.

Physiologic changes during puerperium in blood vessels:
1. Circulating blood volume return to non-pregnant levels by the 10th day.
2. Dilated blood vessels supplying the uterus during pregnancy undergo involution, and extrauterine vessels decrease their dimension to nonpregnant dimension.

Cardiological changes during puerperium:
1. CO increases immediately after delivery, but then slowly declines, aching late pregnancy levels 2days postpartum, and decreasing only by 16% after 2 weeks of the puerperium.
2. This occurs as a consequence of increased stroke volume from increased venous return, despite a quick fall in pulse rate by about 10 beats per minute in the early pueriperium.

Urinary system change during puerperium:
1. Bladder gets increased capacity, decreased volume sensitivity
2. May result in transiet urinary retention. Also increased urine production as a consequence of infused fluid during labor and withdrawal of Antidiuretic effect of oxytocin and in large doses after delivery.
3. Renal function decreases to non-pregnancy levels by 6 weeks of postpartum. A postpartum diuresis occur within 1-2 weeks after delivery and compensate for water retention during pregnancy.
4. Anatomic changes of pregnancy; such as ureteral and calyceal dilation may persist for several months.

Thyroid change in the puerperium:
1. The enlarged thyroid gland returns to prepregnancy dimension over a 12-week period.
2. Increased thyroid-binding globulin, thyroxine and triiodithyronine return to normal levels by 4-6 weeks postpartum.

c. Explain role of midwife in postnatal care:

The midwife provides important physical and emotional care and recovery for both the new mom and the newborn baby following a delivery. They are trained to educate the new mother and watch for signs of postpartum depression, and may work in tandem with a lactation consultant to assist with breastfeeding. A large part of their role is providing support for the mother in any way that's needed.

1. Assess and monitor the new mother after delivery to ensure proper recovery and healing
2. Clean and monitor the newborn baby
3. Check vital signs
4. Check cesarian incisions if applicable
5. Remove catheters after delivery
6. Dispense pain medication and/or antibiotics as needed
7. Provide education to new parents regarding how to care for an infant
8. Help the new mother with the emotional aspects of the birth recovery
9. Work with lactation consultants to help the new mother breastfeed.

SECTION-II

VI. State whether the following is *true* or *false*:
a. Implantation and development of fertilized ovum outside the normal uterine cavity is called hydatidiform mole: **FALSE**
b. In breech presentation denominator is occiput: **FALSE**
c. Leg exercise and early ambulation are encouraged to prevent deep vein thrombosis in puerperium: **TRUE**
d. Tocolytic drugs are used to produce uterine contractions: **FALSE**

VII. Choose the correct answer from the following:
a. During abdominal palpation midwife can suspect polyhydramnios by feeling:
   i. Fluid thrill   ii. Position of fetus   iii. Breech
   Ans: i. Fluid thrill
b. Brandt Andrews manoveure means:
   i. Bimanual contractions   ii. Delivering the placenta by cord traction
   iii Expel the fetus
   Ans: ii. Delivering the placenta by cord traction
c. Tenderness of calf muscle on deep pressure in deep vein thrombosis is:
   i. Hegars signs   ii. Osianders sign   iii Homans sign
   Ans: iii Homans sign

VIII. Write the short notes on any *four* of the following:
a. Forceps delivery. (2013-IX-a)

b. Management of obstetrical shock.

Shock is a condition resulting from inability of the circulatory system to provide the tissues requirements from oxygen and nutrients and to remove metabolites.

Management

1. Detect the cause and arrest hemorrhage.
2. Establish an airway and give oxygen by mask or endotracheal tube.
3. Elevate the legs to encourage return of blood from the limbs to the central circulation.
4. Two or more intravenous ways are established for blood, fluids and drugs infusion which should be given by IV route in shocked patient. If the veins are difficult to find a venous cut down or intrafemoral canulation is done.
5. Restoration of blood volume by:
   a. Whole blood: Cross-matched from the same group if not available group O-ve may be given as a life-saving.
   b. Crystalloid solutions: As ringer lactate, normal saline or glucose 5%. They have a short half life in the circulation and excess amount may cause pulmonary edema.
   c. Colloid solutions: As dextran 40 or 70, plasma protein fraction or fresh frozen plasma.
6. Drug therapy:
   a. Analgesics: 10-15 mg morphine IV if there is pain, tissue damage or irritability.
   b. Corticosteroids: Hydrocortisone 1g or dexamethasone 20 mg slowly IV. Its mode of action is controversial; it may decrease peripheral resistance and potentiate cardiac response so it improves tissue perfusion.
   c. Sodium bicarbonate: 100 mEq IV if metabolic acidosis is demonstrated.
   d. Vasopressors: To increase the blood pressure so maintain renal perfusion.
7. Dopamine: 2.5m g/kg/minute IV is the drug of choice.
8. β-adrenergic stimulant: Isoprenaline 1mg in 500 mL 5% glucose slowly IV infusion.
9. Monitoring:
   a. Central venous pressure (CVP): Normal 10–12 cm water.
   b. Pulse rate.
   c. Blood pressure.
   d. Urine output: Normal 60 mL/hour.
   e. Pulmonary capillary wedge pressure: Normal 6–18 Torr.
   f. Clinical improvement in the: Pallor, cyanosis, air hunger, sweating and consciousness.

c. Indications of prostaglandins and role of midwife in drug administration.

Chief Indications:

1. Maintains patency of ductus arteriosus in neonates with ductal-dependant congenital heart lesions until surgery can be done.
2. Improve shunting after balloon septostomy has failed to improve oxygenation in certain cases of complete transposition of the great arteries.

Contraindications and Precautions:

1. Hypersensitivity to prostaglandin E
2. PPHN
3. Total anomalous pulmonary venous return with obstruction
4. Caution use in presence of bleeding tendencies or seizure disorders.

Nursing Implications:
1. Obtain baseline vital signs, monitor ECG and BP closely
2. Assess for ductal patency and for improvement in oxygenation
3. Monitor for respiratory depression and be prepared for intubation
4. Monitor infant's temperature closely
5. Maintain patient's IV at all times. Have two IV sites to avoid interruption of PGE infusion
6. Solution compatibility: D5W, NS
7. Two RN signatures are required to verify that physician order is calculated within guidelines and that the infusion rate is accurate
8. All meds mixed by pharmacy have 24 hour sterility expiration
9. Standard concentration prepared by pharmacy is 10 mcg/mL in D5W or NS.

d. Teenage pregnancy

Teenage pregnancy is defined as an unintended pregnancy during adolescence. Approximately 750,000 of 15 -to 19-year-old become pregnant each year, according to The American College of Obstetricians and Gynecologists, though many teenagers do not believe that they will get pregnant if they engage in sexual activity.

Causes of Teenage Pregnancy:
1. Peer pressure: During adolescence, teenagers often feel pressure to make friends and fit in with their peers.
2. Absent parents: Teen girls are more likely to get pregnant if they have limited or no guidance from their parents.
3. Glamorization of pregnancy
4. Lack of knowledge
5. Sexual abuse or rape
6. Teenage drinking.

Effects or consequences: The following are some of the effects or consequences: School dropout, fatherless children, street children, arm robbery, dependency burden, death, increase of economic hardship, spread of diseases, abortion, and family conflicts.
1. School dropout: Many teenagers who get pregnant are not able to complete their education.
2. Fatherless or bastard children: Many children born by teenage mothers do not know their biological fathers because the guy or man responsible did not accept to be the impregnator.
3. Street children: Some children born by teenage mothers may end up being street children. This happens because; the teenage parent(s) may not take proper care or cannot afford to provide for the children.
4. Arm robbery: Many arm robbers were born by teenage parent(s). Some of the street children grew up to become arm robbers.
5. Dependency burden: Teenage mothers or parents and babies put their burden on their relatives hence adding to the relatives problems.
6. Death: Some teenagers do not return from hospital when they visit maternity ward to give birth. Meaning some die during child delivery.
7. Increase in economic hardship: Teenage pregnancy increases the population in a nation and may bring economic hardship. The government has to increase infrastructure development, social amenities etc.
8. Spread of diseases: Teenage mothers or parents usually spread sexual transmitted diseases (STD). When the relationship starts, the guy may have indiscriminate sex likewise the girl hence increase in spread of STDs may occur.

9. **Abortion:** Teenage girls usually makes the attempt to abort their babies. Abortion is not accepted in many nations and also immoral according to the bible. The effects of abortion are childlessness in future, death, deformities of the teenager or the baby, etc.
10. **Family conflicts**—usually teenage pregnancy results in conflicts between the girl's parents and the guy or boy's parents. This may be due to tribal issues, finances, religious beliefs, etc.

e. Contracted pelvis. (2016-VIII-a)

f. Hydatidiform mole

A hydatidiform mole is a growing mass of tissue inside the womb (uterus) that will not develop into a baby. It is the result of abnormal conception. It may cause bleeding in early pregnancy and is usually picked up in an early pregnancy ultrasound scan. It needs to be removed and most women can expect a full recovery.

1. There are two types of molar pregnancy: Complete molar pregnancy and partial molar pregnancy.
2. In a complete molar pregnancy, the placental tissue is abnormal and swollen and appears to form fluid-filled cysts
3. In a partial molar pregnancy, there may be normal placental tissue along with abnormally forming placental tissue.

Causes

1. A molar pregnancy is caused by an abnormally fertilized egg. Human cells normally contain 23 pairs of chromosomes. One chromosome in each pair comes from the father, the other from the mother.
2. In a complete molar pregnancy, an empty egg is fertilized by one or two sperm, and all of the genetic material is from the father. In this situation, the chromosomes from the mother's egg are lost or inactivated and the father's chromosomes are duplicated.
3. In a partial or incomplete molar pregnancy, the mother's chromosomes remain but the father provides two sets of chromosomes. As a result, the embryo has 69 chromosomes instead of 46. This most often occurs when two sperm fertilize an egg, resulting in an extra copy of the father's genetic material.

Clinical manifestations: A molar pregnancy may seem like a normal pregnancy at first, but most molar pregnancies cause specific signs and symptoms, including:

1. Dark brown to bright red vaginal bleeding during the first trimester
2. Severe nausea and vomiting
3. Sometimes vaginal passage of grapelike cysts
4. Pelvic pressure or pain.

Management and treatment: Treatment of moles consists of ultrasound-guided suction evacuation. Evacuation must be scheduled rapidly due to the risk of complications, which increases with gestational age.

IX. Answer the following:

a. Define uterine prolapse. (2016-IX-a)

b. Enumerate causes, signs and symptoms of uterine prolapse. (2016-IX-b)

c. Explain the management of uterine prolapse. (2016-IX-c)

OR
a. Define obstructed labor.
Obstructed labor is the failure of the fetus to descend through the birth canal, because there is an impossible barrier (obstruction) preventing its descent despite strong uterine contractions. The obstruction usually occurs at the pelvic brim, but occasionally it may occur in the pelvic cavity or at the outlet of the pelvis. When labor is prolonged because of failure to progress, there is a high-risk that the descent of the fetus will become obstructed. There is no single definition of prolonged labor, because what counts as 'too long' varies with the stage of labor.

b. List out the causes and clinical features of obstructed labor.
Causes of obstructed labor:
1. **Powers:** Inadequate power, due to poor or uncoordinated uterine contractions, is a major cause of prolonged labor. Either the uterine contractions are not strong enough to efface and dilate the cervix in the first stage of labor, or the muscular effort of the uterus is insufficient to push the baby down the birth canal during the second stage.
2. **Passenger:** The fetus is the 'passenger' travelling down the birth canal. Prolonged labour may occur if the fetal head is too large to pass through the mother's pelvis, or the fetal presentation is abnormal.
3. **Passage:** The birth canal is the passage, so labor may be prolonged if the mother's pelvis is too small for the baby to pass through or the pelvis has an abnormal shape, or if there is a tumor or other physical obstruction in the pelvis.

Clinical Features of Obstructed Labor
Assessment of clinical signs of obstruction:
1. The labor has been prolonged (lasting more than 12 hours)
2. The mother appears exhausted, anxious and weak
3. Rupture of the fetal membranes and passing of amniotic fluid was premature (several hours before labor began)
4. The mother has abnormal vital signs: Fast pulse rate, above 100 beats/minute; low blood pressure; respiration rate above 30 breaths/minute; possibly also a raised temperature.

Any of the following additional signs would suggest the presence of obstruction:
1. Foul-smelling meconium draining from the mother's vagina.
2. Concentrated urine, which may contain meconium or blood.
3. Edema (swelling due to collection of fluid in the tissues) of the vulva (female external genitalia, including the labias), especially if the woman has been pushing for a long time. Vagina feels hot and dry to your gloved examining finger because of dehydration.
4. Edema of the cervix.
5. A large swelling over the fetal skull can be felt.
6. Malpresentation or malposition of the fetus.
7. Poor cervical effacement; as the result the cervix feels like an 'empty sleeve'.
8. Bandl's ring may be seen.

Bandl's ring is the name given to the depression between the upper and lower halves of the uterus, at about the level of the umbilicus. It should not be seen or felt on abdominal examination during a normal labor, but when it becomes visible and/or palpable. Bandl's ring is a late sign of obstructed labor. Above this ring is the grossly thickened, upper uterine segment which is pulled

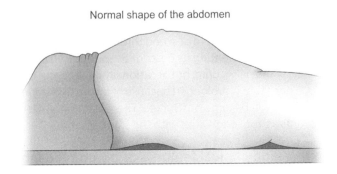

Normal shape of the abdomen

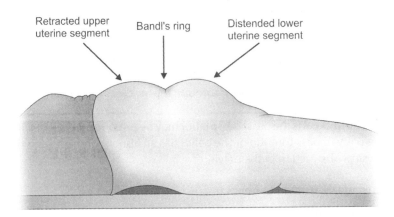

Retracted upper uterine segment | Bandl's ring | Distended lower uterine segment

upwards (retracted) towards the mother's ribs. Below the Bandl's ring is the distended (swollen), dangerously thinned, lower uterine segment. The lower abdomen can be further distended by a full bladder and gas in the intestines.

c. Explain role of midwife in management of obstructed labor.

Management of Prolonged Latent Phase

1. Avoid admission to the labor and delivery area until active labor is established.
2. A plan must be established to meet the woman's needs either at home or in a non-laboring hospital unit.
3. Observation, rest and therapeutic analgesia are favored over a more active approach of amniotomy and oxytocin induction.
4. Support and information from caregivers to provide coping strategies for what to do at home.
5. Prepared childbirth there is little high-quality data on the effect of prepared childbirth on the pain of labor.

Creating a Mother-Friendly Birth Environment

1. Provide a comfortable, clean birth environment.
2. Provide seating for birth companions.
3. Encourage birth companions to provide physical support, such as rubbing back, cool wash cloths, etc.

3. Remain with the woman as much as possible.
4. Talk to the woman, ask about her needs, keep her informed about her progress and any procedures that may become necessary.
5. Avoid routine procedures.
6. Explain the reason for performing all interventions.
7. Encourage the woman to move around and adopt a variety of positions during labor and birth.
8. Encourage the woman to drink and eat lightly in labor to keep her energy up.
9. Deliver the baby onto the mother's abdomen or place the baby in her arms; provide immediate and continued skin-to-skin contact.
10. Allow the mother and family time with their new baby and delay non-urgent procedures, such as measurements and weight.
11. Initiate immediate breastfeeding within the first hour.
12. If baby is ill and needs to be separated from mother, ensure information about baby is provided quickly to the mother and family.
13. Encourage the mother and her family to participate in the care of, and to have contact with, an ill baby.

Emotional support: Continuous presence, reassurance by supportive family members, relatives, or friends. Information: Labour progress and advice regarding coping techniques. Comfort measures: Comforting touch, massage, warm baths or showers, promoting adequate fluid intake.

X. a. Define post-term pregnancy.

Post-term pregnancy is defined as a pregnancy that lasts longer than 42 weeks; 2 weeks past the normal 40-week gestation period. Since a post-term pregnancy is linked with both fetal and maternal health complications, doctors usually do everything they can to ensure that an infant is delivered as close to the due date as possible, which in some cases means that labor is induced, which comes with its own set of complications.

b. Enumerate the causes and clinical features and management of women in post-term pregnancy.

Fetal Macrosomia
1. Fetal macrosomia is defined as an infant who is over 8 pounds, 13 ounces when born. This may cause childhood diabetes, obesity, and metabolic syndrome.
2. Mothers are also as risk when delivering a large baby, including the uterine ruptures, genital tract lacerations, and excessive bleeding after delivery.

Placental Insufficiency
1. Placental insufficiency, also known as uteroplacental vascular insufficiency, occurs when the placenta fails to deliver adequate oxygen and nutrients to the infant.
2. After 37 weeks of pregnancy, the placenta reaches its maximum size and its functions begin to reduce afterwards.
3. The longer an infant goes without proper nutrition and oxygen, the more at risk they become for a host of health problems, including oxygen deprivation that can lead to cerebral palsy, and learning disorders.
4. Since the placental cord may compress in post-term pregnancies, there is a heightened risk of placental insufficiency.

Meconium Aspiration

1. Meconium aspiration is marked by an infant breathing in amniotic fluid and meconium (newborn feces) shortly after birth.
2. Infants who are born post-term are more likely to have a bowel movement while still in utero.
3. Meconium aspiration is considered extremely dangerous and can lead to oxygen deprivation, lung inflammation, and lung infection. Although rare, it can also lead to persistent pulmonary hypertension of the newborn (PPHN) and permanent brain damage.
4. Mothers are also at risk for developing dangerous medical issues, including postpartum hemorrhaging, bacterial infections, perineum injuries, and increased chance of a cesarean section (C-section) surgery.

Clinical Features

The following are the most common symptoms of postmaturity. However, each baby may show different symptoms of the condition. Symptoms may include:
1. Dry, loose, peeling skin
2. Overgrown nails
3. Abundant scalp hair
4. Visible creases on palms and soles of feet
5. Minimal fat deposits
6. Green, brown, or yellow coloring of skin from meconium staining (the first stool passed during pregnancy into the amniotic fluid)
7. More alert and "wide-eyed".

Post-term Pregnancy Treatment

Treatment is imperative for post-term pregnancy and if done properly, may help prevent many of the aforementioned risks. Typical treatment options may include:
1. **Antenatal fetal monitoring:** An infant may be monitored closely once the due date has passed in order to detect any signs of distress. AAFP does not recommend antenatal fetal monitoring until the 42nd week pregnancy.
2. **Contraction stress test:** A contraction stress test will provide Oxycontin to the mother in an attempt to start contractions. The medicine is usually administered intravenously.
3. **Biophysical profile:** A biophysical profile (BPP) is a test that will determine an infant's overall physical score in regards to movement, breathing, fetal tone, and the volume of amniotic fluid.
4. **Labor induction:** It is often difficult to determine the best time to induce labor, but if the results of the previously mentioned treatment options indicate fetal distress, physicians will normally induce labor. Labor induction can include a scheduled C-section or medication applied to the cervix that promotes contractions.

OR

a. Define puerperal sepsis?

Puerperal infection occurs when bacteria infect the uterus and surrounding areas after a woman gives birth. it is also known as a postpartum infection. The mortality rates are thought to be higher in areas that lack proper sanitation.
There are several types of postpartum infections, including:
1. **Endometritis:** An infection of the uterine lining.
2. **Myometritis:** An infection of the uterine muscle.
3. **Parametritis:** An infection of the areas around the uterus.

b. Explain predisposing factors and management of woman with puerperal sepsis.

Predisposing factors: There are factors that may make a woman more at risk for developing an infection. These can include:
1. Anemia
2. Obesity
3. Bacterial vaginosis, a sexually transmitted infection
4. Multiple vaginal exams during labor
5. Monitoring the fetus internally
6. Prolonged labor
7. Delay between amniotic sac rupture and delivery.
8. Colonization of the vaginal tract with Group *B Streptococcus* bacteria
9. Having remains of the placenta in the uterus after delivery
10. Excessive bleeding after delivery
11. Young age
12. Low socioeconomic group.

Symptoms and signs may include:
1. Fever
2. Pain in the lower abdomen or pelvis caused by a swollen uterus
3. Foul-smelling vaginal discharge
4. Pale skin, which can be a sign of large volume blood loss
5. Chills
6. Feelings of discomfort or illness
7. Headache
8. Loss of appetite
9. Increased heart rate

Management of woman with puerperal sepsis:
1. Administration of intravenous broad-spectrum antibiotics within 1 hour of suspicion of severe sepsis, with or without septic shock, is recommended as part of the surviving sepsis resuscitation care bundle.
2. If genital tract sepsis is suspected, prompt early treatment with a combination of high-dose broad-spectrum intravenous antibiotics may be life saving.
3. A combination of either piperacillin/tazobactam or a carbapenem plus clindamycin provides one of the broadest ranges of treatment for severe sepsis.
4. MRSA may be resistant to clindamycin, hence if the woman is or is highly likely to be MRSA-positive, a glycopeptide such as vancomycin or teicoplanin may be added until sensitivity is known.
5. Breastfeeding limits the use of some antimicrobials; hence the advice of a consultant microbiologist should be sought at an early stage.
6. Surgical treatment should be utilized in certain types of puerperal sepsis in conjunction with medical treatment. The operations employed were colpotomy, abdominal drainage and removal of diseased structures and hysterectomy, each operation being employed in certain pathological states. Vein ligation has been done so rarely in this hospital and the mortality in these people so low that the tendency is entirely towards conservative management with repeated blood transfusions.

2016
Midwifery and Gynecology

SECTION-I

I. Give the meaning of the following:
   a. Chorion
   b. Colostrum
   c. Embryo
   d. Lie

II. Fill in the blanks
   a. _____ Suture lies between the two parietal bones.
   b. The normal weight of the placenta is _____
   c. _____ is the dark line running from symphysis pubis to umbilicus during pregnancy.
   d. _____ is the discharge from the uterus following childbirth.

III. Write short notes on any *four* of the following:
   a. Episiotomy
   b. Amniotic fluid
   c. Immediate care of newborn
   d. Antenatal advice
   e. Minor ailments during puerperium and its management

IV. a. Define mechanism of labor
   b. Explain the mechanism of normal labor

V. a. What is preterm baby?
   b. What are the clinical features of a preterm baby?
   c. Explain the nursing management of a preterm baby

SECTION-II

VI. Write whether the following statements are *true* or *false*
   a. Atonic uterus is one of the causes of PPH
   b. Absence of menstruation is known as menopause
   c. Salpingitis is the inflammation of the Fallopian tube
   d. Oxytocin is the drug used for the suppression of lactation.

VII. Choose the correct answer and write
   a. Labor is termed as precipitate labor if it occurs within
      i. 06 hours   ii. 1–2 hours   iii. 08 hours

b. The organ which is affected first in IUGR is
   i. Brain   ii. Liver   iii. Bones
c. The destructive operation performed in hydrocephalus to save the life of the mother is known as
   i. Decapitation   ii. Craniotomy   iii. Cleidotomy

VIII. Write short notes on any *three* of the following:
a. Contracted pelvis
b. Polyhydramnios
c. Retained placenta
d. Carcinoma of the cervix

IX. a. Define uterine prolapse
b. List the causes, signs and symptoms of uterine prolapse
c. Explain the nursing management of mother with uterine prolapse

X. a. Define breech presentation
b. Explain the causes and types of breech presentation
OR
a. Define postpartum hemorrhage
b. Explain the types and nursing management of mother with postpartum hemorrhage

SECTION-I

I. Give the meaning of the following:

a. Chorion

Chorionic villi are villi that sprout from the chorion to provide maximum contact area with maternal blood. They are an essential element in pregnancy from a histomorphologic perspective, and are, by definition, a product of conception. Branches of the umbilical arteries carry embryonic blood to the villi.

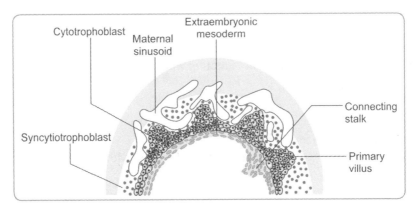

Function of the chorionic villi-day 14. The primery villi appear as cytotrophoblastic stems

The chorion is formed by mesoderm tissue from the mother and trophoblast cells derived from the forming fetus. The **chorionic villi** emerge from this chorion and enter the **endometrium**. The villi are microscopic, finger-like projections that contain capillaries for blood to flow through. The endometrium is the inner membrane of the uterus. It is here that the chorionic villi allow the transfer of nutrients from the mother's blood to the fetus.

Embryonic blood is carried to the villi by the various branches of the umbilical arteries. Here, the blood circulates through the capillaries of the villi and is then returned to the fetus through the umbilical veins. Oxygen and nutrients from the mother's blood diffuse through the walls of the villi to, and provide nourishment for, the growing fetus. Carbon dioxide and waste products from the fetus circulate through the villi back into the mother's blood.

b. Colostrum

Colostrum is a milky fluid that comes from the breasts of humans, cows, and other mammals the first few days after giving birth, before true milk appears. It contains proteins, carbohydrates, fats, vitamins, minerals, and proteins (antibodies) that fight disease-causing agents such as bacteria and viruses.

Colostrum provides over 100 times the amount of immunoglobulins as regular milk. Colostrum is also rich in transfer factors that educate and modulate the immune system and successfully teach it to recognize specific antigens. These transfer factors also help coordinate the immune system to be able to recognize the difference between normal tissue and pathological microbes or abnormal tissue growth. These important transfer factors include hydrogen peroxide and immunoglobulin G (IgG).

The transfer factors from colostrum are able to boost natural killer cell (NK) activity and calm a hyperactive immune system through activating suppressor T cells. This improves the intelligence of the immune system and allows it to function with greater efficiency. These transfer factors also act as a catalytic memory agent for the immune system to alert naive immune cells of an impending danger.

c. Embryo

The term embryo applies to the earliest form of life, produced when an egg (female reproductive cell) is fertilized by a sperm (male reproductive cell; semen). The fertilized egg is called a zygote. Shortly after fertilization, the zygote begins to grow and develop. It divides to form two cells, then four, then eight, and so on. As the zygote and its daughter cells divide, they start to become specialized, meaning they begin to take on characteristic structures and functions that will be needed in the adult plant or animal.

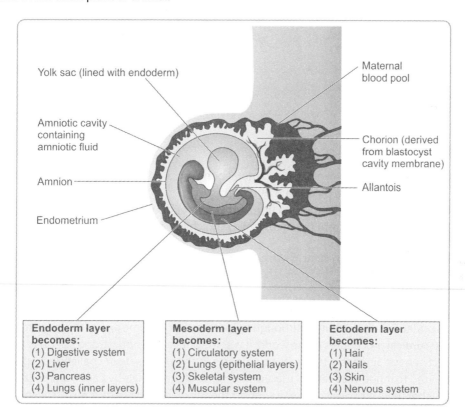

An embryo is a living organism, like a full-grown rose bush, frog, or human. It has the same needs—food, oxygen, warmth, and protection—that the adult organism has. These needs are provided for in a variety of ways by different kinds of organisms.

d. Lie

Fetal **lie** refers to the relationship between the long axis of the fetus with respect to the long axis of the mother. The possibilities include a longitudinal **lie**, a transverse **lie**, and, on occasion, an oblique **lie**.

The lie is the relation of the long axis of the fetus to that of the mother, and is either longitudinal or transverse. Occasionally, the fetal and the maternal axes may cross at a 45-degree angle, forming an oblique lie, which is unstable and always becomes longitudinal or transverse during the course of labor. Fetal attitude or posture: In the later months of pregnancy the fetus assumes a characteristic posture described as attitude or habitus As a rule, the fetus forms an ovoid mass that corresponds roughly to the shape of the uterine cavity. The fetus becomes folded or bent upon itself in such a manner that the back becomes markedly convex; the head is sharply flexed so that the chin is almost in contact with the chest.

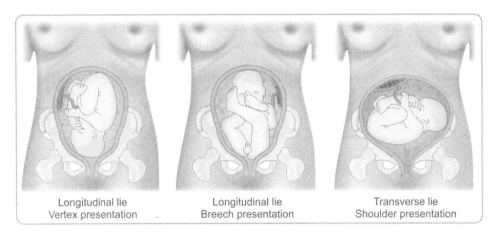

Longitudinal lie
Vertex presentation

Longitudinal lie
Breech presentation

Transverse lie
Shoulder presentation

II. Fill in the blanks

a. **Sagittal** Suture lies between the two parietal bones.
b. The normal weight of the placenta is **600 grams**
c. **Linea Nigra** is the dark line running from symphysis pubis to umbilicus during pregnancy.
d. **Lochia** is the discharge from the uterus following childbirth.

III. Write short notes on any *four* of the following:

a. Episiotomy

Episiotomy is the term for a surgical incision of the perineum made to increase the diameter of the vulval outlet during childbirth. Although episiotomy has become one of the most commonly performed surgical procedures in the world, it was introduced without strong scientific evidence of its effectiveness. Since the 1970s, its routine use in the UK has been challenged. Episiotomy was submitted to randomize clinical trials, and reviews of these trials by Caroli and Belizan, 2004, concluded that there is only evidence to support the selective, and not routine use of episiotomy. Adverse effects of routine episiotomies:

1. An increase in the overall rate of posterior perineal trauma
2. Increased risk of anal sphincter damage
3. Weakened pelvic floor muscles, decreasing sexual function postpartum
4. Increased pain and perineal infection postpartum
5. Increased intrapartum maternal blood loss.

Definition: An episiotomy is a surgical incision made in the perineum, the area between the vagina and anus. Episiotomies are done during the second stage of labor to expand the opening of the vagina to prevent tearing of the area during the delivery of the baby.

Purpose: An episiotomy is usually done during the birthing process in order to deliver a baby without tearing the perineum and surrounding tissue. Reasons for an episiotomy include:

1. Evidence of maternal or fetal distress (i.e. no time to allow perineum to stretch)
2. The baby is premature or in breech position, and his/her head could be damaged by a tight perineum
3. The baby is too large to be delivered without causing extensive tearing
4. The delivery is being assisted by forceps
5. The mother is too tired or unable to push
6. Existing trauma to the perineum.

Types of incision: There are 2 main types of incision.
1. **Mediolateral/Posterolateral:** The incision starts midline at the frenulum of the labia minora, avoiding damage to the Bartholin's gland. It is then directed diagonally to the left over the right side of the posterior perineum to a point midway between the anus and ischial tuberosity, avoiding the anal sphincter.
2. **Midline:** The incision starts in the midline position and is made vertically towards the anus.
3. **Mediolateral versus Midline:** Midline incisions bleed less and are easier to repair. However, the incision carries a greater risk of extension into the rectum, hence it should only be used by the experienced. After reviewing clinical trials, Caroli and Belizan (2004) concluded that there was insufficient evidence to indicate which method was superior.

Procedure: In episiotomy is a surgical incision, usually made with sterile scissors, in the perineum as the baby's head is being delivered. This procedure may be used if the tissue around the vaginal opening begins to tear or does not seem to be stretching enough to allow the baby to be delivered. In most cases, the physician makes a midline incision along a straight line from the lowest edge of the vaginal opening toward the anus. In other cases, the episiotomy is performed by making a diagonal incision across the midline between the vagina and anus (called a mediolateral incision). This method is used much less often, may be more painful, and may require more healing time than the midline incision. After the baby is delivered through the extended vaginal opening, the incision is closed with stitches. A local anesthetic may be applied or injected to numb the area before it is sewn up (sutured).

Episiotomies are classified according to the depth of the incision:
1. A first-degree episiotomy cuts through skin only (vaginal/perineal).
2. A second-degree episiotomy involves skin and muscle and extends midway between the vagina and the anus.
3. A third-degree episiotomy cuts through skin, muscle, and the rectal sphincter.
4. A fourth-degree episiotomy extends through the rectum and cuts through skin, muscle, the rectal sphincter, and anal wall.

After care: The area of the episiotomy may be uncomfortable or even painful for several days. Several practices can relieve some of the pain. Cold packs can be applied to the perineal area to reduce swelling and discomfort. Use of a sitz bath can ease the discomfort. This unit circulates warm water over the area. A squirt bottle with water can be used to clean the area after urination or defecation rather than wiping with tissue. Also, the area should be patted dry rather than wiped. Cleansing pads soaked in witch hazel (such as the brand tucks) are very effective for soothing and cleaning the perineum.

b. Amniotic fluid

Amniotic fluid: The amniotic fluid is formed from the following sources:
1. A secretion from the amniotic epithelium or as a transudate across the umbilical cord or from fetal circulation in the placenta.

2. As a transudate from the maternal serum across the fetal membrane or from maternal circulation.
3. Any at term and equal amount is excreted in the urine.
4. The secretion from the tracheo-bronchial tree across the fetal skin before the skin gets keratinized at the 20th week.

Volume of the amniotic fluid

1. At 12 weeks—50 mL
2. At 20 weeks—400 mL
3. At 36–38 weeks—1000 mL

The specific gravity of the is amniotic fluid low and is about-1.010. The osmolarity of the amniotic fluid is of 250 mOsmol\L—it is suggestive of fetal maturity.

Characteristics of the amniotic fluid

Sl. No.	Amniotic fluid	Normal value	Abnormality	Remarks
1.	Specific gravity	1.016–1.025	1.010-normally seen at term	Low specific gravity is seen at term
2.	Osmolarity	250 mOsmol/L	< 250 or >250	Suggestive of immaturity
3.	Color	Colorless in early pregnancy-pale straw color at term	Meconium stained (green), Golden color, Greenish yellow (yellow), Dark red colored, Dark brown tobacco juice	Fetal distress Rh incompatibility Postmaturity Concealed accidental hemorrhage IUD
	Normal volume	1000 mL	More than 2000 mL Less than 200 mL	Polyhydramnios Oligohydramnios

Suspended particles:
1. Lanugo
2. Foliated squamous epithelial cells from the fetal skin
3. Vernix caseosa
4. Cast of amniotic cells
5. Cells from the respiratory tract, urinary bladder and vagina of the fetus.

Chemical composition:
1. The composition of the amniotic fluid changes with gestation in early pregnancy it is similar to maternal and fetal serum.
2. 98–99% of the amniotic fluid is water.
3. A large number of dissolved substances such as: creatinine, urea, bile pigments, renin, glucose, fructose, proteins (albumin and globulin), lipids, hormones (estrogen and progesterone), enzymes, minerals (N_a^+, K^+ Cl^-).
4. Un-dissolved substances like fetal epithelial cells.
5. During the second half of gestation its osmolarity decreases and is close to dilute fetal urine with added phospholipids and other substances from fetal lung and other metabolites.

c. Immediate care of newborn

Immediate care at birth: The radiant warmer should be put on 15 minutes before the birth of the baby. The baby should be received in pre-warmed linen and dried from top to bottom immediately after birth. The wet linen should be removed and baby should be covered with a dry and warm towel. The baby should be placed in a head low position to facilitate drainage of oropharyngeal secretions. The mouth should be suctioned first followed by suctioning of the nose using a bulb sucker. Suction should be done gently and intermittently. Suctioning should not be more than 5 seconds at a time. The heart rate should be monitored for possible bradycardia. These steps take around 20 to 30 seconds. By this time most babies are vigorously crying, actively moving and pink.

Care after birth: A sterile disposable delivery kit should be used for each baby to prevent cross infection. The eyes should be cleaned with sterile normal saline using one swab for each eye from inner canthus toward outer canthus.
1. The umbilical cord should be tied using umbilical cord clamp, 2 or 3 cm beyond the base of the cord.
2. Do not apply anything on the cord.
3. The patency of the anus should be checked by passing a stiff rubber catheter into the anal orifice.

Essential postnatal care:
1. The bay should be warm to touch and soles should be pink.
2. The umbilical stump should be clean and dry.
3. The tie should be tight. There should be no bleeding.
4. Check that the baby has good suckling. If suckling is poor, assure correct positioning and attachment to breast. Initiate breastfeeding within half an hour in normal delivery.
5. Check that the baby is crying well and has no breathing difficulty. If found the difficulty refer to pediatrician.

d. Antenatal advice

The antenatal education should be include.
I. Diet: The diet during pregnancy should be adequate to provide for
   a. The maintenance of maternal health.
   b. The needs of the growing fetus.
   c. The strength and vitality required during labor.
   d. The successful lactation.

   The pregnancy diet should be light, nutritious and easily digestible. It should be rich in protein, minerals vitamins and fibres and of the required calories. Dietary advice should be given with due consideration to the socioeconomic condition, food habits and taste of the individual. Supplementary iron therapy is needed for all pregnant mothers from 20 weeks onwards.
II. Personal hygiene:
   1. **Rest and sleep:** The woman may continue her usual activities throughout pregnancy. Hard and strenuous work should be avoided. On an average, a patient should have 10 hours of sleep (8 hours at night and 2 hours at noon).
   2. **Bowel:** As there is a tendency of constipation during pregnancy, regular bowel movement may be facilitated by regulation of diet taking plenty of fluids, vegetables and milk.
   3. **Bathing:** Daily baths and preferably twice a day are advised.
   4. **Clothing:** The patient should wear loose but comfortable dresses. High heel shoes are better avoided.
   5. **Dental hygiene:** The dentist should be consulted at the earliest, if necessary.
   6. **Care of the breasts:** Cleanliness of the breasts is maintained. If anatomical defects are present advise to seek medical help.

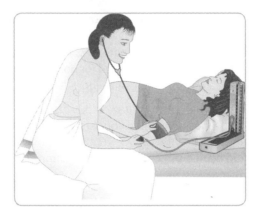

7. **Coitus:** Contact with the husband to be avoided during the first trimester and last 6 weeks.
8. **Travel:** Long distance travel better to be avoided. Rail route is preferable.
9. **Smoking and alcohol:** Smoking and alcohol are to be avoided totally during pregnancy as both cause variable injuries to the fetus.
10. The pregnant women should avoid over-the counter drugs (drugs without medical prescription). The drugs may have teratogenic effects on the growing fetus especially during the first trimester. (The first three months is the period of organogenesis. Teratogens will cause gross malformation or defects to the fetus. The common teratogens are drugs caffeine, exposure to X-rays, alcohol, nicotine, etc).

III. General advice: The patient should be persuaded to attend for antenatal checkup positively on the scheduled date of visit. She is instructed to report to the doctor even at an early date and if the following untoward (warning signs and symptoms) symptoms arise:
1. Intense persistent headache
2. Severe edema
3. Disturbed sleep with restlessness
4. Low urine output (less than 500 mL per day)
5. Epigastric pain
6. Persistent vomiting
7. Painful uterine contractions
8. Sudden gush of watery fluid per vaginum
9. Active vaginal bleeding, etc.

Report the following:
1. Vaginal bleeding
2. Reduced fetal movements
3. Frontal or recurring headaches
4. Sudden swelling
5. Rupture of the membranes
6. Premature onset of contractions, etc.

e. Minor ailments during puerperium and its management

I. Mastitis: Distinction needs to be made between true mastitis and localized inflammation of the breasts resulting from a blocked milk duct. A blocked milk duct responds readily to breast massage. In mastitis there is a bacteria caused infection that needs vigorous intervention. Almost always unilateral and develops well after the flow of milk is established.

Types:
1. Mammary cellulitis—inflammation of the connective tissue between the lobes in the breast
2. Mammary adenitis—infection in the ducts and lobes of the breasts.

Signs and symptoms:
1. Marked engorgement and pain.
2. Chills, fever, tachycardia, hardness and reddening of breasts.
3. Enlarged and tender lymph nodes.

Treatment of mastitis:
1. Rest
2. Appropriate antibiotics—usually cephalosporins
3. Hot and/or cold packs
4. Don't stop breastfeeding because:
   - If the milk contains the bacteria, it also contains the antibiotic
   - Sudden cessation of lactation will cause severe engorgement which will only complicate the situation
   - Breastfeeding stimulates circulation and moves the bacteria containing milk out of the breast.

Preventative measures:
1. Meticulous hand washing by all personnel.
2. Frequent feedings of infant. If the mother finds that one area of breasts feel distended, several methods may help:
   a. Rotate position of baby for nursing so that baby's gums compress different sinuses each time.
   b. If breast not emptied at feeding—manual expression or breast pump can assure that breast is emptied.
   c. As infant nurses, mother should massage distended area to help emptying.

II. Puerperal mastitis

Etiology and pathophysiology: Diuresis is a normal physiological function during the immediate post-partum period. The body uses this mechanism to begin to eliminate the extra fluid volume that has accumulated during pregnancy.

Stretching or trauma to the base of the bladder occurs to some degree in any vaginal delivery, the resulting edema of the trigone is great enough to obstruct the urethra and to cause acute retention. Anesthesia can inhibit normal neural control of the bladder and lead to overdistention and decrease bladder sensitivity. So, residual urine and Bladder trauma can lead to *cystitis*.

Prevention: Diligent monitoring of the bladder during the recovery period and preventive health measures greatly reduces the number of women who get overdistention.
a. Encourage mother to void—regular and complete emptying, proper wiping techniques and good perineal care.
b. Catheterize with extreme gentleness and sterility.

Signs and symptoms:
1. Frequency, urgency
2. Dysuria
3. Nocturia.

Treatment and nursing care:
1. Cath urine for C and S
2. Antibiotics—Ampicillin
3. Urinary tract antispasmodic
4. Force fluids.

III. Thromboembolic disease:
Superficial thrombophlebitis is limited to the superficial saphenous veins, whereas deep thrombophlebitis generally involves most of deep venous system.

Predisposing factors
1. Slowing of blood flow in legs—usually in moms who have a cesarean delivery.
2. Trauma to the vessels during delivery.

Signs and symptoms
1. Sudden onset of pain, tenderness of calf, redness and an increase in skin temp.
2. Positive Homan's sign.

Treatment and nursing care: Heparin—it does not cross into breast milk.

Complication: Pulmonary emboli—substernal chest pain, sudden and intense; dyspnea; pallor and cyanosis; increased jugular pressure; confusion; hypotension; sudden apprehension; hemoptysis.

IV. Localized infection:
A less severe complication of the puerperium is localized infection of the episiotomy, perineal lacerations, vaginal or vulva lacerations. Wound infection of abdominal incision site following cesarean birth. With a localized infection, there is no foul smelling lochia.

Signs and symptoms
1. Reddened, edematous, firm, tender edges of the skin.
2. Edges separate and purulent material mixed with serosanguineous liquid drains from the wound.

Treatment and nursing care
1. Antibiotics
2. Wound care

V. Hematoma
Etiology and pathophysiology: Bleeding into the tissues of the perineal area can cause hematoma formation. May have at least 500 cc. Pooled in the hematoma. May be around the episiotomy site.

Signs and symptoms
1. Pain–perineal. More than normal amount of pain. Mild analgesics are not sufficient to decrease the amount of pain.
2. Hard, firm, area on the perineum.

Treatment and nursing care
1. I and D—incision and drainage. May leave in a penrose drain
2. Dressing changes
3. Replace the blood loss
4. Comfort measures.

VI. Placenta accreta

Etiology and pathophysiology: Placenta accreta is a condition that occurs when all or part of the decidua basalis is absent and the placenta grows directly onto the uterine muscle. This may be partial where only a portion abnormally adhered or it may be complete where all adhered.

Signs and symptoms
1. During the third stage of labor, the placenta does not want to separate.
2. Attempts to remove the placenta in the usual manner are unsuccessful, and lacerations or perforation of the uterus may occur.

Treatment
1. If it is only small portions that are attached, then these may be removed manually
2. If large portion is attached-—a hysterectomy is necessary!

IV. a. Define mechanism of labor. b. Explain the mechanism of normal labor:

It is a series of passive movements of the fetus in its passage through the birth canal. Such movements are essential because the canal is cylindrical with an inlet and outlet differing in size and shape, and a forward curve at its lower end. The fetus is a flexible cylindrical body which during the process of birth is made to accommodate itself to the diameters and the curve of the pelvis.

It is important that these natural movements are thoroughly understood, for the skilful management of normal delivery is based on the knowledge of mechanism.

Mechanism of Normal Vertex Presentation (Left Occiput Anterior—LOA)

1. The lie is longitudinal
2. The attitude is universal flexion
3. The presentation is vertex
4. Position is LOA
5. Denominator is the occiput
6. The presenting part is the posterior area of the right parietal bone.

The engaging diameter of the fetal head fits into the largest diameter of the pelvis. The engaging diameter in LOA is suboccipitobregmatic 9.5 cm. Head can engage in transverse diameter of the pelvis also, i.e. LOT or ROT. The following movements take place as a result of the expulsive action of the uterine and abdominal muscle and diaphragm and the resistance offered by the pelvis, cervix and pelvic floor.

1. Flexion of the head
2. Internal rotation of the head
3. Crowning of the head
4. Extension of the head
5. Restitution of the head
6. Internal rotation of the shoulders
7. External rotation of the head
8. Lateral flexion of the body.

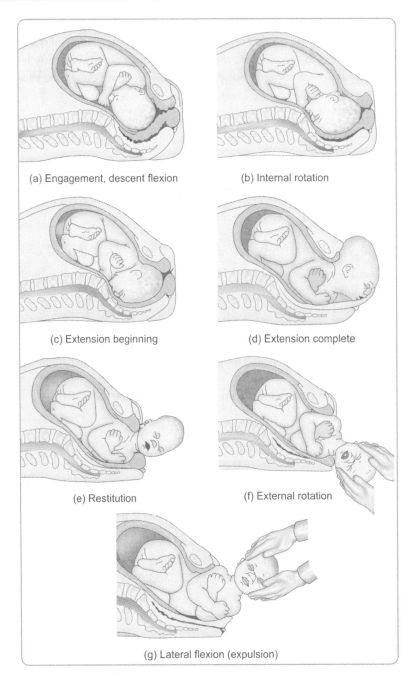

(a) Engagement, descent flexion
(b) Internal rotation
(c) Extension beginning
(d) Extension complete
(e) Restitution
(f) External rotation
(g) Lateral flexion (expulsion)

Descent: It begins in most primigravida two weeks before the onset of labor, when engagement of head occurs, unless there is disproportion. Further descent takes place during the first stage due to the force of uterine contractions. When the head meets resistance, flexion is increased and dilatation allows sink down. During the second stage descent is more rapid, because the abdominal muscle and diaphragm coming into action and the fetus is being expelled

Flexion of the head: The head is usually flexed at the beginning of the labor with the suboccipitofrontal diameter 10 cm engaging at the brim. But when the flexion is increased the suboccipitobregmatic 9.5 cm engages. This increased flexion helps the descents and the occiput becomes the leading part.

Causes of flexion: (1) Exaggeration of the existing attitude. (2) The liver theory when the head meets with the resistance of the pelvis and pelvic floor the flexion is increased. (3) The wedge shape of the head. Descent takes place throughout.

Internal rotation: It is the turning forward of whatever part of the fetus reaches the gutter shaped pelvic floor first. This movement causes the larger diameter of the head, shoulders and buttock to come under the pubic arch, in the anteroposterior diameter of the outlet.

Factors which bring about internal rotation: (1) The passive recoil of one lateral half of the pelvic floor. When the leading part reaches the level of ischial spine it comes in contact with the left half of the pelvic floor. The force of uterine contractions causes the occiput to stretch the left half of the pelvic floor and push it downwards and outwards, when the contraction passes off the pelvic floor recoils because it slips forwards to the left side of the pelvis. If there is no leading part and the head comes and contacts with the both part of the pelvic floor and rotation does not take place. (2) The gutter shaped of the pelvic floor which directs the leading part towards front.

Crowning of the head: It is the term used when the occipital prominence escapes under the symphysis pubis and the head no longer receeds between uterine contractions.

Extension of the head: It is the movement by which the flexion of the head is undone. The nape of the neck (is under the symphysis pubis) pivots on the lower border of the symphysis pubis, while the chin, face and the sinciput sweep the perineum. Extension results from the action of two forces: the uterine and abdominal muscle exert downward pressure and the pelvic floor and perineum resist the above pressure and tend to push head forward and upward.

Restitution: This is the turning of the head to undo the twist in the neck that took place during the internal rotation of the head. This movement reveals whether the position is right or left and midwife is more likely to manage the birth of the shoulders without perineal laceration.

Internal rotation of the shoulders: It is a similar movement as the internal rotation of the head. The shoulders in an LOA position are in the left oblique diameter of the pelvic cavity. The anterior shoulder reaches the right side of the pelvic floor and rotates forwards into the anteroposterior diameter of the outlet. This should take place with the uterine contraction which occurs after the head has been born. Now the anterior shoulder is under the symphysis pubis and it is born and then the post shoulder.

External rotation of the head: It is the turning of the head which accompany with internal rotation of the shoulders, always in the same direction as in restitution. When the head rotates externally, it indicates that the shoulders are in the anteroposterior and is ready to expel.

Lateral flexion of the body: It is a sideway bending of the spine of the baby so that it confirms to the curve of the birth canal. After the expulsion of the shoulders the body is carried forwards over the symphysis pubis towards the mother's abdomen to facilitate the lateral flexion.

V. a. What is preterm baby? b. What are the clinical features of a preterm baby? c. Explain the nursing management of a preterm baby

In humans preterm birth (Latin: *partus praetemporaneus or partus praematurus*) refers to the birth of a baby of less than 37 weeks gestational age. The cause for preterm birth is in many situations elusive and unknown; many factors appear to be associated with the development of preterm birth, making the reduction of preterm birth a challenging proposition.

Definition: Preterm labor is defined as the presence of uterine contractions of sufficient frequency and intensity to effect progressive effacement and dilation of the cervix prior to term gestation (between 20 and 37 weeks).

Causes of preterm labor
1. **Infection:** About 40–50% of all preterm labor can be traced to infection. Many women do not show classic signs of infection, like fevers.
2. **Bleeding:** This does include placental abruption, where the placenta tears away from the uterine wall too early. It also includes bleeding disorders that may be genetic or acquired
3. **Stretching of the uterus:** The stretching or over distension of the uterus has also been linked to preterm labor and birth. This can be caused by fibroids, multiple pregnancies (twins, triplets, etc.), or even having too much amniotic fluid (Polyhydramnios).
4. **Maternal factors:** Low socioeconomic status, maternal age ≤18 or ≥40 years, low prepregnancy weight, smoking, substance abuse
5. **Maternal history:** Previous history of preterm delivery and second-trimester abortion
6. **Uterine factors:** Uterine volume increased, uterine anomalies Trauma and Infection

Signs and symptoms
1. **More than 6 contractions per hour:** It is normal for the uterus to contract, or tightens, as the pregnancy progresses. Contractions that happen more than about every 10 minutes, though, could be a sign of premature labor.
2. **Change in vaginal discharge:** Mother notices that there is leaking clear, watery fluid or if has any bloody discharge later weeks of pregnancy, inform the doctor know right away, mother may have preterm premature rupture of membranes (PPROM) or bloody show from early labor.
3. **Cramping:** Early labor mother may feel like the abdominal cramps (with or without diarrhea) may also be a sign of premature labor.
4. **Backache:** A low backache may be a sign of premature labor. The backache may come and go or be steady, and is usually a dull ache.
5. **Pelvic pressure:** Women in premature labor may feel low-down pelvic pressure, as if the baby is pressing down on the cervix.
    a. Low back pain
    b. Suprapubic pressure
    c. Vaginal pressure
    d. Rhythmic uterine contractions
    e. Cervical dilation and effacement
    f. Possible rupture of membranes
    g. Expulsion of the cervical mucus plug
    h. Bloody show.

Warning signs
1. Contractions every 10 minutes or more often
2. Change in vaginal discharge (leaking fluid or bleeding from your vagina)
3. Pelvic pressure-the feeling that your baby is pushing down
4. Low, dull backache

5. Cramps that feel like menstrual period pain
6. Abdominal cramps with or without diarrhea.

Factors Associated with Increasing Rates of Preterm Birth
1. Increasing rates of multifetal pregnancies
2. Greater percentage of births to women of advanced maternal age
3. Increasing rates of asymptomatic infections, labor inductions, cesarean births and scheduled births
4. Advances in maternal-fetal management.

Management of Preterm Labor
Labor is judged to have started when the woman experiences regular, painful uterine contractions accompanied by either show, rupture of membranes or complete effacement of the cervix. The principles in the management of preterm labor are: (1) To prevent asphyxia, which makes the neonate more susceptible to RDS (2) To prevent birth trauma.

First Stage
1. The woman is put to bed to prevent early rupture of membranes.
2. Oxygen is given by mask to ensure adequate fetal oxygenation.
3. Strong sedatives or acceleration of labor is to be avoided. Epidural analgesia is the choice.
4. Progress of labor should be monitored clinically or (preferably) by electronic monitoring.
5. In case of delay or anticipating a tedious traumatic vaginal delivery, it is better to deliver by cesarean section.

Second Stage
1. The birth should be gentle and slow to avoid rapid compression and decompression of fetal head.
2. Liberal episiotomies should be done under local anesthesia, especially in primigravidae to minimize head compression.
3. Tendency to delay must be curtailed by low forceps.
4. The cord must be clamped immediately at birth to prevent the development of hypervolemia and hyperbilirubinemia.
5. To place the baby in the intensive neonatal care unit under the care of a neonatologist. Preterm fetuses before 34th week presented by breech are generally delivered by cesarean section.

Immediate Management of the Preterm Baby Following Birth
1. The cord is to be clamped quickly to prevent hypervolemia and development of hyperbilirubinemia.
2. The cord length should be about 10–12 cm in case exchange transfusion will be required due to hyperbilirubinemia.
3. The air passage should be cleared of mucus promptly and gently. The stomach contents are also to be sucked out.
4. Adequate oxygenation must be provided.
5. The baby should be wrapped in a sterile warm blanket or towel or laid in the warmer with the head slightly lowered (Temperature 36.5–37.5°C).
6. Vitamin K_1 mg to be injected intramuscularly to prevent hemorrhagic manifestations.
7. Bathing is not appropriate for the preterm baby.
Preterm babies are functionally immature and need special care for their survival.

SECTION-II

VI. Write whether the following statements are *true* or *false*

a. Atonic uterus is one of the causes of PPH: **TRUE**
b. Absence of menstruation is known as menopause: **TRUE**
c. Salpingitis is the inflammation of the Fallopian tube: **TRUE**
d. Oxytocin is the drug used for the suppression of lactation: **FALSE**

VII. Choose the correct answer and write

a. Labor is termed as precipitate labor if it occurs within: **Ans: ii**
   i. 06 hours   ii. 1-2 hours   iii. 08 hours
b. The organ which is affected first in IUGR is: **Ans: i**
   i. Brain   ii. Liver   iii. Bones
c. The destructive operation performed in hydrocephalus to save the life of the mother is known as: **Ans: ii**
   i. Decapitation   ii. Craniotomy   iii. Cleidotomy

VIII. Write short notes on any *three* of the following

a. Contracted Pelvis

The pelvis usually is not contracted in cases of unilateral lameness. With bilateral lameness, the pelvis is wide and short, but most women are able to deliver vaginally. In poliomyelitis, now extremely rare, the pelvis may be asymmetric, but most patients can deliver vaginally. In dwarfism, cesarean delivery is generally the rule because of marked fetopelvic disproportion. Cesarean sections occur more frequently in women with a history of a pelvic fracture, especially bilateral fracture of the pubic rami, before pregnancy.

Definition

1. **Anatomical definition:** It is a pelvis in which one or more of its diameters is reduced below the normal by one or more centimeters.
2. **Obstetric definition:** It is a pelvis in which one or more of its diameters are reduced so that it interferes with the normal mechanism of labor.

Factors influencing size and shape of pelvis

1. Developmental factor: Hereditary or congenital.
2. Racial factor.
3. Nutritional factor: Malnutrition results in small pelvis.
4. Sexual factor: As excessive androgen may produce android pelvis.
5. Metabolic factor: As rickets and osteomalacia.
6. Trauma, diseases or tumors of the bony pelvis, legs or spines.

b. Polyhydramnios

Polyhydramnios: Acute polyhydramnios may occur as early as 18–20 weeks. It is more likely to be due to the fetofetal transfusion syndrome (FFTS) also known as twin-to-twin transfusion syndrome (TTS).

Fetal abnormality: This is particularly associated with monozygotic twins.
1. **Conjoined twins:** Cardiac malformation, fetus in fetus, malpresentations
   Premature rupture of the membranes, prolapse of the cord, prolonged labor.
   Monoamniotic twins. Locked twin
2. **Delay in the birth of the second twin:** The risks of such delay are intrauterine hypoxia, birth asphyxia following premature separation of the placenta and sepsis as a result of ascending infection from the first umbilical cord which lies outside the vulva.
3. **Premature expulsion of the placenta:** In dichorionic twins with separate placentae, one placenta may be delivered separately; in monochorionic twins the shared placenta may be expelled. Postpartum hemorrhage; undiagnosed twins.
   This is also common and is particularly associated with monochorionic twins and with fetal abnormalities. If acute polyhydramnios occurs it can lead to miscarriage or premature labor.

C. Retained Placenta

In humans, **retained placenta** is generally defined as a **placenta** that has not undergone **placental** expulsion within 30 minutes of the baby's birth where the third stage of labor has been managed actively. Risks of **retained placenta** include hemorrhage and infection.

Causes of retained placenta: The primary causes of retained placenta are as follows:
1. **Uterine atony:** In this case, the uterus ceases contraction or does not contract enough to separate the placenta from the walls of the uterus.
2. **Adherent placenta:** In rare cases, a part or the entire placenta is deeply embedded in the uterine wall and fails to detach itself from the uterus.
3. **Placenta accreta:** Placenta Accreta is a rare but serious condition where a part of the placenta adheres to a scar on the uterine muscle instead of the lining. This condition could happen in women who have scars on the uterine muscle from the previous caesarean births. Placenta percreta happens if the placenta has spread through the wall of the uterus.
4. **Trapped placenta:** Trapped placenta is a condition when the placenta successfully separates itself from the uterine wall but fails to pass through cervix that is semi-closed. A trapped placenta would also happen during a controlled cord contraction in the third stage. The umbilical cord may snap if pulled too hard or is too thin, leaving the placenta inside the uterus.

   Some other rare causes of retained placenta are:
5. **Full bladder:** A full bladder will not allow the uterus to contract adequately, eventually preventing placenta delivery. In such a case, the doctor will help to drain out the bladder through a catheter.
6. **'Fiddling' with the uterus:** Action, such as massaging or rubbing the uterus before the third stage will cause weaker, irregular contractions leading to partial separation of the placenta.
7. **Bicornuate uterus:** Bicornuate uterus is a heart-shaped uterus. Tissue present prior pregnancy stretches itself within the uterus giving it a heart shape. If the placenta is attached to the tissue, it will not be able to disconnect itself from the uterine wall.
8. **Succenturiate lobe:** A succenturiate lobe is a tiny piece of placenta that is attached to the actual placenta through a blood vessel. This lobe is usually left behind the placenta which could lead to a possible retained placenta.
9. **Emotional reactions:** Overwhelming emotional reactions like fear or helplessness during childbirth would trigger the release of adrenaline and cease the release of oxytocin, eventually stopping the contractions to release the placenta.

d. Carcinoma of the Cervix

Definition: Cancer of cervix caused mainly by human papilloma virus (HPV). Most common female cancer in developing countries and can be prevented by screening and vaccination against HPV.

Cause/Risk factors
1. Infection with human papilloma virus
2. Early age of first sexual intercourse
3. Multiple sexual partners (unprotected)
4. Multiparity
5. Smoking
6. Age ≥35 to <45.

Signs and Symptoms
1. Very often asymptomatic in early stages
2. Abnormal vaginal bleeding
3. Post coital bleeding
4. Exclude cervix cancer in any postmenopausal bleeding
5. Foul smelling vaginal discharge
6. Symptoms of metasis
7. Hydronephrosis and renal failure
8. By speculum examination, lesions infiltrating the cervix.

Complications
1. Anemia
2. Cachexia
3. Pain
4. Hematuria and dysuria
5. Ureteral obstruction and renal failure
6. Edema of legs
7. Bowel invasion: Diarrhea, tenesmus, rectal bleeding
8. Sepsis
9. Metastasis.

Investigations
1. For invasive cancer, consider stages of cancer
2. Speculum examination: Cervical lesion that easily bleeds on contact
3. PAP smear
4. VIA
5. VILI
6. HPV/DNA testing
7. Colposcopy
8. Biopsy
9. FBC
10. ESR
11. Renal function
12. Intravenous pyelography

13. X-rays: CXR, skeletal X-rays, CT-scan
14. MRI lymphatic metastasis.

Staging
Stage 0: Carcinoma *in situ*
Stage Ia1: Stromal invasion <3 mm (microinvasive)
Stage Ia2: Stromal invasion 3–5 mm
Stage Ib1: Stromal invasion >5 mm, or gross cervical lesion <4cm
Stage Ib2: Gross cervical lesion > 4 cm
Stage IIa: Extending to upper 2/3 vagina
Stage IIIa: Extending to lower 1/3 vagina
Stage IIIb: Extending into parametrium to pelvic sidewall or hydronephrosis
Stage IVa: Extending to bladder/ bowel mucosa
Stage IVb: Distant metastasis.

Management
Principle of treatment
1. Provide general supportive care, e.g., correction of anemia.
2. Undertake examination under anesthesia for staging, biopsy.
3. Provide supportive treatment, surgery, and or radio therapy according to staging.

General measures
1. It is important to clinically assess the extent of disease prior to the onset of treatment.
2. Surgery can be utilized in early stage- disease Ia1-IIa.
3. Radiotherapy+/- chemotherapy can be utilized in all stages I-IV.

Surgery
Stage Ia1: Cold knife cone or LEEP cone in young patients, in old women hysterectomy.
Stage Ib1, Ib2, IIa: radical hysterectomy with bilateral pelvic lymphadenectomy (Para aortic nodes optional)
Stage III and IV: Inoperable (radiotherapy)

Recommendations
1. HPV vaccine is more important for the prevention of cancer cervix
2. Cervical cancer screening (HPV, pap smear, VIA, VILI, Colposcopy, biopsy)
3. Treatment of precancerous lesion (cryotherapy, LEEP, cervical conization)
4. Treatment of invasive cancer (radiotherapy, surgery, chemotherapy)
5. Psychological and financial support in advanced stage of cervical cancer

IX. a. Define uterine prolapse. b. List the causes, signs and symptoms of uterine prolapse. c. Explain the nursing management of mother with uterine prolapse

Genital prolapse is oldest and most common gynecological operative problem.
The exact incidence in our country is not known, but from published data—13% of total women have pelvic organ prolapse. Among these only 20% undergo surgery.

Definition:
1. Pelvic organ prolapse is the downward displacement of the structures that are normally located adjacent to the vaginal vault.
2. Prolapse is a downward descent of the female pelvic organs due to weakness of the structures which normally retain them in position. Both descent and prolapse are relative terms and perceived differently, but are more frequently encountered in women who have borne children and rarely in nulliparous women. Prolapse does not usually become apparent until after the menopause when there is general shrinking and weakening of the supports of the pelvic organs.

Patient history: The following history given by the patient should arouse a suspicion of prolapse of the uterus:
1. Mass coming down per vaginum, weakness in the perineal region, dragging sensation, bearing down sensation.
2. Urinary symptoms—incomplete voiding of urine, frequency of micturition, stress incontinence
3. Vaginal discharge—leucorrhea, blood stained discharge
4. Incomplete evacuation of the feces
5. Sexual dysfunction and dyspareunia—a huge prolapse may interfere with coites
6. Lower back pain—relieved by lying down
7. Systemic symptoms of precipitating diseases
    a. Chronic bronchitis and asthma
    b. Mass per abdomen, ascites
    c. Constipation
    d. Retention of urine

Examination
1. Local examination of external genitalia
2. Per speculum examination
3. Degree of prolapse—level of descent in relation to introitus
4. Check for cervical changes
    a. Elongation and hypertrophy of cervix, atrophy
    b. Decubitus ulcer or ulcer suspicious of malignancy.
    c. Keratinization
    d. Discharge—white/blood stained
5. Anterior/posterior vaginal wall defects
6. Stress in continence
7. Per vaginum examination—size, mobility of uterus, any other palpable mass
8. Rectovaginal examination
9. Abdominal examination—mass per abdomen/free fluid
10. Spine—to rule out neurological and anatomical defect

Differential diagnosis
1. Congenital elongation of cervix
2. Fibroid polyp
3. Gartner's cyst
4. Chronic inversion of uterus
5. Local mass in vagina

Diagnosis

Clinical diagnosis: Confirm the diagnosis by per speculum, per vaginal and rectovaginal examination.

Investigation

Routine Investigation
1. CBC, blood grouping and RH typing
2. FBS, PPBS
3. Blood urea, serum creatinine
4. ECG, chest X-ray
5. Stool for ova, cyst and worms.

Special Investigations
1. USG of abdomen and pelvis to rule out associated pelvic pathology and renal problems due to pressure effect on ureter
2. Pap smear
3. D and C—if menstrual disturbances are present
4. Cervical biopsy—done when malignancy is suspected
5. IVP—where kinking of ureter is suspected in long standing cases and residual volume of urine is more than 100 mL

Treatment Approach: Types of management of prolapse
1. Expectant management
2. Nonsurgical pessaries
3. Surgical.

Expectant Management

Physiotherapy: Useful in minor degrees of uterovaginal prolapse
During 6 months following delivery.
Pelvic floor muscle training (PFMT)—Kegel's exercise: Patient is taught to voluntarily contract the sphincters- initially 15 times each of 3 seconds, duration 6 times per day for 3 weeks and then less frequently for 6 months.

Pessary Treatment

It is non-surgical and palliative. Ring and round pessaries are used.

Indications
Pregnancy
Medical disorder which make operation unsafe
- Patient refuses operation
- To help healing of decubitus ulcer.

Surgery

Preoperative Preparation

1. Daily vaginal douching to prevent the infection and sterilize the vagina.
2. Tampon to reduce to the prolapse and replace the organ back.
3. It helps to prevent kinking of ureter and congestion of organs and also increase the blood flow.

4. If the vaginal walls are senile and atropic, estrogen can be given in the form of cream twice daily.
5. Correction of anemia.
6. Treatment of UTI.
7. Treat diabetes and hypertension
8. Treat other systemic infection

Factors determining the choice of surgery

Type of operation selected depends upon:
1. Age of the patient, her desire to preserve the menstrual and reproductive functions and a functioning vagina.
2. Degree, type, components of prolapse
   Presence of adnexal or uterine pathology in the form of TO mass, myomas, ovarian tumors
   Innumerable surgeries have been designed; most suitable method for each patient is selected.

Surgical Principles: Management of advanced and symptomatic prolapse is primarily surgical.

Anterior compartment defect: Anterior colporrhaphy

Central compartment defect: Includes uterine prolapse, enterocele, eversion of vault
The choice of operation to this defect ranges from Hysterectomy with colporrhaphy and colpopexy
Colpocleisis or colpectomy

Hysterectomy

1. Transabdominal surgery
2. Transvaginal surgery

Transabdominal surgery: This route is useful when the abdomen is open for an unrelated reason such as removal of an ovarian tumor. In selected patients - Abdominal sacrocolpopexy in conjunction with TAH.

Transvaginal Surgery

Vaginal hysterectomy

Enterocele repair
1. Mild and moderate degrees of prolapse—posterior culdoplasty is done for closing cul-de-sac.
2. **Advanced prolapse**—posterior culdoplasty + suspension procedures + posterior colpoperineorrhaphy

Posterior compartment defect: Posterior colpoperineorraphy—it is correction of rectocele with restoration of perineal body.

X. a. Define breech presentation. b. Explain the causes and types of breech presentation

Definition: It is a longitudinal lie in which the buttocks is the presenting part with or without the lower limbs.

Incidence: 3.5% of term singleton deliveries and about 25% of cases before 30 weeks of gestation as most cases undergo spontaneous cephalic version up to term.

Etiology: In general, the fetus is adapted to the pyriform shape of the uterus with the larger buttock in the fundus and smaller head in the lower uterine segment. Any factor that interferes

with this adaptation, allows free mobility or prevents spontaneous version, can be considered a cause for breech presentation as:
1. Prematurity—due to relatively small fetal size, relatively excess amniotic fluid, and more globular shape of the uterus.
2. Multiple pregnancies—one or both will present by the breech to adapt with the relatively small room.
3. Poly- and oligohydramnios.
4. Hydrocephalus.
5. Intrauterine fetal death.
6. Bicornuate and septate uterus.
7. Uterine and pelvic tumors.
8. Placenta previa.

Types
1. **Complete breech:** The feet present beside the buttocks as both knees and hips are flexed and more common in multiparas.
2. **Incomplete breech**: Frank breech: It is breech with extended legs where the knees are extended while the hips are flexed and More common in primigravida.

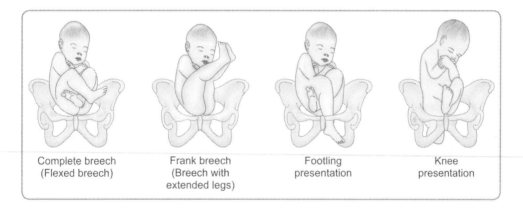

Complete breech (Flexed breech)   Frank breech (Breech with extended legs)   Footling presentation   Knee presentation

3. **Footling presentation**: The hip and knee joints are extended on one or both sides. More common in preterm singleton breeches.
4. **Knee presentation**: The hip is partially extended and the knee is flexed on one or both sides.

Positions
1. Left sacroanterior.
2. Right sacroanterior.
3. Right sacroposterior.
4. Left sacroposterior.
5. Left and right sacrotransverse (lateral).
6. Direct sacroanterior and posterior.

Sacroanterior positions are more common than sacroposterior as in the first the concavity of the fetal front fits into the convexity of the maternal spines.

OR

a. Define postpartum hemorrhage. b. Explain the types and nursing management of mother with postpartum hemorrhage

It is the bleeding from the genital tract after the birth of the baby and is one of the greatest emergencies occurring in childbirth; and if treatment is inadequate, it may have fatal results. PPH is bleeding after the birth of the child and up to 6 weeks after the expulsion of the placenta. The actual amount that constitutes postpartum loss is doubtful and tends to depend on the general condition of the woman.

Definition: Postpartum hemorrhage defined as any amount of bleeding from or into the genital tract following birth of the baby up to the end of the puerperium which adversely affects the general condition of the patient evidenced by rise in pulse rate and falling blood pressure is called postpartum hemorrhage.

Types of PPH: Traditionally, PPH has been classified as early or late with respect to the birth. Early, acute, or primary PPH occurs within 24 hours of the birth. Late or secondary PPH occurs more than 24 hours but less than 6 weeks postpartum. Today's health care environment encourages shortened stays after birth, thereby increasing the potential for acute episodes of PPH to occur outside the traditional hospital or birth center setting.

1. **Primary postpartum hemorrhage:** It occurs within the first 24 hours after delivery of the baby.
2. **Second postpartum hemorrhage:** It occurs at any time after 24 hours and up to 6 weeks following delivery of the baby. The midwife caring the patient should encounter either of these, the first, shortly after transfer from the delivery room and the second; commonly during the second postnatal week.

Predisposing factors: Predisposing factors, which might increase the risk of atonic postpartum hemorrhage include:

1. **Previous history of postpartum** hemorrhage or retained placenta-in such women there is a risk in subsequent pregnancies.
2. **High parity:** With each successive pregnancy, fibrous tissue replaces muscle fibers in the uterus, reducing its contractility and the blood vessels become more difficult to compress. Women, who have had five or more deliveries, are at increased risk.
3. **Fibroids:** These benign tumors may impede efficient uterine action.
4. **Anemia:** Women who enter labor with reduced hemoglobin concentration (below 10 g/dl) may succumb more quickly.
5. **Traumatic:** Hemorrhage in third stage.

2015

Midwifery and Gynecology

SECTION-I

I. Give the meaning of the following:
   a. Nullipara
   b. Conception
   c. Morula
   d. twin.

II. Fill in the blanks
   a. The biparietal diameter measures about: _____
   b. The process of formation of matured ovum in the ovary is: _____
   c. The anterior fontanel is otherwise known as: _____
   d. The endometrium after implantation is known as: _____

III. Write short notes on any *three* of the following:
   a. APGAR score
   b. Partograph
   c. True labor
   d. Postnatal assessment.

IV. a. Define mechanism of labor
   b. Explain the normal mechanism of labor
      OR
   a. Define normal newborn
   b. Explain the clinical features of normal newborn

V. a. Define pregnancy. b. Explain the physiological changes during pregnancy.

SECTION-II

VI. State whether the following statement are *true* or *false*
   a. The normal position of the uterus is retroverted and anteflexed
   b. Internal podalic version is done under general anesthesia
   c. The vault of foetal skull is made-up of 7 bones
   d. Seminal fluid contains 50 million sperms per mL.

VII. Write difference between the following:
   a. Salpingitis and cervicitis
   b. True pelvis and false pelvis
   c. Para and gravida.

VIII. Write short notes on any *three* of the following:
   a. Induced abortion
   b. Postpartum hemorrhage
   c. Postnatal exercise
   d. Nursing management of eclampsia
   e. Cancer cervix.

IX. a. Define eclampsia
   b. Explain the stages of eclampsia
   c. Discuss the nursing management of a patient with eclampsia.

X. a. Define family planning
   b. Write the objectives of family planning
   c. Explain the temporary methods of family planning.

Midwifery and Gynecological Nursing: 2015

SECTION-I

I. Give the meaning of the following:

a. Nullipara

Nulliparous is the medical term for a woman who has never given birth either by choice or for any other reason. This term also applies to women who have given birth to a stillborn or nonviable infant. Many women in the United States are **nulliparous** and the number of women without children is at an all-time high.

b. Conception

Biologically, **conception** is the moment when a sperm cell from a male breaches the **ovum**, or egg, from a female. The process is also known as **fertilization** and is the initial stage of development for human growth. This is a key stage of sexual reproduction, which is a form of reproduction that is necessary for genetic diversity. This is the reproduction method employed by humans.

In order for sexual reproduction to be successful, something called meiosis must take place. The process of **meiosis**, or sex cell division, is necessary for the production of **gametes**, or sex cells. Most cells in the body have 46 chromosomes, which is a full complement of DNA. However, the goal of meiosis is to reduce this number of gametes by half, down to 23 chromosomes. During fertilization, the sperm cell and the ovum, which are the gametes, will have 23 chromosomes apiece. When they combine, the total chromosomal number of the new structure is 46; this is now called a **zygote**, or a fertilized egg cell.

c. Morula

A morula is an embryo at an early stage of embryonic development, consisting of cells in a solid ball contained within the zona pellucida. The morula is produced by embryonic cleavage, the division of the zygote It is the alteration of the shape of the fetal skull that takes place during labor due to the pressure to which it is subjected during its passage through the pelvis. This is permitted by the incomplete ossification of the bones of the vault. The parietal bones overlap the frontal and occiput, while one of the parietal bones slips under the other. The engaging diameter is decreased and the diameter at right angles to it is increased. Moulding occur to a certain degree in all the babies, unless delivered by cesarean section. The overriding the skull bones at the sutures are the most important factor in moulding. Premature babies have very soft skull bones and wide sutures which give no protection to the vital structures of the brain. Post-mature babies have very hard skull, the sutures being almost closed, thus preventing moulding and giving rise to difficulties.

d. Twin

Nobody knows what causes identical (monozygotic) twins. All pregnant women have approximately the same chance of having identical twins – about 1 in 250. Identical twins do not run in families. However, there are some factors that make having nonidentical twins more likely:
1. Nonidentical twins are more common in some ethnic groups, with the highest rate among Nigerians and the lowest among Japanese.
2. Older mothers are more likely to have nonidentical twins because they are more likely to release more than one egg during ovulation.
3. Nonidentical twins run on the mother's side of the family, probably because of an inherited tendency to release more than one egg.

Different types of twins: One-third of all twins will be identical and two-thirds, nonidentical.
1. **Identical twins:** Identical (monozygotic) twins happen when a single egg (zygote) is fertilized. The egg then divides in two, creating identical twins who share the same genes. Identical twins are always the same sex, so if your twins are identical, you'll have two girls or two boys and they'll look very alike.
2. **Non-identical twins:** Non-identical (dizygotic) twins happen when two separate eggs are fertilized and then implant into the woman's womb (uterus). These non-identical twins are no more alike than any other two siblings. Non-identical twins are more common. The babies may be of the same sex or different sexes.

II. Fill in the blanks

a. The biparietal diameter measures about: **9.5 CM**
b. The process of formation of matured ovum in the ovary is: **OOGENESIS**
c. The anterior fontanelle is otherwise known as: **BREGMA**
d. The endometrium after implantation is known as: **DECIDUA**

III. Write short notes on any *three* of the following:

a. Apgar score

Provided the baby is seen to be making some respiratory effort, a quick assessment of its general condition is made which includes the following factors: 1. Heart rate, 2. Respiratory rate, 3. Muscle tone., 4. Reflex response to stimulus, 5. Color. The scoring system is called as the **Apgar** scoring system.

	Score 0	Score 1	Score 3
Appearance			
Pulse	No pulse	<100/min	>100/min
Grimace			
Activity			
Respirations	No respirations	Weak, slow	Strong, cry

Apgar score: Apgar score is developed by Virginia Apgar in 1952. This assessment starts immediately at the birth to assess the resuscitation of the newborn. Apgar scores to check for 5th minutes, 10th minutes and 20 h minutes and also observe the baby's color, mucus membrane of the mouth, conjunctivae, sole and feet. Each item is give grading score like 0, 1, and 2. These score based on the baby's response. Following factors are involved in this observation:1. Appearance 2. Pulse/ Heart rate, 3. Grimace/reflex response, 4. Activity/muscle tone, 5. Respirations.

Babies normally have a score of 8–9 within first minute after the birth. If the score is between 8 and 10 means newborn is easily adjusting to the extra uterine life. Neonate and condition is good. The score of 5–7 shows moderate difficulty of the newborn to adjust to the extra uterine life. The condition is fair but the baby needs assistance with the oxygen and the Ambu bag. The score of four or below four shows severe distress and may require an endotracheal intubation.

Transitional assessment: After birth, neonate tries to adjust with the environment. During the first 24 hours, changes in the vital functions, such as heart rate, respiration, motor activity, color mucus production, and bowel activity occur in orderly manner. This is the period of reactivity.

b. Partograph

Managerial tool for the prevention of prolonged labor: Measuring progress of labor in relation to time. Observations charted on pantograph

The progress of labor with time
1. Cervical dilatation
2. Descent of fetal head: Descent: abdominal palpation of fifths of head felt above the pelvic brim.

Uterine contraction
1. Frequency per 10 min
2. Duration/shown by different shading.

The fetal condition
1. Fetal heart rate
2. Membranes and liquor
3. Moullding of the fetal skull.

Grading
1. **Normal:** Space felt between the edged of parital bone in the sagital suture.
2. **Mild:** The edge of partial bone comes very closer at the sagital suture.
3. **Moderate:** The edge of the partial bone over lap at sagital suture but can be easily separated.
4. **Severe:** Overlap of the bones and not separable.

The maternal condition
1. Pulse, B/P temperature
2. Drug and IV fluids
3. Urine /volume, protein, acetone/
4. Oxytoin regime.

The progress of labor: The 1st stage is divided in to the latent and active phases

Latent phase: Slow period of cervical dilatation from 0 to 2 cm and also it is the period of gradual shortening of the cervix.

Active phase: faster period of cervical dilatation from 3 to 10 cm or full cervical diltation.

c. True labor

True pelvis: The true or "lesser" pelvis is bounded in front and below by the pubic symphysis and the superior rami of the pubis; above and behind, by the sacrum and coccyx; and laterally, by a broad, smooth, quadrangular area of bone, corresponding to the inner surfaces of the body and superior ramus of the ischium, and the part of the ilium below the arcuate line.

True labor pains have the following features:
1. The woman complains of intermittent abdominal pain which can start any time after 22 weeks of gestation.
2. The pain is often associated with a blood-stained mucus discharge known as "show".
3. The woman might have a watery vaginal discharge or a sudden gush of water.
4. On vaginal examination, you will find:
   a. **Cervical effacement:** This refers to the progressive shortening and thinning of the cervix during labor.
   b. **Cervical dilatation:** This refers to an increase in the diameter of the cervical opening. It is measured in centimeters. A fully dilated cervix has a cervical opening that is 10cm in diameter, which means that the cervix is no longer felt on vaginal examination Sometimes the patient may not be in true labor but she does experience pain. This means that she has false labor pains. The following table will help you in differentiating true labor pains from false labor pains.

d. Postnatal assessment

The 1st day after the first couple hours is when it expresses the difficulty after given birth. The nurse this assessment after doing a regular assessment of lungs, bowels, skin and pulses. Vital signs are check q 15 min. for the 1st hr plus fundus (uterus).

B – Breast
U – Uterus
B – Bladder
B – Bowel Sounds
L – Lochia
E – Episiotomy
H – Hemorrhoids and Homan's sign
E – Education and edema.

I. Breast
1. Gently palpate each breast
2. If you feel nodules in the breast, the ducts may not have been emptied at last.
3. Stroke downward towards the nipple and then gently release the milk by manual.
4. If nodules remain, notify the doctor.
5. Take this opportunity to explain the process of milk production, what to do about engorgement, how to perform self breast examinations, and answer any questions she may have about breastfeeding.
6. What is the contour?
7. Are the breast full, firm, tender, shiny?
8. Are the veins distended?
9. Is the skin warm?
10. Does the patient complain of sore nipples?
11. Are breasts so engorged that she requires pain medication?

II. Uterus
1. Palpate the uterus
2. Have the patient feel her uterus as you explain the process of involution
3. If uterus is not involution properly, check for infection, fibroids and lack of tone.
4. Uterus should the firm decrease approximately one finger breath below
5. Unsatisfactory involution may result if there are retained secundines or the bladder not completely empty.

III. Bladder
1. Inspect and palpate the bladder simultaneously while checking the height of the fundus.
2. An order from the physician is necessary cauterization may be done. An order for culture and sensitivity test since definitive treatment may be required.
3. Talk to mother about proper perineal care. Explain that she should wipe from front to back after voiding and defecating.
4. Bladder distention should not be present after recent emptying.
5. When bladder distention does occur, a pouch over the bladder area is observed, felt upon palpation; mother usually feels need to urinate.
6. It is imperative that the first three postpartum voiding be measured and should be at least 150 cc. Frequent small voiding with or without pain and burning may indicate infection or retention.

IV. Bowel Function
1. Question patient daily about bowel movements. She must not become constipated. If her bowels have not functioned by the second postpartum day, the doctor may start her on a mild laxative
2. Encourage patient to drink extra fluids.
3. Have patient select fruits and vegetables from her menu.

V. Lochia
1. Assess the amount and type of lochia on pad in relations to the number of postpartum days. First 3 days of postpartum, you should find a very red lochia similar to the menstrual flow (lochia ruba).
2. During the next few days, it should become watery serous (lochia serosa). On the tenth day, it
3. Should become thin and colorless (lochia alba).
4. Inform the mother about what changes she should expect in the lochia and when it should cease.
5. Tell the mother when her next menstrual period will probably begin and when she can resume sexual relations.
6. Discuss family planning at this time.
7. Notify the doctor if the lochia looks abnormal in to color or contains clogs other than small ones.

VI. Episiotomy
1. Inspect episiotomy thoroughly using flashlight if necessary, for better visibility.
2. Check rectal area. If hemorrhoids are present, the doctor may want to start on sitz bath and local analgesic medication. Reassure patient and answer questions she may have regarding pain, cleanliness, and coitus.
3. Check episiotomy for proper wound healing, infection, inflammation and suture sloughing.
4. Is the surrounding skin warm to touch?
5. Does the patient complain of discomfort? Notify the doctor if any occurs.

VII. Homan's Sign
1. Press down gently on the patient's knee (legs extended flat on bed) ask her to flex her foot.
2. Pain or tenderness in the calf is a positive Homan's sign and indication of thrombophlebitis. Physician should be notified immediately.

VIII. Emotional Status
1. Throughout the physical assessment, notice and evaluate the mother's emotional status.
2. Explain to the mother and to her family that she may cry easily for a while and that her emotions may shift from high to low. The changes are normal and are probably caused by the tremendous hormonal changes occurring in her body and by her realization of new responsibilities that accompany each child's birth.
3. Does the patient appear dependent or independent? Is she elated or despondent? What does she say about family? Are there other nonverbal responses?

IV. a. Define mechanism of labor. b. Explain the normal mechanism of labor:
See 2016-IV

OR

a. Define normal newborn. b. Explain the clinical features of normal newborn.

Newborn period encompasses the first four weeks of extrauterine life. It is an important link in the chain of events from conception to adulthood. The physical and mental wellbeing of an individual depends on the correct management of events in the perinatal period. In India average weight of a normal newborn infant born after 40 weeks of gestation is around 2.8 kg, whereas it is 3.4 kg. or more among affluent societies. Care of the newborn at birth is primarily aimed at helping the newborn to adapt to the extra-uterine environment. Physiological adaptation includes: 1. Initiating respiration and oxygenation of the arterial blood, 2. Temperature adaptation, 3. Initiation of feeding.

Definition: A healthy infant born at term (38–42 weeks) should have an average birth weight of 2500–3000 g.
1. It cries immediately following birth.
2. It establishes independent respiration.
3. It quickly adapts to changed environment.

The newborn is otherwise called as the neonate (between 0-28 days). After 28 days to one year, it is called as an **infant**.

Physical features of newborn at birth

Weight: The weight is variable from country to country but usually exceeds 2500 g. In India, the weight varies between 2.7 kg and 3.1 kg.

Length: Usually, length is between 50 cm and 52 cm.

Posture: The newborn assumes the attitude of its intrauterine existence-extremities flexed and fists clenched.

Skin: Initially slightly blue, but soon become pink. Vernix caseosa may be present.

Head: Head is larger in relation to the rest of the body.

Face: The face is comparatively smaller in relation to the head. The eyes remain closed most of the times. Pupils react to light. The cheeks are full due to brown fat.

Neck and trunk: The neck is short the circumference of the chest is slightly less than that of the head.

Genitalia: In the males, the testes are in the scrotum, the rugae cover the scrotum. In females, labia minora and clitoris are covered by labia majora.

Temperature: The body temperature may fall to as low as 97°F because the newborn is very thermolabile due to immature hypothalamus.

Urine: Small amount of urine is passed. A neonate passes urine 6–8 times a day.

Stool: The first stools passed are called as the meconium (sticky, dark colored) may be passed soon after birth.

V. a. Define pregnancy. b. Explain the physiological changes during pregnancy

Pregnancy is a chronological event that occurs traditionally during the stage of early adulthood. The duration of an average pregnancy is 38 weeks from conception or 40 weeks from the last menstrual period which is divided into 3 trimesters of 3 months each. Pregnancy (gestation) is the maternal condition of having a developing fetus in the body.

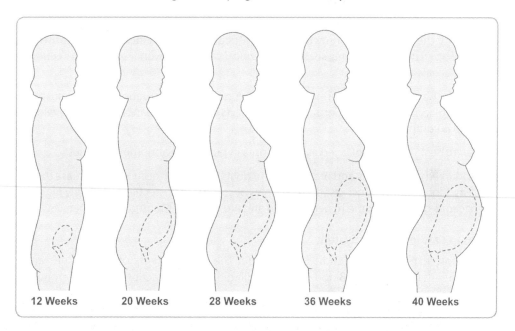

The human conceptus from fertilization through the eight weeks of pregnancy is termed as embryo, from eight week until delivery, it is a fetus. For obstetric purposes the duration of pregnancy is based on gestational age, the estimated age of the fetus calculated from the first day of the last (normal) menstrual period (LMP), assuming a 28 days cycle.

Physiological changes during pregnancy: During pregnancy there are progressive anatomical and physiological changes, not only confined to the genital organs but also to all systems of the body. This principally is a phenomenon of maternal adaptation to the increasing demands of the growing fetus.

Reproductive organs

Vulva: Vulva becomes hyperemic. Labia minora are hyperpigmented and hypertrophied.

Vagina: Vaginal walls become hypertrophied and more vascular. Increased blood supply gives the bluish discolouration of the mucosa. The vaginal secretions become copious, thin and white.

Uterus: There is enormous growth of the uterus during pregnancy. The uterus in non-pregnant state weighs about 60 g and measures about 7.5 x 5 x 2.5 cm in size. At term, it weighs 900–1000 g and measures 35 x 22 x 13 cm in size. The changes occur in all the parts of the uterus that is the body, isthmus and cervix.

Body of the uterus: There is an increase in growth and enlargement of the body of the uterus. The muscle fibres undergo both hypertrophy and hyperplasia [both increase in length and breadth and addition of new muscle fibers]. The uterus feels soft and elastic in contrast to firm feel of the nongravid uterus.

Decidua: Decidua is the name given to the endometrium during pregnancy. It becomes thick and spongy and blood supply is also increased. The upper and lower uterine segments are formed towards the later weeks of pregnancy. The shape of the uterus changes from pear shaped to ovoid. Uterus rises out of the pelvic cavity by 12th week of pregnancy.

Cervix: Cervix softens and loosens in preparation for labor and delivery. There is hypertrophy and hyperplasia of the elastic and connective tissues. Mucus production increases and forms a thick plug (called operculum) effectively sealing the cervical canal to prevent ascending infection from the vaginal canals.

Ovary: Both the ovarian and uterine cycles of the normal menstruation remains suspended. Hence, no ovulation takes place. Corpus luteum persists in early pregnancy until the development of placenta is completed.

Fallopian tubes: They get enlarged as uterus rises in pelvic and abdominal cavities.

Breasts: Marked hypertrophy and proliferation of ducts and alveoli occurs that increase the size of the breasts. Blood supply is increased. The nipples become larger, erectile and deeply pigmented. The sebaceous glands become hypertrophied and are called as Montgomery tubercles.

Changes in Cardiovascular System

Blood volume expands as much as 50% to meet the requirements of new tissues and the increasing needs of all systems. Blood vessels are dilated due to the action of progesterone, which predisposes the woman to varicose veins and hemorrhoids (caused by abnormal dilation of blood vessels). The plasma volume increases 40% and the red blood cells increases only 20% that leads to hemodilution, which causes physiological anemia in healthy women. The heart rate is slightly increased to improve blood flow to the fetus and placenta.

Changes in the respiratory system: As the uterus grow, it presses on the diaphragm and causes shallow and more frequent respiration. Hence, respiratory rate is slightly increased and oxygen consumption is increased by 15%.

Changes in digestive system: Nausea and vomiting occur in the morning usually in early pregnancy. Heart burn and mild indigestion may occur. Constipation may occur probably due to the action of progesterone. Increased salivation occurs, called as **ptyalism.** Cravings or desires to nonnutritive substances may occur. After that condition is called as **pica.** Bleeding gums and tooth loss due to demineralization are common.

Changes in the skin: There is an increased pigmentation occurring around the nipples and areola of the breasts, the center line of abdomen (linea nigra), in the face especially on forehead and cheek (chloasma). Stretch marks (striae gravidarum) occur in abdomen, thighs and breasts.

Changes in skeletal system: Alternations in posture, walking and gait occur due to change in center of gravity as the uterus enlarges in size. Joint mobility is increased as a result of action of relaxin, an ovarian hormone on connective tissue. Backache is common. Occasional calf muscle cramps may occur due to calcium deficiency.

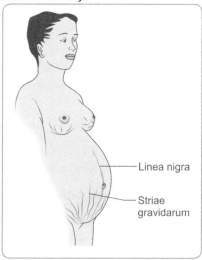

Changes in skin

Changes in urinary system: Frequency of urination is common in early pregnancy as the gravid uterus pressing on the bladder when it is in the pelvic cavity. Again frequency increases in the last few weeks of pregnancy due to pressure from the enlarged uterus. When the fetal head enters into the pelvic cavity, lightening will occur. The pregnant woman will have easy breathing as the pressure on the diaphragm is relieved.

Weight gain in pregnancy: The total weight gain during pregnancy averages 10–12 kg. The total weight gain is distributed approximately as follows:

Weight gain
Up to 20 weeks—2 kg.
After 20 weeks till term—10 kg

Distribution of weight gain during pregnancy
Fetus 3.4 kg
Placenta 0.6 kg
Amniotic fluid 0.6 kg
Fat deposit and protein 3.5 kg
Uterus 0.9 kg
Breasts 0.5 kg
Increase in blood volume 1.5 kg
Increase in extracellular fluid 1.0 kg

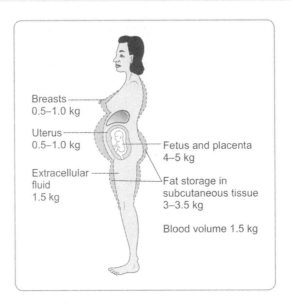

Total weight gain 12.0 kg
Periodic and regular weight checking is of high importance to detect abnormality.

Changes in endocrine system: Corticosteroid production is increased. The anterior pituitary gland is enlarged. Adrenocorticotrophic hormone, melanocyte stimulating hormone and thyrotrophic hormone increase their activities.

SECTION-II

VI. State whether the following statement are *true* or *false*

a. The normal position of the uterus is retroverted and anteflexed.   **FALSE**
b. Internal podalic version is done under general anesthesia.   **TRUE**
c. The vault of foetal skull is made up of 7 bones.   **TRUE**
d. Seminal fluid contains 50 million sperms per mL.   **FALSE**

VII. Write difference between the following:

a. Salpingitis and cervicitis

Salpingitis is an infection of fallopian tube.

Cervicitis: The term cervicitis is reserved to infection of the endocervix including the glands and the stroma, it may be acute or chronic.

b. True pelvis and false pelvis

True pelvis: The true or "lesser" pelvis is bounded in front and below by the pubic symphysis and the superior rami of the pubis; above and behind, by the sacrum and coccyx; and laterally, by a broad, smooth, quadrangular area of bone, corresponding to the inner surfaces of the body and superior ramus of the ischium, and the part of the ilium below the arcuate line.

True labor pain	False labor pain
Regular	Irregular
Increase progressively in frequency, duration and intensity	Do not
Pain is felt the abdomen and radiating to the back.	Pain is felt mainly in the abdomen
Progressive dilatation and effacement of the cervix.	No effect on the cervix
Membranes are bulging during contractions	No bulging of the membranes
Note relived by antispasmodics or sedatives	Can be relived by antispasmodics and sedatives

False pelvis: The false "greater" pelvis is bounded on either side by the ilium; in front it is incomplete, presenting a wide interval between the anterior borders of the ilia; behind is a deep notch on either side between the ilium and the base of the sacrum.

c. Para and gravida

Gravidity is defined as the number of times that a woman has been pregnant and parity is defined as the number of times that she has given birth to a fetus with a gestational age of 24 weeks or more, regardless of whether the child was born alive or was stillborn.

The term **gravida** comes from the Latin word *gravidus*. It is used to describe a woman who is pregnant and is also a medical term for the total number of confirmed pregnancies a woman has had, regardless of the outcome of the pregnancy. For example, a woman who is pregnant for the first time will be termed a **primigravida**, which means first pregnancy.

Para refers to the total number of pregnancies that a woman has carried past 20 weeks of pregnancy. This number includes both live births and pregnancy losses after 20 weeks, such as stillbirths. The term **primipara** may be used to describe a woman who has had one delivery after 20 weeks, and **multipara** is used for a woman who has had two or more births. **Nulliparous** is the term that describes a woman who has never given birth after 20 weeks of pregnancy.

VIII. Write short notes on any *three* of the following:

a. Induced abortion

Deliberate termination of pregnancy before the viability of the fetus is called induction of abortion. Deliberate induction of abortion, by a registered medical practitioner in the interest of mother's health and life is protected under the Medical Termination of Pregnancy (MTP) Act, 1975.

The following provisions are laid down:
1. The continuation of pregnancy would involve serious risk of life
2. There is a substantial risk of the child being born with serious physical and mental abnormalities, so is to handicapped in life.
3. Pregnancy caused as a result of failure of a contraceptive.
4. Pregnancy caused by a rape, both in cases of major and minor girl and in mentally imbalanced women.

Indications for medical termination of pregnancy
1. To save the life of the mother
2. Social indications—this is almost the sole indication and is covered under the provision prevent grave injury to the physical and mental health of the pregnant woman.

Eugenic
1. Structural, chromosomal, genetic abnormalities of the fetus.
2. When the fetus is likely to be deformed due to action of teratogenic drugs.

Methods of Medical Termination of pregnancy

A. First trimester (up to 12 weeks)

I. Surgical
1. Manual vacuum aspiration (MVA)
2. Section evacuation and or curettage
3. Dilatation and evacuation
    a. Rapid method
    b. Slow method.

II. Medical
1. Mifepristone
2. Mifepristone and misoprostol
3. Methotrexate and misoprostol
4. Tamoxifen and misoprostol.

B. Second trimester
1. Dilation and evacuation
2. Intrauterine instillation of hyperosmotic solutions.
    a. Intra-amniotic hypertonic urea, saline
    b. Extra-amniotic ethacridine lactate
        i. Prostaglandins
        ii. Oxytocin infusion
        iii. Hysterotomy.

Complications of MTP

A. Immediate
1. Trauma to the cervix and uterus leading to hemorrhage and shock.
2. Hemorrhage and shock due to trauma, incomplete abortion, atonic uterus or rarely coagulation failure,
3. Thrombosis or embolism
4. Post abortal pain, bleeding, and low grade fever due to retained clots or products.
5. Related to the methods employed.

Saline: Hypernatremia, pulmonary edema, DIC, renal failure, etc.
Prostaglandin—diarrhea, fever, vomiting
Oxytocin—convulsions, water intoxication.

B. Remote
I. Gynecological
1. Menstrual disturbances
2. Chronic pelvic inflammation
3. Infertility due to cornual block.
4. Scar endometriosis
5. Secondary amenorrhea.

II. Obstetrical
1. Recurrent mid-trimester abortion due to cervical incompetence
2. Ectopic pregnancy
3. Preterm labor
4. Dysmaturity
5. Increased perinatal loss
6. Rupture uterus
7. Rh ISO immunization in Rh-ye women
8. Failed abortion and continued pregnancy.

B. Postpartum hemorrhage

Postpartum hemorrhage is bleeding from the genital tract during the 3rd stage of labor, or within 24 hours after delivery of the placenta to the amount of 500 mL or any amount that will change the patient's condition.

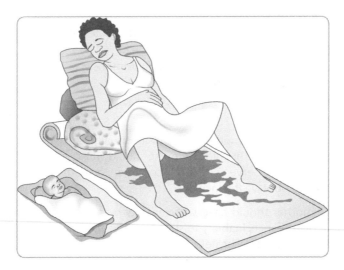

It is responsible for maternal deaths and is one of the emergencies in which if the nurse/mid wife does not know how or fails to play the part the doctor may be Unable to save the mother's life as shock gets in quickly and can become irreversible. The rate of flow that is more important than the amount Anemia is a predisposing cause. It is occurs within 24 hours at delivery it is caused primary while after 24 hours of Delivery is secondary PPH.

Cause of Primary PPH
1. Retained Placenta
2. Retained Cotyledon
3. Genital trauma
4. Disseminated intramuscular coagulation (DIC)
5. Inversion of uterus.

Cause of secondary PPH
1. Chorioamnionitis
2. Retained products.

Type of PPH
1. Atonic postpartum hemorrhage
2. Traumatic postpartum hemorrhage
3. Hypofibrinogenemia.

Management of PPH
Three basic principle are applied as:
1. Call an obstetrician
2. Stop the bleeding
3. Resuscitate the mother.

c. Postnatal exercise

An important aspect of the midwife/nurse works whether in hospital or at home is her educational role. Advice the mother to care for herself and for her baby covering a wide range of subjects like hygiene nutrition, immunization, family planning, etc.

The basic principles of postnatal care include:
1. Promotion of physical well-being by good nutrition, adequate fluid intake, comfort, cleanliness, and sufficient exercises to ensure good muscle tone.
2. Early ambulation is insisted to prevent deep vein thrombosis.
3. Establishment of emotional wellbeing.
4. Promotion of breastfeeding.
5. Prevention of complications.

Admission to postnatal ward: The mother and baby are usually transferred to the postnatal word within an hour or 2 after delivery. The midwife/nurse should well come the mother and help her to settle in the ward. She will observe her general condition, palpate the uterus to note whether it is contracted or not and observe the lochia.

Sleep and rest: The mother should have sufficient sleep and rest. Keep a quiet comfortable atmosphere without disturbance. Inability to sleep must be regarded with concern and Doctor should be consulted. Hypnotics may be needed and it is given without hesitation. Undue anxiety, sleeplessness and loss of appetite should be rewarded as serious. Rest is usually encouraged during the day preferably in prone position as this aids drainage from the uterus and vagina.

Ambulation: Mothers benefit a feeling of wellbeing from this early activity and this reduces the incidence of thrombi embolic disorders.

Diet: A good balanced diet should be taken as advised in pregnancy the woman's appetite usually returns very quickly after labor is ended and has had some sleep. Protein foods are important particularly if she is breast feeding. Excess fruit should be avoided as substances from this will pass to the baby in the milk & may cause diarrhea. The daily fluid intake should be from 2.5–3 liters of which at least 600 mL should be milk.

Postnatal exercises—Advantages
1. Gives the women a sense of well-beingness
2. Maintains good circulation, lessens possibility of venous thrombosis.
3. Restores muscle tone of the abdominal wall and pelvic floor.
4. Promotes for normal drainage of lochia
5. Prevents hypostatic pneumonia.

6. Helps in emptying the bladder, bowels and uterus.
7. Permits her to enjoy a daily bath.
8. Enables her to take early care of her baby.
9. Restores her body figure.

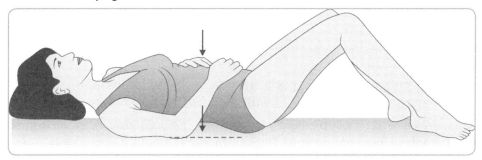

Pelvic tilt

Pelvic Floor Exercises (Kegel exercise): The pelvic floor muscles have been under strain during pregnancy and stretched during delivery, and it may be both difficult and painful to contract these muscles postnatally. Mothers should be encouraged to do the exercise (as explained in the antenatal section) as often as possible in order to regain full bladder control, prevent uterine prolapsed and ensure normal sexual satisfaction in future.

The contraction should be held for ten seconds (to a count of six) and repeated up to ten times at any one session, breathing normally throughout. The mother should continue to do this exercise for 2–3 months. After three months if the mother is able to cough deep deeply with a full bladder without leaking urine (stress incontinuance), she may stop the exercise. If leaking occurs, she may to continue the exercise for the rest of her life.

Role of the nurse: During this period now a days is largely for advice and educate the mother in the care of her baby and herself, to listen patiently to her fears and expression, to answer her questions and through out to given her encouragement and reassurance. This is an exchanging and highly responsible task for a competent and thoughtful midwife/nurse.

d. Nursing management of eclampsia

An eclamptic convulsion is frightening to behold. First, the woman's face becomes distorted, and her eyes protrude. Then her face acquires a congested expression, and foam may exude from her mouth. Breathing stops. Because eclampsia is so frightening, the natural tendency is to try to stop a convulsion, but this is not the wisest strategy.

Eclampsia is defined as the development of convulsions and/or coma unrelated to other cerebral pathology during pregnancy or in the postpartum period in patients with signs and symptoms of preeclampsia. It is a life-threatening obstetrical emergency that is not limited to occurrence in tertiary care centers. Obstetricians and perinatal nurses in every facility therefore must be familiar with the diagnosis and management of this complication of pregnancy. Astute care by the obstetrical team is of paramount importance in eclampsia management because of increased risks of maternal trauma, volume overload, gastric aspiration, and fetal distress. Basic principles in the management of eclampsia are maternal support of vital functions, protection of mother from injury, prevention of recurrent convulsions, correction of maternal hypoxemia or acidemia, control of severe hypertension, and initiation of the delivery process. Parenteral magnesium sulfate remains the anticonvulsant agent of choice in eclamptic patients. Administration of magnesium sulfate requires personnel to be familiar with its pharmacology, side effects, and appropriate antidote in the event of over dosage. With a well-formulated management plan, improved maternal and fetal outcome is achievable in this infrequent but severe complication of pregnancy.

e. Cancer cervix
See 2016-VIII-D

IX. a. Define eclampsia. b. Explain the stages of eclampsia. c. Discuss the nursing management of a patient with eclampsia.

Eclampsia is rarely seen. Usually pregnancy-induced hypertension is diagnosed and treatment is instituted in order to prevent eclampsia. The incidence of eclampsia is approximately 1 in 1500 pregnancies and of these about 20% occurs in the antenatal period, 25% occur intrapartum and 35% within the first few hours after delivery. Eclampsia is characterized by convulsions and coma.

Eclampsia is characterized by epileptiform fits associated with hypertension of a moderate-to-severe degree. Worldwide, it is usually preceded by preeclampsia, but the quality of antenatal care in the UK now is such that three-quarters of cases of eclampsia occur without preexisting recorded evidence of hypertension.

Etiology
1. Cerebral edema.
2. Cerebral vasoconstriction.
3. Cerebral hypoxia.

These lead to cerebral ischemia and hence fit.

Clinical course: At present in the UK about 25% of women with eclampsia will have a fit before labor; most of the rest are likely to have a fit in the postpartum period. The character of the fit is very similar to an epileptic fit with a typical fit consisting of:
1. Twitching: 30 seconds.
2. Tonic phase: 30 seconds.
3. Clonic phase: 2 minutes.
4. Coma: 10–30 minutes.

Such fits may repeat frequently.

Treatment
Aims
1. Keep the woman alive during the fit.
2. Prevent more fits.
3. Deliver the baby.

Prevention: Magnesium sulfate reduces the incidence and severity of fits.
During fit:
1. Turn the woman on her side.
2. Maintain the airway.
3. Stop the fit by giving IV diazepam and magnesium sulfate.

After the fit:
1. Prevent further fits. This is usually done by giving a continuous infusion of magnesium sulfate or diazepam.
2. If the woman is not in hospital, arrange an emergency transfer giving adequate anticonvulsants to cover the journey.
3. Lower the blood pressure by use of IV hydralazine, labetalol or magnesium sulfate.
4. Deliver the baby. As with fulminating PIH, such women are best if the baby is delivered vaginally, as these speeds the recovery process. The indications for cesarean section are those listed in the section on preeclampsia.

Prognosis

Maternal mortality: In the UK death from eclampsia is rare with the woman more likely to die from the hypertensive effects on the cerebral circulation from a cerebrovascular accident.

Fetal mortality: During an eclamptic fit: 300/1000. Overall: 150/1000 intrauterine deaths from hypoxia or neonatal death from prematurity.

X. a. Define family planning. b. Write the objectives of family planning. c. Explain the temporary methods of family planning.

Family planning is defined as a way of thinking and living that is adopted voluntarily, upon the basis of knowledge, attitude and responsible decisions by individuals and couples in order to promote the health and welfare of the family group and thus contribute effectively to the social development of a country. This is the WHO definition of family planning.

Definition: According to WHO Expert Committee in 1971 defined and described: "Family planning refers to practices that help individuals and couples to attain certain objectives like, to avoid unwanted births, at which births occur in relation to the ages of the patient and to determine the number of children in the family." Family planning is the way of thinking and living that it is adopted voluntarily upon the basis of knowledge attitude and responsible decisions by individuals and couples in order to promote the health and welfare of the health and welfare of the family group and thus contribute effectively to the social development of a country.

Objectives
1. To avoid unwanted births.
2. To bring about wanted births.
3. To regulate intervals between pregnancies.
4. To control the time at which births occur in relation to the age of the parent.
5. To determine the number of children in the family.

Importance: Family planning avoids and also prevents a variety of adverse effects on the health of mother, fetus and child.

Mother: The adverse effects prevented are:
1. Maternal depletion
2. Maternal morbidity
3. Maternal mortality
4. Lowered nutritional status
5. Complications of pregnancy.

Fetus: Preventable effects are:
1. Fetal undernutrition
2. Fetal mortality.

Child: The following can be prevented:
1. Mortality of children
2. Protein energy malnutrition (PEM)
3. Inadequate child care
4. Emotional consequences of inadequate care.

Scope of family planning services: A WHO Expert Committee (1970) has stated that family planning includes the following services:
1. The proper spacing and limitation of birth.
2. Advice of sterility.
3. Education for parenthood.
4. Sex education.
5. Screening for pathological conditions related to the reproductive system.
6. Genetic counseling.
7. Premarital consultation and examination.
8. Carrying out pregnancy tests.
9. Marriage counseling
10. The preparation of couple for the arrival of their first child.
11. Providing services for unmarried mothers.
12. Teaching home economics and nutrition.

Classification of Contraceptive Methods

A. Temporary methods (Spacing methods)
1. Barrier methods: Physical methods, chemical methods
2. Intrauterine devices
3. Hormonal methods
4. Postconceptional methods
5. Miscellaneous.

B. Permanent methods (Terminal methods)
1. Male sterilization
2. Female sterilization.

Health Education in Family Planning
1. It can create awareness in the community regarding the availability of various family planning services.
2. It can produce a positive attitude to family planning by motivating eligible couples to adopt the small family norm.
3. It allays fears and removes misconcepts about family planning.
4. It ensures that people utilize family planning programs optimally.

5. Health education efforts are directed at conducting orientation camps. These camps can motivate local leaders to undertake activities at gross roots. So, it can be made a movement of the people, by the people and for the people.
6. Health education also involves mass communication programs through modern media (radio, TV and cinema) and cultural media (folk songs, puppet shows, etc).

2014
Midwifery and Gynecology

SECTION-I

I. Give the meaning of the following:
   a. Midwife.
   b. Lightening.
   c. Presentation.
   d. Vernix caseosa.

II. Fill in the blanks
   a. Intermittent painless uterine contractions are called: ―――――――
   b. The process by which the reproductive organ return to the pregravid state is called: ―――――――
   c. ――――― sign is made out by feeling increased pulsation in lateral vaginal fornices.
   d. ――――― is the first stool of the baby.

III. Write short notes on any *three* of the following:
   a. Antenatal advice.
   b. Fetal skull and its diameter.
   c. Advantages of breastfeeding.
   d. Preparation of women for labor.
   e. Minor disorders in pregnancy.

IV. a. Define fertilization.
   b. What are the abnormalities of placenta?
   c. Write in detail about functions of placenta.

V. a. What is puerperium?
   b. Write in detail the postnatal care for a primi mother after labor up to 10 days.

SECTION-II

VI. Write whether the following statements are *true* or *false*
   a. Implantation of placenta in the lower uterine segments is called abruption placenta.
   b. Bandi's ring is seen near symphysis pubis.
   c. Labor which exceeds 10 hours is called prolonged labor.
   d. Destructive operations are done only when the fetus is dead.

VII. Fill in the blanks
a. Inflammation of the breast is called: ───────
b. Absence of menstruation is called: ───────
c. Inflammation of fallopian tube is called: ───────

VIII. Write short notes on any *three* of the following:
a. Thrombophlebitis.
b. Types of cesarian section.
c. Uterine prolapsed.
d. Puerperal psychosis.
e. Responsibility of the nurse when oxytocin is administered.

IX.
a. What is hysterectomy?
b. List the indications for hysterectomy.
c. Write the pre- and postoperative nursing care of women posted for hysterectomy.

X.
a. What is postpartum hemorrhage?
b. Write the difference between atonic and traumatic postpartum hemorrhage (PPH).
c. Explain the management for atonic PPH and traumatic PPH.

SECTION-I

I. Give the meaning of the following:

a. Midwife

A midwife is a person who has successfully completed a midwifery education program that is recognized in the country; who has acquired the requisite qualifications to be registered and/or legally licensed to practice midwifery and use the title 'midwife'; and who demonstrates competency in the practice of midwifery.

The midwife is recognized as a responsible and accountable professional who works in partnership with women to give the necessary support, care and advice during pregnancy, labor and the postpartum period, to conduct births on the midwife's own responsibility and to provide care for the newborn and the infant. This care includes preventative measures, the promotion of normal birth, the detection of complications in mother and child, the accessing of medical care or other appropriate assistance and the carrying out of emergency measures.

The midwife has an important task in health counseling and education, not only for the woman, but also within the family and the community. This work should involve antenatal education and preparation for parenthood and may extend to women's health, sexual or reproductive health and child care.

A midwife may practice in any setting, including the home, community, hospitals, clinics or health units.

b. Lightening

Lightening is the sensation the mother feels when the baby "drops" down or gradually settles into the pelvis. At the end of the third trimesters, the baby settles, or drops lower, into the mother's pelvis. This is known as dropping or lightening. Dropping is not a good predictor of when labor will begin. In first-time mothers, dropping usually occurs 2–4 weeks before delivery, but it can happen earlier. In women who have already had children, the baby may not drop until labor begins.

c. Presentation

In obstetrics, the **presentation** of a fetus about to be born refers to which anatomical part of the fetus is leading, that is, is closest to the pelvic inlet of the birth canal. According to the leading part, this is identified as a cephalic, breech, or shoulder presentation. A malpresentation is any other presentation than a vertex presentation (with the top of the head first). Breech presentation of the fetal buttocks or feet in labor; the feet may be alongside the buttocks (complete breech presentation); the legs may be extended against the trunk and the feet lying against the face (frank breech presentation); or one or both feet or knees may be prolapsed into the maternal vagina (incomplete breech presentation).

d. Vernix caseosa

Vernix caseosa, also known as vernix, is the waxy or cheese-like white substance found coating the skin of newborn human babies. Vernix starts developing on the baby in the womb around 18 weeks into pregnancy. Vernix caseosa is a white cheesy substance that covers and protects the skin of the fetus and is still all over the skin of a baby at birth. Vernix caseosa is composed of sebum (the oil of the skin) and cells that have sloughed off the fetus' skin. "Vernix" is the Latin word for "varnish." The vernix varnishes the baby. "Caseosa" is "cheese" in Latin.

II. Fill in the blanks

a. Intermittent painless uterine contractions are called: **False labor.**
b. The process by which the reproductive organ return to the pregravid state is called: **Involusion of uterus.**
c. **Osiander's** sign is made out by feeling increased pulsation in lateral vaginal fornices.
d. **Meconium** is the first stool of the baby.

III. Write short notes on any *three* of the following:

a. Antenatal advice

The antenatal period is an extremely important time during pregnancy. It is well recognized that good antenatal care improves maternal, perinatal and neonatal outcomes. Most women will progress through pregnancy in an uncomplicated fashion and deliver a healthy infant with little medical intervention. However, a significant number will develop medical or fetal complications. The current challenge in antenatal care is to identify those women who will require specialist support while allowing uncomplicated pregnancy to proceed with minimal interference.

The aims of antenatal care are to:
1. Provide high-quality information that can be easily understood in the current climate of ethnic and social diversity.
2. Provide an informed choice about the pathways of antenatal care.
3. Identify and screen for maternal complications.
4. Identify and screen for fetal complications.
5. Assess maternal and fetal wellbeing throughout pregnancy.
6. Provide advice and education on the normal symptoms of pregnancy.

At the initial antenatal care visit and with the aid of a special booking checklist the pregnant women become classified into either normal risk or high risk.

b. Fetal skull and its diameters

The **fetal skull**, from an obstetrical viewpoint, and in particular its size, is important because an essential feature of labor is the adaptation between the fetal head and the maternal bony pelvis. Only a comparatively small part of the head at term is represented by the face. The rest of the head is composed of the firm skull, which is made up of two frontal, two parietal, and two temporal bones, along with the upper portion of the occipital bone and the wings of the sphenoid.

These bones are separated by membranous spaces, or sutures. The most important sutures are the frontal, between the two frontal bones; the sagittal, between the two parietal bones; the two

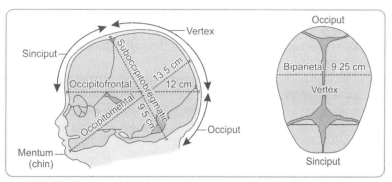

coronal, between the frontal and parietal bones; and the two lambdoid, between the posterior margins of the partial bone and upper margin of the occipital bone. Where several sutures meet, an irregular space forms, which is enclosed by a membrane and designated as a fontanel. The greater, or anterior fontanel, is a lozenge-shaped space that is situated at the junction of the sagittal and the coronal sutures. The lesser, or posterior fontanel, is represented by a small triangular area at the intersection of the sagittal and lambdoid sutures. The localization of these fontanels gives important information concerning the presentation and position of the fetus. The temporal, or casserian fontanels, have no diagnostic It is customary to measure certain critical diameters and circumferences of the newborn head. The diameters most frequently used, and the average lengths thereof, are:

1. The occipitofrontal (11.5 cm), which follows a line extending from a point just above the root of the nose to the most prominent portion of the occipital bone.
2. The biparital (9.5 cm), the greatest transverse diameter of the head, which extends from one parietal boss to the other.
3. The bitemporal (8.0 cm), the greatest distance between the two temporal sutures.
4. The occipitomental (12.5 cm), from the chin to the most prominent portion of the occiput.
5. The suboccipitobregmatic (9.5 cm), which follows a line drawn from the middle of the large fontanel to the undersurface of the occipital bone just where it joins the neck.

The greatest circumference of the head, which corresponds to the plane of the occipitofrontal diameter, averages 34.5 cm, a size too large to fit through the pelvis without flexion. The smallest circumference, corresponding to the plane of the suboccipitobregmatic diameter, is 32 cm. The bones of the cranium are normally connected only by a thin layer of fibrous tissue that allows considerable shifting or sliding of each bone to accommodate the size and shape of the maternal pelvis. This intrapartum process is termed molding. The head position and degree of skull ossification result in a spectrum of cranial plasticity from minimal to great and, in some cases, undoubtedly contribute to fetopelvic disproportion, a leading indication for cesarean delivery.

c. Advantages of breastfeeding

Breast milk is best for your baby, and the benefits of breastfeeding extend well beyond basic nutrition. In addition to containing all the vitamins and nutrients your baby needs in the first 6 months of life, breast milk is packed with disease-fighting substances that protect your baby from illness.

1. Research shows that breastfed infants have fewer and shorter episodes of illness.
2. Breastfeeding is the most natural and nutritious way to encourage your baby's optimal development.
3. Colostrum (the first milk) is a gentle, natural laxative that helps clear baby's intestine, decreasing the chance for jaundice to occur.
4. The superior nutrition provided by breast milk benefits your baby's IQ.
5. Breastfeeding is a gentle way for newborns to transition to the world outside the womb.
6. The skin-to-skin contact encouraged by breastfeeding offers babies greater emotional security and enhances bonding.
7. The activity of sucking at the breast enhances development of baby's oral muscles, facial bones, and aids in optimal dental development.
8. Breastfeeding appears to reduce the risk of obesity and hypertension.
9. Breastfeeding delays the onset of hereditary allergic disease, and lowers the risk of developing allergic disease.
10. Breastfeeding helps the baby's immune system mature, protecting the baby in the meantime from viral, bacteria, and parasitic infections.

11. Breastfeeding increases the effectiveness of immunizations, increasing the protection against polio, tetanus, and diphtheria vaccines.
12. Breastfeeding protects against developing chronic diseases, such as celiac disease, inflammatory bowel disease, asthma, and childhood cancers.

d. Preparation of women for labor

Preparing for childbirth is one of the most exciting times for a woman; however, it may also be a time of fear and anxiety for a mom-to-be. During this transitional period as a woman may start preparing for the special new addition to her family, she may also have to come to terms with the many adjustments that will have to be made. Staying organized, positive, relaxed and planning properly can help make the childbirth process easier. Ensure that early and regular prenatal care is put into place and that you are consulting with your physician and following the prescribed dietary and nutritional requirements. Maintain an emotional connection with your unborn child during the pregnancy period by massaging your belly, through meditation or music to strengthen the bond with you and your baby.

In the eighth month of pregnancy, you and your partner will most likely be sorting out some last minute details. To eliminate additional stress on the day of the delivery, you may want to preregister at the hospital before you go into labor. Here you can read and sign the necessary preadmission and medical consent forms in your own time. Arrange another tour of your birthing center, so that you can check on visiting hour schedules, find out about parking passes, etc.

More and more women are choosing natural and holistic treatments, such as herbal remedies to help prepare them physically and emotionally for natural birth. Herbs such as Squaw Vine (Mitchella repens), Raspberry leaves (Rubus idaeus) and Passiflora incarnate help prepare the body for labor and childbirth as well as relieve fear, anxiety and nervousness about the delivery. In addition, Glycyrrhiza glabra (licorice) acts as a powerful anti-inflammatory and tonic for the uterus to stimulate contractions. Natural remedies formulated for childbirth and labor are side effect free and won't cause harm to mom and baby.

e. Minor disorders in pregancy

1. **Edema:** Swelling of the feet and ankles is very common in pregnancy, especially in the afternoon, or in hot weather. It is due to **edema**, the retention of fluids in the body tissues. Under the force of gravity, the retained fluid tends to sink down the body and collect in the feet. Advise the woman to sit with her feet raised as often as possible, to allow the fluid to be absorbed back into the circulatory system. Swelling of the feet is usually not dangerous, but severe swelling when the woman wakes up in the morning, or swelling of the hands and face at any time, can be signs of preeclampsia, which is a very serious (even life-threatening) condition.

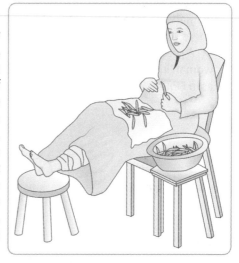

Management: Swelling in the feet may improve if the woman puts her feet up for a few minutes at least two or three times a day, avoids eating packaged foods that are very salty, and drinks more water or fruit juices.

2. **Frequency of urination:** Urinary frequency is a common complaint throughout pregnancy, especially in the first and last months. This happens because the growing fetus and uterus presses against the bladder. It will stop once the baby is born. If urinating hurts, itches, or burns, the woman may have a bladder infection.
3. **Vaginal discharge:** Discharge is the wetness all women have from the vagina. A woman's body uses this discharge to clean itself from the inside. For most women, the discharge changes during their monthly cycle. Pregnant women often have a lot of discharge, especially near the end of pregnancy. It may be clear or yellowish. This is normal. However, the discharge can be a sign of an infection if it is white, gray, green, lumpy, or has a bad smell, or if the vagina itches or burns.
4. **Feeling hot or sweating a lot:** Feeling hot is very common in pregnancy, and as long as there are no other warning signs (such as signs of infection), the woman should not worry. She can dress in cool clothes, bathe frequently, use a paper fan or a large leaf, and drink plenty of water and other fluids.
5. **Dyspnea (shortness of breath):** Many women get short of breath (can not breathe as deeply as usual) when they are pregnant. This condition is called dyspnea.

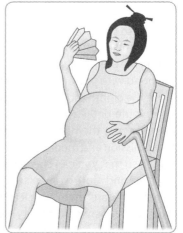

    Management: Reassure women who are breathless near the end of pregnancy that this is normal. But if a woman is also weak and tired, or if she is short of breath all of the time, she should be checked for signs of sickness, heart problems, anemia, or poor diet. Get medical advice if you think she may have any of these problems.
6. **Difficulty in getting up and down:** It is better if a pregnant woman does not lie flat on her back, because it can be difficult for her to get up again, and because when a woman is on her back, the weight of the uterus presses on the big blood vessels that return blood to her heart. This can temporarily reduce the supply of oxygen to her brain, and she may feel dizzy. If the woman wants to be on her back, she should put something behind her back and under her knees so she is not lying completely flat.

    A pregnant woman should also be careful how she gets up. She should not sit up like the woman in Figure (A). Instead, she should roll to the side and push herself up with her hands, as in Figure (B).

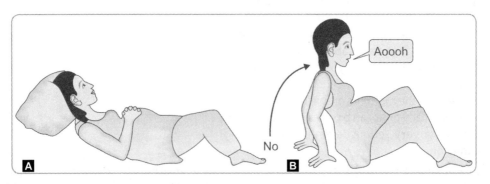

(A) Getting up without turning onto one side first can tear the muscles of the abdomen; (B) Turning to the side and pushing up with the hands is much safer and more comfortable

IV. a. Define fertilization

Human fertilization is the union of a human egg and sperm, usually occurring in the ampulla of the uterine tube. The result of this union is the production of a zygote, or fertilized egg, initiating prenatal development. Scientists discovered the dynamics of human fertilization in the nineteenth century. The process of fertilization involves a sperm fusing with an ovum. The most common sequence begins with ejaculation during copulation, follows with ovulation, and finishes with fertilization. Various exceptions to this sequence are possible, including artificial insemination, *in vitro* fertilization, external ejaculation without copulation, or copulation shortly after ovulation. Upon encountering the secondary oocyte, the acrosome of the sperm produces enzymes which allow it to burrow through the outer jelly coat of the egg. The sperm plasma then fuses with the egg's plasma membrane, the sperm head disconnects from its flagellum and the egg travels down the fallopian tube to reach the uterus.

b. What are the abnormalities of placenta?

Placental disease, also known as **placental pathology**, is a broad term describing any single number of diseases affecting the placenta. The article also covers placentation abnormalities, which is often used synonymously for placental disease.

Abnormalities of the Placenta

a. Abnormal Shape

1. Placenta bipartite.
2. Placenta succenturiata.
3. Placenta circumvallata.
4. Placenta fenestrata.

The placenta consists of two equal lobes connected by placental tissue.

I. *Placenta bipartite*
1. The placenta consists of two equal parts connected by membranes.
2. The umbilical cord is inserted in one lobe and branches from its vessels cross the membranes to the other lobe.
3. Rarely, the umbilical cord divides into two branches, each supplies a lobe.
4. The placenta consists of a large lobe and a smaller one connecting together by membranes.
5. The umbilical cord is inserted into the large lobe and branches of its vessels cross the membranes to the small succenturiate (accessory) lobe.

II. *Placenta succenturiata*
1. The accessory lobe may be retained in the uterus after delivery leading to postpartum hemorrhage.
2. This is suspected if a circular gap is detected in the membranes from which blood vessels pass towards the edge of the main placenta.
3. A whitish ring composed of decidua, is seen around the placenta from its fetal surface.
4. This may result when the chorion frondosum is too small for the nutrition of the fetus, so the peripheral villi grow in such a way splitting the decidua basalis into a superficial layer (the whitish ring) and a deep layer.

III. *Placenta circumvallata*: It can be a cause of—abortion, antepartum hemorrhage, preterm labor and intrauterine fetal death.

IV. *Placenta fenestrata*: A gap is seen in the placenta covered by membranes giving the appearance of a window.

V. *Placenta membranacea*
   1. A great part of the chorion develops into placental tissue.
   2. The placenta is large, thin and may measure 30–40 cm in diameter.
   3. It may encroach on the lower uterine segment, i.e. placenta previa.

b. Abnormal Weight

The placenta increases in size and weight as in:
   1. Congenital syphilis.
   2. Hydrops fetalis.
   3. Diabetes mellitus.

Placenta praevia: The placenta is partly or completely attached to the lower uterine segment In this gravid uterus, the placenta implanted over the os. This is called placenta previa. Implantation in this low lying position can lead to extensive hemorrhage as the dilation of the cervix disrupts the placenta.

c. Abnormal Adhesion
   1. *Placenta accreta*: The chorionic villi penetrate deeply into the uterine wall to reach the myometrium, due to deficient decidua basalis.
   2. *Placenta increta*: When the villi penetrate deeply into the myometrium, it is called "placenta increta"
   3. *Placenta percreta*: When they reach the peritoneal coat it is called "placenta percreta".

d. Placental Lesions

Seen in placenta at term, mainly in hypertensive states with pregnancy.
   1. *White infracts*: Due to excessive fibrin deposition (Normal placenta may contain white infracts in which calcium deposition may occur).
   2. *Red infarcts*: Due to hemorrhage from the maternal vessels of the decidua (Old red infarcts finally become white due to fibrin deposition).

Placental Tumor

Chorioangioma: It is a rare benign tumor of the placental blood vessels which may be associated with hydramnios.

c. Write in detail about functions of placenta

The placenta is the highly specialized organ of pregnancy that supports the normal growth and development of the fetus. Growth and function of the placenta are precisely regulated and coordinated to ensure the exchange of nutrients and waste products between the maternal and fetal circulatory systems operates at maximal efficiency. The main functional units of the placenta are the chorionic villi within which fetal blood is separated by only three or four cell layers (placental membrane) from maternal blood in the surrounding intervillous space. After implantation, trophoblast cells proliferate and differentiate along two pathways described as villous and extravillous. Non-migratory, villous cytotrophoblast cells fuse to form the multinucleated syncytiotrophoblast, which forms the outer epithelial layer of the chorionic villi. It is at the terminal branches of the chorionic villi that the majority of fetal/maternal exchange occurs. Extravillous trophoblast cells migrate into the decidua and remodel uterine arteries. This facilitates blood flow to the placenta via dilated, compliant vessels, unresponsive to maternal vasomotor control. The placenta acts to provide oxygen and nutrients to the fetus, whilst removing carbon dioxide and other waste products. It metabolises a number of substances and can release metabolic products into maternal and/or fetal circulations. The placenta can help to protect the fetus against certain xenobiotic molecules, infections and maternal diseases. In addition, it releases hormones into both the maternal and fetal circulations to affect pregnancy, metabolism, fetal growth, parturition and other functions. Many placental functional changes occur that accommodate the increasing metabolic demands of the developing fetus throughout gestation.

V. a. What is puerperium?

Puerperium, the period of adjustment after childbirth during which the mother's reproductive system returns to its normal prepregnant state. It generally lasts 6 to 8 weeks and ends with the first ovulation and the return of normal menstruation. Puerperal changes begin almost immediately after delivery, triggered by a sharp drop in the levels of estrogen and progesterone produced by the placenta during pregnancy. The uterus shrinks back to its normal size and resumes its prebirth position by the sixth week. During this process, called involution, the excess muscle mass of the pregnant uterus is reduced, and the lining of the uterus (endometrium) is reestablished, usually by the third week. While the uterus returns to its normal condition, the breasts begin lactation. Colostrum, a high-protein form of milk, is produced by the second day after the birth and is gradually converted to normal breast milk, which has less protein and more fat, by the middle of the second week.

The chief medical problems associated with the puerperium include usually mild, transient depression, resulting from emotional letdown and discomfort associated with puerperal changes; clotting disorders, caused by blood stasis and prevented by an early return to normal activity; bleeding from a retained placenta; and puerperal fever, a major cause of maternal death until the 19th century. A combination of improved sanitary measures and modern antibiotics has now greatly reduced the mortality associated with puerperal fever.

b. Write in detail the postnatal care for a primi mother after labor up to 10 days

The first few hours following the successful birth of the baby and afterbirth are sometimes known as the 4th stage of birth or labor. Immediately after its delivery, the placenta should be examined carefully to detect abnormalities (infarcts, hematomas, abnormal insertion of the umbilical cord), but above all to ensure that it is complete. If there is a suspicion that part of the placenta is missing, the uterine cavity needs to be explored.

The mother should be also observed carefully during the first hour postpartum. The most important observations include the amount of blood lost, and uterine contraction, since if the uterus contracts insufficiently, blood may accumulate in the uterine cavity. If the blood loss is abnormal and the uterus is contracting poorly, gentle abdominal massage of the uterus can be helpful. It is essential to ensure that uterine contraction is not inhibited by the presence of a full bladder. Postpartum hemorrhage, defined by the WHO as abnormal blood loss more than 500 mL, should be treated with oxytocics. The mother's blood pressure, pulse and temperature, and general wellbeing should be assessed.

At this stage, any tears in the cervix or vagina and the episiotomy incision (if performed) are stitched. The mother, baby and partner are now moved to the recovery room and for the next few hours are closely monitored, as many complications may arise in this period.

A woman delivering in a hospital may leave the hospital as soon as she is medically stable and chooses to leave, which can be as early as a few hours postpartum, though the average for spontaneous vaginal delivery (SVD) is 1–2 days, and the average cesarean section postnatal stay is 3–4 days. During this time, the mother is monitored for bleeding, bowel and bladder function, and baby care. The infant's health is also monitored.

Mother's health: The first few days after birth are consumed with the joy of being a mother. After the 'blues', typically around day 3 (feeling weepy because of the big drop in hormones), the job of motherhood gets underway in earnest. While all this is happening the body is rapidly returning to normal. Whether the delivery is by cesarean or vaginal the vaginal bleeding should start to settle and reduce in the first week. Although it may last for 4–6 weeks, it should gradually reduce with time. If it increases in the first weeks you should return to your doctor for assessment. This is called a secondary post (= after) partum (= delivery) hemorrhage (= blood loss) and may indicate that there is some infection in the womb.

Wound healing and infection: Whether the wound is from a cesarean or vaginal delivery, it tends to heal rapidly as the mother is young. If infection occurs (about 5%), it is usually the patient's own bugs taking advantage of the healing skin. The body delays healing, so that it can deal with the infection. It is important therefore to control any infection sooner rather than later. This is often by local means (keeping the area clean, washing), but will sometimes require antibiotics. Bruising can also cause some extra pain. Arnica may help the body to absorb the bruise and quicken healing. Bladder infections are also common; you should contact your doctor if you have symptoms (wanting to go often, pain passing urine). Breast infection (mastitis) occurs when the bugs on mother's skin get in through the nipple and infects the gland. Antibiotics are usually necessary to help with this problem.

SECTION-II

VI. Write whether the following statements are *true* or *false*

a. Implantation of placenta in the lower uterine segments is called abruption placenta: **FALSE**
b. Bandi's ring is seen near symphysis pubis: **TRUE**
c. Labor which exceeds 10 hours is called prolonged labor: **TRUE**
d. Destructive operations are done only when the fetus is dead: **FALSE**

VII. Fill in the blanks

a. Inflammation of the breast is called: **Mastitis.**
b. Absence of menstruation is called: **Amenorrhea.**
c. Inflammation of fallopian tube is called: **Salpingitis.**

VIII. Write short notes on any *three* of the following:

a. Thrombophlebitis

Thrombophlebitis is inflammation of a vein (usually in an extremity, especially one of the legs) that occurs in response to a blood clot in the vessel. When it occurs in a vein near the surface of the skin, it is known as superficial thrombophlebitis, a minor disorder commonly identified by a red, tender vein.

Deep-vein thrombophlebitis (affecting the larger veins farther below the skin's surface) is more serious. It may produce less-pronounced symptoms at first (half of all cases are asymptomatic) but carries the risks of pulmonary embolism (when the clot detaches from its place of origin and travels to the lung) and chronic venous insufficiency (impaired outflow of blood through the veins), resulting in dermatitis, increased skin pigmentation and swelling.

b. Types of cesarean section

There are several types of cesarean section (CS). An important distinction lies in the type of incision (longitudinal or latitudinal) made on the uterus, apart from the incision on the skin.

1. **The classical cesarean section** involves a midline longitudinal incision which allows a larger space to deliver the baby. However, it is rarely performed today, as it is more prone to complications.
2. **The lower uterine segment section** is the procedure most commonly used today; it involves a transverse cut just above the edge of the bladder and results in less blood loss and is easier to repair.
3. **An unplanned cesarean section** is performed once labor has commenced due to unexpected labor complications.
4. **A crash/emergent/emergency cesarean section** is performed in an obstetric emergency, where complications of pregnancies onset suddenly during the process of labor, and swift action is required to prevent the deaths of mother, child(ren) or both.
5. **A planned cesarean (or elective/scheduled cesarean),** arranged ahead of time, is most commonly arranged for medical reasons and ideally as close to the due date as possible.
6. **A cesarean hysterectomy** consists of a cesarean section followed by the removal of the uterus. This may be done in cases of intractable bleeding or when the placenta cannot be separated from the uterus.
7. **Traditionally, other forms of cesarean section** have been used, such as extraperitoneal cesarean section or porro cesarean section.
8. **A repeat cesarean section** is one that is done when a patient had a previous cesarean section. Typically, it is performed through the old scar.

c. Uterine prolapsed

Uterine prolapse is a form of female genital prolapse. It is also called pelvic organ prolapse or prolapse of the uterus (womb). The uterus (womb) is normally held in place by a hammock of muscles and ligaments. Prolapse happens when the ligaments supporting the uterus become so weak that the uterus cannot stay in place and slips down from its normal position. These ligaments are the round ligament, uterosacral ligaments, broad ligaments and the ovarian ligament. The uterosacral ligaments are by far the most important ligaments in preventing uterine prolapse. The most common cause of uterine prolapse is trauma during childbirth, in particular multiple or difficult births. About 50% of women who have had children develop some form of pelvic organ prolapse in their lifetime. It is more common as women get older, particularly in those who have gone through menopause. This condition is surgically correctable.

d. Puerperal psychosis

Postpartum psychosis (or **puerperal psychosis**) is a term that covers a group of mental illnesses with the sudden onset of psychotic symptoms following childbirth. A typical example is for a woman to become irritable, have extreme mood swings and hallucinations, and possibly need psychiatric hospitalization. Often, out of fear of stigma or misunderstanding, women hide their condition.

Some women have typical manic symptoms, such as euphoria, over activity, decreased sleep requirement, loquaciousness, flight of ideas, increased sociability, disinhibition, irritability, violence and delusions, which are usually grandiose or religious in content; on the whole these symptoms are more severe than in mania occurring at other times, with highly disorganized speech and extreme excitement. Others have severe depression with delusions, auditory hallucinations, mutism, stupor or transient swings into hypomania. Some switch from mania to depression (or vice versa) within the same episode.

Atypical features include perplexity, confusion, emotions like extreme fear and ecstasy, catatonia or rapid changes of mental state with transient delusional ideas; these are so striking that some authors have regarded them as a distinct, specific disease, but they are the defining features of acute polymorphic (cycloid) psychoses, and are seen in other contexts (for example, menstrual psychosis) and in men.

e. Responsibility of the nurse when oxytocin is administered

1. Ensure fetal position and size and absence of complications that are contraindicated with oxytocin before therapy.
2. Ensure continuous observation of patient receiving IV oxytocin for induction or stimulation of labor; fetal monitoring is preferred. A physician should be immediately available to deal with complications if they arise.
3. Regulate rate of oxytocin delivery to establish uterine contractions that are similar to normal labor; monitor rate and strength of contractions; discontinue drug and notify physician at any sign of uterine hyperactivity or spasm.
4. Monitor maternal BP during oxytocin administration, discontinue drug and notify physician with any sign of hypertensive emergency.
5. Monitor neonate for the occurrence of jaundice.

Drug-specific teaching points: The patient receiving parenteral oxytocin is usually receiving it as part of an immediate medical situation, and the drug teaching should be incorporated into the teaching about the procedure, labor, or complication of delivery that is involved. The patient needs to know the name of the drug and what she can expect once it is administered.

IX. a. What is hysterectomy?

A hysterectomy is an operation to remove a woman's uterus. A hysterectomy is surgery to remove a woman's uterus or womb. The uterus is the place where a baby grows when a woman is pregnant. After a hysterectomy, you no longer have menstrual periods and cannot become pregnant. Sometimes, the surgery also removes the ovaries and fallopian tubes. If you have both ovaries taken out, you will enter menopause.

b. List the indications for hysterectomy

A woman may have a hysterectomy for different reasons, including:
1. Uterine fibroids that cause pain, bleeding, or other problems.
2. Uterine prolapse, which is a sliding of the uterus from its normal position into the vaginal canal.
3. Cancer of the uterus, cervix, or ovaries.
4. Endometriosis.
5. Abnormal vaginal bleeding.
6. Chronic pelvic pain.
7. Adenomyosis, or a thickening of the uterus.

Hysterectomy for non-cancerous reasons is usually considered only after all other treatment approaches have been tried without success.

c. Write the pre- and postoperative nursing care of women posted for hysterectomy

Hysterectomy preoperative procedures: No matter which type of hysterectomy procedure is performed, hysterectomy requires hospitalization for one to five days. Preparation for a hysterectomy typically involves several steps, including the following:

1. Physical examination to determine overall health.
2. Pelvic examination.
3. Blood and urine tests.
4. Preoperative meeting with the surgeon to discuss the procedure and receive presurgery instructions.
5. Preoperative meeting with the anesthesiologist to discuss the type of anesthesia that will be used (general or local).

In many cases, patients are advised to quit smoking 2–6 weeks before surgery. Smoking may cause breathing problems during surgery and has been shown to delay healing.

If a pain reliever is needed in the week prior to surgery, acetaminophen is recommended over aspirin, ibuprofen, or naproxen, to reduce the risk for heavy bleeding during surgery.

In general, **no food or drink** is to be taken after midnight on the day of the procedure. In some cases, a laxative or enema is indicated to empty the bowels before surgery.

Postoperative care after hysterectomy: Immediately after surgery, the patient remains in the recovery room for a few hours. She is monitored for discomfort, and is given medications to prevent pain and infection.

Hysterectomy requires at least one overnight stay in the hospital, and may require hospitalization for as many as 5 days. After the first night, patients are up and walking. Sanitary pads are used to manage bleeding and discharge, which can last for several days.

Full recovery can take from 4–8 weeks for open abdominal hysterectomy, and from 1–2 weeks for vaginal and laparoscopic hysterectomies. During this time, patients should get plenty of rest. She should avoid heavy lifting and tub baths for a full 6 weeks.

Depending on the type of procedure used and on the patient's rate of recovery, light chores, some driving, and even returning to work during this period of time may be possible. In general, patients can resume sexual relations after 6 weeks.

X. a. What is postpartum hemorrhage?

Hemorrhage after delivery, or **postpartum hemorrhage** (PPH), is the loss of blood following a delivery resulting in hypovolemia or otherwise causing the patient to become symptomatic due to the blood loss. Some practitioners measure PPH by a blood loss of greater than 500 mL of blood following vaginal delivery, or 1000 mL of blood following cesarean section. It is the most common cause of perinatal maternal death in the developed world and is a major cause of maternal morbidity worldwide.

b. Write the difference between atonic and traumatic PPH

Atonic PPH: Any condition that interferes with uterine contraction, such as a retained placenta, remnants of placental tissue, or retained amniotic membranes or blood clots, increases the risk of excessive bleeding. If the placenta has separated but is still, even partially, in the uterus, it can prevent the uterus from contracting. Even a small piece of placenta or a blood clot left inside the uterus can keep it in the atonic condition. When the uterus is not contracted, the mother's blood vessels continue to pump blood out and the woman will quickly lose blood. The real problem with atonic PPH is that you cannot predict who will bleed excessively after the birth, and this is because two-thirds of women who develop atonic PPH have no known risk factors. This is why it is important to remember that *all* women must be considered at risk and prevention of PPH must be a part of every birth. The most important known risk factors are summarized below.

Traumatic PPH: In traumatic postpartum hemorrhage, excessive bleeding occurs as a result of trauma (injury) to the reproductive tract following delivery of the baby. Trauma can occur to the cervix, vagina, perineum or anus. It could also be from a ruptured uterus. Signs of traumatic postpartum hemorrhage are when there is bleeding from the vagina but the uterus is well contracted (hard). Trauma to the reproductive tract is preventable through skilled and gentle management during delivery, and referring the mother in good time if the labor is prolonged, or if the fetus is in an abnormal presentation or malposition.

c. Explain the management for atonic PPH and traumatic PPH

Medical Management of Atonic PPH

The treatment of patients with PPH has 2 major components: (1) resuscitation and management of obstetric hemorrhage and, possibly, hypovolemic shock and (2) identification and management of the underlying cause(s) of the hemorrhage. For the purpose of discussion, these components are discussed separately; however, remember that successful management of PPH requires that both components be simultaneously and systematically addressed.

Pharmacologic management of atonic PPH includes the use of oxytocin, ergometrine and prostaglandins. Intravenous oxytocin is the preferred initial agent in PPH treatment, regardless of whether a prophylactic dose was administered. If bleeding continues after oxytocin administration or if oxytocin is unavailable, IV ergometrine, ergometrine-oxytocin fixed dose (syntometrine) or a prostaglandin such as misoprostol 800 μg sublingual can be administered. Simultaneous administration of misoprostol with treatment doses of oxytocin is not recommended. Carboprost is may be useful when bleeding is resistant to other agents.

If bleeding proves unresponsive to uterotonics, consideration may be given to tranexamic acid (TXA), a synthetic derivative of lysine with antifibrinolytic properties, or recombinant activated factor VII (rvFIIa), the latter of which is discussed later. A 2010 Cochrane Review of TXA reported decreased blood loss after vaginal and cesarean birth but called for further investigation around efficacy and safety. Two more recent randomized controlled trials (RCT) concurred, yet were underpowered to evaluate safety concerns such as thrombolytic events. The World Maternal Antifibrinolytic (WOMAN) Trial is currently evaluating TXA for PPH treatment. WHO provides a weak recommendation for TXA where oxytocin and prostaglandins fail to control atonic PPH; however, RCOG reports that fibrinolytic inhibitors seldom have a place in PPH management.

Management for Traumatic PPH

Emergency management for traumatic PPH: Try to slow the bleeding from an injury (e.g. a tear in the perineum or vagina) by applying pressure over the source of the hemorrhage. Roll up 10–15 pieces of sterile gauze or a small, sterile cloth into a thick pad and push it firmly against the bleeding part of the tear. Hold it there for 10 minutes. Carefully remove the gauze and check for bleeding. If the tear is still bleeding, press the gauze against the source of the hemorrhage again and take the woman to the nearest health facility. Do not stop pressing on the tear until you get to there. If the woman has a long or deep tear, even if it is not bleeding much, take her to a health facility where it can be repaired.

2013
Midwifery and Gynecology

SECTION-I

I. Give the meaning of the following:
   a. Midwife.
   b. Morula.
   c. Perculum plug.
   d. Attitude.
   e. Milia.

II. Fill in the blanks
   a. Neuromuscular harmony between the upper and lower uterine segment is called: _____
   b. A women who has never given birth to a viable child is known as: _____
   c. Anterior fontanel closes by: _____

III. Write short notes on any *three* of the following:
   a. Development of maternity services in India.
   b. Fetal circulation.
   c. Genetic counseling.
   d. Vaginal examination.
   e. Minor disorders of newborn.

IV. a. Define labor.
   b. Write the physiological changes during the 3rd stage of labor.
   c. Explain the role of a nurse in the management of 3rd stage of labor.

V. a. What is an episiotomy?
   b. List the indications for episiotomy.
   c. Explain the nursing care of a mother with right mediolateral episiotomy.

OR

   a. List the equipments necessary for normal delivery.
   b. How will you prepare women in labor?

SECTION-II

VI. State whether the following statements are *true* or *false*
   a. Pelvic inflammatory disease is a disease of the lower genital tract.
   b. Twin-to-twin transfusion syndrome is a complication of monozygotic twin.
   c. Inflammation of the ovaries is called oophoritis.
   d. Concealed menstruation is known as cryptomenorrhea.

VII. Choose the correct answer and write:
   a. Implantation occurs at a site other than the utrine cavity is known as:
      (i. Molar pregnancy, ii. Ectopic pregnancy, iii. Multiple pregnancy)
   b. A brownish vaginal discharge is present during pregnancy in case of:
      (i. Missed abortion, ii. Septic abortion, iii. Threatened abortion)
   c. The denominator in breech presentation is:
      (i. Mentum, ii. Occiput, iii. Sacrum)

VIII. Write short notes on any *three* of the following:
   a. Polyhydramnios.
   b. Care of an elderly primigravida.
   c. Preterm labor.
   d. Laparoscopic sterilization.
   e. Vulvitis.

IX. a. Define postpartum hemorrhage.
   b. List the causes of atonic postpartum hemorrhage.
   c. Explain the nursing management of a mother with atonic postpartum hemorrhage.

OR

   a. Define forceps delivery.
   b. List the indications for forceps delivery.
   c. Explain the management of a mother following forceps delivery.

X. a. What is breast cancer?
   b. List the causes, signs and symptoms.
   c. Explain in detail about the surgical and nursing management of a women with breast cancer.

SECTION-I

I. Give the meaning of the following:

a. Midwife

A midwife is a person who has successfully completed a midwifery education program that is recognized in the country; who has acquired the requisite qualifications to be registered and/or legally licensed to practice midwifery and use the title 'midwife'; and who demonstrates competency in the practice of midwifery.

The midwife is recognized as a responsible and accountable professional who works in partnership with women to give the necessary support, care and advice during pregnancy, labor and the postpartum period, to conduct births on the midwife's own responsibility and to provide care for the newborn and the infant. This care includes preventative measures, the promotion of normal birth, the detection of complications in mother and child, the accessing of medical care or other appropriate assistance and the carrying out of emergency measures. The midwife has an important task in health counseling and education, not only for the woman, but also within the family and the community. This work should involve antenatal education and preparation for parenthood and may extend to women's health, sexual or reproductive health and child care. A midwife may practice in any setting including the home, community, hospitals, clinics or health units.

b. Morula

A morula is an embryo at an early stage of embryonic development, consisting of cells in a solid ball contained within the zona pellucida. The morula is produced by embryonic cleavage, the division of the zygote. It is the alteration of the shape of the fetal skull that takes place during labor due to the pressure to which it is subjected during its passage through the pelvis. This is permitted by the incomplete ossification of the bones of the vault. The parietal bones overlap the frontal and occiput, while one of the parietal bones slips under the other. The engaging diameter is decreased and the diameter at right angles to it is increased. Moulding occur to a certain degree in all the babies, unless delivered by cesarean section. The overriding the skull bones at the sutures are the most important factor in moulding. Premature babies have very soft skull bones and wide sutures which give no protection to the vital structures of the brain. Post-mature babies have very hard skull, the sutures being almost closed, thus preventing moulding and giving rise to difficulties.

c. Operculum plug

A cervical mucus plug (operculum) is a plug that fills and seals the cervical canal during pregnancy. It is formed by a small amount of cervical mucus.

The mucus plug acts as a protective barrier by deterring the passage of bacteria into the uterus, and contains a variety of antimicrobial agents, including immunoglobulin, and similar antimicrobial peptides to those found in nasal mucus. Normally during human pregnancy, the mucus is cloudy, clear, thick, and sticky. Toward the end of the pregnancy, when the cervix thins, some blood is released into the cervix which causes the mucus to become bloody. As the woman gets closer to labor, the mucus plug discharges as the cervix begins to dilate. The plug may come out as a plug, a lump, or simply as increased vaginal discharge over several days. The mucus may be tinged with brown, pink, or red blood, which is why the event is sometimes referred to as "bloody show". Loss of the mucus plug by no means implies that delivery or labor is imminent.

d. Attitude

Attitude is the relationship of the fetal head and limbs to its trunk. The attitude of the fetus varies according to its presentation. For example, a fetus in a vertex presentation has a well-flexed head, flexion of the extremities over the thorax and abdomen, and a convex curved back; while a fetus with a face presentation has a head, which is acutely extended, flexion of the extremities on the thorax and abdomen, and a vertebral column which not only is straightened but also has some degree of arching.

e. Milia

A milium (*plural* milia), also called a **milk spot** or an **oil seed**, is a keratin-filled cyst that can appear just under the epidermis or on the roof of the mouth. Milia are commonly associated with newborn babies but can appear on people of all ages. They are usually found around the nose and eyes, and sometimes on the genitalia, often mistaken by those affected as warts or other sexually transmitted diseases. Milia can also be confused with stubborn whiteheads. In children, milia often disappear within two to four weeks. For adults, they can be removed by an esthetician or physician (a dermatologist will have specialist knowledge in this area).

II. Fill in the blanks

a. Neuromuscular harmony between the upper and lower uterine segment is called: **Polarity.**
b. A women who has never given birth to a viable child is known as: **Nullipara.**
c. Anterior fontanelle closes by: **12 Months.**

III. Write short notes on any *three* of the following:

a. Development of maternity services in India

Mothers and children not only constitute a large group, but they are also vulnerable or special risk group. The risk is connected with child bearing in the case of women and growth, development and survival in the case of infants and children. A pregnant woman is a dyad a unit of two individuals consisting of the mother and the fetus. Maternal child health services are directed towards mothers and children under nutrition to attain total well being of the children within the framework of family and community. Every aspect of community health programs in India has marked effects on the health of infants and children. Global observations show that in developed regions maternal mortality ratio averages at 30 per 100,000 live births. In developing regions, the figure is 480 for the same number of live births. The problems affecting the health of mother and child are multifactorial. The present strategy is to provide mother and child health services as an integrated package of "essential health care. **Maternal and child health services** were first organized in India in 1921 by a committee of "**The lady Chelmsford League**", which collected funds for child welfare and established demonstration services on an all India basis. Other voluntary agencies took up this work and in 1932 the Indian Red Cross society established a maternal child welfare bureau.

- 1921—The maternal and child health services started by lady Chelmsford League.
- 1931—The maternal and child health bureau was established by Indian Red Cross Society.

The Victoria memorial scholarship fund was established and provided to the trainees.

It was again the Madras state which first attempted to replace dais by the better qualified personnel, such as midwives and nurse midwives.

- 1938—The maternal morbidity and mortality cause were investigated in Indian Research Fund Association.
- Sri AL Ambedkar was the key person of this committee. Investigation revealed that the institutional midwifery services were limited.
- 1946—The Bhore Committee stated in his report that India was having the problem of high maternal and infant mortality.
- 1954—First five year plan continued. Central Drug Research Institute was started at Lucknow. BCG vaccine was introduced.
- 1960—School Health Committee was formed.
- 1971—Medical Termination of Pregnancy (MTP) bill was passed by the parliament and it came into force in that year itself.
- 1975—Integrated Child Development Scheme (CDS) was launched in India.
- 1979—A healthy child—a safe future.
- 1984—Children's health—Tomorrow's wealth—WHO theme.
- 1985—Universal Immunization Program was launched.
- 1987—Immunization—A chance for every child—WHO theme.
- A worldwide safe motherhood "campaign" was launched by the World Bank.
- 1992—Child Survival and safe Motherhood Program (SSM) was launched on 20th August.
- Safe Motherhood Initiative (SMI).
- Infant Food Act 1992 came into force (Regulation of production supply and distribution).
- 1995—ICDS renamed as Integrated Mother and Child Development Services (IMCD).
- 1996—Pulse Polio Immunization (PPI), the largest single day public health event took place on the 9th December 1995 and 20th January 1996.
- 1997—Family Welfare Program made target free from 1st April 1996.
- Prenatal Diagnostic Techniques Act, 1994 came into force from 1996 (Regulation and Prevention).

b. Fetal circulation

The key to understand fetal circulation is that oxygen is derived from the placenta and placenta is the source of nutrition and the site of elimination of waste. There are several temporary structures in addition to the placenta. The umbilical vein leads from the umbilical cord to the under surface of the liver and carries blood rich in oxygen and nutrients. It has a branch which joins the portal vein and supplies the liver.

The important four temporary structures are:
1. The ductus venosus (drain from vein to vein) connects the umbilical vein to the inferior vena cava.
2. The foramen ovale (an oval opening between the right to left atrium) the blood entering from the inferior vena cava to the right atrium and to the left atrium through the foramen ovale.
3. The ductus arteriosus (form an artery to an artery) leads from the bifurcation of the pulmonary artery to the descending aorta entering just beyond the point where the subclavian and carotid arteries leave.
4. The hypogastric arteries branch off from the internal iliac arteries and become the umbilical arteries when they enter the umbilical cord and return the blood to the placenta.

The blood takes about half a minute to circulate and to start the following course.

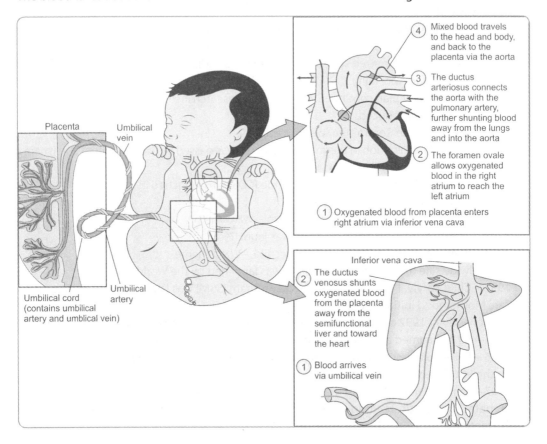

The actual circulation from the placenta blood passes through the umbilical vein along the abdominal wall to the under surface of the liver, which is the only vessel in the fetus carrying unmixed blood. The ductus venosus carries to the inferior vena cava when mixes with the blood from the lower body. Then the blood is carried to the right atrium and most of it is passed to the left atrium through foramen ovale. From the left atrium to the left ventricle and pass into the aorta. As the coronary and carotid arteries are the easily branches from the aorta the heart and brain get relatively well-oxygenated blood. The arms also get the benefit via the subclavian arteries and that is the reason why arms are more developed than legs at birth.

The blood collected from the upper body is collected in the superior vena cava which is depleted of oxygen and nutrients. It mixes with the blood of inferior vena cava in the right atrium. Even through the two streams remain separate due to the shape of atrium 25% of mixing occurs allowing a little oxygen and food to the lungs through the pulmonary artery which is necessary for their development. After supplying blood to the lungs the remaining blood is passed to the aorta through ductus arteriosus. Though low in oxygen blood is supplied to the other organs of the body and legs through the aorta. The internal iliac arteries lead to hypogastric arteries which return the blood to the placenta via umbilical arteries. The remaining blood supplies the lower limbs and returns to the inferior vena cava.

c. Genetic counseling

Genetic counseling is the process by which patients or relatives at risk of an inherited disorder are advised of the consequences and nature of the disorder, the probability of developing or transmitting it, and the options open to them in management and family planning. This complex process can be separated into diagnostic (the actual estimation of risk) and supportive aspects The goals of genetic counseling are to increase understanding of genetic diseases, discuss disease management options, and explain the risks and benefits of testing. Counseling sessions focus on giving vital, unbiased information and non-directive assistance in the patient's decision making process. Seymour Kessler, in 1979, first categorized sessions in five phases: an intake phase, an initial contact phase, the encounter phase, the summary phase, and a follow-up phase. The intake and follow-up phases occur outside of the actual counseling session. The initial contact phase is when the counselor and families meet and build rapport. The encounter phase includes dialogue between the counselor and the client about the nature of screening and diagnostic tests. The summary phase provides all the options and decisions available for the next step. If counselees wish to go ahead with testing, an appointment is organized and the genetic counselor acts as the person to communicate the results.

d. Vaginal examination

The functions of a vaginal examination are to:
1. Determine if true labor has begun and the stage it has reached, based on measuring the dilatation of the cervix.
2. Assess the progress of labor in terms of the rate of increase in cervical dilatation and the descent of the fetus down the birth canal.
3. Identify the fetal presentation and position.
4. Detect any moulding of the fetal skull bones (the extent to which they overlap under pressure from the birth canal).
5. Assess the size of the mother's pelvis and its adequacy for the passage of the fetus.
6. Check the color of the amniotic fluid.

e. Minor disorders of newborn

The minor disorders are most common among newborns, neglecting the minor health problem is one of the factor contributing to the newborn mortality rate. In India, most the mothers are not aware of management regarding minor disorders of newborn (vomiting, constipation, diarrhea, physiological jaundice, conjunctivitis, umbilical cord infection, pseudo menstruation, breast engorgement, and skin rashes).

IV. a. Define labor

Labor is a physiologic process during which the fetus, membranes, umbilical cord, and placenta are expelled from the uterus. The process of expulsion of the fetus and the placenta from the uterus. The stages of labor include: first stage, beginning with the onset of uterine contractions through the period of dilation of the os uteri; second stage, the period of expulsive effort, beginning with complete dilation of the cervix and ending with expulsion of the infant; third stage or placental stage, the period beginning at the expulsion of the infant and ending with the completed expulsion of the placenta and membranes.

b. Write the physiological changes during the 3rd stage of labor

The third stage of labor commences with the completed delivery of the fetus and ends with the completed delivery of the placenta and its attached membranes. The clinician immediately recognizes that from a practical perspective, the risk of complications continues for some period after delivery of the placenta. For this reason, many authorities have advocated a so-called fourth stage of labor, which begins with the delivery of the placenta and lasts for an arbitrary period afterward. The most commonly chosen duration is 1 hour; however, periods as long as 4 hours have been suggested. The length of the third stage itself is usually 5–15 minutes. The absolute time limit for delivery of the placenta, without evidence of significant bleeding, remains unclear. Periods ranging from 30–60 minutes have been suggested.

During labor the muscle fibers of the uterus cause it to contract and get smaller. The baby moves down the birth canal and once it is born, the uterus continues contracting naturally. As the uterus gets smaller the placenta begins to detach from where it has been attached to the uterus wall throughout the pregnancy.

At the same time, the muscle fibers in the uterus close around the woman's blood vessels, effectively sealing them and reducing further bleeding. In addition, the blood clotting system is activated to limit blood loss. The flow of blood through the placenta is approximately over 500 mL (more than a pint) per minute, but during third stage it reduces to virtually nothing.

Once the placenta has separated it will come out of the uterus, through the birth canal and be expelled. This may require gravity (upright positions) and possibly some maternal effort (pushing) but the contractions of the uterus themselves do most of the work. Skin-to-skin contact with the baby or breastfeeding can also make the uterus contract to help this process.

Once the placenta has been delivered, the uterus continues to contract and gradually returns to its pre-pregnancy size.

c. Explain the role of a nurse in the management of 3rd stage of labor

a. Continue observation. Following delivery of the placenta, continue in your observation of the fundus. Ensure that the fundus remains contracted. Retention of the tissues in the uterus can lead to uterine atony and cause hemorrhage. Massaging the fundus gently will ensure that it remains contracted.
b. Allow the mother to bond with the infant. Show the infant to the mother and allow her to hold the infant.

Record the following Information
a. Time the placenta is delivered.
b. How delivered (spontaneously or manually removed by the physician).
c. Type, amount, time and route of administration of oxytocin. Oxytocin is never administered prior to delivery of the placenta because the strong uterine contractions could harm the fetus.
d. If the placenta is delivered complete and intact or in fragments.

V. a. What is an episiotomy?

An **episiotomy** also known as **perineotomy**, is a planned, surgical incision on the perineum and the posterior vaginal wall during second stage of labor.

The incision, which can be done at a 90° angle from the vulva towards the anus or at an angle from the posterior end of the vulva (mediolateral episiotomy), is performed under local anesthetic (pudendal anesthesia), and is sutured closed after delivery. It is one of the most common medical procedures performed on women.

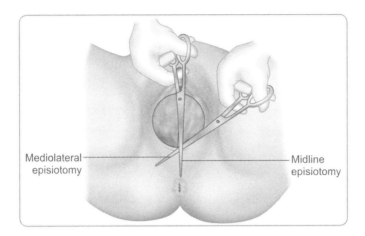

b. List the indications for episiotomy
1. There is a serious risk to the mother of second- or third-degree tearing.
2. In cases, where a natural delivery is adversely affected, but a cesarean section is not indicated.
3. "Natural" tearing will cause an increased risk of maternal disease being vertically transmitted.
4. The baby is very large.
5. When perineal muscles are excessively rigid.
6. When instrumental delivery is indicated.
7. When a woman has undergone female genital mutilation (FGM), indicating the need for an anterior and or mediolateral episiotomy.
8. Prolonged late decelerations or fetal bradycardia during active pushing.
9. The baby's shoulders are stuck (shoulder dystocia), or a bony association (Note that the episiotomy does not directly resolve this problem, but it is indicated to allow the operator more room to perform maneuvers to free shoulders from the pelvis).

c. Explain the nursing care of a mother with right mediolateral episiotomy

A right mediolateral episiotomy begins at the vaginal opening in the midline with the incision directed toward the right buttocks at a 45 degree angle. The main advantage of the mediolateral episiotomy is that it is less likely to extend into or involve the anal sphincter and the rectum. Disadvantages of the medio-lateral episiotomy are significant and include increased blood loss, increased pain, difficult repair, and an increased risk of long-term discomfort, especially during intercourse.

Both midline and mediolateral episiotomies are easy to perform. They involve the simple incision of the opening of the vagina. The episiotomy should be performed when 3 or 4 centimeters (cm) of the baby's head is visible at the vaginal opening. If the mother has not received anesthesia in the form of an epidural block, local anesthesia may be given at the site of the episiotomy. The area is cleaned with soap. The provider then inserts two fingers into the vaginal opening to protect the baby's head (the fingers should be inserted between the baby's head and the tissue of the vaginal opening). One blade of the scissors is then inserted between the two fingers and a small incision, approximately 2–3 cm in length, is made. The incision may be made in the midline or mediolaterally.

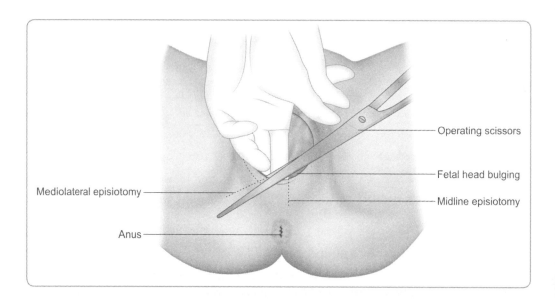

After the incision has been made, the physician gently supports the episiotomy site to prevent further tearing by pinching the tissue just below the incision. Gentle pressure is also placed against the top of the baby's head to prevent the head from rapidly or abruptly delivering. A controlled delivery is preferred because it is easier to prevent tearing during a slow and steady delivery of the baby's head.

OR

a. List the equipments necessary for normal delivery

1. Clean water, soap and hand towel.
2. Apron, goggle, face mask and gown.
3. Sterile gloves.
4. Sterile or very clean new string to tie the cord.
5. New razor blade or sterilized scissors.
6. Two sterile clamp forceps, for clamping the umbilical cord before you cut it.
7. Mucus traps or suction bulb to suck mucus from the baby's airways (if needed).
8. Sterile gauze, cotton swab and sanitary pad for the mother.
9. Two dry, clean baby towels and two drapes.
10. Blood pressure cuff and stethoscope.
11. Antiseptic solution for cleaning the mother's perineum and genital area.
12. 10 IU (International units) of the injectable drug called oxytocin, or 600 µg (micrograms) tablets of misoprostol. These drugs are used for the prevention of postpartum hemorrhage. Oxytocin is the preferred drug for this purpose, but if you do not have it then misoprostol can be used.
13. Tetracycline eye ointment (antibiotic eye ointment used for the prevention of eye infection in the newborn.
14. Three buckets or small bowls each with 0.5% chlorine solution, or soap solution and clean water (To prepare 0.5% chlorine solution you can use the locally available Berekina. Read the

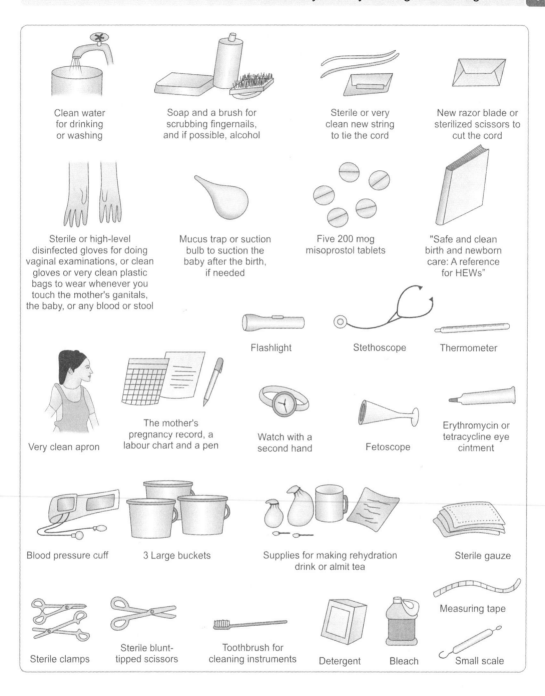

concentration from the bottle—if it is 5% you can make a solution of 0.5% strength by mixing one cup of Berekina with nine cups of clean water.)
15. Plastic bowl to receive the placenta.

b. How will you prepare women in labor?

Preparing the birthing place: Once the onset of the second stage has been confirmed you should make preliminary preparations for the delivery. The room should be warm and well lit, so that the perineum and vulva can be easily observed. A clean surface should be prepared to receive the baby using the infection control procedures described in Section 3.5. Spread waterproof covers to protect the bed and the floor. Make sure there is a warm coat and clothes for the baby.

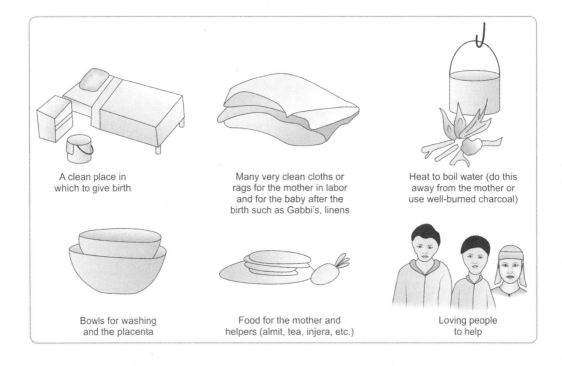

Figure: Supplies to conduct the delivery include making a safe and clean place for the mother to give birth.

Preparing for childbirth is one of the most exciting times for a woman; however, it may also be a time of fear and anxiety for a mom-to-be. During this transitional period as a woman may start preparing for the special new addition to her family, she may also have to come to terms with the many adjustments that will have to be made. Staying organized, positive, relaxed and planning properly can help make the childbirth process easier. Ensure that early and regular prenatal care is put into place and that you are consulting with your physician and following the prescribed dietary and nutritional requirements. Maintain an emotional connection with your unborn child during the pregnancy period by massaging your belly, through meditation or music to strengthen the bond with you and your baby.

In the eighth month of pregnancy, to eliminate additional stress on the day of the delivery, you may want to preregister at the hospital before get into labor. Here you can read and sign the necessary pre-admission and medical consent forms in your own time. Arrange another tour of your birthing center, so that you can check on visiting hour schedules, find out about parking passes, etc.

More and more women are choosing natural and holistic treatments, such as herbal remedies to help prepare them physically and emotionally for natural birth. Herbs, such as Squaw Vine (Mitchella repels), Raspberry leaves (Rubus idaeus) and Passiflora incarnate help prepare the body for labor and childbirth as well as relieve fear, anxiety and nervousness about the delivery. In addition, Glycyrrhiza glabra (licorice) acts as a powerful anti-inflammatory and tonic for the uterus to stimulate contractions. Natural remedies formulated for childbirth and labor are side effect free and would not cause harm to mom and baby.

SECTION-II

VI. State whether the following statements are *true* or *false*

a. Pelvic inflammatory disease is a disease of the lower genital tract: **FALSE**
b. Twin-to-twin transfusion syndrome is a complication of monozygotic twin: **TRUE**
c. Inflammation of the ovaries is called oophoritis: **TRUE**
d. Concealed menstruation is known as cryptomenorrhea: **TRUE**

VII. Choose the correct answer and write

a. Implantation occurs at a site other than the utrine cavity is known as: **Ectopic pregancy.**
   (i. Molar pregnancy, ii. Ectopic pregnancy, iii. Multiple pregnancy)
b. a Brownish vaginal discharge is present during pregnancy in case of: **Missed abortion**.
   (i. Missed abortion, ii. Septic abortion, iii. Threatened abortion)
c. The denominator in breech presentation is: **Mentum.**
   (i. Mentum, ii. Occiput, iii. Sacrum)

VIII. Write short notes on any *three* of the following:

a. Polyhydramnios

This term is applied to excessive fluid.

Signs and Symptoms

1. **Inspection:** Uterus is larger than the date of gestation. The abdominal girth over 1 m at term. Shape globular rather than avoid. If there is marked distention, abdominal wall is very thin; skin shines with marked veins and sterile gravidarum. These are cases with abdominal girth over 1 m (100 cm) at term even up to 130 cm.
2. **Palpation:** It is very difficult through sometimes ballottement is possible. A fluid thrill can be felt by placing the palm of the left hand on the side of the abdomen and giving the abdomen a sharp flik.
3. **Auscultation:** FHS are muffled and sometimes inaudible, X-ray shows a blurred outline and a large uterine cavity. Twins and fetal abnormalities are also shown.

Effect of Hydramnios

1. Pressure symptoms are very severe and distressing especially in acute hydramnios edema of the vulva, and lover limbs, dyspnea and

2. Palpitation during night, vague abdominal discomfort particularly under the ribs. Indigestion and constipation, weight of the uterus produces difficulty in moving about and hence requires rest in bed.

Complications
1. Cord presentation and cord prolapse.
2. Malpresentation.
3. Uterine inertia.
4. Premature labor.
5. Postpartum hemorrhage (PPH).
6. Premature rupture of membranes.
7. Placental abruption when the membranes rupture.

Treatment: Hospitalization because of the possible complications. Artificial rupture of membranes (high rupture) after ensuring that the lie and presentation are normal.

Objective of ARM
1. To reduce the size of the uterus.
2. To ensure the uterine contractions.
3. To allow the presenting part to sink into the lower part of the uterus.
4. Method 'Drew Smith' catheter is used and the hind water is ruptured.

Advantage
1. It prevent prolapse of the cord.
2. Allow slow drainage and prevent.
a. Maternal and fetal distress.
b. Intrauterine infection is prevented.
c. Fore-water assists for dilatation.
d. Reduces the risk of premature separation of the placenta.

b. Care of elderly primigravida

Elderly primigravida is a woman who becomes pregnant for the first time after the age of 34. Although an elderly primigravida was in the past at greater risk of adverse complications of a pregnancy, newer techniques and drugs have eliminated most of the risk and made it possible even for women of menopausal age to bear children. A residence for individuals of advancing years which provides a room and meals and is staffed with personnel who help with activities of daily living and recreation. Nursing interventions are focused on determining the nature of the problem, assessing the family's ability to deal with it, and identifying available resources for assistance. Plans for utilizing available resources are developed with family members. These might include procuring a part-time homemaker, obtaining supportive assistance such as legal aid or nutritional care, or providing therapeutic care by nurses, speech therapists, physical therapists or other professionals who are involved in home health care.

c. Preterm labor

Premature labor is also called preterm labor. It is when the body starts getting ready for birth too early in the pregnancy. Labor is premature if it starts more than three weeks before your due date.

Premature labor can lead to an early birth. Premature birth is defined either as the same as preterm birth or the birth of a baby before the developing organs are mature enough to allow normal postnatal survival. Premature infants are at greater risk for short- and long-term complications, including disabilities and impediments in growth and mental development. Significant progress has been made in the care of premature infants, but not in reducing the prevalence of preterm birth. Preterm birth is among the top causes of death in infants worldwide.

d. Laproscopic sterilization

Sterilization by laparoscopy is a common procedure used to perform tubal ligation in women. Tubal ligation is a method of sterilization that involves obstruction of the fallopian tubes. The

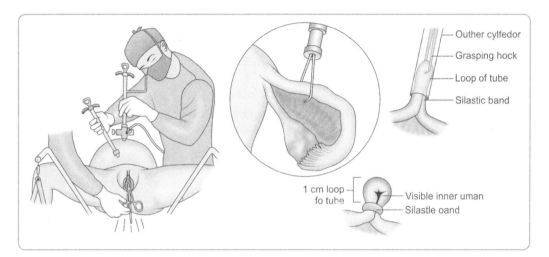

fallopian tubes are on either side of the uterus and extend toward the ovaries. They receive eggs from the ovaries and transport them to the uterus. Once the fallopian tubes are closed, the man's sperm can no longer reach the egg.

Laparoscopy enables the physician to complete tubal ligation by making a small incision near the navel. This smaller incision reduces recovery time after surgery and the risk of complications. In most cases, the woman can leave the surgery facility within 4 hours after laparoscopy.

e. Vulvitis

Vulvitis is inflammation of the external genital organs of the female (the vulva). The vulva includes the labia, clitoris, and entrance to the vagina (the vestibule of the vagina). An inflammation of the vulva is referred to as vulvitis. Vulvitis like vaginitis, may be caused by a number of different infections. Because the vulva is also often inflamed when there is inflammation of the vagina; vaginitis is sometimes referred to as vulvovaginitis.

IX. a. Define postpartum hemorrhage. b. List the causes of atonic postpartum hemorrhage. c. Explain the nursing management of a mother with atonic postpartum hemorrhage.

Postpartum hemorrhage is defined as excessive bleeding from the genital tract at anytime following the baby's birth up to 6 weeks after delivery.

If it occurs during the third stage of labor or within 24 hours of delivery it is termed primary postpartum hemorrhage.

If bleeding occurs subsequent to the first 24 hours following birth up until the sixth week postpartum, it is termed secondary postpartum hemorrhage.

Primary Postpartum Hemorrhage

1. If measured blood loss reaches 500 mL it must be treated as a postpartum hemorrhage, irrespective of maternal condition.
2. Any blood loss, however, small which adversely affects the mother's condition constitutes a postpartum hemorrhage.

Causes of Atonic Uterine Action

1. Incomplete separation of the placenta.
2. Retained cotyledon, placental fragment or membranes.
3. Precipitate labor.
4. Prolonged labor resulting in uterine inertia.
5. Polyhydramnios or multiple pregnancies causing over distension of uterine muscle.
6. Placenta previa.
7. Placental abruption.
8. General anesthesia especially halothane or cyclopropane.
9. Mismanagement of the third stage of labor.
10. A full bladder.
11. Etiology unknown.

Predisposing factors that causes that increase the likelihood of excessive bleeding:
1. Previous history of postpartum hemorrhage or retained placenta.
2. High parity resulting in uterine sacred tissue.
3. Presence of fibroids.
4. Maternal anemia.
5. Ketoacidosis.

Traumatic: Hemorrhage may occur from the cervical, vaginal and vestibular tear-rarely by the rupture of the uterus.

Symptoms

1. Bleeding per vagina—heavy or slow oozing.
2. Intermittent gushes occur in atony.
3. Traumatic bleeding—bright red color blood.

Signs

1. *Hypovolemia*: Slow pulse rate BP is raised or normal or slight fall. No pallor.
2. *Late features*: Hypotension tachycardia, severe pallor, cold clammy skin, air hunger per abdomen uterus is soft and flaccid to feel. Height is at higher level. Hard uterus in presence of continuous vaginal bleeding suggests trauma at birth canal.

Treatment of Postpartum Hemorrhage

Three basic principles apply.
 I. Call a doctor or call for help.
 II. Stop the bleeding
   1. Rub up a contraction.
   2. Give an oxytocic.
   3. Empty the uterus.
 III. Resuscitate the mother
   1. Call for emergency obstetric unit.
   2. The emergency obstetric unit should be called.
   3. Stop the bleeding.
   4. Rub up a contraction.
   5. The fluid is massaged with a smooth, circular motion, applying without pressure when a contraction occurs, the hand is held still.
   6. Give an oxytocic to sustain the contraction.
   7. Syntocinon 5 units or 10 units or syntometrine 1 mL has already been administered and this may be repeated.
   8. Alternatively, ergometrine 0.25–0.5 mg may be injected intravenously which will be effective in 45 seconds.
   9. Note: No more than two doses of ergometrine should be given (including any dose of syntometrine) as it may cause pulmonary hypertension.
   10. Empty the uterus: Once the uterus is well contracted—the uterus is emptied.

Resuscitate the Mother

1. Catheterize the bladder to exclude a full bladder as a precipitating cause of further bleeding before emptying the uterus—
   Note: The foot of the bed should not be raised as this encourage.
   Pooling of blood in the uterus, which prevents the uterus contracting.
2. Can not account must a woman in a collapsed condition be moved prior to resuscitation.

OR

a. Define forceps delivery. b. List the indications for forceps delivery. c. Explain the management of a mother following forceps delivery.

Forceps delivery is a means of extracting the fetus with the aid of obstetric forceps when it is inadvisable or impossible for the mother to complete the delivery by her own efforts. Forceps are also used to assist the delivery of the after coming head of the breech and on occasion to withdraw the head up and out of the pelvis at cesarean section. Ever since the invention of obstetric forceps around 1,600 AD by the Chamberlen family, many designs were invented and modified.

Forceps deliveries were formerly classified by the level of the head at the time the forceps were applied, i.e. high-cavity, mid-cavity and low-cavity. Low-cavity forceps is the one frequently performed, as cesarean section is usually preferred to the more traumatic high and mid-cavity operations. Low-cavity forceps can be divided into rotational and non-rotational. Rotational forceps delivery refers to a maneuver of the fetal head from a malposition into a more favorable position

with the aid of specially designed forceps usually Kielland's examples of non-rotational forceps are:
- Wrigley's forceps and Simpson's forceps (low cavity)
- Neville-Barne's and Haig Ferguson's forceps (high and mid-cavity forceps).

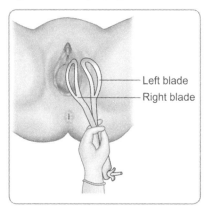

Basic Construction of the Forceps

Obstetric forceps consist of two separate blades, each with a handle. Each blade is marked 'L' (left) or 'R' (right). They are inserted separately on either side of the fetal head and locked together by English or Smellie lock (rotational forceps have a sliding lock). The blades are spoon shaped to accommodate the fetal head and fenestrated to minimize trauma and for lightness. The spoon shape of the blade is called the cephalic curve. When the blades are articulated it holds the fetal head. The blades are attached to the handle at an angle, which corresponds to the curve of Carus (curve on the axis of birth canal). This is termed as the pelvic curve of the blade. When the blades are correctly placed on the fetal head, the handles will be neatly aligned.

Indications of forceps operation: Delay in the second stage due to uterine inertia. If the head is on the perineum for 20–30 minutes without advancement, forceps application may be decided.
1. Maternal indications.
2. Maternal distress.
3. Preeclampsia, eclampsia.
4. Vaginal birth after cesarean section (VBAC).
5. Heart disease.
6. Failure to bear down during the second stage of labor due to regional blocks, paraplegia or psychiatric disturbance.
7. Fetal indications.
8. Appearance of fetal distress in the second stage.
9. Cord prolapse.
10. After coming head of breech.
11. Low birth weight baby.
12. Postmaturity.

Prerequisites for forceps delivery: There are certain conditions which must exist before forceps delivery can be performed.
1. The cervix must be fully dilated and effaced.
2. Membranes must be ruptured.

3. Presentation and position must be suitable to apply the blades correctly to the sides of the head.
4. The head must be engaged with no parts of the head palpable abdominally.
5. No appreciable cephalopelvic disproportion.
6. The bladder must be emptied.
7. Presence of good uterine contractions as a safeguard to postpartum hemorrhage.

Preparation of the woman: The woman should be prepared in advance for the possibility of a forceps delivery if this looks likely. Full explanation of the procedure and the need for it must be given to the woman.

Once the decision has been made, adequate and appropriate analgesia must be offered. When analgesia has been instituted and the obstetrician is ready to proceed, the woman's legs are placed in lithotomy position. Both legs must be placed simultaneously to avoid strain on the woman's back and hips.

The woman should be tilted towards the left at an angle of 15° by the use of a pillow or a rubber wedge under the mattress to prevent aortocaval occlusion.

Preparations must also be done for the baby including equipment for resuscitation. In some hospitals, a pediatrician will also be present.

Procedure of low forceps operation: The woman's vulval area is thoroughly cleaned and draped with sterile towels using aseptic technique. The bladder is emptied using a straight catheter.
1. A vaginal examination is performed by the obstetrician to confirm the station and exact position of the fetal head.
2. A pudental block, supplemented by perineal and labial infiltration with 1% lignocaine hydrochloride, is given to produce effective local anesthesia.
3. An episiotomy may be done prior to introduction of the blades or during traction when the perineum becomes bulged and thinned out by the advanced head.
4. The forceps are identified as left or right by assembling them briefly before proceeding.

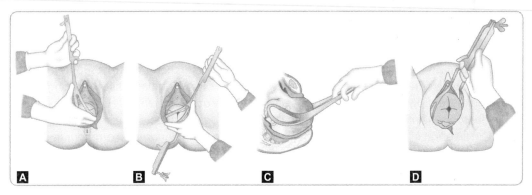

(A) Introduction of the left blade; (B) Introduction of the right blade; (C) Traction of the head; (D) Change of the one in the final stage

Complications of Forceps Operation

The hazards of the forceps operation are mostly related to the faulty technique and to the indications for which the forceps are applied.

In the Mother

Immediate
1. Injury.
2. Extension of the episiotomy towards rectum or upwards up to the vault of vagina.
3. Vaginal lacerations.
4. Cervical tear especially when applied through an incompletely dilated cervix.
5. Bruising and trauma to the urethra.
6. Postpartum hemorrhage due to trauma, or atonic uterus related to prolonged labor or effect of anesthesia.
7. Shock due to blood loss, prolonged labor and dehydration.
8. Sepsis due to devitalization of local tissues and improper asepsis.

Late Complications
1. Chronic low backache due to tension imposed on softened ligaments of lumbosacral or sacroiliac joints during lithotomy position.
2. Genital prolapses or stress incontinence.

In the Infant

Immediate
1. Asphyxia due to intracranial stress out of prolonged compression.
2. Intracranial hemorrhage due to mal-application of the blades.
3. Cephalhematoma.
4. Facial palsy due to damage to facial nerve.
5. Abrasions on the soft tissues of the face and forehead by the forceps blade, severe bruising will cause marked jaundice.
6. Tentorial tear from compression of the fetal head by the forceps.

X. a. What is breast cancer?

Breast cancer affects one in eight women during their lives. Breast cancer kills more women in the United States than any cancer except lung cancer. No one knows why some women get breast cancer, but there are a number of risk factors. Breast cancer is a type of cancer originating from breast tissue, most commonly from the inner lining of milk ducts or the lobules that supply the ducts with milk. Cancers originating from ducts are known as ductal carcinomas, while those originating from lobules are known as lobular carcinomas. Breast cancer occurs in humans and other mammals. While the overwhelming majority of human cases are in women, breast cancer can also occur in men. The first sign of breast cancer often is a breast lump or an abnormal mammogram. Breast cancer stages range from early, curable breast cancer to metastatic breast cancer, with a variety of breast cancer treatments. Male breast cancer is not uncommon and must be taken seriously.

b. List the causes, signs and symptoms

Breast cancer is a kind of cancer that develops from breast cells. Breast cancer usually starts off in the inner lining of milk ducts or the lobules that supply them with milk. A malignant tumor can spread to other parts of the body. A breast cancer that started off in the lobules is known as lobular carcinoma, while one that developed from the ducts is called ductal carcinoma.

Experts are not sure what **causes breast cancer**. It is hard to say why one person develops the disease while another does not. We know that some risk factors can impact on a woman's likelihood of developing breast cancer.

1. **Getting older:** The older a woman gets, the higher is her risk of developing breast cancer; age is a risk factor. Over 80% of all female breast cancers occur among women aged 50+ years.
2. **Genetics:** Women who have a close relative who has/had breast or ovarian cancer are more likely to develop breast cancer. If two close family members develop the disease, it does not necessarily mean they shared the genes that make them more vulnerable, because breast cancer is a relatively common cancer. The majority of breast cancers are not hereditary. Women who carry the BRCA1 and BRCA2 genes have a considerably higher risk of developing breast and/or ovarian cancer. These genes can be inherited. TP53, another gene, is also linked to greater breast cancer risk.
3. **A history of breast cancer:** Women who have had breast cancer, even non-invasive cancer, are more likely to develop the disease again, compared to women who have no history of the disease.
4. **Having had certain types of breast lumps:** Women who have had some types of benign (non-cancerous) breast lumps are more likely to develop cancer later on. Examples include atypical ductal hyperplasia or lobular carcinoma in situ.
5. **Dense breast tissue:** Women with more dense breast tissue have a greater chance of developing breast cancer.
6. **Estrogen exposure:** Women who started having periods earlier or entered menopause later than usual have a higher risk of developing breast cancer. This is because their bodies have been exposed to estrogen for longer. Estrogen exposure begins when periods start, and drops dramatically during the menopause.
7. **Obesity:** Postmenopausal obese and overweight women may have a higher risk of developing breast cancer. Experts say that there are higher levels of estrogen in obese menopausal women, which may be the cause of the higher risk.
8. **Height:** Taller-than-average women have a slightly greater likelihood of developing breast cancer than shorter-than-average women. Experts are not sure why.
9. **Alcohol consumption:** The more alcohol a woman regularly drinks, the higher her risk of developing breast cancer is.
10. **Radiation exposure:** Undergoing X-rays and CT scans may raise a woman's risk of developing breast cancer slightly.
11. **Hormone replacement therapy (HRT):** Both forms, combined and estrogen—only HRT therapies may increase a woman's risk of developing breast cancer slightly. Combined HRT causes a higher risk.
12. **Cosmetic implants may undermine breast cancer survival:** Women who have cosmetic breast implants and develop breast cancer may have a higher risk of dying prematurely form the disease compared to other females.

Symptoms of breast cancer may include a lump in the breast, a change in size or shape of the breast or discharge from a nipple. Breast self-exam and mammography can help find breast cancer early when it is most treatable.

1. A lump in a breast.
2. A pain in the armpits or breast that does not seem to be related to the woman's menstrual period.
3. Pitting or redness of the skin of the breast like the skin of an orange.

4. A rash around (or on) one of the nipples.
5. A swelling (lump) in one of the armpits.
6. An area of thickened tissue in a breast.
7. One of the nipples has a discharge; sometimes it may contain blood.
8. The nipple changes in appearance; it may become sunken or inverted.
9. The size or the shape of the breast changes.
10. The nipple-skin or breast-skin may have started to peel, scale or flake.

c. Explain in detail about the surgical and nursing management of women with breast cancer.

A multidisciplinary team will be involved in a breast cancer patient's treatment. The team may consist of an oncologist, radiologist, specialist cancer surgeon, specialist nurse, pathologist, radiographer, and reconstructive surgeon. Sometimes, the team may also include an occupational therapist, psychologist, dietitian, and physical therapist.

Surgical Interventions
1. Surgeries include lumpectomy (breast-preventing procedure), mastectomy (breast removal), and mammoplasty (reconstructive surgery).
2. Endocrine related surgeries to reduce endogenous estrogen as a palliative measure.
3. Bone marrow transplantation may be combined with chemotherapy.

Lumpectomy: Surgically removing the tumor and a small margin of healthy tissue around it. In breast cancer, this is often called breast-sparing surgery. This type of surgery may be recommended if the tumor is small and the surgeon believes it will be easy to separate from the tissue around it.

Mastectomy: Surgically removing the breast. Simple mastectomy involves removing the lobules, ducts, fatty tissue, nipple, areola, and some skin. Radical mastectomy means also removing muscle of the chest wall and the lymph nodes in the armpit.

Sentinel node biopsy: One lymph node is surgically removed. If the breast cancer has reached a lymph node it can spread further through the lymphatic system into other parts of the body.

Axillary lymph node dissection: If the sentinel node was found to have cancer cells, the surgeon may recommend removing several lymph nodes in the armpit.

Breast reconstruction surgery: A series of surgical procedures aimed at recreating a breast, so that it looks as much as possible like the other breast. This procedure may be carried out at the same time as a mastectomy. The surgeon may use a breast implant, or tissue from another part of the patient's body.

Radiation therapy (radiotherapy): Controlled doses of radiation are targeted at the tumor to destroy the cancer cells. Usually, radiotherapy is used after surgery, as well as chemotherapy to kill off any cancer cells that may still be around. Typically, radiation therapy occurs about one month after surgery or chemotherapy. Each session lasts a few minutes; the patient may require three to five sessions per week for three to six weeks.

Nursing Interventions
1. Monitor for adverse effects of radiation therapy such as fatigue, sore throat, dry cough, nausea, anorexia.

2. Monitor for adverse effects of chemotherapy; bone marrow suppression, nausea and vomiting, alopecia, weight gain or loss, fatigue, stomatitis, anxiety, and depression.
3. Realize that a diagnosis of breast cancer is a devastating emotional shock to the woman. Provide psychological support to the patient throughout the diagnostic and treatment process.
4. Involve the patient in planning and treatment.
5. Describe surgical procedures to alleviate fear.
6. Prepare the patient for the effects of chemotherapy, and plan ahead for alopecia, fatigue.
7. Administer antiemetics prophylactically, as directed, for patients receiving chemotherapy.
8. Administer IV fluids and hyperalimentation as indicated.
9. Help patient identify and use support persons or family or community.
10. Suggest to the patient the psychological interventions may be necessary for anxiety, depression, or sexual problems.
11. Teach all women the recommended cancer-screening procedures.

2012
Midwifery and Gynecology

SECTION-I

I. **Give the meaning of the following:**
   a. Decidua.
   b. Partograph.
   c. Lie.
   d. Menarche.

II. **Choose the correct answers and write:**
   a. Weight of a non-pregnant uterus:_____ (i. 20–30 g, ii. 50–60 g, iii. 80–90 g)
   b. Planned surgical incision made on posterior wall of perineum: _____
      (i. Encirclage, ii. Episiotomy, iii. Perineal tear)
   c. Women in labor is called: _____ (i. Para, ii. Gravid, iii. Parturient)
   d. Fetal period begins from: _____ (i. 8th week, ii.18th week, iii. 28th week)

III. **Differentiate between the following:**
   a. Quickening and lightening.
   b. Tonic neck reflex and rooting reflex.
   c. Fertilization and ovulation.
   d. Caput succedaneum and caphalhematoma.
   e. Symmetrical IUGR and asymmetrical IUGR.

IV. **Write short notes any *three* of the following:**
   a. Features of placenta at term.
   b. USG in antenatal period.
   c. 5 Ps of labor.
   d. Breastfeeding.

V. **Surabhi an antenatal mother with previous history of 2 abortions, now at 28th week GA, visits antenatal clinic for check-up, if her LMD = 28.1.2012:**
   a. Calculate the expected date of delivery.
   b. Write obstetrical score.
   c. Plan the health education.

   OR

   a. What is preterm baby?
   b. What are the characteristic features of preterm baby?
   c. Explain the management of preterm baby.

SECTION-II

VI. State whether the following statements are *true* or *false*:
   a. Collection of pus in the uterine cavity is called polymetra.
   b. Syphilis is caused by human papillomavirus.
   c. Displacement of functional endometrium other than uterine mucosa is called endometriosis.

VII. Fill in the blanks:
   a. The denominator in face presentation is:_____
   b. Bimanual compression is used in:_____
   c. Fetal macrosomia is when birth weight exceeds:_____
   d. Downy hair in the neonates is named as:_____

VIII. Write the action and indication of the following drugs:
   a. Oxytocin.
   b. Betamethasone.
   c. Lasix.

IX. Write short notes on any *three* of the following:
   a. Types and causes of infertility.
   b. Temporary methods of family planning.
   c. Placenta previa.
   d. Assisted breech delivery.

X. a. Define eclamsia.
   b. Write the signs and symptoms of eclampsia.
   c. Management of mother getting admitted with one episodes of seizures.

XI. Mrs X, a 54-year-old lady, diagnosed to have multiple fibroids and she is very anxious about it:
   a. Classify the fibroids.
   b. Write the signs and symptoms of fibrosis.
   c. Give her brief idea about the management modalities available for fibroid uterus.

SECTION-I

I. Give the meaning of the following:

a. Decidua

At the implantation location, the maternal endometrium is changed by the decidual reaction (epithelial transformation of the fibroblasts of the uterine stroma, in that lipids and glycogen accumulate) and is called the **decidua**. The decidua consists of various parts, depending on its relationship with the embryo:

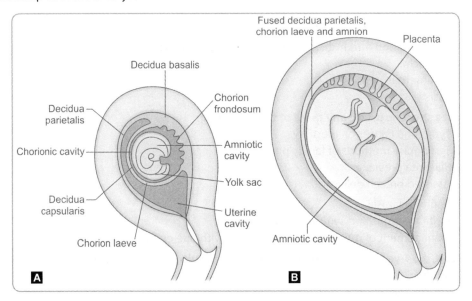

Decidua basalis, where the implantation takes place and the basal plate is formed. This can be subdivided into a zona compacta and a zona spongiosa (where the detachment of the placenta takes place following birth).
1. Decidua capsularis lies like a capsule around the chorion.
2. Decidua parietalis, on the opposite uterus wall.

At around the 4th month, the fetus is so large that the decidua capsularis comes into contact with the decidua parietalis. The merging of these two deciduae causes the uterine cavity to obliterate.

b. Partograph

Partograph or partogram is a graphic recording of the salient features of labor status. In the management of women in labor program serves to validate the normal progress of labor and to facilitate early identification of deviations from normal pattern.

Uses of partogram:
1. Provides a predictive value of labor progress.
2. Transfer of information becomes easy when labor status changes.
3. Saves writing time of staff against writing in long hand.
4. It is of educational value as it indicated the nature of labor.

c. Lie

Lie is the relationship of the long axis of the fetus to the long axis of the uterus. There are three possible lies—longitudinal, transverse and oblique.

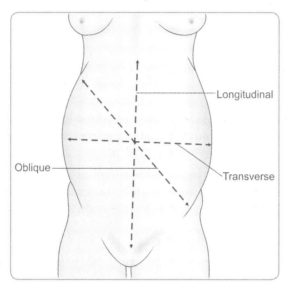

In 95% of cases, the lie is longitudinal owing to the ovoid shape of the uterus; the remainders are oblique or transverse. Oblique lie that results when the fetus is diagonally across the uterus must be distinguished from obliquity of the uterus, when the whole uterus is tilted to one side (usually right) and the fetus lies longitudinally within it. When the lie is transverse the fetus lies at right angles across.

d. Menarche

Menarche is the name given to the time when a girl has her first period. The age at which this happens varies from person to person. Most girls experience the menarche between the ages of 10 and 14 years. This age has been dropping for several years, probably due to improved nutrition and better social conditions. Before their first period arrives, most girls will have shown the early signs of puberty—the beginnings of breast development and fine hair growth in the pubic region and axilla (armpit). If signs of puberty begin much earlier, before age 8 for girls, it is called precocious puberty. This may be normal for that individual, or it may be a sign of underlying hormonal problems, so it is best to get children with very early puberty reviewed by their doctor.

It is uncommon for a regular menstrual cycle to follow the first period. Periods tend to occur in a haphazard way for the first year or 2 before settling into a regular pattern, which is usually once every 24 to 30 days. Some girls experience their first period without knowing what it is, which can be a frightening experience. For this reason, it is important for parents to prepare their daughters in advance for the changes associated with growing up.

II. Choose the correct answers and write.
a. Weight of a non-pregnant uterus: **50–60 g.**
   (i) 20–30g, (ii) 50–60g, (iii) 80–90 g

b. Planned surgical incision made on posterior wall of perineum: **Episiotomy.**
   (i.) Encirclage, (ii.) Episiotomy, (iii) Perineal tear
c. Women in labor is called: **Parturient.**
   (i.) Para, (ii) Gravid, (iii) Parturient
d. Fetal period begins from: **8th Week.**
   (i) 8th week, (ii)18th week, (iii) 28th week

III. Differentiate between the following:

a. Quickening and lightening

Quickening: The first natural sensation of quickening may feel like a light tapping, or the fluttering of a butterfly. These sensations eventually become stronger and more regular as the pregnancy progresses. Sometimes, the first movements are mis-attributed to gas or hunger pangs

Lightening: The process of your baby settling or lowering into your pelvis just before labor is called lightening. Lightening can occur a few weeks or a few hours before labor. Because the uterus rests on the bladder more after lightening, you may feel the need to urinate more frequently.

b. Tonic neck reflex and rooting reflex

Tonic neck reflex occurs when you move the head of a child who is relaxed and lying on his back to the side. The arm on the side where the head is facing reaches straight away from the body with the hand partly open. The arm on the side away from the face is flexed and the fist is clenched tightly. Turning the baby's face in the other direction reverses the position. The tonic neck position is often described as the fencer's position because it looks like a fencer's stance.

Rooting reflex occurs when you stroke the baby's cheek. The infant will turn toward the side that was stroked and begin to make sucking motions with the mouth.

c. Fertilization and ovulation

Fertilization: If one sperm does make its way into the fallopian tube and burrow into the egg, it fertilizes the egg. The egg changes so that no other sperm can get in. At the instant of fertilization, your baby's genes and sex are set. If the sperm has a Y chromosome, your baby will be a boy. If it has an X chromosome, the baby will be a girl.

Ovulation: Each month inside the ovaries, a group of eggs starts to grow in small, fluid-filled sacs called follicles. Eventually one of the eggs erupts from the follicle (ovulation). It usually happens about 2 weeks before your next period.

d. Caput succedaneum and cephalohematoma

Caput succedaneum: Localized edema occurring just under the presenting part of the fetal scalp during labor disappears within 36–48 hours of life.

Cephalohematoma: It is a collection of blood under the periosteum of a skull bone "very tough tissue covering that encapsulates bones". Because of its location, it is impossible for cephalhematoma to cross suture lines. If more than one bone is affected, there will be a separation between the two areas at the suture line as seen in the photo at the left where the sagittal suture separates the bilateral parietal cephalhematomas.

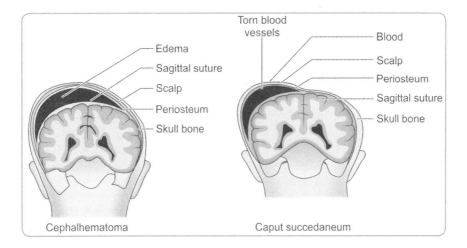

Cephalhematoma | Caput succedaneum

e. Symmetrical IUGR and Asymmetrical IUGR

There are 2 major categories of IUGR—symmetrical and asymmetrical. Some conditions are associated with both symmetrical and asymmetrical growth restriction.

Asymmetrical IUGR is more common. In asymmetrical IUGR—there is restriction of weight followed by length. The head continues to grow at normal or near-normal rates (head sparing). A lack of subcutaneous fat leads to a thin and small body out of proportion with the head. This is a protective mechanism that may have evolved to promote brain development. In these cases, the embryo/fetus has grown normally for the first two trimesters but encounters difficulties in the third, sometimes secondary to complications such as preeclampsia. Other symptoms than the disproportion include dry, peeling skin and an overly-thin umbilical cord. The baby is at increased risk of hypoxia and hypoglycemia. This type of IUGR is most commonly caused by extrinsic factors that affect the fetus at later gestational ages. Specific causes include:
1. Chronic high blood pressure
2. Severe malnutrition
3. Genetic mutations, Ehlers-Danlos syndrome.

Symmetrical IUGR is less common and more worrisome. It is less commonly known as **global growth restriction**, and indicates that the fetus has developed slowly throughout the duration of the pregnancy and was thus affected from a very early stage. The head circumference of such a newborn is in proportion to the rest of the body. Since most neurons are developed by the 18th week of gestation, the fetus with symmetrical IUGR is more likely to have permanent neurological sequela. Common causes include:
1. Early intrauterine infections, such as cytomegalovirus, rubella or toxoplasmosis.
2. Chromosomal abnormalities
3. Anemia
4. Maternal substance abuse (prenatal alcohol use can result in fetal alcohol syndrome).

IV. Write short notes any *three* of the following:

a. Features of placenta at term

The usual term placenta is about 22 cm in diameter and 2.0–2.5 cm thick. It generally weighs approximately 470 g (about 1 lb). However, the measurements can vary considerably, and placentas generally are not weighed in the delivery room.

The maternal surface of the placenta should be dark maroon in color and should be divided into lobules or cotyledons. The structure should appear complete, with no missing cotyledons. The fetal surface of the placenta should be shiny, gray and translucent enough that the color of the underlying maroon villous tissue may be seen.

At term, the typical umbilical cord is 55–60 cm in length, with a diameter of 2.0–2.5 cm. The structure should have abundant Wharton's jelly, and no true knots or thromboses should be present. The total cord length should be estimated in the delivery room, since the delivering physician has access to both the placental and fetal ends.

The normal cord contains two arteries and one vein. During the placental examination, the delivering physician should count the vessels in either the middle third of the cord or the fetal third of the cord, because the arteries are sometimes fused near the placenta and are therefore difficult to differentiate.

Fetal membranes are usually gray, wrinkled, shiny and translucent. The membranes and the placenta have a distinctive metallic odor that is difficult to describe but is easily recognized with experience. Normally, the placenta and the fetal membranes are not malodorous.

b. USG in antenatal period

Obstetric ultrasonography is the application of medical ultrasonography to obstetrics, in which sonography is used to visualize the embryo or fetus in its mother's uterus (womb). The procedure is a standard part of prenatal care, as it yields a variety of information regarding the health of the mother and of the fetus, the progress of the pregnancy, and further information on the baby.

Traditional obstetric sonograms are done by placing a transducer on the abdomen of the pregnant woman. One variant, a transvaginal sonography, is done with a probe placed in the woman's vagina. Transvaginal scans usually provide clearer pictures during early pregnancy and in obese women. Also used is Doppler sonography which detects the heartbeat of the fetus. Doppler sonography can be used to evaluate the pulsations in the fetal heart and bloods vessels for signs of abnormalities.

c. 5 Ps of labor

Factors affecting labor (the **5 Ps** of labor):
- **P**assenger
- **P**assageway
- **P**owers
- **P**osition
- **P**sychological response.

d. Breastfeeding

Breast milk is best for your baby, and the benefits of breastfeeding extend well beyond basic nutrition. In addition to containing all the vitamins and nutrients your baby needs in the first 6 months of life, breast milk is packed with disease-fighting substances that protect your baby from illness.

1. Research shows that breastfed infants have fewer and shorter episodes of illness.
2. Breastfeeding is the most natural and nutritious way to encourage your baby's optimal development.
3. Colostrum (the first milk) is a gentle, natural laxative that helps clear baby's intestine, decreasing the chance for jaundice to occur.
4. The superior nutrition provided by breast milk benefits your baby's IQ.

5. Breastfeeding is a gentle way for newborns to transition to the world outside the womb.
6. The skin-to-skin contact encouraged by breastfeeding offers babies greater emotional security and enhances bonding.
7. The activity of sucking at the breast enhances development of baby's oral muscles, facial bones, and aids in optimal dental development.
8. Breastfeeding appears to reduce the risk of obesity and hypertension.
9. Breastfeeding delays the onset of hereditary allergic disease, and lowers the risk of developing allergic disease.

V. Surabhi an antenatal mother with previous history of 2 abortions, now at 28th week GA, visits antenatal clinic for check-up, if her LMP = 28.1.2012

a. Calculate the expected date of delivery
LMP +9 months ± 7 days
The expected data of delivery is: 21/09/2012 to 5/10/2012.

b. Write obstetrical score
An evaluation of a newborn's physical condition, usually performed 1 minute and again 5 minutes after birth, based on a rating of five factors that reflect the infant's ability to adjust to extrauterine life. The system rapidly identifies infants requiring immediate intervention or transfer to a neonatal intensive care unit.

Method: The infant's heart rate, respiratory effort, muscle tone, reflex irritability, and color are scored from a low value of 0 to a normal value of 2. The five scores are combined, and the totals at 1 minute and 5 minutes are noted; for example, Apgar 9/10 is a score of 9 at 1 minute and 10 at 5 minutes.

Nursing considerations: A low 1-minute score requires immediate intervention, including administration of oxygen, clearing of the nasopharynx, and usually transfer to a neonatal intensive care unit. A baby with a low score that persists at 5 minutes requires expert care, which may include assisted ventilation, umbilical catheterization, cardiac massage, blood gas analysis, correction of acid-base deficit, or medication to reverse the effects of maternal medication.

Outcome criteria: A score of 0–3 represents severe distress, a score of 4–7 indicates moderate distress, and a score of 7–10 indicates an absence of difficulty in adjusting to extrauterine life. The 5-minute total score is normally higher than the 1-minute score. Because a normal, vigorous, healthy newborn almost always has bluish hands and feet at 1 minute, the first score for color will include a 1 rather than a perfect 2; however, at 5 minutes the blueness may have passed, and a score of 2 may be given. A 5-minute overall score of 0–1 correlates with a 50% neonatal mortality rate; infants who survive exhibit three times as many neurologic abnormalities at 1 year of age as do children with a 5-minute score of 7 or more.

c. Plan the health education
The antenatal period is an extremely important time during pregnancy. It is well recognized that good antenatal care improves maternal, perinatal and neonatal outcomes. Most women will progress through pregnancy in an uncomplicated fashion and deliver a healthy infant with little medical intervention. However, a significant number will develop medical or fetal complications. The current challenge in antenatal care is to identify those women who will require specialist support while allowing uncomplicated pregnancy to proceed with minimal interference.

The aims of antenatal care are to:
1. Provide high-quality information that can be easily understood in the current climate of ethnic and social diversity.
2. Provide an informed choice about the pathways of antenatal care.
3. Identify and screen for maternal complications.
4. Identify and screen for fetal complications.
5. Assess maternal and fetal wellbeing throughout pregnancy.
6. Provide advice and education on the normal symptoms of pregnancy.

At the initial antenatal care visit and with the aid of a special booking checklist the pregnant women become classified into either normal risk or high risk.

OR

a. What is preterm baby?

In humans **preterm birth** (Latin: *partus praetemporaneus* or *partus praematurus*) is the birth of a baby of less than 37 weeks gestational age. The cause of preterm birth is in many situations elusive and unknown; many factors appear to be associated with the development of preterm birth, making the reduction of preterm birth a challenging proposition.

Premature birth is defined either as the same as preterm birth, or the birth of a baby before the developing organs are mature enough to allow normal postnatal survival. Premature infants are at greater risk for short-and long-term complications, including disabilities and impediments in growth and mental development. Significant progress has been made in the care of premature infants, but not in reducing the prevalence of preterm birth. Preterm birth is among the top causes of death in infants worldwide.

b. What are the characteristic features of preterm baby?

Premature babies have a number of characteristics depending on their gestational age:
1. **Skin:** May be reddened. The skin may be thin so blood vessels are easily seen.
2. **Lanugo:** There is a lot of fine hair all over the baby's body.
3. **Limbs:** The limbs are thin and may be poorly flexed or floppy due to poor muscle tone.
4. **Head size:** Appears large in proportion to the body. The fontanelles (open spaces where skull bones join) are smooth and flat.
5. **Chest:** No breast tissue before 34 weeks of pregnancy.
6. **Sucking ability:** Weak or absent.
7. **Genitals:** In boys the testes may not be descended and the scrotum may be small; in girls the clitoris and labia minora may be large.
8. **Soles of feet:** Creases are located only in the anterior (front) of the sole, not all over, as in the term baby.

c. Explain the management of preterm baby

Babies who are born preterm need the same care that other babies get and a little more. This includes:

Good Pregnancy Care

1. All pregnant women should receive good care, including at least four antenatal visits with a health worker.
2. Mothers at risk of preterm birth (e.g. those who have had a preterm birth before) need to be aware that it may happen again, and plan accordingly.

3. Health workers caring for pregnant women need to assess their risk of delivering preterm and be able to recognize and manage conditions that can lead to preterm birth (e.g. preeclampsia, a condition in pregnancy that causes the mother to have high blood pressure).
4. Women in preterm labor should give birth at a health facility where they and their babies can get the care they need. They may need to be referred to a hospital where more advanced care is available, and the safest time to do this is when the baby is still in the womb.
5. Delivery by cesarean section or early induction of labor that is not medically necessary should be avoided.
6. Women in preterm labor, before 34 weeks of pregnancy have been completed, should receive steroid injections to speed up the development of the baby's lungs.

Essential Newborn Care

1. All babies need to be protected from infections: Everyone who touches the mother or the baby should have clean hands. Medical examinations and procedures should only be done if necessary. Sterile gloves and cutting devices should be used for clamping and cutting the umbilical cord.
2. All babies need to be kept warm: Right after birth, they should be dried thoroughly and placed on their mother's abdomen. If they breathe normally, and after the umbilical cord has been clamped and cut, they should be put on their mother's chest, with skin-to-skin contact, until after the first breastfeed. They should not be bathed right away.
3. Most babies will breathe normally after thorough drying. Those who do not start breathing on their own need help: ventilation with a bag and mask will usually put them back on track.
4. Breast is best: just like full-term babies, breast milk is the best nutrition for preterm babies. Babies should be breastfed as soon as possible after birth. Most premature babies who are unable to coordinate the suck and swallow reflex can be fed their mother's expressed breast milk by cup, spoon or nasogastric tube.

Extracare for Small Babies

1. Preterm babies, and full-term babies with low birth weight need extra warmth and support for feeding.
2. Kangaroo Mother Care is a good way of doing this.

SECTION-II

VI. State whether the following statements are *true* or *false*:
a. Collection of pus in the uterine cavity is called polymetra: **FALSE.**
b. Syphilis is caused by human pepilloma virus: **FALSE.**
c. Displacement of functional endometrium other than uterine mucosa is called endometriosis: **TRUE.**

VII. Fill in the blanks
a. The denominator in face presentation is: **Cephalic.**
b. Bimanual compression is used in: **Postpartum hemorrhage.**
c. Fetal macrosomia is when birth weight exceeds: **4 kg.**
d. Downy hair in the neonates is named as: **Lanugo.**

VIII. Write the action and indication of the following drugs:

a. Oxytocin

Oxytocin is a protein produced by the pituitary gland of mammals including man. Pitocin is a man-made version of oxytocin used for stimulating contraction of the uterus. Oxytocin works by increasing the concentration of calcium inside muscle cells that control contraction of the uterus. Increased calcium increases contraction of the uterus. The FDA approved oxytocin in November 1980. Pitocin is indicated for the initiation or improvement of uterine contractions, where this is desirable and considered suitable for reasons of fetal or maternal concern, in order to achieve vaginal delivery. It is indicated for (1) induction of labor in patients with a medical indication for the initiation of labor, such as Rh problems, maternal diabetes, preeclampsia at or near term, when delivery is in the best interests of mother and fetus or when membranes are prematurely ruptured and delivery is indicated; (2) stimulation or reinforcement of labor, as in selected cases of uterine inertia; (3) as adjunctive therapy in the management of incomplete or inevitable abortion. In the first trimester, curettage is generally considered primary therapy. In second trimester abortion, oxytocin infusion will often be successful in emptying the uterus.

b. Betamethasone

Treating certain conditions associated with decreased adrenal gland function. It is used to treat severe inflammation caused by certain conditions, including severe asthma, severe allergies, rheumatoid arthritis, ulcerative colitis, certain blood disorders, lupus, multiple sclerosis, and certain eye and skin conditions. It may be used for certain types of cancer (e.g. leukemia). It may also be used for other conditions as determined by your doctor. Betamethasone is a corticosteroid. It works by modifying the body's immune response to various conditions and decreasing inflammation. Betamethasone comes in ointment, cream, lotion, and aerosol (spray) in various strengths for use on the skin. It is usually applied one to four times a day. Follow the directions on your prescription label carefully, and ask your doctor or pharmacist to explain any part you do not understand. Use betamethasone exactly as directed. Do not use more or less of it or use it more often than prescribed by your doctor.

c. Lasix

Lasix® is a diuretic which is an anthranilic acid derivative. Lasix tablets for oral administration contain furosemide as the active ingredient and the following inactive ingredients: lactose monohydrate NF, magnesium stearate NF, starch NF, talc USP, and colloidal silicon dioxide NF. Chemically, it is 4-chloro-N-furfuryl-5-sulfamoyl anthranilic acid. Lasix is available as white tablets for oral administration in dosage strengths of 20, 40 and 80 mg. Furosemide is a white to off-white odorless crystalline powder. It is practically insoluble in water, sparingly soluble in alcohol, freely soluble in dilute alkali solutions and insoluble in dilute acids.

IX. Write short notes on any *three* of the following:

a. Types and causes of infertility

The causes of infertility are varied and complex. According to studies from around the world, both men and women are affected by infertility: about 40–60% of causes are linked to female factors, and 20–40% are related to male factors.

It is important for you to understand the anatomical, physiological and psychological conditions affecting fertility in women and men, both of whom should normally be able to conceive. Firstly, a man has to have normal functioning reproductive organs capable of producing normal sperm in sufficient numbers, and he has to be able to transfer them successfully to the woman's reproductive system through sexual intercourse.

Similarly, the woman's reproductive system should function normally and be able to produce healthy eggs, have normal fallopian tubes and uterus and produce normal cervical mucus.

To achieve normal physiological functions and processes, the endocrine (hormone-producing) glands of both the man and woman involved in reproduction must function normally. In addition, psychological and social conditions can influence the timing and frequency of sexual intercourse, which in turn can influence the chance of getting pregnant.

Age is an important factor in both women and men. In many women fertility declines as they age, especially over 35 years of age when the quality of eggs remaining in the ovaries is lower than when the women were younger. In men, sperm motility is reduced as they age, but overall fertility is not affected as much. There are many case reports describing men having children even after the age of 90 years.

There are two types of infertility—primary and secondary.
- **Primary infertility** is when a couple have never had children, or have been unable to achieve pregnancy after one year of living together despite having unprotected sexual intercourse.
- **Secondary infertility** is when a couple have had children or achieved pregnancy previously, but are unable to conceive at this time, even after one year of having unprotected sexual intercourse. Secondary infertility occurs more commonly than primary infertility, especially in developing countries where sexually transmitted infections are common. In many countries, induced abortion (intentionally done) contributes much to secondary infertility. Generally, it accounts for 60% of the total number of infertility cases.

b. Temporary methods of family planning

Temporary methods are divided into:
1. Natural methods: Abstinence, lactation, withdrawal, and safe period methods.
2. Barrier methods: Condoms with/without spermicide, diaphragm, cervical cap, sponge, vaginal spermicides.
3. Hormonal methods: Oral pills, injectables, implants.
4. Others: Intrauterine devices, e.g. Cu T.

c. Placenta previa

Placenta previa is the most common cause of painless bleeding in the later stages of pregnancy (after the 20th week). The placenta is a temporary organ that joins the mother and fetus and transfers oxygen and nutrients from the mother to the fetus. The placenta is disk-shaped and at full term measures about seven inches in diameter. The placenta attaches to the wall of the uterus (womb). Placenta previa is a complication that results from the placenta implanting either near to, or overlying, the outlet of the uterus (the opening of the uterus, the cervix). The types of placenta previa include:
1. **Complete placenta previa** occurs when the placenta completely covers the opening from the womb to the cervix.
2. **Partial placenta previa occurs** when the placenta partially covers the cervical opening.

3. **Marginal placenta previa occurs** when the placenta is located adjacent to, but not covering, the cervical opening.

Placenta previa occurs in 1 out of 200 pregnancies. It is more common in women who have:
1. Abnormally shaped uterus.
2. Many previous pregnancies.
3. Multiple pregnancy (twins, triplets, etc.).
4. Scarring on the lining of the uterus, due to history of surgery, c-section, previous pregnancy, or abortion.

Women who smoke or have their children at an older age may also have an increased risk.

The main symptom of placenta previa is sudden bleeding from the vagina. Some women have cramps, too. The bleeding often starts near the end of the second trimester or beginning of the third trimester. Bleeding may be severe. It may stop on its own but can start again days or weeks later. Labor sometimes starts within several days of heavy bleeding. Sometimes, bleeding may not occur until after labor starts.

d. Assisted breech delivery

Breech presentation is defined as a fetus in a longitudinal lie with the buttocks or feet closest to the cervix. This occurs in 3–4% of all deliveries. The percentage of breech deliveries decreases with advancing gestational age from 22% of births prior to 28 weeks' gestation to 7% of births at 32 weeks' gestation to 1-3% of births at term. There are many methods which have been attempted with the aim of turning breech babies, with varying degrees of success:

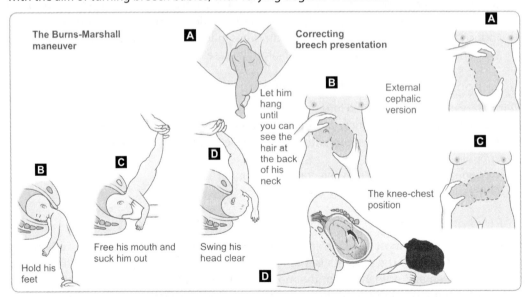

External cephalic version (ECV) where a midwife or doctor turns the baby by manipulating the baby through the mother's abdomen. ECV has a success rate between 40% and 70% depending on practitioner. The fetal heart is monitored after the turn attempt, usually in the context of an institutional protocol. Studies show that turning the baby at term (after 36 weeks) is effective in reducing the number of babies born in the breech position. Complications from external cephalic version are rare. Studies have also shown that attempting to turn the baby prior to this point has no impact on the presentation at term. Using hypothetical scenarios, a small study in the Netherlands found that few obstetric practitioners would attempt ECV in the presence of oligohydramnios. A case report of treating oligohydramnios with amnioinfusion, followed by ECV, was successful in turning the fetus.

Various maneuvers are suggested to assist spontaneous version of a breech presenting pregnancy. These include maternal positioning or other exercises. A study has shown that there is insufficient evidence as to the benefit of maternal positioning in reducing the incidence of breech presentation.

X. a. Define eclampsia

Eclampsia, which is considered a complication of severe preeclampsia, is commonly defined as new onset of grand mal seizure activity and/or unexplained coma during pregnancy or postpartum in a woman with signs or symptoms of preeclampsia. Eclampsia is a rare but severe condition that causes seizures during pregnancy. Seizures are periods of disturbed brain activity that can cause episodes of staring, decreased alertness, and violent shaking (convulsions). Eclampsia affects about one in every 2,000–3,000 pregnancies, and it can affect you even if you do not have a history of seizures.

b. Write the signs and symptoms of eclampsia

Because preeclampsia can lead to eclampsia, you may have the symptoms of both conditions. However, some of your symptoms may be caused by other conditions, such as kidney disease or diabetes. It is important to tell your doctor, so that he or she may rule out other possible causes.

Most women with mild preeclampsia do not have any symptoms. The hallmark signs, as mentioned previously, are the presence of protein in the urine and elevated blood pressure. Swelling of the feet, legs, and hands is also common, but this can occur in normal pregnancy and

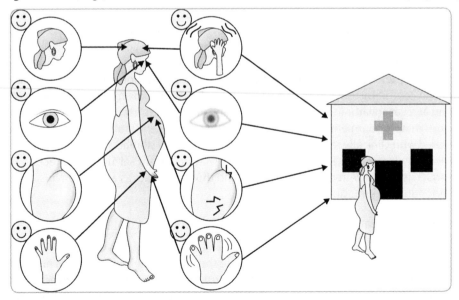

is not necessarily related to preeclampsia. Women with preeclampsia may experience sudden weight gain over 1–2 days.

Other symptoms and signs that can occur with severe preeclampsia are dizziness, headaches, nausea, vomiting, abdominal pain, vision changes, changes in reflexes, altered mental state, fluid in the lungs (pulmonary edema), and a decrease in urine output. Symptoms of eclampsia include those of preeclampsia along with the development of seizures. When seizures occur, they are most often preceded by neurologic symptoms like headache and vision disturbances. Women with severe preeclampsia may have a reduced platelet count (below 100,000).

c. Management of mother getting admitted with one episode of seizures

The mainstays of management of the neurological symptoms of severe preeclamptic and eclamptic patients are the rapid lowering of blood pressure, administration of $MgSO_4$ and delivery of the fetus. Mean arterial blood pressure should be lowered in patients with severe hypertension by 15–20%. Intravenous labetalol, hydralazine, or nicardipine work rapidly and safely. Nitroprusside and nitroglyercine contain cyanide and thus can cause fetal toxicity. Angiotensin-converting enzyme (ACE) inhibitors are contraindicated during pregnancy (category D). Fluid therapy can be beneficial to eclamptic patients and those with severe preeclampsia because of the associated volume contraction (or lack of expansion of plasma volume associated with normal pregnancy), however, this should be monitored closely in women with severe and persistent hypertension, oliguria and pulmonary edema.

Prevention of the eclamptic seizure in a woman with preeclampsia is obvious and justified. Traditionally, obstetricians have favored the use of $MgSO_4$ for the prevention of the eclamptic convulsion whereas neurologists have favored antiepileptic agents, such as phenytoin. A single first-onset seizure that occurs during pregnancy and resolves within minutes can usually be managed without anti-convulsant agents. $MgSO_4$ therapy has been shown to be more effective than anti-convulsant agents, including phenytoin, and is now considered the treatment of choice for preventing eclampsia in preeclamptic women. Therapy can start with a loading dose of 4–6 g $MgSO_4$ followed by 2 g/h infusion. A supplemental dose of 2 g can be given if seizure recurs.

Mechanisms of $MgSO_4$ for seizure prevention $MgSO_4$ is the therapy of choice for preventing eclamptic convulsions. The mechanisms by which $MgSO_4$ is effective at preventing eclamptic convulsions are likely multifactorial and have been recently reviewed in 16 and will only be summarized here. $MgSO_4$ is a calcium antagonist and as such could inhibit vascular smooth muscle contraction. $MgSO_4$ is a potent vasodilator, however, its effects in the cerebral circulation are considerably less effective than systemic vasculature. In addition, the sensitivity to $MgSO_4$ is decreased in cerebral arteries from late-pregnant and postpartum animals, suggesting $MgSO_4$ is not acting as a vasodilator in the cerebral circulation. $MgSO_4$ has been shown to protect the BBB, likely through its calcium antagonistic effects in the cerebral endothelium. When pregnant rats were treated with clinically relevant doses of $MgSO_4$, they had significantly less BBB permeability during acute hypertension. Thus, $MgSO_4$ could prevent recurrent seizure by protecting the BBB. Lastly, $MgSO_4$ is an NMDA receptor antagonist and thus would act as an anticonvulsant if it were in high enough concentration in the brain.

X. Mrs X, a 54-year-old lady, diagnosed to have multiple fibroids and she is very anxious about it.

Fibroids are not cancerous. Drugs that manipulate the levels of steroid hormones are effective in treating fibroids, but side effects limit their long-term use. Fibroids may be removed if they cause appreciable discomfort or if they are associated with uterine bleeding. Surgery is the mainstay of fibroid treatment. In addition to hysterectomy and abdominal myomectomy, various minimally invasive procedures have been developed to remove fibroids from the uterus.

Fibroids are abnormal growths that develop in or on a woman's uterus. Sometimes, these tumors become quite large and cause severe abdominal pain and heavy periods. In other cases, they cause no signs or symptoms at all. The growths are typically benign (noncancerous). The cause of fibroids is unknown.

a. Classify the fibroids

Growth and location are the main factors that determine if a fibroid leads to symptoms and problems. A small lesion can be symptomatic if located within the uterine cavity while a large lesion on the outside of the uterus may go unnoticed. Different locations are classified as follows:

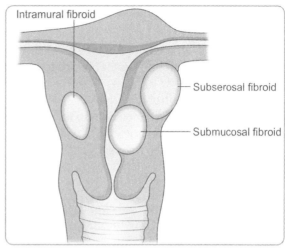

1. **Intramural fibroids** are located within the wall of the uterus and are the most common type; unless large, they may be asymptomatic. Intramural fibroids begin as small nodules in the muscular wall of the uterus. With time, intramural fibroids may expand inwards, causing distortion and elongation of the uterine cavity.
2. **Subserosal fibroids** are located underneath the mucosal (peritoneal) surface of the uterus and can become very large. They can also grow out in a papillary manner to become pedunculated fibroids. These pedunculated growths can actually detach from the uterus to become a parasitic leiomyoma.
3. **Submucosal fibroids** are located in the muscle beneath the endometrium of the uterus and distort the uterine cavity; even small lesions in this location may lead to bleeding and infertility. A pedunculated lesion within the cavity is termed an intracavitary fibroid and can be passed through the cervix.
4. **Cervical fibroids** are located in the wall of the cervix (neck of the uterus). Rarely, fibroids are found in the supporting structures (round ligament, broad ligament, or uterosacral ligament) of the uterus that also contain smooth muscle tissue.

Fibroids may be single or multiple. Most fibroids start in an intramural location that is the layer of the muscle of the uterus. With further growth, some lesions may develop towards the outside of the uterus or towards the internal cavity. Secondary changes that may develop within fibroids are hemorrhage, necrosis, calcification, and cystic changes.

b. Write the signs and symptoms of fibrosis

Fibroids, particularly when small, may be entirely asymptomatic. Symptoms depend on the location of the lesion and its size. Important symptoms include abnormal gynecological hemorrhage, heavy or painful periods, abdominal discomfort or bloating, painful defecation, backache, urinary frequency or retention, and in some cases, infertility. There may also be pain during intercourse, depending on the location of the fibroid. During pregnancy, they may also be the cause of miscarriage, bleeding, premature labor, or interference with the position of the fetus.

While fibroids are common, they are not a typical cause for infertility accounting for about 3% of reasons why a woman may not be able to have a child. The majority of women with uterine fibroids will have normal pregnancy outcomes. In cases of intercurrent uterine fibroids in infertility, a fibroid is typically located in a submucosal position and it is thought that this location may interfere with the function of the lining and the ability of the embryo to implant. Also larger fibroids may distort or block the fallopian tubes.

c. Give her brief idea about the management modalities available for fibroid uterus

Most fibroids do not require treatment unless they are causing symptoms. After menopause fibroids shrink and it is unusual for fibroids to cause problems. Symptomatic uterine fibroids can be treated by:

1. Medication to control symptoms.
2. Medication aimed at shrinking tumors.
3. Ultrasound fibroid destruction.
4. Myomectomy or radio frequency ablation.
5. Hysterectomy.
6. Uterine artery embolization.

Treatment for the symptoms of fibroids may include:

1. Birth control pills (oral contraceptives) to help control heavy periods.
2. Intrauterine devices (IUDs) that release the hormone progestin to help reduce heavy bleeding and pain.
3. Iron supplements to prevent or treat anemia due to heavy periods.
4. Nonsteroidal anti-inflammatory drugs (NSAIDs) such as ibuprofen or naprosyn for cramps or pain.
5. Short-term hormonal therapy injections to help shrink the fibroids.

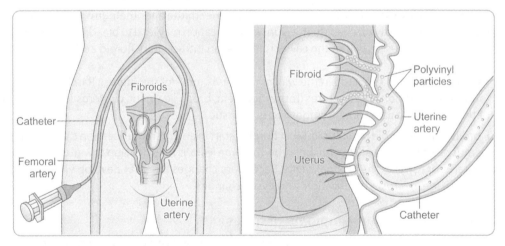

Surgery and procedures used to treat fibroids include:

1. **Hysteroscopic resection of fibroids:** Women who have fibroids growing inside the uterine cavity may need this outpatient procedure to remove the fibroid tumors.
2. **Uterine artery embolization:** This procedure stops the blood supply to the fibroid, causing it to die and shrink. Women who may want to become pregnant in the future should discuss this procedure with their healthcare provider.
3. **Myomectomy:** This surgery removes the fibroids. It is often the chosen treatment for women who want to have children, because it usually can preserve fertility. More fibroids can develop after a myomectomy.
4. **Hysterectomy:** This invasive surgery may be an option if medicines do not work and other surgeries and procedures are not an option.

2011
Midwifery and Gynecology

SECTION-I

I. Give the meaning of the following:
  a. Nullipara.
  b. Langue.
  c. Surrogate mother.
  d. Quickening.
  e. Bandl's ring.

II. Fill in the blanks:
  a. The term used for abnormal labor:_____
  b. Anterior fontanel is otherwise known as:_____
  c. Craving for non-nutritional substance is known as:_____

III. Write short notes on any *four* of the following:
  a. Fetal skull.
  b. Episiotomy.
  c. Placenta.
  d. Diet during puerperium.
  e. Physiological changes during pregnancy.

IV. Differentiate between the following:
  a. True pelvis and false pelvis.
  b. Lie and attitude.
  c. Menarche and menopause.

V. a. Define eutocia.
  b. Explain the management of third stage of labor.

SECTION-II

VI. State whether the following statements are *true* or *false*.
  a. The android pelvis resembles the male pelvis.
  b. In septic abortion, shock is due to neurogenic shock.
  c. Fetal macrosomia is when birth weight exceeds 3 kg.

VII. Write the indications of the following drugs:
  a. Ergometrine. b. Folic acid. c. Oxytocin. d. Magnesium sulfate.

VIII. Write short notes on any *four* of the following:
   a. Care following cesarian section.
   b. Sexually transmitted diseases.
   c. Infertility.
   d. Postpartum hemorrhage.
   e. Carcinoma of cervix.

IX. a. What is hysterectomy?
   b. List the indications for hysterectomy.
   c. Write the pre- and postoperative nursing care of women posted for hysterectomy.

X. a. What is breech presentation?
   b. List the types of breech presentation.
   c. Explain the management of breech delivery.

Midwifery and Gynecological Nursing: 2011

SECTION-I

I. Give the meaning of the following:
a. **Nullipara:** Having never given birth to a viable infant.
b. **Lanugo:** Downy hair on the body of a fetus or newborn baby. Lanugo is the first hair to be produced by the fetal hair follicles, and it usually appears on the fetus at about 5 months of gestation. Lanugo is very fine, soft, and usually unpigmented. Although lanugo is normally shed before birth, around 7 or 8 months of gestation, it is sometimes present at birth. This is not a cause for concern. Lanugo disappears of its own accord within a few days or weeks.
c. **Surrogate mother:** A surrogacy arrangement or surrogacy agreement is the carrying of a pregnancy for intended parents. There are two main types of surrogacy, gestational surrogacy and traditional surrogacy. In gestational surrogacy, the pregnancy results from the transfer of an embryo created by IVF, in a manner so the resulting child is genetically unrelated to the surrogate. Gestational surrogates are also referred to as gestational carriers. In traditional surrogacy, the surrogate is impregnated naturally or artificially, but the resulting child is genetically related to the surrogate. In the US, gestational surrogacy is more common than traditional surrogacy and is considered less legally complex.
d. **Quickening:** The first natural sensation of quickening may feel like a light tapping, or the fluttering of a butterfly. These sensations eventually become stronger and more regular as the pregnancy progresses. Sometimes, the first movements are mis-attributed to gas or hunger pangs.
e. **Bandl's ring:** Bandl's ring (also known as pathological retraction ring) is the abnormal junction between the two segments of the human uterus, which is a late sign associated with obstructed labor, Prior to the onset of labor, the junction between the lower and upper uterine segments is a slightly thickened ring. In abnormal and obstructed labors, after the cervix has reached full dilatation further contractions cause the upper uterine segment muscle fibers myometrium to shorten, so that the actively contracting upper segment becomes thicker and shorter. The ridge of the pathological ring of Bandl's can be felt or seen rising as far up as the umbilicus. The lower segment becomes stretched and thinner and if neglected may lead to uterine rupture.

II. Fill in the blanks.
a. The term used for abnormal labor: **Dystocia.**
b. Anterior fontanel is otherwise known as: **Bregma.**
c. Craving for non-nutritional substance is known as: **Pica.**

III. Write short notes on any *four* of the following:

a. Fetal skull
The skull bones encase and protect the brain, which is very delicate and subjected to pressure when the fetal head passes down the birth canal. Correct presentation of the smallest diameter of the fetal skull to the largest diameter of the mother's bony pelvis is essential if delivery is to proceed normally. But if the presenting diameter of the fetal skull is larger than the maternal pelvic diameter, it needs very close attention for the baby to go through a normal vaginal delivery.

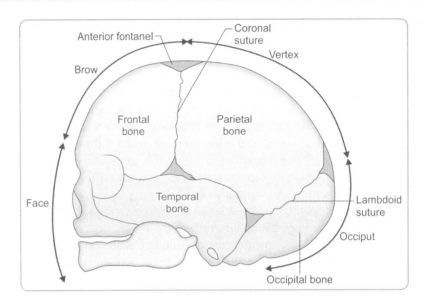

The fetal skull bones are as follows:
1. The frontal bone, which forms the forehead. In the fetus, the frontal bone is in two halves, which fuse (join) into a single bone after the age of 8 years.
2. The two parietal bones, which lie on either side of the skull and occupy most of the skull.
3. Parietal is pronounced 'parr eye ett al'. Occipital is pronounced 'ox ipp itt al'.
4. The occipital bone, which forms the back of the skull and part of its base. It joins with the cervical vertebrae (neck bones in the spinal column, or backbone).
5. The two temporal bones, one on each side of the head, closest to the ear.
6. Understanding the landmarks and measurements of the fetal skull will help you to recognize normal and abnormal presentations of the fetus during antenatal examinations, labor and delivery.

Sutures are joints between the bonessss of the skull. In the fetus they can 'give' a little under the pressure on the baby's head as it passes down the birth canal. During early childhood, these sutures harden and the skull bones can no longer move relative to one another, as they can to a small extent in the fetus and newborn. It is traditional for their names and locations to be taught in midwifery courses. You may be able to tell the angle of the baby's head as it 'presents' in the birth canal by feeling for the position of the main sutures with your examining fingers.

b. Episiotomy

This is an incision through the perineal tissues which is designed to enlarge the vulval outlet during delivery. The rationale for its use depends largely on the need to minimize the risk of severe, spontaneous, maternal trauma and to expedite the birth when there is evidence of fetal distress.

Indications
1. To speed up delivery if there is fetal distress.

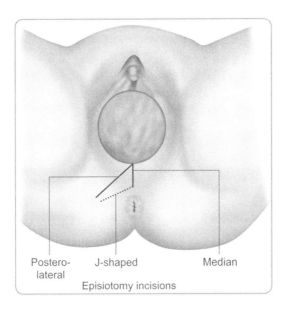

Episiotomy incisions: Postero-lateral, J-shaped, Median

2. Prior to an assisted delivery, such as forceps or ventouse extraction.
3. To minimize the risk of intracranial damage during preterm and breech delivery.

Dubious Indications
1. To prevent overstretching of the perineal muscles with the intention of preventing the longer terms problem of prolapse and stress incontinence.
2. To reduce the risk of spontaneous explosive trauma to the perineum.

The timing of the incision episiotomy involves incision of the fourchette, the superficial muscles and skin of the perineum and the posterior vaginal wall. So, it can successfully speed up delivery only when the presenting part is directly applied to these tissues. If episiotomy is performed early it will fail to release the presenting part and hemorrhage from the cut vessel may ensure. In addition, the levator and muscles will not have had time to be displaced laterally and may be incised. If performed too late there will not be enough time to infiltrate with a local anesthesia. Episiotomy should not be done if a tear has already begun.

c. Placenta
Placenta is the mechanical and physiological connection between fetal and maternal tissues for the nutrition, respiration and excretion of the fetus. The surface of the blastocyst gives rise to finger-like outgrowths called chorionic villi which penetrate into depressions on the wall of the uterus called crypts. The intimate connection between the fetal membranes and the uterine wall is known as placenta. The part of the placenta contributed by the fetal (chorion) membranes of the fetus is called the fetal placenta and that contributed by the uterine wall of the mother (decidua basalis) is called the maternal placenta. The degree of intimacy between the fetal placenta and maternal placenta is so strong, that, eventually the blood vessels of the chorionic villi are literally bathed in the mother's blood. This type of placenta is known as hemochorial placenta.

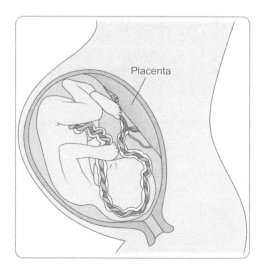

Fetal Membranes and Placenta

In the placenta, the fetal blood comes into close contact with the maternal blood, resulting in exchange of materials. Food and oxygen pass from the maternal blood into the fetal blood and the wastes from the fetus pass into the maternal blood.

There is no mixing up of maternal and fetal blood. The umbilical cord connects the fetus to the placenta.

Functions of Placenta

1. **Nutrition:** Placenta helps transport nutrients from maternal blood into fetus.
2. **Respiration:** It helps in getting oxygen from the maternal blood into the fetus and CO_2 from fetus blood into the maternal blood.
3. **Excretion:** Nitrogenous waste products produced in the embryo diffuse through the placenta into the maternal bloodstream.
4. **Immunity:** Antibodies developed in the mother against certain diseases like measles, smallpox, diphtheria pass from mother into the fetal blood through the placenta.
5. **Transport of pathogens:** Pathogenic organisms like viruses diffuse through the placenta. Viruses causing syphilis, measles, rubella, smallpox may infect the fetus, if the mother gets the disease during pregnancy. Some of these diseases may even cause congenital deformities.
6. **Transport of drugs:** Some of the drugs taken by the mother during pregnancy cross the placental barrier and may even cause developmental deformities. For example, the drug thalidomide used to avoid nausea and morning sickness during early pregnancy by some women resulted in the child born to such mothers to have deformities in the limb development and heart. The children had flipper like limbs, a condition called as phocomelia. Children born to drug addicts are born with addiction and withdrawal symptoms.
7. **Storage:** Placenta stores some fats, glycogen and iron.
8. **Secretion of hormones:** Placenta secretes many hormones like estrogen, progesterone, gonadotropin and placental lactogen, thus functioning as an endocrine gland.

d. Diet during puerperium

Eating right after delivery is not that complex. Just continue eating a good quality diet just as you did during pregnancy. If you are not breastfeeding, your nutrient and calorie needs are the same as they were before you became pregnant. If you are breastfeeding, or if you are anemic or recovering from a cesarean delivery, you require special nutritional management. Take a creative approach to nutrition, choosing foods that require little or no preparation. Quick, nutritious foods include fresh fruit, raw vegetables, melted cheese on toast, cottage cheese, and yogurt with raisins, sunflower seeds, nugget-type cereal, or low-fat granola. Broiled meats and fish are faster to prepare than casseroles.

e. Physiological changes during pregnancy

During pregnancy, your body goes through many emotional and physiological changes. These changes are a natural part of pregnancy and a better understanding will help you cope with them. Pregnancy is more than just the growth of the uterus and the embryo. Some of the physiological changes during pregnancy are listed in the table below.

Physiologic changes in pregnancy	
Cardiovascular	Increased cardiac output Increased blood volume Increased resting heart rate Decreased peripheral resistance Decreased blood pressure (second trimester)
Pulmonary	Increased respiratory rate Decreased functional residual capacity Increased tidal volume Increased minute ventilation Respiratory alkalosis
Gastrointestinal	Decreased gastric motility Decreased esophageal sphincter tone
Musculoskeletal	Increased ligament laxity

Fertilization and early embryo formation cause significant changes in all of your body's systems. This is how your body prepares and helps the pregnancy develop into successful childbirth. Each woman is affected differently. Understanding the changes and effects on the various body systems helps the burden during pregnancy, reduces anxiety and unnecessary tensions. Some of the symptoms go away immediately after birth and most of them disappear within six weeks of delivery.

Normally, the uterus weighs 60 g and is as large as a chicken egg. By the end of a pregnancy it will weigh 1 kilogram and contain a baby, a placenta and more than a quart of water.

As the uterus grows it presses against the woman's abdominal organs. The uterus presses against the bladder, stomach and lungs, the arteries, veins and nerves and stretches the abdominal skin. This results in frequent urination, heartburn, congestion in the veins, difficulty breathing and other conditions that will pass after birth as the uterus returns to its prepregnancy size.

IV. Differentiate between the following:

a. True pelvis and false pelvis

True pelvis: The true or "lesser" pelvis is bounded in front and below by the pubic symphysis and the superior rami of the pubis; above and behind, by the sacrum and coccyx; and laterally, by a broad, smooth, quadrangular area of bone, corresponding to the inner surfaces of the body and superior ramus of the ischium, and the part of the ilium below the arcuate line.

False pelvis: The false "greater" pelvis is bounded on either side by the ilium; in front it is incomplete, presenting a wide interval between the anterior borders of the ilia; behind is a deep notch on either side between the ilium and the base of the sacrum.

b. Lie and attitude

Fetal lie: The lie is the relation of the long axis of the fetus to that of the mother, and is either longitudinal or transverse. Occasionally, the fetal and the maternal axes may cross at a 45 degree angle, forming an oblique lie, which is unstable and always becomes longitudinal or transverse during the course of labor.

Fetal attitude or posture: In the later months of pregnancy the fetus assumes a characteristic posture described as attitude or habitus As a rule, the fetus forms an ovoid mass that corresponds roughly to the shape of the uterine cavity. The fetus becomes folded or bent upon itself in such a manner that the back becomes markedly convex; the head is sharply flexed, so that the chin is almost in contact with the chest.

c. Menarche and menopause

The start: Menarche is the name given to the first menstrual period, which usually occurs between the ages of 11 and 16.

The end: Menopause is that point in time when periods stop permanently. It is also called the "change of life" or "climacteric".

V. a. Define eutocia
b. Explain the management of third stage of labor

Definition of labor: Series of events that take place in the genital organs in an effort to expel the viable products of conception out of the uterus through the vagina into the outer world is called labor.

Normal labor (eutocia): Labor is called normal if it fulfills the following criteria:
1. Spontaneous in onset and at term.
2. With vertex presentation.
3. Without undue prolongation.
4. Natural termination with minimal aids.
5. Without having any complications affecting the health of the mother or the baby.

Contraction and Retraction of Uterine Muscle

a. Uterine contractions are involuntarily controlled by the nervous system and indirectly by endocrines.
b. Contractions are intermittent, occurring every 1–15 minutes and increases gradually to 1–2 minutes.
c. Contractions are painful. This is probably due to squeezing of the nerve endings, between the muscle fibers and partly due to the resistance in the cervix and soft parts. If the patient is tensed this will increase the resistance and thus the pain is more.
d. Contractions last for several seconds but rarely exceed 60–70 seconds. This prevents prolonged compression on the uterine arteries and interference with the oxygen supply to the fetus.

A uterine contraction consists of the following:
a. **Contractional:** Temporary shortening of the muscle fibers.
b. **Relaxation:** When the contraction is absent.
c. **Retraction:** Instead of complete relaxation when the muscle fibers should return to its previous size there is some permanent shortening of the fibers.

Formation of the Upper and Lower Uterine Segment

At the end of pregnancy the uterus is divided into two:
a. The upper uterine segment, which is the thick, muscular contractile part.
b. The lower uterine segment, which is relaxed, thin, distensable area. It is about 8–10 cm long and is formed from the isthmus.

Development of the retraction ring: The contractions and retractions of the upper uterine segment cause it to become thicker and shorter, as it attempts to push the fetus out into the birth canal. This stretches lower uterine segment causing it to become thinner. At the junction of the upper and lower segment a ridge forms this is the retraction ring.

Formation of retraction ring

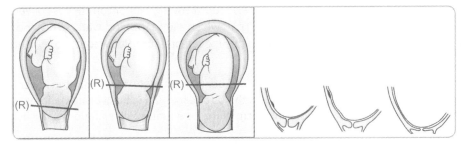

When the retraction ring is exaggerated, it is visible over the abdomen.

The term Bandl's ring is applied. The retraction ring is perfectly normal providing it remains below the symphysis pubis, but should the fetus not be able to pass through the os as in obstructed labor the lower uterine segment, stretches further to accommodate it as it is being pushed out of the upper uterine segment, and the retraction ring becomes visible and palpable as a depressed ridge running transversely or slightly oblique across the abdomen above the symphysis pubis. This is serious for, the uterus is in danger of rupturing.

Polarity: This is the term used to describe the harmonious neuromuscular action between the upper and lower uterine segment. The upper uterine segment contracts and retracts, and this is controlled by the parasympathetic nervous system. The lower uterine segment mainly passive and therefore relaxes and dilates. This is controlled by the sympathetic nervous system. During contraction the upper uterine segment contracts and retracts to expel the fetus and the lower uterine segment relaxes and dilates to allow the fetus to escape. This harmonious action is called polarity. When the polarity is disorganized the progress of labor is inhibited or prolonged fear during labor will cause the lower segment to go into spasm. Thus, slowing labor and causing greater pain.

Taking-up of the cervix: This occurs as the result of the retraction of the upper segment and the relaxation and dilatation of the lower uterine segment when the fetus is pushed into it. This causes the internal os to open and the cervical canal to be drawn up into the lower uterine segment. As the canal widens it resembles a funnel.

Dilatation of the os: It is the opening up of the external os. In a primigravida, it occurs after whole cervical canal has been drawn up into the lower uterine segment. In a multigravida, it usually occurs at the same time as the taking up of the cervix. Dilatation of the os is assisted by the bag of fore-waters; it acts as a fluid wedge that protrudes into the cervical canal slightly aids the dilatation. But a well-flexed head has a similar effect.

Show: It is the escape of the plug of mucus from the cervical canal as it dilates. It is slightly stained with blood from decidua vera when the chorion become detached.

Formation of fore-waters: During each contraction in the first stage of labor, the sac of fluid in front of the presenting part is cut off from the water behind. And it is forced into the cervical canal and thus helping the cervix to take up. When a well-flexed head is presented, it fits into the cervix and acts as a valve and prevents the hind-waters from joining the fore-waters.

This causes an even pressure on the membrane and keeps them intact during the first stage. While the membranes are intact the placenta cannot be compressed between the uterine wall and the fetus. So the oxygen supply to the fetus is well-maintained, also there is less risks of infection and thus while the membranes are intact, the mother and the baby are reasonable safe.

Rupture of membranes: Usually, the membranes rupture towards the end of first stage of labor because the support from the cervix has been removed by dilatation and the uterine contractions are very much stronger. The membranes may also rupture before labor commences or very early.

This may be due to badly fitting presenting part which allows the hind-water to distend the sac of fore-waters causing them to rupture due to the uneven pressure. But in some cases, it happens for no apparent reason.

Full dilatation of the cervix: Now the cervix has been completely drawn into the lower uterine segment and the presenting part passes into the birth canal. On vaginal examination the cervix is not felt all around (a normal condition) 10 cm of the os equates full dilatation of the os.

Secondary powers: As the head distends the vagina, character of contraction is altered and the mother begins to push which make the abdominal muscles and diaphragm into action.

Swing door action of the pelvic floor: As the head dilates the vagina, the anterior segment of the pelvic floor is drawn up the post; segments is pushed downwards and backwards, the advancing head presses on the rectum and expels the fecal matters out. This pressure makes the anus to spout, the perineum stretches and the head is seen at the vulva. Progressing with each contraction until crowning takes place, then the head is born followed by the rest of the body.

SECTION-II

VI. State whether the following statements are *true* or *false*.
a. The android pelvis resembles the male pelvis: **TRUE.**
b. In septic abortion shock is due to neurogenic shock: **TRUE.**
c. Fetal macrosomia is when birth weight exceeds 3 kg: **FALSE.**

VII. Write the indications of the following drugs:

a. Ergometrine
Ergometrine is a type of medicine called an ergot alkaloid. It is used to help prevent and control bleeding after childbirth. Ergometrine acts on three different types of receptors found in the walls of the blood vessels and in the uterus. When these receptors are stimulated by ergometrine

they cause the blood vessels to constrict and the uterus to contract. The contractions help the placenta to be pushed out. Both actions reduce blood flow to the uterus, which helps reduce blood loss as the placenta comes away from the wall of the uterus. Ergometrine can be used to control excessive bleeding following childbirth. Ergometrine helps the uterus contract back and controls blood loss as it does this.

b. Folic acid

Folic acid is a type of B vitamin. It is the man-made (synthetic) form of folate that is found in supplements and added to fortified foods. Folate is a generic term for both naturally occurring folate found in foods and folic acid. Folic acid is water-soluble. Water-soluble vitamins dissolve in water. Leftover amounts of the vitamin leave the body through the urine. That means your body does not store folic acid and you need a continuous supply of the vitamin in the foods you eat.

c. Oxytocin

Oxytocin is a protein produced by the pituitary gland of mammals including man. Pitocin is a man-made version of oxytocin used for stimulating contraction of the uterus. Oxytocin works by increasing the concentration of calcium inside muscle cells that control contraction of the uterus. Increased calcium increases contraction of the uterus. The FDA approved oxytocin in November 1980. Pitocin is indicated for the initiation or improvement of uterine contractions, where this is desirable and considered suitable for reasons of fetal or maternal concern, in order to achieve vaginal delivery. It is indicated for (1) induction of labor in patients with a medical indication for the initiation of labor, such as Rh problems, maternal diabetes, preeclampsia at or near term, when delivery is in the best interests of mother and fetus or when membranes are prematurely ruptured and delivery is indicated; (2) stimulation or reinforcement of labor, as in selected cases of uterine inertia; (3) as adjunctive therapy in the management of incomplete or inevitable abortion. In the first trimester, curettage is generally considered primary therapy. In second trimester abortion, oxytocin infusion will often be successful in emptying the uterus.

d. Magnesium sulfate

Action: Decreases acetylcholine in motor nerve terminals, which is responsible for anti-convulsant properties, thereby reduces neuromuscular irritability. It also decreases intracranial edema and helps in diuresis. Its peripheral vasodilatation effect improves the uterine blood supply. Has depressant action on the uterine muscle and CNS.

Use: It is a valuable drug lowering seizure threshold in women with pregnancy-induced hypertension. The drug is used in preterm labor to decrease uterine activity.

Dosage and route: For control of seizures, 20 mL of 20% solution IV slowly in 3–4 minutes; to be followed immediately by 10 mL of 50% solution IM, and continued 4 hourly till 24 hours postpartum. Repeat injections are given only if the knee jerks are present, urine output exceeds 100 mL in previous 4 hours and the respirations are more than 10/min. The therapeutic level of serum magnesium is 4–7 mEq/L.

4 g IV slowly over 10 mm, followed by 2 g/h, and then 1 g/h in drip of 5% dextrose for tocolytic effect.

Side effects

1. *Maternal*: Severe CNS depression (respiratory depression and circulatory collapse), evidence of muscular paresis (diminished knee jerks).
2. *Fetal*: Tachycardia, hypoglycemia.

VIII. Write short notes on any four of the following:

a. Care following ceserean section

Immediate care (4–6 hours): In the immediate recovery period, the blood pressure is recorded every 15 minutes. Temperature is recorded every two hours. The wound must be inspected every half hour to detect any blood loss. The lochia are also inspected and drainage should be small initially. Following general anesthesia, the woman is nursed in the left lateral or 'recovery' position until she is fully conscious, since the risks of airway obstruction or regurgitation and silent aspiration of stomach contents are still present. Analgesia is given as prescribed.

First 24 hours: IV fluids (5% dextrose or Ringer's lactate) are continued. Blood transfusion is helpful in anemic mothers for speedy postoperative recovery. Injection methergine 0.2 mg may be repeated intramuscularly. Parenteral antibiotic is usually given for the first 48 hours. Analgesics in the form of pethidine 75–100 mg are administered as required. Ambulation is encouraged on the day following surgery and baby is brought to her.

After 24 hours: The blood pressure, pulse and temperature are usually checked every four hours. Oral feeding is started with clear liquids and then advanced to light and regular diet. TV fluids are continued for about 48 hours. Urinary catheter may be removed on the following day when the woman is able to get up to the toilet. The woman is helped to get out of bed as soon as possible and encouraged to become fully mobile.

The mother must be encouraged to rest as much as possible and needed help is to be given with care for the baby. This should preferably take place at the mother's bedside and should include support with breastfeeding. The mother is usually discharged with the baby after the abdominal skin stitches are removed by the 4th or 5th day.

b. Sexually transmitted diseases

Sexually transmitted diseases (STDs) are infections that you can get from having sex with someone who has the infection. The causes of STDs are bacteria, parasites and viruses. There are more than 20 types of STDs. Most STDs affect both men and women, but in many cases the health problems they cause can be more severe for women. If a pregnant woman has an STD, it can cause serious health problems for the baby. Sexually transmitted diseases (STDs) are caused by infections that are passed from one person to another during sexual contact. These infections often do not cause any symptoms. Medically, infections are only called diseases when they cause symptoms. That is why STDs are also called "sexually transmitted infections." But it is very common for people to use the terms "sexually transmitted diseases" or "STDs," even when there are no signs of disease. Sexually transmitted diseases (STDs), or sexually transmitted infections (STIs), are generally acquired by sexual contact. The organisms that cause sexually transmitted diseases may pass from person to person in blood, semen, or vaginal and other bodily fluids. Sexually transmitted infections (STIs) have a range of signs and symptoms. That is why they may go unnoticed until complications occur or a partner is diagnosed.

Sexually transmitted infections can be caused by:
1. Bacteria (gonorrhea, syphilis, chlamydia).
2. Parasites (trichomoniasis).
3. Viruses (human papillomavirus, genital herpes, HIV).

Sexual activity plays a role in spreading many other infectious agents, although it is possible to be infected without sexual contact. For examples, include the hepatitis A, B and C viruses, *Shigella*, and *Cryptosporidium* and *Giardia lamblia*.

Signs and symptoms that might indicate an STI include:
1. Sores or bumps on the genitals or in the oral or rectal area.
2. Painful or burning urination.
3. Discharge from the penis.
4. Vaginal discharge.
5. Unusual vaginal bleeding.
6. Sore, swollen lymph nodes, particularly in the groin but sometimes more widespread.
7. Lower abdominal pain.
8. Rash over the trunk, hands or feet.

Signs and symptoms may appear a few days to years after exposure, depending on the organism. They may resolve in a few weeks, even without treatment, but progression with later complications, or recurrence, sometimes occurs.

c. Infertility

The causes of infertility are varied and complex. According to studies from around the world, both men and women are affected by infertility: about 40–60% of causes are linked to female factors, and 20–40% is related to male factors.

It is important for you to understand the anatomical, physiological and psychological conditions affecting fertility in women and men, both of whom should normally be able to conceive. Firstly, a man has to have normal functioning reproductive organs capable of producing normal sperm in sufficient numbers, and he has to be able to transfer them successfully to the woman's reproductive system through sexual intercourse.

Similarly, the woman's reproductive system should function normally and be able to produce healthy eggs, have normal fallopian tubes and uterus and produce normal cervical mucus.

To achieve normal physiological functions and processes, the endocrine (hormone-producing) glands of both the man and woman involved in reproduction must function normally. In addition, psychological and social conditions can influence the timing and frequency of sexual intercourse, which in turn can influence the chance of getting pregnant.

Age is an important factor in both women and men. In many women fertility declines as they age, especially over 35 years of age when the quality of eggs remaining in the ovaries is lower than when the women were younger. In men, sperm motility is reduced as they age, but overall fertility is not affected as much. There are many case reports describing men having children even after the age of 90 years.

There are two types of infertility: primary and secondary:
- **Primary infertility** is when a couple have never had children, or have been unable to achieve pregnancy after one year of living together despite having unprotected sexual intercourse.
- **Secondary infertility** is when a couple have had children or achieved pregnancy previously, but are unable to conceive at this time, even after one year of having unprotected sexual intercourse. Secondary infertility occurs more commonly than primary infertility, especially in developing countries where sexually transmitted infections are common. In many countries, induced abortion (intentionally done) contributes much to secondary infertility. Generally, it accounts for 60% of the total number of infertility cases.

c. Postpatrum hemorrhage

Hemorrhage after delivery, or postpartum hemorrhage (PPH), is the loss of blood following a delivery resulting in hypovolemia or otherwise causing the patient to become symptomatic due to the blood loss. Some practitioners measure PPH by a blood loss of greater than 500 mL of blood following vaginal delivery, or 1000 mL of blood following cesarean section. It is the most common cause of perinatal maternal death in the developed world and is a major cause of maternal morbidity worldwide.

The treatment of patients with PPH has 2 major components: (1) resuscitation and management of obstetric hemorrhage and, possibly, hypovolemic shock and (2) identification and management of the underlying cause(s) of the hemorrhage. For the purpose of discussion, these components are discussed separately; however, remember that successful management of PPH requires that both components be simultaneously and systematically addressed.

Pharmacologic management of atonic PPH includes the use of oxytocin, ergometrine and prostaglandins. Intravenous oxytocin is the preferred initial agent in PPH treatment, regardless of whether a prophylactic dose was administered. If bleeding continues after oxytocin administration or if oxytocin is unavailable, IV ergometrine, ergometrine-oxytocin fixed dose (Syntometrine) or a prostaglandin such as misoprostol 800 μg sublingual can be administered. Simultaneous administration of misoprostol with treatment doses of oxytocin is not recommended. Carboprost is may be useful when bleeding is resistant to other agents.

d. Carcinoma of the cervix

Cervical cancer is a malignant neoplasm arising from cells originating in the cervix uteri. One of the most common symptoms of cervical cancer is abnormal vaginal bleeding, but in some cases, there may be no obvious symptoms until the cancer has progressed to an advanced stage.

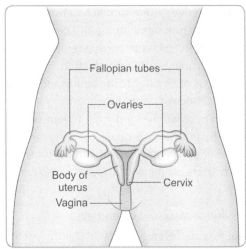

Cancer of the cervix (also called cervical cancer) begins in the cells lining the cervix. These cells do not suddenly change into cancer. Instead, the normal cells of the cervix first slowly change into pre-cancer cells that can then turn into cancer. These changes may be called dysplasia. The change can take many years, but sometimes it happens faster. They can be found by the Pap test and treated to prevent cancer. There are 2 main types of cancer of the cervix. About 8–9 out of 10 are squamous cell carcinomas. Under the microscope, this type of cancer is made up of cells that are like squamous cells that cover the surface of the cervix.

Most of the rest are adenocarcinomas. These cancers start in the gland cells that make mucus. Less often, the cancer has features of both types and is called adenosquamous or mixed carcinoma. Other types of cancer also can develop in the cervix. These other types (such as melanoma, sarcoma, and lymphoma) happen most often in other parts of the body. If you have cervical cancer, ask your doctor to explain exactly what type of cancer you have.

Treatment usually consists of surgery (including local excision) in early stages, and chemotherapy and/or radiation in more advanced stages of the disease. Cancer screening using the pap smear can identify precancerous and potentially precancerous changes in cervical cells and tissue. Treatment of high-grade changes can prevent the development of cancer in many cases. In developed countries, the widespread use of cervical screening programs has dramatically reduced the incidence of invasive cervical cancer.

IX. a. What is hysterectomy?

A hysterectomy is an operation to remove a woman's uterus. A hysterectomy is surgery to remove a woman's uterus or womb. The uterus is the place where a baby grows when a woman is pregnant. After a hysterectomy, you no longer have menstrual periods and can not become pregnant. Sometimes the surgery also removes the ovaries and fallopian tubes. If you have both ovaries taken out, you will enter menopause.

b. List the indications for hysterectomy

A woman may have a hysterectomy for different reasons, including:
1. Uterine fibroids that cause pain, bleeding, or other problems.
2. Uterine prolapse, which is a sliding of the uterus from its normal position into the vaginal canal.
3. Cancer of the uterus, cervix, or ovaries.
4. Endometriosis.
5. Abnormal vaginal bleeding.
6. Chronic pelvic pain.
7. Adenomyosis, or a thickening of the uterus.

Hysterectomy for noncancerous reasons is usually considered only after all other treatment approaches have been tried without success.

c. Write the pre- and postoperative nursing care of women posted for hysterectomy

Hysterectomy preoperative procedures: No matter which type of hysterectomy procedure is performed, hysterectomy requires hospitalization for one to five days. Preparation for a hysterectomy typically involves several steps, including the following:
1. Physical examination to determine overall health.
2. Pelvic examinations.
3. Blood and urine tests.
4. Preoperative meeting with the surgeon to discuss the procedure and receive pre-surgery instructions.
5. Preoperative meeting with the anesthesiologist to discuss the type of anesthesia that will be used (general or local).

In many cases, patients are advised to quit smoking 2–6 weeks before surgery. Smoking may cause breathing problems during surgery and has been shown to delay healing.

If a pain reliever is needed in the week prior to surgery, acetaminophen is recommended over aspirin, ibuprofen, or naproxen, to reduce the risk for heavy bleeding during surgery.

In general, no food or drink is to be taken after midnight on the day of the procedure. In some cases, a laxative or enema is indicated to empty the bowels before surgery.

Postoperative care after hysterectomy: Immediately after surgery, the patient remains in the recovery room for a few hours. She is monitored for discomfort, and is given medications to prevent pain and infection.

Hysterectomy requires at least one overnight stay in the hospital, and may require hospitalization for as many as 5 days. After the first night, patients are up and walking. Sanitary pads are used to manage bleeding and discharge, which can last for several days.

Full recovery can take from 4 to 8 weeks for open abdominal hysterectomy, and from 1 to 2 weeks for vaginal and laparoscopic hysterectomies. During this time, patients should get plenty of rest. She should avoid heavy lifting and tub baths for a full 6 weeks.

Depending on the type of procedure used and on the patient's rate of recovery, light chores, some driving, and even returning to work during this period of time may be possible. In general, patients can resume sexual relations after six weeks.

X. a. What is breech presentation?
   b. Lists the types of breech presentation
   c. Explain the management of breech delivery

Breech presentation is defined as a fetus in a longitudinal lie with the buttocks or feet closest to the cervix. This occurs in 3–4% of all deliveries. The percentage of breech deliveries decreases with advancing gestational age from 22% of births prior to 28 weeks' gestation to 7% of births at 32 weeks' gestation to 1–3% of births at term. There are many methods which have been attempted with the aim of turning breech babies, with varying degrees of success:

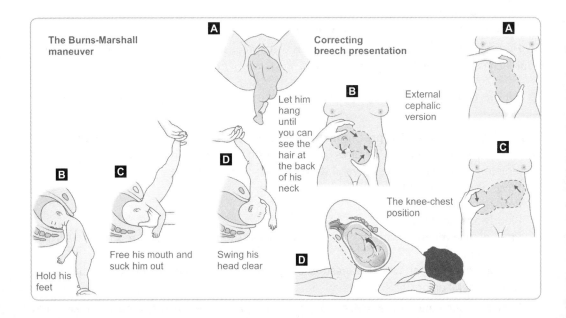

External cephalic version, where a midwife or doctor turns the baby by manipulating the baby through the mother's abdomen. ECV has a success rate between 40–70% depending on practitioner. The fetal heart is monitored after the turn attempt, usually in the context of an institutional protocol. Studies show that turning the baby at term (after 36 weeks) is effective in reducing the number of babies born in the breech position. Complications from external cephalic version are rare. Studies have also shown that attempting to turn the baby prior to this point has no impact on the presentation at term. Using hypothetical scenarios, a small study in the Netherlands found that few obstetric practitioners would attempt ECV in the presence of oligohydramnios. A case report of treating oligohydramnios with amnioinfusion, followed by ECV, was successful in turning the fetus.

Various maneuvers are suggested to assist spontaneous version of a breech presenting pregnancy. These include maternal positioning or other exercises. A study has shown that there is insufficient evidence as to the benefit of maternal positioning in reducing the incidence of breech presentation.

2010
Midwifery and Gynecology

SECTION-I

I. Give the meaning of the following:
   a. True labor.
   b. Puberty.
   c. Caput succedaneum.
   d. Pseudocyesis.
   e. Partograph.

II. Fill in the blanks with suitable answers:
   a. _____ denotes the perception of active fetal movements by pregnant women.
   b. _____ is the cessation of breathing for more than 20 seconds.
   c. Women having their first pregnancy at or above the age of 30 years are called: _____

III. Write short notes on any *four* of the following:
   a. Fetal circulation.
   b. True pelvis and its diameters.
   c. Breastfeeding techniques.
   d. Weight gain during pregnancy.
   e. Management of birth asphyxia.

IV. a. Explain the preparations needed for a woman in labor.
   b. Write the physiological changes in first stage of labor.

   OR

   a. Define puerperium.
   b. Write detail the postnatal care for primi women after labor up to 10 days.

SECTION-II

V. State whether the following statements are *true* or *false*:
   a. Choriocarcinoma is a highly malignant tumor arising from the chorionic epithelium.
   b. The labor is said to be precipitate when the combined duration of the first and second stage is more than two hours.
   c. An infection of the genital tract which occurs as a complication of delivery is termed puerperal sepsis.
   d. Removal of the body of the uterus or corpus leaving the cervix is said as total hysterectomy.

Midwifery and Gynecological Nursing: 2010

VI. Select the suitable answers and write.
   a. Premature separation of abnormally situated placenta is called: _____
      (i. Placenta previa, ii. Abruptio placenta, iii. Velamentous placenta, iv. Placenta accreta)
   b. Physiological anemia during pregnancy is the result of _____
      (i. Increase in blood volume demand of the mother, ii. Decreased dietary intake of iron, iii. Decreased erythropoietin after the first trimesters, iv. Increased detoxification demands on the mother's liver
   c. The embryotomy measures which is adopted in hydrocephalus to save the life of the mother is said _____
      (i. Decapitation, ii. Craniotomy, iii. Cleidotomy, iv. Evisceration)

VII. Write the difference between the following:
   a. Cryptomenorrhea and dysmenorrhea.
   b. Retroversion and retroflexion of uterus.
   c. Primary infertility and secondary infertility.
   d. Salpingitis and cervicitis.

VIII. Short notes on any *four* of the following:
   a. Indications and criteria to be fulfilled before application of forceps.
   b. Uses of analgesics in normal pregnancy.
   c. Puerperal psychosis.
   d. Effects of syphilis on pregnancy and its prevention.
   e. Unstable lie.

IX. a. Define antepartum hemorrhage.
   b. What are the causes and signs and symptoms of APH.
   c. Explain the management of placenta previa.

   OR

   a. What is malposition and abnormal presentation, give example.
   b. List the causes of occipitoposterior position.
   c. Explain the management of second stage of labor in occiput posterior position (OPP).
   d. Write the complications

SECTION-I

I. Give the meaning of the following:

a. True labor
When uterine contractions are regular with increasing intensity and occur with greater frequency; contractions that effect a change in the dilatation and effacement of the cervix.

b. Puberty
Puberty is the period in which the reproductive organs develop and reach maturity. The first signs are breast development and appearance of pubic hair. The body grows considerably and takes on the female space. Puberty culminates in the onset of menstruation, the first period being called menarche. The first few cycles are not usually accompanied by ovulation, so conception is unlikely before a girl has been menstruating for years or two.

c. Caput succedaneum
Localized edema occurring just under the presenting part of the fetal scalp during labor disappears within 36–48 hours of life.

d. Pseudocyesis
Characterized by irregular Braxton–Hicks contractions which do not change the cervix and do not increase in intensity, duration or frequency.

e. Partograph
Patrogram is a graphic recording of the salient features of labor status. In the management of women in labor program serves to validate the normal progress of labor and to facilitate early identification of deviations from normal pattern.

Uses of partogram
1. Provides a predictive value of labor progress.
2. Transfer of information becomes easy when labor status changes.
3. Saves writing time of staff against writing in long hand.
4. It is of educational value as it indicated the nature of labor.

II. Fill in the blanks with suitable answers.
a. **Quickening** denotes the perception of active fetal movements by pregnant women.
b. **Apnea** is the cessation of breathing for more than 20 seconds.
c. Women having their first pregnancy at or above the age of 30 years are called: **Elderly primi**.

III. Write short notes on any four of the following.

a. Fetal circulation
See 2013-III-b.

b. True pelvis and its diameter

The true pelvis constitutes the bony passage through which the fetus must maneuver to be born vaginally. Therefore, its construction planes and diameters are of utmost interest in obstetrics.

The true pelvis has the following as its boundaries:
1. **Superiorly:** The sacral promontory, linea terminalis and the upper margin of pubic bones.
2. **Inferiorly:** The inferior margins of the ischial tuberosities and the tip of coccyx.
3. **Laterally:** The sacroiliac notches and ligaments, and the inner surface of ischial bones.
4. **Anteriorly:** The obturator foramina and the posterior surface of the symphysis pubis, pubic bones and the ascending rami of ischial bones.

The true pelvis has a brim, a cavity and an outlet.

The pelvic brim: The brim is also termed as the inlet. Its boundaries are the sacral promontory and wings of the sacrum behind the iliac bones on the sides and the pubic bones in front.

Landmarks of the brim: These are the fixed anatomical points on the brim.
1. Sacral promontory.
2. Sacral ala or sacral wing.
3. Sacroiliac joint.
4. Iliopectineal line: The edge formed at the inward aspect of the ilium.
5. Iliopectineal eminence: A roughened area where the superior ramus of the pubic bone meets the ilium.
6. Superior ramus of the pubic bone.
7. Upper inner border of the body of pubic bone.
8. Upper inner border of the symphysis pubis.

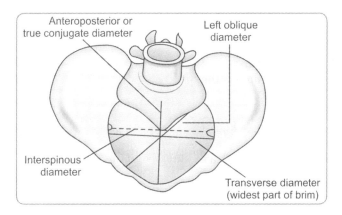

Diameters of the brim

1. **The anteroposterior diameter of the brim:** It is a line from the sacral promontory to the upper border of the symphysis pubis. When the anteroposterior diameter is measured from the sacral promontory to the uppermost point of the symphysis pubis, it is called the anatomical conjugate and measures 12 cm. When it is taken to the posterior border of the upper surface, it is called the obstetrical conjugate and measures 11 cm. It is the anteroposterior diameter available for childbirth. The term true conjugate may be used to refer to either of these measurements.

2. **The transverse diameter of the brim of the inlet:** It is the maximum transverse diameter that can be found between similar points on opposite sides of the pelvic brim. In other words, it is a line between the furthest points on the iliopectineal lines. It measures 13.5 cm.
3. **The oblique diameter:** It is a line from one sacroiliac joint to the iliopectineal eminence on the opposite side of the pelvis and measures 12.75 cm. There are two oblique diameters—right and left. Each takes its name from the sacroiliac joint from which it arises.
4. **The diagonal conjugate:** It is also measured anteroposteriorly from the lower border of the symphysis pubis to the sacral promontory. It may be estimated per vagina and should measure 12–13 cm.

c. Breastfeeding techniques

Breastfeeding: The baby should be put to the mother's breast within half an hour of birth or as soon as possible the mother has recovered from the exertion of labor. No prelacteal feeds to be given and colostrum feeding must be offered. All babies should invariably receive the colostrum during first three days of life. Mother should be informed about the importance and technique of breastfeeding. Initially the feeding should be given in short interval of 1–2 hours and then every 2–3 hours. Most babies regularize their feeding pattern by the end of first week and self demand feeding is established in every 3–4 hours interval. Nurse should assist the mother to feed her baby adequately for the maintenance of hydration and optimum nutrition. Exclusive breastfeeding procedure should be explained to the mother and family members.

d. Weight gain during pregancy

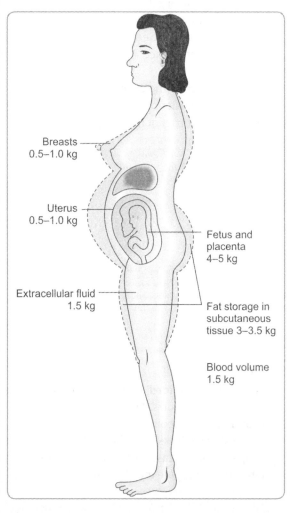

A continuing weight increase in pregnancy is considered to be a favorable indicator for maternal adaptation and fetal growth. Analysis of studies on weight gain in pregnancy suggests the following as the expected increase in primigravida.
- 4.0 kg in first 20 weeks
- 8.5 kg in second 20 weeks (0.4 kg per week in the last trimester)
- 12.5 kg approximate total (Murray, 1999).

The average weight gain in multigravida is approximately 1 kg less than in the primigravida.

There is a wide range of normality in weight gain and many factors influence it which includes maternal edema, maternal metabolic rate, dietary intake, vomiting or diarrhea, amount of amniotic fluid and size of the fetus. Maternal age, pre-pregnancy body size, parity and diseases like diabetes and hypertension also seem to influence the pattern of weight gain.

e. Management of birth hypoxia

As soon as the baby is born the clock timer should be started. Apgar score is assessed in the normal manner at 1 minute. In the absence of any respiratory effort resuscitative measures are started without delay. The upper airways should be deared by gentle suction. Baby is quickly transferred to the resuscitation unit, kept in a flat surface at comfortable working height and under the radiant heat source to prevent hypothermia. The baby's shoulder must be elevated on a small towel of straighten the trachea by slight extension of the head. Hyperextension is unnecessary. It is not desirable to hold the baby upside down as this causes a sharp rise in cerebral venous pressure, hyperextends and stretches the spine which is painful and risks the infant being dropped.

The aims of birth asphyxia are:
1. To establish and maintain a clear airway, ventilation and oxygenation
2. To correct acidosis
3. To prevent hypothermia, hypoglycemia and hemorrhage.

The points of management of asphyxia are:
1. Clearing the airway
2. Stimulation
3. Warmth
4. Ventilation and oxygenation
5. Neonatal bag and mask
6. Endotracheal intubation
7. Mouth to mouth resuscitation
8. External cardiac massage
9. Use of drugs
10. Observation and after care.

Throughout the resuscitation procedure the baby should be monitored and recorded making special notes on the time when spontaneous respirations are established. The endotracheal tube should be left in place for a few minutes after the baby starts to breathe spontaneously. Suction may be applied when it is removed. Recording of the drugs given and serial Apgar scores is essential.

A baby whose Apgar score is less than 6 at 5 minutes or who has slow response to resuscitation should be transferred to the neonatal unit for a period of observation in order to monitor the behavior and correction if needed. Babies who respond quickly to resuscitation can be reunited with their parents remaining in the delivery room until the usual time of transfer to the postnatal ward where their care continues as normal.

IV. a. Explain the preparations needed for a woman in labor.

Preparation of the patient in labor: The pubic area must be shaved or clipped because it is difficult to keep the vulva clean throughout labor or during the puerperal period; in some centers, neither shaving nor clipping is done. The principle of swabbing technique is to cleanse the vulva of secretions and organisms without contaminating the birth canal. The equipment used and the method employed may vary from hospital to hospital depending on whether.
a. Sterile gloves
b. The non-touch method or
c. Disposable equipment is used.

Swabbing is done for the comfort of the woman and for its aseptic value and merely cleansing the vulva is not enough. In all cases, swabbing must be proceeded by washing the pubis, groins, inner thighs, and buttocks with soap and water, unless a good bath has been taken recently. The vulva is swabbed on admission and at six hourly intervals during labor as well as immediately preceding vaginal examination and delivery.

Evaluation of lower bowel: If the woman is suffering from eclampsia or antepartum hemorrhage an enema or suppository is not given. It is advisable that the lower bowel is emptied at the beginning of labor. Suppositories are slow in action and it does not empty the bowel effectively as a plain water or disposable enema. There is some connection between the nerve supply of uterus and bowel, so that the stimulation of the bowel will stimulate the uterine action. But a woman in strong labor should not be given enema as the baby maybe born during the expulsion of an enema. A primigravida woman can be given enema whose cervix is 6 cm dilated, but it should not be given to a multiparous patient at this stage. In doubt, a vaginal examination is done to ascertain the dilatation before giving the enema and the strength of uterine contraction also should be watched. An empty rectum allows more room for descent of the fetal head. A bath or thorough wash is given following the shaving or clipping the hair and giving the enema worked and cleansing the pubic area is done with antiseptic lotion. A full bladder should be recognized and emptied at the end of first stage or of the beginning of second stage. Hair combed, nail polish or lipsticks removed if any, to observe the natural color of nails and lips. Nails cut if long. The use of cosmetics may keep her morale but obstetric precautions must be observed. Patient is dressed in labor room dress according to the custom of the hospital.

Psychological preparation of mother and family: It has been proved that the emotions of a woman in labor has great influence on her reaction to discomfort and pain and contributory factors in determining the amount of physical and mental exhaustion she will experience.

The fear of labor: The onset of labor gives rise to various emotions particularly for primi patient. Some women will be glad and others will be apprehensive about the process of labor and the outcome. Anxiety culminates in fear. A home like atmosphere should be prevailed as the hospital situation suggests preparation for operation rather than a natural event.

Emotional support: It is the meeting of the emotional needs of the patient in labor. The doctor and midwife should give confidence to the patient by soothing words and action. Providing competent physical care during labor, giving a feeling of safety are the valuable sources of emotional support. Her emotional requirements must be met in order to prevent labor from becoming the nerve wracking experience with emotionally traumatizing effects.

Companionship is needed; loneliness breeds fear: The comforting companionship of the midwife who will listen, explain, encourage and assure to keep silent when required is of immense value to a woman in labor. When labor is established the midwife should remain in constant attendance with the patient. When left for longer time, the woman's confidence in her attendants is lost. In Western countries, husbands are allowed to stay with the patient in labor. But in our set-up, it is not practiced. Their presence is of social companionship and emotional support but not a substitute for the midwife. The patient needs the professional presence of the midwife for the intelligent observation and skilled professional administration of the midwife.

Adequate communications is essential for the peace of mind of most of the woman that they are kept informed of the progress they are making. Woman who screams during labor, do so, more from fear than from pain and the midwife should communicate confidence by her calm competent bearing and kindly actions. Woman responds soon to a word of praise and explanations for doing every procedure. The atmosphere of the labor ward should be as quiet as possible and the midwife in charge should set the tone for the same. An attitude of reverence should always prevail while in attendance on woman during childbirth.

b. Write the physiological changes in first stage of labor.

Contraction and Retraction of Uterine Muscle

a. Uterine contractions are involuntarily controlled by the nervous system and indirectly by endocrines.
b. Contractions are intermittent, occurring every 1–15 minutes and increases gradually to 1–2 minutes.
c. Contractions are painful. This is probably due to squeezing of the nerve endings, between the muscle fibers and partly due to the resistance in the cervix and soft parts. If the patient is tensed this will increase the resistance and thus the pain is more.
d. Contractions last for several seconds but rarely exceed 60–70 seconds. This prevents prolonged compression on the uterine arteries and interference with the oxygen supply to the fetus.

A uterine contraction consists of the following:
a. **Contraction:** Temporary shortening of the muscle fibers.
b. **Relaxation:** When the contraction is absent.
c. **Retraction:** Instead of complete relaxation when the muscle fibers should return to its previous size there is some permanent shortening of the fibers.

Formation of the upper and lower uterine segment.

At the end of pregnancy the uterus is divided into two:
a. The upper uterine segment, which is the thick, muscular contractile part.
b. The lower uterine segment, which is relaxed, thin, distensable area. It is about 8–10 cm long and is formed from the isthmus.

Development of the retraction ring: The contractions and retractions of the upper uterine segment cause it to become thicker and shorter, as it attempts to push the fetus out into the birth canal. This stretches lower uterine segment causing it to become thinner. At the junction of the upper and lower segment a ridge forms this is the retraction ring.

Formation of retraction ring

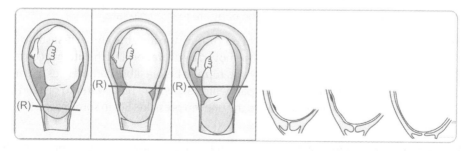

When the retraction ring is exaggerated, it is visible over the abdomen.
The term Bandl's ring is applied. The retraction ring is perfectly normal providing it remains below the symphysis pubis but should the fetus not be able to pass through the os as in obstructed

labor the lower uterine segment, stretches further to accommodate it as it is being pushed out of the upper uterine segment, and the retraction ring becomes visible and palpable as a depressed ridge running transversely or slightly oblique across the abdomen above the symphysis pubis. This is serious for, the uterus is in danger of rupturing.

Polarity: This is the term used to describe the harmonious neuromuscular action between the upper and lower uterine segment. The upper uterine segment contracts and retracts and this is controlled by the parasympathetic nervous system. The lower uterine segment mainly passive and therefore relaxes and dilates. This is controlled by the sympathetic nervous system. During contraction the upper uterine segment contracts and retracts to expel the fetus and the lower uterine segment relaxes and dilates to allow the fetus to escape. This harmonious action is called polarity. When the polarity is disorganized the progress of labor is inhibited or prolonged fear during labor will cause the lower segment to go into spasm. Thus slowing labor and causing greater pain.

Taking-up of the cervix: This occurs as the result of the retraction of the upper segment and the relaxation and dilatation of the lower uterine segment when the fetus is pushed into it. This causes the internal os to open and the cervical canal to be drawn up into the lower uterine segment. As the canal widens it resembles a funnel.

Dilatation of the os: It is the opening up of the external os. In a primigravida, it occurs after whole cervical canal has been drawn up into the lower uterine segment. In a multigravida, it usually occurs at the same time as the taking up of the cervix. Dilatation of the os is assisted by the bag of fore-waters; it acts as a fluid wedge that protrudes into the cervical canal slightly aids the dilatation. But a well-flexed head has a similar effect.

Show: It is the escape of the plug of mucus from the cervical canal as it dilates. It is slightly stained with blood from decidua vera when the chorion become detached.

Formation of fore-waters: During each contraction in the first stage of labor the sac of fluid in front of the presenting part is cut off from the water behind. And it is forced into the cervical canal and thus helping the cervix to take up. When a well-flexed head is presented, it fits into the cervix and acts as a valve and prevents the hind-waters from joining the fore-waters. This causes an even pressure on the membrane and keeps them intact during the first stage. While the membranes are intact the placenta cannot be compressed between the uterine wall and the fetus. So, the oxygen supply to the fetus is well maintained, also there is less risks of infection and thus while the membranes are intact, the mother and the baby are reasonable safe.

Rupture of membranes: Usually, the membranes rupture towards the end of first stage of labor because the support from the cervix has been removed by dilatation and the uterine contractions are very much stronger. The membranes may also rupture before labor commences or very early. This may be due to badly fitting presenting part which allows the hind-water to distend the sac of fore-waters causing them to rupture due to the uneven pressure. But in some cases, it happens for no apparent reason.

Full dilatation of the cervix: Now the cervix has been completely drawn into the lower uterine segment and the presenting part passes into the birth canal. On vaginal examination, the cervix is not felt all around (a normal condition) 10 cm of the os equates full dilatation of the os.

Secondary powers: As the head distends the vagina, character of contraction is altered and the mother begins to push which make the abdominal muscles and diaphragm into action.

Swing door action of the pelvic floor: As the head dilates the vagina, the anterior segment of the pelvic floor is drawn up the post; segments is pushed downwards and backwards, the advancing head presses on the rectum and expels the fecal matters out. This pressure makes the anus to spout, the perineum stretches and the head is seen at the vulva. Progressing with each contraction until crowning takes place, then the head is born followed by the rest of the body.

OR

a. Define puerperium. b. Write detail the postnatal care for primi women after labor up to 10 days.

Puerperium is the period immediately following labor during which the reproductive organs return to their prepregnant stage, lactation is initiated and the mother recovers from the physical and emotional experiences of parturition. This takes between 6 weeks and 8 weeks. The lying in period is the time that the mother spends in the hospital or attended by the midwife in her own home immediately after delivery for 10–14 days. The progress of returning the reproductive organs to its normal size is called involution. After delivery the uterus weighs about 1 kg. At the end of puerperium it weighs about 60 g only. The greater reduction being in the first week when it is half the size on the 7th day.

Basic Principles (Aim)

1. Promotion of physical well-being by good nutrition, comfort, cleanliness, and sufficient exercise to ensure good muscle tone.
2. Establishment of emotional well-being by quietness, freedom from worry and excitement.
3. Promotion of breastfeeding.
4. Prevention of avoidable complications.

Observations during the First Week of Puerperium

1. Fundal height—to note the involution.
2. Bladder—to get the proper fundal height and to aid involution.
3. Bowel—to aid the involution.
4. Lochia—to note the color.
5. Breast—to note the engorgement, secretion mastitis, etc.
6. General condition of the patient, TPR, etc.
7. Micturition.
8. Perineum vulva and anus.
9. Condition of the baby.

Important Points of Postnatal Care (Puerperium)

Rest and sleep: Adequate rest and sleep are required because of the nervous exhaution that result from strain of labor. To ensure a good sleep, the first night a sedative may be necessary. Any discomfort, after pains, such as hemorrhoids, or engorged breast should be treated before giving sedatives. Rest and sleep during the day must be encouraged, e.g. midmorning and afternoon. Persistant insomnia in the absence of pain should be viewed as a warning sign of coming insanity.

Micturition: Large amounts of urine are secreted during the first few days due to the discarding of extra-blood plasma present during pregnancy. Difficulty with micturition is quite common during the first few clays due to trauma. The midwife must ensure that the bladder should be emptied completely; if necessary catheterize the patient. An over distended bladder predisposes to cystitis and prevent involution.

Bowels: There is a tendency for the bowels to be sluggish during the puerperium because:
1. The woman is losing fluid from her body as milk and large quantities of urine secreted.
2. The abdominal walls are laxed.
3. The anus does not respond to stimulation, having been forcibly dilated by the baby's head during labor.
4. Bed pans are not accustomed.

It is usual to give a laxative after 36 hours. If this fails enema can be given. Never give purgative or castor oil. Senna or cascara are good and no effect on baby. Early ambulation may overcome from the disadvantage of bed pans.

Diet: A good wholesome diet containing sufficient protein (90 g), minerals and vitamins should be given. Adequate supply of milk is needed by the amount of protein and vitamin B intake should be increased. Additional fluid is required at least 4 pints a day. A glass of water should be taken just before breastfeeding. Milk drink in the midmorning and evening and further milk in cooking. One and a half pint is an ideal amount. Fresh fruits and vegetables should be included in the main meals.

Position and exercise: After delivery the position is recumbent to promote good drainage, the mother should be encouraged to sit up during a part of the day and to lie down in prone position for 15 minutes twice daily, as this promotes good drainage and the prone position also encourage the anteversion and anteflexion of the uterus. The postnatal exercise must commence from the second day onwards. Ambulation is encouraged for all normal cases from the first day onwards and is increased gradually each day, but never overdone.

Advantages of Early Ambulation
1. It promotes good drainage and rapid involution.
2. Possibility of chest complications are reduced.
3. Cases of thrombosis are minimized.
4. A more rapid resumption, for bladder and bowel action takes place.
5. The mother appears brighter and stronger and learns to handle the baby with confidence.
6. Records to be kept:
   a. **TPR twice daily:** This is an excellent guide for noting the patient's condition. The midwife should call for medical aid for a reading of temperature above 37. 30° C. A steady rising or rapid pulse also should be informed to the doctor.
   b. **Fundal height:** It must be recorded daily as it is a means of estimating involution; also it draws attention to a full bladder. Before taking it, ensure that the bladder is empty, and it should be done at the same time everyday (morning).
   c. **Lochia:** It must be observed and any abnormalities to be reported to the doctor.

SECTION-II

V. State whether the following statements are *true* or *false*.
a. Choriocarcinoma is a highly malignant tumor arising from the chorionic epithelium: **True.**
b. The labor is said to be precipitate when the combined duration of the first and second stage is more than two hours: **False.**
c. An infection of the genital tract which occurs as a complication of delivery is termed puerperal sepsis: **True.**

d. Removal of the body of the uterus or corpus leaving the cervix is said as total hysterectomy: **True.**

VI. Select the suitable answers and write.

a. Premature separation of abnormally situated placenta is called: **Abruptio placenta.**
   (i. Placenta previa, ii. Abruption placenta, iii. Velamentous placenta, iv. Placenta accreta)
b. Physiological anemia during pregnancy is the result of: **Decreased erythropoietin after the first trimesters.**
   (i. increase in blood volume demand of the mother, ii. Decreased dietary intake of iron, iii. Decreased erythropoietin after the first trimesters, iv. Increased detoxification demands on the mother's liver)
c. The embryotomy measures which is adopted in hydrocephalus to save the life of the mother is said: **Craniotomy.**
   (i. Decapitation, ii. Craniotomy, iii. Cleidotomy, iv. Evisceration)

VII. Write the difference between the following:

a. Cryptomenorrhea and dysmenorrhea.

Cryptomenorrhea, there is periodic shadding of the endometrium and bleeding but the menstrual blood fails to come out from the genital tract due to obstruction in the passage.

Dysmenorrhea, there is a painful menstruation but more realistic and practical definition includes cases of painful menstruation of sufficient magnitude so as incapacities day to day activities.

b. Retroversion and retroflexion of uterus.

Retroversion is the term used when the long axes of the corpus and cervix are in line and whole organ turns backwards in relation to the long axis of the birth canal.

Retroflexion signifies a bending backward level of internal os. The two conditions are usually present together and are loosely called retroversion or retrodisplacement.

c. Primary infertility and secondary infertility.

Primary infertility denotes these patients who have never conceived.

Secondary infertility indicates previous pregnancy but failure to conceive subsequent with one or more years of unprotected regular intercourse.

d. Salpingitis and cervicitis.

Salpingitis is an infection of fallopian tube.

Cervicitis—the term cervicitis is reserved to infection of the endocervix, including the glands and the stroma; it may be acute or chronic.

VIII. Short notes on any *four* of the following:

a. Indications and criteria to be fulfilled before application of forceps.

Indications of forceps operation: Delay in the second stage due to uterine inertia. If the head is on the perineum for 20–30 minutes without advancement, forceps application may be decided.

Maternal Indications
1. Maternal distress.
2. Preeclampsia, eclampsia.
3. Vaginal birth after cesarean section (VBAC).
4. Heart disease.
5. Failure to bear down during the second stage of labor due to regional blocks, paraplegia or psychiatric disturbance.

Fetal Indications
1. Appearance of fetal distress in the second stage.
2. Cord prolapse.
3. After-coming-head of breech.

Low birth-weight baby: Postmaturity.

Prerequisites for Forceps Delivery
There are certain conditions which must exist before forceps delivery can be performed.
1. The cervix must be fully dilated and effaced.
2. Membranes must be ruptured.
3. Presentation and position must be suitable to apply the blades correctly to the sides of the head.
4. The head must be engaged with no parts of the head palpable abdominally.

No appreciable cephalopelvic disproportion.

The bladder must be emptied: Presence of good uterine contractions as a safeguard to postpartum hemorrhage.

Preparation of the Woman
The woman should be prepared in advance for the possibility of a forceps delivery if this looks likely. Full explanation of the procedure and the need for it must be given to the woman.

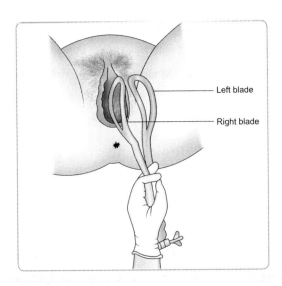

Once the decision has been made, adequate and appropriate analgesia must be offered. When analgesia has been instituted and the obstetrician is ready to proceed, the woman's legs are placed in lithotomy position. Both legs must be placed simultaneously to avoid strain on the woman's back and hips.

The woman should be tilted towards the left at an angle of 15° by the use of a pillow or a rubber wedge under the mattress to prevent aortocaval occlusion.

Preparations must also be done for the baby including equipment for resuscitation. In some hospitals, a pediatrician will also be present.

Procedure of low forceps operation: The woman's vulval area is thoroughly cleaned and draped with sterile towels using aseptic technique. The bladder is emptied using a straight catheter.
1. A vaginal examination is performed by the obstetrician to confirm the station and exact position of the fetal head.
2. A pudental block, supplemented by perineal and labial infiltration with 1% lignocaine hydrochloride, is given to produce effective local anesthesia.
3. An episiotomy may be done prior to introduction of the blades or during traction when the perineum becomes bulged and thinned out by the advanced head.
4. The forceps are identified as left or right by assembling them briefly before proceeding.

b. Uses of analgesics in normal pregnancy.

labor may be easy and trouble free with good psychological approach. Unprepared and untreated patient feel more pain during uterine contractions. Drugs are useful for the relief of pain but they are not much important than the proper preparation and training for childbirth. The intensity of labor pain depends on the intensity and duration of uterine contractions, the degree of dilatation of cervix, the distension of perineal tissue, the parity and pain threshold of the woman. The most distressing time during the whole labor is just prior to full dilatation of the cervix.

The ideal procedure should produce efficient relief from pain without depressing the respiration of the fetus and should not depress the uterine activity causing prolonged labor. The drug must be non-toxic and safe to the mother and fetus. But there is no such drugs are available fulfilling all these conditions. Every cases of labor do not require analgesia and only sympathetic explanation may be all that is required.

Methods to Relief of Pain
1. Hypnosis, this method is not reliable. So not proved popular for general use.
2. Sedatives and analgesics.
3. Inhalation agents.
4. Regional analgesics.
5. Psychoprophylaxis.

Sedatives and analgesics: There are certain factors to control the dose of sedative and analgesics.
1. The threshold of pain, varies in individuals. Some patients may feel pain though the uterine contractions are weak. In such patients, pain must be controlled even if this involves a temporary depression in uterine action.
2. Primigravida or multigravida, multiparous woman need less analgesics due to added relaxation of the birth canal and rapid delivery.
3. Maturity of the fetus, minimal dose is indicated while the fetus is thought to be premature to avoid asphyxia.

Sedatives chloral hydrate, barbiturates benzodiazepines, etc. may be employed in the early part of the first phase. That is up to 8 cm dilatation of cervix to primigravida and up to 6 cm dilatation of cervix to multigravida.

Pethidine (Meperidine)

It is synthetic narcotic analgesic agent, well absorbed by all routes of administration.

Action: Inhibits ascending pain pathways in central nervous system, increases pain threshold and alters pain perception.

Indications: Moderate to severe pain in labor, postoperative pain, abruptio placenta, pulmonary edema.

Dosage and route of administration: Injectable preparation contains 50 mg/mL, can be administered SC, IM, IV. Its dose is 50–100 mg IM combined with pro-methazine mg.

Contraindication: Pethidine should not be used intravenously within 2 hours and intramuscularly within 3 hours of the expected time of delivery of the baby, for fear of birth asphyxia. It should not be used in cases of preterm labor and when the respiratory reserve of the mother is reduced.

c. Puerperal psychosis.

The onset of puerperal psychosis is usually rapid, occurring within the first few days of delivery and rarely beyond the first 2–3 weeks. The condition is more common in primiparous women and in those who have suffered previous psychosis. No defined cause has been identified.

Diagnosis: Puerperal psychosis may have an acute onset. The woman may appear to be experiencing normal emotional adaptive responses to childbirth and may exhibit symptoms similar to those of maternal blues which is a psychological phenomenon manifested as unexplainable sadness and frequent bouts of crying.

These become more profound with extreme mood swings during which feelings of guilt or anxiety may be expressed. The euphoria following childbirth is seen extended and exaggerated in puerperal psychosis. The onset of symptoms may be heralded by a time of acute restlessness and inability to sleep. Subsequently the behavior of the woman may become bizarre. She may do or say inappropriate things or react out of character. She may experience delusions or hallucinations and become detached from the reality of her situation. She may state that her baby is abnormal, believe it to be possessed and may avoid the baby.

There may be periods of normal behavior and at other times, she may appear depressed. She may experience suicidal impulses or desires to harm her baby.

Treatment: Because of extreme nature of the illness, medical help is required as a matter of emergency. The woman must be kept under constant observation until appropriate psychiatric help is obtained.

Heavy sedation is given at the time of onset.

Early treatment with antipsychotic drugs under the care of a psychiatric team is usually instituted. Admission to a psychiatric unit and treatment with lithium and/or electroconvulsive therapy is given. Psychosis may persist for 8–10 weeks even with prompt treatment, especially when the woman has a pre-existing history of schizophrenia or manic-depressive illness.

Prognosis: Whilst complete recovery is often achieved, it is possible that further episodes of illness will occur throughout the woman's life and there is an increased risk of recurrence in subsequent pregnancies.

Role of the midwife: The community midwife should continue to visit both mother and baby to undertake the nonpsychiatric aspects of postnatal care. Family support also needs consideration. The midwife needs to offer advice and support to women during subsequent pregnancies and to alert the physician regarding psychiatric care when appropriate, in order to initiate prompt referral, should it become necessary.

The community midwife should be able to help the mother re-establish the mother-baby relationship and to rebuild self-esteem by encouraging care of the baby within a safe environment.

d. Effects of syphilis on pregnancy and its prevention.

Syphilis is an infection caused by *Treponema pallidum*. In pregnancy, its particular significance is the devastating effect it has on fetal well-being. The Natural course of adult infection is divided into stages.

Early infectious stage

- Primary stage: 9–60 days after exposure
- Secondary stage: 6 weeks to 6 months after exposure
- Early latent stage: 2 years after exposure.

Late non-infectious stage: Late latent stage: more than 2 years after exposure.

Neurosyphilis, cardiovascular syphilis or gummatous syphilis.

Most pregnant women diagnosed are in the primary or secondary stages and untreated infection will affect almost all fetuses. Depending upon the intensity and time of occurrence of the infiltration, the fate of the fetus will be as follows:

1. Abortion or intrauterine death 20%.
2. Preterm deliveries 20%.
3. Delivery of highly infected baby with neonatal death 20%.
4. Survival with congenital syphilis with resulting disability 40%.

Prenatal diagnosis and treatment through routine serological testing in early pregnancy is the key to prevention of congenital syphilis. This should be done as a routine in the first antenatal visit. VDRL (Venereal Disease Research Laboratory) is commonly done. A positive VDRL test has to be confirmed by Fluorescent Treponemal Antibody (FTA) test, which is a specific test. Husband's blood should also be tested for VDRL. Detection of spirochetes from the cetaceous lesion, if any is done by dark field examination. Fetal infection could be diagnosed by demonstration of *T. Pallidum* in the amniotic fluid.

Congenital syphilis: The syphilitic baby may appear normal at birth but shows signs of infection within one or two weeks after birth. Purulent nasal discharge—often hemorrhagic, hoarse cry, maculopapular rash and pemphigus (highly contagious vesicles) on the soles and palms are common manifestations. Ulcers can occur on the lips and mouth and, if on the larynx, the baby's cry may be thin or soundless.

Poor feeding and weight loss may be features of infection. Periostitis produces swelling of the long bones and the resulting pain may cause the baby to behave as if he or she has a fracture. The baby may also present with patchy alopecia, hepatosplenomegaly and mild jaundice.

Late signs may develop at any time from second to thirtieth year of life even if none of the early signs was exhibited. These include eighth nerve deafness, saddle nose (depression on the nasal bridge), corneal scarring causing impaired vision or blindness, and mental disability. Prognosis depends on the damage, which has occurred prior to treatment.

Treatment

Mother: Treatment should be started as soon as the diagnosis is established. The baby may have the chance of protection even if the treatment is begun late in pregnancy. For primary, secondary or latent syphilis (of less than one year duration), Benzathine penicillin 2.4 million units intramuscularly as a single dose is administered. When the duration is more than a year, Benzathine penicillin 2.4 million units weekly for 3 weeks is given. If the woman is allergic to penicillin, oral erythromycin 2 g daily for 15 days is given. If the treatment is given in early pregnancy, the treatment should be repeated in late pregnancy. Irrespective of the serological report, treatment should be repeated in subsequent pregnancies.

e. Unstable lie.

An unstable lie is a condition in which, at any time after 36 completed weeks of pregnancy, the fetal lie is oblique or transverse, and the presentation changes from one examination to another.

Causes: Any condition in late pregnancy that increases the mobility of the fetus or prevents the head from entering the pelvic brim, may cause this:
1. Lax uterine muscles in multigravidae.
2. Contracted pelvis.
3. Polyhydramnios.

Management: The woman is admitted to the hospital to avoid unsupervised onset of labor with a transverse lie.

After hospitalization, the lie may stabilize. If it does not, labor may be induced after 38th week of gestation, provided there is no placenta previa. The woman's bladder and rectum are emptied and an external cephalic version is done if the fetus is in a malpresentation. When the fetus is in a vertex presentation, labor is induced with an oxytocin infusion. Fetal oxytocin infusion is continued and the woman is encouraged to empty her bladder frequently. Forewaters is not ruptured until the head is deeply engaged and labor is well advanced. Labor is regarded as a trial presentation is checked in every five minutes. Once regular contractions are established, a vaginal examination is done to rule out cord presentation. The membranes are then stripped and a high rupture of membranes is done, removing as much of amniotic fluid as possible, so that the head enters the pelvis.

IX. a. Define antepartum hemorrhage.

Antepartum hemorrhage is defined as the hemorrhage from the genital tract occurring after twenty eighth week of pregnancy but before birth of the baby.

Causes

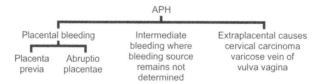

b. What are the causes and signs and symptoms of APH.

Causes

1. Toxemia of pregnancy: Usually associated with preeclamptic toxemia and eclampsia.
2. Trauma: (a) Physical: Any accident, fall, forceful ECV, etc. (b) Psychological: Emotional shock.

3. **Hypertension:** Spasms of blood vessels—ischemia—choriodecidual apoplexy.
4. **Traction:** Any pull upon the cord, especially when short, can cause detachment of placenta.
5. **Torsion:** Uterus is usually dextrorotated. If it is more—venous congestion—bleeding.
6. Chronic nephritis.
7. Vitamin E and folic acid—deficiency.
8. Implantation of placenta on a tumor: The chorionic attachment is poor, so placenta gets separated easily.
9. Rupture of membranes in hydramnios or birth of first twin. Sudden decompression and diminutions of the size of the uterus. Separation of placenta.
10. Idiopathic causes.

c. Explain the management of placenta previa.

Definition: A low implantation of the placenta in the uterus causing it to lie alongside or in front of the presenting part.

Incidence: Placenta previa occurs approximately one of every 250 births. It is one in 200 in India. One-third of all antepartum hemorrhage occurs due to placenta previa.

Causes

The exact cause of implantation of the placenta in the lower segment is not known. Following are the postulated theories.

Dropping down theory: The fertilized ovum drops down to the lower uterine segment. Poor decidual reaction in the upper segment may be the cause.

Multiple pregnancies: The large placental bed of the twin placenta is prone to low implantation of at least a part of the placenta.

Diagnosis

1. Clinical diagnosis is reached by an ultrasound examination in which the placenta is localized in relation to the cervix.
2. The placenta may be visualized by means of an examination with a sterile speculum. This should be done only with a "double setup" with personnel and equipment available for immediate cesarean delivery, should a sudden hemorrhage occur.
3. The midwife should not attempt to do a vaginal examination as this could precipitate severe hemorrhage.

Management: After a diagnosis of placenta previa is established by ultrasonography, the gestational age is calculated. Management depends on the gestation of pregnancy.

1. If the gestational age is early, an attempt is made to prolong the pregnancy with the intention of optimizing the neonatal outcome. The woman is usually hospitalized to try and avoid preterm labor or hemorrhage.
2. Her mobility is usually restricted to bed-rest at first.
3. Activity may be gradually increased as the pregnancy progresses to term.
4. The hemoglobin and hematocrit values are monitored.
5. Blood replacement therapy or iron therapy is instituted if anemia is present.
6. The pulmonary maturity of the fetus is monitored at appropriate intervals.
7. Unless an emergency situation arises, delivery is planned for some point after the fetus has reached 37 weeks gestation and lung maturity is assured.

A vaginal delivery would be considered only if the placenta previa were 1st degree or very marginal, the fetal head has descended low enough to act as a tampon placing pressure against the placenta, active labor has begun and no other complications were evident. Vaginal delivery would also be considered if the fetus were dead. In most situations however, surgical intervention is the delivery method of choice.

The women are at increased risk of postpartum hemorrhage because the lower uterine segment, where the placenta was attached, does not have the number of interlacing muscle fibers found in the upper portion of the uterus and thus is not as efficient in contraction to control bleeding in the early postpartum period.

OR

a. What is malposition and abnormal presentation?

1. Occipitoposterior position
2. Face presentation
3. Brow presentation
4. Breech presentation
5. Shoulder presentation
6. Compound presentation
7. Shoulder dystocia
8. Unstable lie.

b. List the causes of occipitoposterior position.

Occipito-posterior position is a malposition of the head and occurs in about 13% of all head positions. The presenting part is the vertex and the denominator is the occiput. Right occiput posterior (ROP) is three times as common as left occiput posterior (LOP).

Postulated Causes of Occipito-posterior Positions

1. Pendulous abdomen, common in multiparous women.
2. Anthropoid pelvic brim.
3. Android pelvic brim. The transverse diameter of the brim being nearer the sacrum encourages the biparietal diameter to accommodate posteriorly.
4. A flat sacrum with a poorly flexed head leads to further deflexion and occiput-posterior position.
5. The placenta on the anterior uterine wall tends to encourage the fetus to flex round it.

Occipito-posterior Positions of the Vertex

In posterior positions of the vertex, occiput occupies one of the post: quadrant of the mother's pelvis. The ROP position is more common than LOP for the same reason that the LOA is more common than ROA. It occurs about 10% of vertex presentation, and as vertex. It is a normal presentation, but about 1/5 of them tend to have prolonged labor.

Causes are not well understood

1. 60 percent vertex presentation enters into the transverse diameter, i.e. left occiput transverse (LOT) or right occiput transverse (ROT) and it is just a matter of luck as to whether it turns little to anterior or posterior.

2. Male type of pelvis tends to predispose posterior positions of vertex because the biparietal of the fetal head fits more comfortably into the posterior quadrants, into the heard shaped brim.
3. Elongated head.
4. Placenta previa.

Persistent Occipito-posterior or Unreduced Occipito-posterior Position

In this condition the occiput fails to rotate to the front, and instead of that, it goes round to the hollow of the sacrum, and the baby is born to pubis (short internal rotation).

Causes
1. Deflexion of the head in a post position of the head is in the military attitude, the occipitofrontal diameter 11.5 cm in the right oblique diameter of the pelvic brim. The sinciput becomes the leading part, instead of the occiput it reaches the pelvic floor first and rotates to the front, while the occiput goes back to the hollow of the sacrum.
2. Small head or a large pelvis When the head is small in relation to the pelvis, it need not flex before descent can take place, and in that case the sinciput might reach the pelvic floor first and rotate forward.
3. When the pelvis is anthropoid in type. The head can descend via, the antero-posterior diameter of the brim, without flexion taking place, and descent with the occiput in the hollow of the sacrum.

c. Explain the management of second stage of labor in occipitoposterior position.

Second Stage
1. Vaginal exam reveals the anterior fontanelle behind the symphysis pubis. Sometimes, the anterior fontanel covered by a big caput, where the doctor has to introduce the whole hand into the vagina and the pinna of the ear may be felt. If it is directed to the sacrum, it will determine that the occiput is posterior.
2. Excessive bulging of the perineum and anus are often present due to the biparietal diameter distending the perineum instead of the bitemporal.

Management of delivery of the head: Flexion is maintained by holding the sinciput back under the symphysis pubis until the occiput comes over the perineum; the face is then brought from behind the symphysis pubis by grasping the vertex and extending the head.

d. Write the complications.

To the mother often the 3rd degree tears.
Danger to the baby intracranial hemorrhage due to excessive moulding.

Complications associated with occipitoposterior positions:
1. Prolonged labor
2. Obstructed labor
3. Maternal trauma
4. Cord prolapse
5. Cerebral hemorrhage of baby.

PEDIATRIC NURSING

2019
Pediatric Nursing

SECTION-I

I. Give the meaning of the following:
   a. Pica.
   b. Vernix caseosa.
   c. Hypoglycemia.
   d. Growth.

II. Fill in the blanks:
   a. The anterior fontanelle otherwise known as _____
   b. The headquarter of Hind Kusht Nivaran Sangh is situated at _____
   c. Vitamin B is _____ soluble vitamin.
   d. Apgar score was developed by _____

III. Write short notes on any *four* of the following:
   a. Immunization schedule.
   b. Advantages of breastfeeding.
   c. Day care centers.
   d. Phototherapy.
   e. Emerging challenges in pediatric nursing.

IV. a. Define pyloric stenosis.
   b. List the clinical manifestations and complications of pyloric stenosis.
   c. Discuss the pre- and postoperative of a child posted for surgery of pyloric stenosis.

OR

   a. Define tetralogy of Fallot.
   b. List the clinical features of tetralogy of Fallot.
   c. Explain the management of child with tetralogy of Fallot.

V. a. Define child welfare services.
   b. Explain about anganwadi in detail.

SECTION-II

VI. Choose the correct answer and write:
   a. The most common upper respiratory infection in children is: _____
      i. Pneumonia   ii. Bronchitis   iii. Atelectasis

b. Stuttering refers to: _____
   i. Speech disorders   ii. Vision disorders   iii. Hearing disorders
c. Rubella can be prevented by administering: _____
   i. MMR   ii. DPT   iii. BCG

VII. State whether the following statements are *true* or *false*:
   a. Pleural effusion is collection of fluid in pleural space.
   b. Cerebral palsy is the most frequent permanent disability of childhood.
   c. Malaria is an anthropode borne infection caused by *Plasmodium vivax*.
   d. Osteomyelitis is an inflammation of bone.

VIII. Write short notes on any *four* of the following:
   a. Management of a child with leukemia
   b. Nursing intervention of a child with colostomy
   c. Baby friendly hospital concept
   d. Care of child with poliomyelitis and preventive measures
   e. Prevention of home accidents in toddler.

IX. a. Define nephritic syndrome.
   b. List the causes and clinical features of nephritic syndrome.
   c. Explain the nursing management of child with nephritic syndrome.

OR

   a. Define rheumatic fever.
   b. List the causes of rheumatic fever.
   c. Explain the medical and nursing management of rheumatic fever.

X. a. Define appendicitis.
   b. List the causes and clinical features of appendicitis.
   c. Explain the pre and postoperative management of a child admitted for appendectomy.

SECTION-I

I. Give the meaning of the following:

a. Pica. (2016-I.b)

b. Vernix caseosa.

Vernix caseosa, also known as vernix, is the waxy or cheese-like white substance found coating the skin of newborn human babies.

c. Hypoglycemia. (2013-I.b)

d. Growth.

Growth is the progressive increase in the size of a child or parts of a child.

II. Fill in the blanks:

a. The anterior fontanelle otherwise known as **Bregmatic.**
b. The headquarter of Hind Kasht Nivaran Sangh is situated at **New Delhi.**
c. Vitamin B is **Water soluble vitamin**.
d. Apgar score was developed by **Virginia Apgar.**

III. Write short notes on any *four* of the following:

a. Immunization schedule. (2016-VIII.d)

b. Advantages of breastfeeding. (2015-III.c)

c. Day care centers. (2014-I.a)

d. Phototherapy. (2016-III.c)

e. Emerging challenges in pediatric nursing.

Genetic disorders: The recent decoding and sequencing of the human genome has expanded the horizon of possibilities in the diagnosis of genetic disorders. Researchers and scientists are now facing the difficulties of identifying strengths and limitations of the genome versus exome sequencing to identify the genetic causes of primary immunodeficiencies, before making the information available for potential clinical applications.

Prenatal diagnosis: Substantial progress has been made in the prenatal epidemiology in order to identify the congenital heart malformations and facilitate the appropriate treatment as early as possible.

Prematurity: As a consequence of the improvement of pre-natal screening and diagnosis, the recognition of high-risk neonates allowed the referral for delivery in proximity of high level Neonatal Intensive Care Units, with substantial benefits for the neonatal outcomes.

Traumas: Recent studies have shown the unexpected evidence that the burden of permanent disability resulting from traumatic brain injuries among children is primarily accounted for by mild injuries, rather than by severe injuries. As a result, efforts have to be addressed to prevent, not only severe, but also mild injuries to decrease the levels of disability following traumatic brain injuries.

Limited resources: Despite generalized attempts to diffuse globalization, difficulties still exist in providing medical treatment to geographical areas which have difficult access and/or limited resources. This problem has been documented in the diagnosis of posterior urethral valve, where late referral and presentation are associated with high morbidity and mortality rates.

Ambulatory monitoring and care: Since there is an evident trend to develop and manage healthcare services, it is vital to prevent errors in pediatric ambulatory care. The mistakes most frequently reported include failures in medical treatment, communication, monitoring, patient identification, and the laboratory.

Education and training of the caregivers: The importance of training non-technical skills is becoming increasingly prominent in the field of enhancing the safety of patients. So far a recognized educational model to support the design of patient safety is lacking, even though a number of theories have been suggested to guide educators in future instructional designs.

IV. a. Define pyloric stenosis.

Pyloric stenosis is a narrowing of the opening from the stomach to the first part of the small intestine (the pylorus). Symptoms include projectile vomiting without the presence of bile.

b. List the clinical manifestations and complications of pyloric stenosis.

Clinical manifestations: The most common symptoms noted in a baby with pyloric stenosis is forceful, projectile vomiting. This kind of vomiting is different from a "wet burp" that a baby may have at the end of a feeding. Large amounts of breast milk or formula are vomited, and may go several feet across a room. The baby is usually quite hungry and eats or nurses eagerly. The milk is sometimes curdled in appearance, because as the milk remains in the stomach and does not move forward to the small intestine, the stomach acid "curdles" it.

Other symptoms may include:
1. Weight loss
2. Ravenously hungry despite vomiting
3. Lack of energy
4. Fewer bowel movements
5. Constipation
6. Frequent, mucous stools.

Complications:
1. Bleeding (rare) and wound infection (usually managed by antibiotics);
2. Sometimes the cut made in the thickened muscle may be insufficient to relieve the narrowing, resulting in an incomplete pyloromyotomy. If this happens, you baby will continue to vomit and they may need repeat surgery.
3. **Perforation:** This is when the lining of the bowel is damaged during the operation. It is a rare complication, usually noted and repaired at the time of surgery. Occasionally this complication becomes evident when the baby is back to the ward. In this case your baby will need to return to theater to have the lining repaired by a second operation.

c. Discuss the pre- and postoperative of a child posted for surgery of pyloric stenosis.

Before the surgery: The child will not be allowed to have any milk or formula for 6 hours before surgery to reduce the risk of vomiting and aspiration while under anesthesia.

During the surgery: The following events will take place in the event of a surgery:
1. A pediatric anesthesiologist (a physician who specializes in sedation and pain relief in children) gives your child general anesthesia which induces sleep.
2. A small incision is made on the left side of the abdomen, higher than the umbilicus (belly button).
3. The surgeon then performs a "pyloromyotomy," which involves making an incision in the thickened pylorus to allow food to move out of the stomach into the intestines properly. This procedure generally takes less than an hour to complete.

After the surgery: The usual length of stay after surgery is 24–36 hours. Several hours after surgery, your child will be able to eat again. Oral (by mouth) feedings are started very slowly in very small amounts. The volume and concentration of the formula will be increased as your child is able to tolerate the feeding. If you breastfeed your child, breast milk must be given to your child through a bottle for the first few feedings so that it can be accurately measured.

Sometimes, babies will still vomit after surgery, but this does not mean that they have pyloric stenosis again. The child might vomit after surgery because of the anesthesia. The child also might vomit if feedings advance too quickly or if the child is not adequately burped after feedings. If your child continues to vomit for a prolonged periods, he or she may need more tests. Problems with vomiting should be corrected before the child is discharged from the hospital.

OR

a. Define tetralogy of Fallot.

Tetralogy of Fallot caused by a combination of four heart defects that are present at birth (congenital). These defects, which affect the structure of the heart, cause oxygen-poor blood to flow out of the heart and to the rest of the body. Infants and children with tetralogy of Fallot usually have blue-tinged skin because their blood doesn't carry enough oxygen.

b. List the clinical features of tetralogy of Fallot. (2010 [February]-V.a)

c. Explain the management of child with tetralogy of Fallot. (2010 [February]-V.b)

V. a. Define child welfare services.

The child welfare system is a group of public and private services that are focused on ensuring that all children live in safe, permanent and stable environments that support their well-being. Child welfare services may interact with entire families, or they may be focused on direct intervention with children.

b. Explain about anganwadi in detail.

The word Anganwadi means "courtyard shelter" in Indian languages. They were started by the Indian government in 1975 as part of the Integrated Child Development Services program to combat child hunger and malnutrition. Anganwadis are the focal point for implementation of all the health, nutrition and early learning initiatives under ICDS.

Beneficiaries and service details:

S.No.	Beneficiaries	Services
1.	Expectant and nursing mothers, adolescent girls 11–18 years	Health check-up Immunization of expectant mother against tetanus Referral services Supplementary nutrition Nutrition and health education
2.	Other women 15–45 years	Nutrition and health education
3.	Children below 1 year of age	Supplementary nutrition Immunization Health check-up Referral services
4.	Children between 1 and 3 years of age	Supplementary nutrition Immunization Health check Up Referral services
5.	Children between 3 and 6 years of age	Supplementary nutrition Immunization Health check up Referral services Non-formal preschool education

Role and responsibilities of Anganwadi Workers:

The role and responsibilities of AWWs and Helpers envisaged under the ICDS Scheme is as under:
1. To elicit community support and participation in running the program.
2. To weigh each child every month, record the weight graphically on the growth card, use referral card for referring cases of mothers/children to the subcenters/PHC, etc. and maintain child cards for children below 6 years and produce these cards before visiting medical and para-medical personnel.
3. To carry out a quick survey of all the families, especially mothers and children in those families in their respective area of work once in a year.
4. To organise non-formal preschool activities in the Anganwadi of children in the age group 3–6 years of age and to help in designing and making of toys and play equipment of indigenous origin for use in anganwadi.
5. To organize supplementary nutrition feeding for children (0-6 years) and expectant and nursing mothers by planning the menu based on locally available food and local recipes.
6. To provide health and nutrition education and counseling on breastfeeding/infant and young feeding practices to mothers. Anganwadi workers, being close to the local community, can motivate married women to adopt family planning/birth control measures.
7. AWWs shall share the information relating to births that took place during the month with the Panchayat Secretary/Gram Sabha Sewak/ANM whoever has been notified as Registrar/Sub Registrar of Births and Deaths in her village.
8. To make home visits for educating parents to enable mothers to plan an effective role in the child's growth and development with special emphasis on newborn child.
9. To maintain files and records as prescribed.
10. To assist the PHC staff in the implementation of health component of the programme viz. immunisation, health check-up, antenatal and postnatal check etc.
11. To assist ANM in the administration of IFA and Vitamin A by keeping stock of the two medicines in the Centre without maintaining stock register as it would add to her administrative work which would affect her main functions under the Scheme.

12. To share information collected under ICDS Scheme with the ANM. However, ANM will not solely rely upon the information obtained from the records of AWW.
13. To bring to the notice of the Supervisors/ CDPO any development in the village this requires their attention and intervention, particularly in regard to the work of the coordinating arrangements with different departments.
14. To maintain liaison with other institutions (Mahila Mandals) and involve lady school workers and girls of the primary/middle schools in the village which have relevance to her functions.
15. To guide Accredited Social Health Activists (ASHA) engaged under National Rural Health Mission in the delivery of health care services and maintenance of records under the ICDS Scheme.
16. To assist in implementation of Kishori Shakti Yojana (KSY) and motivate and educate the adolescent girls and their parents and community in general by organizing social awareness programmes/campaigns etc.
17. AWW would also assist in implementation of Nutrition Programme for Adolescent Girls (NPAG) as per the guidelines of the Scheme and maintain such record as prescribed under the NPAG.
18. Anganwadi Worker can function as depot holder for RCH Kit/contraceptives and disposable delivery kits. However, actual distribution of delivery kits or administration of drugs, other than OTC (Over the Counter) drugs would actually be carried out by the ANM or ASHA as decided by the Ministry of Health & Family Welfare.
19. To identify the disability among children during her home visits and refer the case immediately to the nearest PHC or District Disability Rehabilitation Centre.
20. To support in organizing Pulse Polio Immunization (PPI) drives.
21. To inform the ANM in case of emergency cases like diahorrea, cholera etc.

SECTION-II

VI. Choose the correct answer and write:
a. The most common upper respiratory infection in children is:
   i. Pneumonia ii. Bronchitis iii. Atelectasis
   Ans: ii. Bronchitis
b. Stuttering refers to:
   i. Speech disorders ii. Vision disorders iii. Hearing disorders
   Ans: i. Speech disorders
c. Rubella can be prevented by administering:
   i. MMR ii. DPT iii. BCG
   Ans: i. MMR

VII. State wether the following statements are *true* or *false*:
a. Pleural effusion is collection of fluid in plural space: **TRUE**
b. Cerebral palsy is the most frequent permanent disability of childhood: **TRUE**
c. Malaria is an anthropode borne infection caused by *Plasmodium vivax*: **TRUE**
d. Osteomyelitis is an inflammation of bone: **TRUE**

VIII. Write short notes on any *four* of the following:
a. Management of a child with leukemia.

Leukemia is cancer of the blood forming tissues and usually involves the white blood cells. The bone marrow produces abnormal white blood cells that do not function properly. The life cycle of the white blood cells is changed and the cells do not die when they should, thus accumulating and taking up space. They eventually crowd out the good cells which impairs the growth and function of healthy cells. There are many types of leukemia. Some types can be cured while others cannot. Treatment is highly dependent upon the type of leukemia.

Treatment: A pediatric oncologists will lead the medical team caring for a child with leukemia. The oncologist works with other specialists, including nurses, social workers, psychologists, and surgeons.

Chemotherapy is the main treatment for childhood leukemia. The dosages and drugs used may differ based on the child's age and the type of leukemia.

Other treatments include:
1. Radiation therapy: High-energy X-rays that kill cancer cells.
2. Targeted therapy: Specific drugs that find and attack cancer cells without hurting normal cells.
3. Stem cell transplants: Putting healthy stem cells into the body.

Nursing Interventions and Rationales:
1. **Initiate bleeding precautions:** Clotting factors are impaired and patients are at a higher risk of bleeding and bruising.
2. **Assess and manage pain appropriately: Massage, Positioning, Cool/heat therapy, Aromatherapy, Guided imagery, Medications as necessary**—pain can be difficult to control and manage and medications may be scheduled with PRN measures for breakthrough pain. Make sure the intervention is appropriate for the patient and avoid extra stressors such as movement. Encourage patient to try non-pharmacological interventions and balance those with medication for more comprehensive pain control.
3. **Monitor for signs/symptoms of infection or sepsis:** Especially during treatment, patients are at higher risk of developing sepsis. Monitor closing for signs and symptoms and notify.
4. **Promote normothermia:** Progressive hyperthermia may occur as the body's response to disease and effects of treatment. Monitor temperature closely, especially during chemotherapy.
5. **Anticipate needs:** Time pain and nausea medications at their peak according to therapy, chemo and meal times to increase their effectiveness.
6. **Monitor Intake and output, and signs/symptoms of dehydration: Skin turgor, dry mucous membranes, capillary refill:** Dehydration and kidney compromise is a potential complication of disease and treatment. Encourage hydration and monitor closely.
7. **Patient and family education: Symptoms and disease process, infection prevention, plan of care**—patients and family members must be knowledgeable of process and what to expect to help reduce anxiety and be prepared for complications as they arise. Educate family members and caregivers of the importance to help reduce risk of infection for the patient by practicing good hand hygiene.
8. **Avoid risk of infection from procedures: Foley catheter insertion, injections, lines and tubes:** Lack of sufficient white blood cells damages the immune system and patients are more prone to infections. Weight risk versus benefit.
9. **Promote self care, independence and ADLs:** Fatigue is a common symptom and can prevent the patient from participating in self care. Provide assistance with ADLs as needed and cluster care to reduce fatigue and promote rest. Prioritize activities to help conserve energy for self care.

b. Nursing intervention of a child with colostomy. (2016-VIII.a)

c. Baby friendly hospital concept.

The Baby-friendly Hospital Initiative (BFHI) was launched by WHO and UNICEF in 1991, following the Innocenti Declaration of 1990. The initiative is a global effort to implement practices that protect,

promote and support breastfeeding. Breastfeeding reduces the risk of babies developing many illnesses like diarrhea, respiratory and middle ear infections, including allergies. Breastfeeding even leads to fewer illnesses in later childhood. It is also important for the mother's health, i.e. it helps the mother to recover more quickly after delivery, reduces the risk of breast, uterine and ovarian cancer, and it promotes emotional health. Enhancing breastfeeding leads to:
1. Better health for children
2. Better health for mother
3. Significant cost saving to the family
4. Significant cost saving to the society.

Ten steps to successful breastfeeding:
1a. Comply fully with the International Code of Marketing of Breast-milk Substitutes and relevant World Health Assembly resolutions.
1b. Have a written infant feeding policy that is routinely communicated to staff and parents.
1c. Establish ongoing monitoring and data-management systems.
2. Ensure that staff has sufficient knowledge, competence and skills to support breastfeeding.
3. Discuss the importance and management of breastfeeding with pregnant women and their families.
4. Facilitate immediate and uninterrupted skin-to-skin contact and support mothers to initiate breastfeeding as soon as possible after birth.
5. Support mothers to initiate and maintain breastfeeding and manage common difficulties.
6. Do not provide breastfed newborns any food or fluids other than breast milk, unless medically indicated.
7. Enable mothers and their infants to remain together and to practise rooming-in 24 hours a day.
8. Support mothers to recognize and respond to their infants' cues for feeding.
9. Counsel mothers on the use and risks of feeding bottles, teats and pacifiers.
10. Coordinate discharge so that parents and their infants have timely access to ongoing support and care.

d. Care of child with poliomyelitis and preventive measures. (2010-X.a, b, c)
e. Prevention of home accidents in toddler. (2010-VIII.a)

IX. a. Define nephrotic syndrome.

Nephrotic syndrome is the name given to a collection of different signs and symptoms that occur as a result of inflammation in the kidneys. This inflammation causes the kidneys to work less effectively. It also causes protein and red blood cells to leak from the bloodstream into the urine.
1. Nephrotic syndrome, or nephrosis, is defined by the presence of nephrotic-range proteinuria, edema, hyperlipidemia, and hypoalbuminemia.
2. While nephrotic-range proteinuria in adults is characterized by protein excretion of 3.5 g or more per day, in children it is defined as protein excretion of more than 40 mg/m^2/h or a first-morning urine protein/creatinine of 2–3 mg/mg creatinine or greater.

b. List the causes and clinical features of nephrotic syndrome.

Causes:
1. **Primary:** Common primary causes of nephrotic syndrome include kidney diseases such as minimal-change nephropathy, membranous nephropathy, and focal glomerulosclerosis.

2. **Secondary:** Secondary causes include systemic diseases such as diabetes mellitus, lupus erythematosus, and amyloidosis.

Clinical features: Typical symptoms include passing less urine than normal, having blood in the urine and swelling of the feet or face (edema). Other possible symptoms are flank pain, back pain, headache, shortness of breath and symptoms related to the underlying cause, for example, a skin rash and joint pain.

Symptoms of acute nephritic syndrome include:
1. **Edema in the face and legs:** Edema is the accumulation of fluids in the body, usually under the skin, leading to a puffy appearance.
2. **Low urine volume:** Known as oliguria, this is defined as less than 500 mL of urine being produced in a 24-hour period.
3. **Hematuria:** Blood in the urine which often, but not necessarily, leads to red discoloration. There are two types of hematuria: microhematuria, which indicates unseen blood, and macrohematuria, in which the blood is visible to the eye.
4. **High blood pressure:** Hypertension, which results from the disruption of kidney function, may also occur. High blood pressure is generally defined as a resting blood pressure of 140/90 mm Hg or higher in adults. In children, what constitutes hypertension depends on the age and size of the child.
5. **Fever, weakness and fatigue**
6. **Appetite loss, vomiting and abdominal pain**
7. **Malaise** (a feeling of general unwellness) and **nausea** may also be present.

Chronic nephritic syndrome usually presents with fairly mild or even undetectable symptoms, which can include:
1. Edema
2. Hypertension/high blood pressure
3. Kidney failure in later stages.

c. **Explain the nursing management of child with nephrotic syndrome.**

Treatment of nephrotic syndrome: Treatment depends on the underlying causes. Medications (such as ramipril, benazepril, candesartan, or valsartan) are typically used to treat the high blood pressure. Medications will also be administered to reduce inflammation in the kidneys.

Generally, doctors will recommend:
1. Bed rest
2. A diet that is restricted in salt, potassium and fluid
3. Medication to control blood pressure, if necessary
4. Medication to reduce inflammation
5. Medication to remove fluids from the body
6. Dialysis to replace kidney function in severe cases.

Nursing Interventions

Nursing interventions for a child with nephrotic syndrome are:
1. **Monitoring fluid intake and output:** Accurately monitor and document intake and output; weigh the child at the same time every day, on the same scale in the same clothing; measure the child's abdomen daily at the level of the umbilicus.

2. **Improving nutritional intake:** Offer a visually appealing and nutritious diet; consult the child and the family to learn which foods are appealing to the child; serving six small meals my help increase the child's total intake better.
3. **Promoting skin integrity:** Inspect all skin surfaces regularly for breakdown; turn and position the child every 2 hours; protect skin surfaces from pressure by means of pillows and padding; protect overlapping skin surfaces from rubbing by careful placement of cotton gauze; bathe the child regularly; a sheer dusting of cornstarchma be soothing to the skin.
4. **Promoting energy conservation:** Bed rest is common during the edema stage of the condition; balance the activity with rest periods and encourage the child to rest when fatigued; plan quiet, age-appropriate activities that interest the child.
5. **Preventing infection:** Protect the child from anyone with an infection—staff, family, visitors, and other children; hand washing and strict medical asepsis are essential; and observe for any early signs of infection.

OR

a. Define rheumatic fever.

Rheumatic fever is a complicated, involved disease that affects the joints, skin, heart, blood vessels, and brain. It is a systemic immune disease that may develop after an infection with streptococcus bacteria, such as strep throat and scarlet fever.

b. List the causes of rheumatic fever.

Rheumatic fever is believed to result from an autoimmune response; however, the exact pathogenesis remains unclear.

1. **GABHS infection:** Rheumatic fever only develops in children and adolescents following group A beta-hemolytic streptococcal (GABHS) pharyngitis, and only infections of the pharynx initiate or reactivate rheumatic fever.
2. **Molecular mimicry:** So-called molecular mimicry between streptococcal and human proteins is felt to involve both the B and T cells of peripheral blood, with infiltration of the heart by T cells; some believe that an increased production of inflammatory cytokines is the final mechanism of the autoimmune reaction that causes damage to cardiac tissue in RHD.
3. **Streptococcal antigens:** Streptococcal antigens which are structurally similar to those in the heart, include hyaluronate in the bacterial capsule, cell wall polysaccharides (similar to glycoproteins in heart valves), and membrane antigens that share epitopes with the sarcolemma and smooth muscle.
4. **Decrease in regulatory T-cells:** Decreased levels of regulatory T-cells have also been associated with rheumatic heart disease and with increased severity.

c. Explain the medical and nursing management of rheumatic fever. (2012-VIII.d)

X. a. Define appendicitis. (2010 [February]-IX-a)
   b. List the causes and clinical features of appendicitis. (2010 [February]-IX-b)
   c. Explain the pre and postoperative management of a child admitted for appendectomy. (2010 [February]-IX-c)

2018

Pediatric Nursing

SECTION-I

I. Give the meaning of the following:
   a. Preschool.
   b. Tetralogy of Fallot.
   c. Preterm baby.
   d. Infant mortality rate.

II. Fill in the blanks:
   a. The child attains the head control at – month of age.
   b. The first stool of the newborn is called as _____
   c. _____ is the process of introducing liquid and solid food into the diet of infant.
   d. The shape of anterior fontanelle is _____

III. Write short notes on any four of the following:
   a. Importance of play therapy in children.
   b. Under-five clinic.
   c. Nursing management of child with cleft lip and cleft palate.
   d. Trends in pediatric nursing.
   e. Advantages of breastfeeding.
   f. Importance of menstrual hygiene.

IV. Define the following:
   a. Define clubfoot.
   b. Mention the causes and types of club foot.
   c. Explain the nursing, surgical management and parenteral education of child with club foot.

V. a. Define growth and development.
   b. Enlist the any five principles of growth and development.
   c. Explain the factors influencing growth and development.

OR

   a. Define anorectal malformation.
   b. Enlist the causes and types of anorectal malformation.
   c. Explain in detail the nursing management of child with anorectal malformation.

SECTION-II

VI. State whtether the following statements are *true* or *false*:
   a. Apgar scoring is first done after the five minutes of birth.
   b. Thumb sucking is psychiatric disorder.
   c. Colostrum is the first milk of the mother.
   d. Kangaroo mother care is used to prevent hypothermia.

VII. Choose the correct answer from the following:
  a. The rickets is caused by deficiency of:
   i. Vitamin A   ii. Vitamin D   iii. Vitamin C   iv. Vitamin E
  b. Involuntary passing of urine is called as:
   i. Enuresis   ii. Encopresis   iii. Tics   iv. Nocturia
  c. Scabies in children is caused by:
   i. Fungus   ii. Mites   iii. Virus   iv. Bacteria

VIII. Write short notes on any *four* of the following:
  a. Management of child with patent ductus arteriosus.
  b. Care of newborn in phototherapy.
  c. Management of child with protein-energy malnutrition.
  d. Pre- and postoperative nursing care of child undergoing surgery.
  e. Integrated child development services programmes.
  f. Universal immunization schedule.

IX. Answer the following:
  a. Define meningitis.
  b. Mention the causes and types of meningitis.
  c. Discuss the nursing and medical management of child with meningitis.

X. a. Define otitis media.
  b. List down the signs and symptoms of otitis media.
  c. Explain the management of otitis media.

OR

  a. Define diarrhea.
  b. Mention the causes and signs and symptoms of diarrhea.
  c. Explain in detail the management of diarrhea.

SECTION-I

I. Give the meaning of the following:

a. Preschool.

Children are most commonly enrolled in preschool between the ages of three and five, though those as young as two can attend some schools.

b. Tetralogy of fallot. (2011-III-a)

Tetralogy of Fallot caused by a combination of four heart defects that are present at birth (congenital). These defects which affect the structure of the heart, cause oxygen-poor blood to flow out of the heart and to the rest of the body. Infants and children with tetralogy of Fallot usually have blue-tinged skin because their blood does not carry enough oxygen.

c. Preterm baby.

Preterm birth, also known as premature birth, is the birth of a baby at fewer than 37 weeks gestational age. These babies are known as preemies or premies. Premature infants are at greater risk for cerebral palsy, delays in development, hearing problems and sight problems.

d. Infant mortality rate.

The infant mortality rate is the number of deaths under 1 year of age occurring among the live births in a given geographical area during a given year, per 1,000 live births occurring among the population of the given geographical area during the same year.

II. Fill in the blanks

a. The child attains the head control at **4th** month of age.
b. The first stool of the newborn is called as **Meconium**.
c. **Weaning** is the process of introducing liquid and solid food into the diet of infant.
d. The shape of anterior fontanelle is **Kite**.

III. Write short notes on any four of the following:

a. Importance of play therapy in children.

1. Therapists strategically utilize play therapy to help children express what is troubling them when they do not have the verbal language to express their thoughts and feelings.
2. In play therapy, toys are like the child's words and play is the child's language.
3. Through play, therapists may help children learn more adaptive behaviors when there are emotional or social skills deficits.
4. The positive relationship that develops between therapist and child during play therapy sessions can provide a corrective emotional experience necessary for healing.
5. Play therapy may also be used to promote cognitive development and provide insight about and resolution of inner conflicts or dysfunctional thinking in the child.

b. Under-five clinic.

Under five clinic **is a** center, where preventive, promotive, curative, referral and educational services are provided in a package manner to under five children under one roof. To overall goal of under five clinic is to provide comprehensive health care to young children in a specialized facility.

The main objectives of the under-fives' clinic are:
1. Supervision of health and promotion of growth;
2. Prevention of common infectious diseases of childhood through immunization;
3. Early diagnosis and management of common illnesses;
4. Health education;
5. The issue of food supplements; and
6. At-risk selection.

Preventive care:
1. Immunization
2. Nutritional surveillance
3. Sub clinical nutrition
4. Food supplementation
5. Health checkups—every 3-6 months
6. The child health card is maintained
7. Oral rehydration solution for diarrhea
8. The child gets 2-6 attacks in a year
9. Family planning
10. Health education.

c. Nursing management of child with cleft lip and cleft palate.

Nursing interventions for the patient with cleft lip and palate are:
1. **Maintain adequate nutrition:** Breastfeeding may be successful because the breast tissue may mold to close the gap; if the newborn cannot be breastfeed, the mother's breast milk may be expressed and used instead of formula; a soft nipple with a cross-cut made to promote easy flow of milk may work well.
2. **Positioning:** If the cleft lip is unilateral, the nipple should be aimed at the unaffected side; the infant should be kept in an upright position during feeding.
3. **Tools for feeding:** Lamb's nipples (extra long nipples) and special cleft palate nipples molded to fit into the open palate area to close the gap may be used; one of the simplest and most effective methods may be the use of an eyedropper or an Asepto syringe with a short piece of rubber tubing on the tip (Breck feeder).
4. **Promote family coping:** Encourage the family to verbalize their feelings regarding the defect and their disappointment; serve as a model for the family caregiver's attitudes toward the child.
5. **Reduce family anxiety:** Give the family information about cleft repairs; encourage them to ask questions and reassure them that any question is valid.
6. **Provide family teaching:** Explain the usual routine of preoperative, intraoperative, and post-operative care; written information is helpful, but be certain the parents understand the information.

d. Trends in pediatric nursing.
1. **Family centered care (FCC):** It is based on philosophy that quality care can be provided in an environment that support family integrity and promote psychological and physiological health of the family. FCC provides a holistic approach than simply providing medical and nursing care. Parents know best about their childs need more, aware of their childs behavior and habits.
2. **High technology care:** Advancement in medical field has created the care of children too technologically versatile. The nurse also needs to be technologically competent enough to meet the nursing care needs of children. The advancement in diagnostic technology has made detection of many disorders even in the fetal period.
3. **Evidence-based practice:** In evidence based practice nurses need to make decisions on the best available evidence. EBP in nursing provides a systematic approach to enable nurse to effectively use. Clinical practice guidelines (CPGs) and patient centered multidisciplinary, multidimensional plans of care will help nursing team move toward evidence-based practice and improve the process of care delivered. The nurse needs to be vigilant in practicing EBP in nursing children.
4. **Prevention and child health promotion:** The pediatric nurse applied health promotion and health maintenance in all setting in which children are served. The nurse possesses a compheransive background on all aspects of children and an understanding of child growth and development. The family is role in the children's health is critical child health depends upon preventive care. Majority of the child health problems are preventable. Modern concept of child health emphasize on continuous care of whole child.

e. Advantages of breastfeeding.

Advantages of breastfeeding for baby:
- Superior nutrition
- There is an increased resistance to infections, and therefore fewer incidents of illness and hospitalization
- Decreased risk of allergies and lactose intolerance
- Breast milk is sterile
- Baby experiences less nappy rash and thrush
- Baby is less likely to develop allergies
- Baby experiences fewer stomach upsets and constipation
- Breastfed infants tend to have fewer cavities
- Breastfeeding promotes the proper development of baby's jaw and teeth
- Breastfed infants tend to have higher IQs due to good brain development early in life
- Babies benefit emotionally, because they are held more
- Breastfeeding promotes mother-baby bonding
- In the long-term, breastfed babies have a decreased risk of malnutrition, obesity and heart disease compared to formula fed babies.

Advantages of breastfeeding for the mother:
- The baby's sucking causes a mothers uterus to contract and reduces the flow of blood after delivery
- During lactation, menstruation ceases, offering a form of contraception
- Mothers who breastfeed tend to lose weight and achieve their prepregnancy figure more easily than mothers who bottle feed
- Mothers who breastfeed are less likely to develop breast cancer later in life

- Breastfeeding is more economical than formula feeding
- There are less trips to the doctor and less money is spent on medications
- Breastfeeding promotes mother-baby bonding
- Hormones released during breastfeeding create feelings of warmth and calm in the mother.

f. Importance of menstrual hygiene.

The approach is to promote awareness among the girls and women and their families and introduce new, low cost, locally appropriate simple solutions. Our work includes:
1. Access to information to understand the menstrual cycle and how to manage menstruation hygienically;
2. Promote better awareness amongst men and boys (father, husband, teachers, brothers and peers) to overcome the embarrassment, cultural practices and taboos around menstruation that impact negatively on women and girls' lives;
3. Adaptation of existing water, sanitation and hygiene services, to ensure their appropriateness to include water for washing clothes used to absorb menstrual blood and having a place to dry them and having a private space to change;
4. Access to hygienic clothes or disposable sanitary pads;
5. Facilities to hygienically dispose off used clothes and pads; and

Basic hygiene measures every girl and woman should take during menstruation:
1. Take a shower or bath at least once a day.
2. Change pads or tampons regularly to prevent infections—it is advisable to change a sanitary pad once every 6 hours, for a tampon, it is every 2 hours.
3. Opt for good sanitary pads—women with sensitive skin may avoid sanitary pads with plastic lining, as they can cause rashes, itchiness, and boils when rubbing against the skin.
4. Use clean underwear and change it everyday.
5. Do not use soaps or vaginal hygiene products to wash the genital area. Instead, clean the vaginal area using warm water regularly, after each use of toilet and even after urination. Washing the vagina with an intimate wash can kill the good bacteria making way for infections.
6. Always pat the vaginal area dry after every wash, else it might cause irritation. Also, keep the area between the legs dry. Use antiseptic powder to help keep the area dry—preferably before wearing the pad and after washing the vagina.
7. Always wash or wipe the genitals from front to back. This is important because cleaning in the opposite direction can make way for bacteria from the anus to the vagina and urethral opening, leading to infection.
8. Make sure that you wash your hands with warm water and soap after changing your pad/tampon/menstrual cup.
9. Never flush used sanitary pad and tampons down the toilet as they can clog plumbing and cause the toilet to overflow. Discard them properly and throw them in the dustbin to prevent the spread of infections.
10. Wear comfortable, loose clothing, rather than jeans or tight-fitting during periods. This will ensure air flow around the sensitive areas as well as prevent sweating to a large extent.

IV. Define the following:
a. Define clubfoot

Clubfoot describes a range of foot abnormalities usually present at birth (congenital) in which your baby's foot is twisted out of shape or position. In clubfoot, the tissues connecting the muscles to the bone (tendons) are shorter than usual. Clubfoot is a fairly common birth defect and is usually an isolated problem for an otherwise healthy newborn.

Symptoms of clubfoot: Clubfoot can usually be seen in a prenatal ultrasound, and is readily visible when a baby is born.
1. The heel points downward, and the front half of the foot turns inward.
2. The calf muscles on the affected side are smaller than on the normal side.
3. The leg on the affected side is slightly shorter than on the other side.
4. The foot itself is usually short and wide.
5. The Achilles tendon is tight.

b. Mention the causes and types of clubfoot.

Causes of clubfoot:
1. Clubfoot is mainly idiopathic which means that the cause is unknown.
2. Genetic factors are believed to play a major role, and some specific gene changes have been associated with it, but this is not yet well understood.
3. Clubfoot is a relatively common deformity, affecting about one of every 1,000 newborns.
4. There have been some indications of a genetic cause, but these have not been confirmed.
5. Most children who are born with a clubfoot do not have a family history of the condition.
6. If a girl baby has a clubfoot, there is a 6.5% chance that her next-born sibling will also have a clubfoot.
7. Clubfoot is serious only if it is left untreated. A child's well-treated clubfoot is very functional, enabling the child to run and play freely. But if left untreated, the condition progresses and limits the child's mobility.

Types of Clubfoot

Idiopathic clubfoot: Also known as talipes equinovarus, idiopathic clubfoot is the most common type of clubfoot and is present at birth. This congenital anomaly is seen in one out of every 1,000 babies, with half of the cases of club foot involving only one foot. There is currently no known cause of idiopathic clubfoot, but baby boys are twice as likely to have clubfoot compared to baby girls.

Neurogenic clubfoot: Neurogenic clubfoot is caused by an underlying neurologic condition. For instance, a child born with spina bifida A clubfoot may also develop later in childhood due to cerebral palsy or a spinal cord compression.

Syndromic clubfoot: Syndromic clubfoot is found along with a number of other clinical conditions, which relate to an underlying syndrome. Examples of syndromes where a clubfoot can occur include arthrogryposis, constriction band syndrome, tibial hemimelia and diastrophic dwarfism.

c. Explain the nursing, surgical management and parenteral education of child with clubfoot.

Surgical management of child with clubfoot:

Stretching and casting: It is also known as the Ponseti method. The foot is manipulated into a correct position and a cast is placed to maintain that position. Repositioning and recasting is repeated for every 1 to 2 weeks for 2 to 4 months, each time bringing the foot toward the normal position. After realignment of the foot, it is maintained through splinting with braces to keep the foot in the corrected position. The brace is worn for 3 months following which it is worn only at night for up to 3 years, to maintain the correction.

Clubfoot repair: It is surgical repair of the birth defect which involves lengthening or shortening the tendons (tissues that help attaches muscles to bones) of the foot.

Osteotomy: It is a surgical procedure where a part of the bone is cut to shorten or lengthen its alignment. The procedure involves removal of a wedge shaped bone located near the damaged joint and the remaining bones are joined together and secured using the staples or pins.

Fusion or arthrodesis: It is a surgical procedure where two or more bones are joined or fused together. Bone for fusion will be taken from other parts in the body. Metal pins or plates may be used to hold the bones in position.

Parenteral education of child with clubfoot

Clinical staff are often too busy to provide detailed education and support to parents. Therefore many clinics now use parent advisors to help improve their effectiveness. In addition to providing education as above, parent advisors can also help with:
1. Encouraging adherence, e.g. through reminder calls or messages before appointment, or home and community visits
2. Problem-solving practical challenges, such as difficulties attending appointments
3. Identifying and working with families at risk of dropout
4. Calling after patients miss appointments
5. Dispelling myths about clubfoot and causes
6. Advocating for families
7. Acting as a communication link between families and medical staff
8. Encouraging discussion and support between parents, e.g. in the waiting area
9. Working in the community to raise awareness
10. Providing encouragement throughout the process
11. Encouraging fathers to get involved
12. Working with community leaders to endorse families seeking and attending treatment
13. Dealing with conflict in the family that may disrupt clinic attendance.

Nursing care of child with clubfoot: As well as providing empathetic support and information throughout the treatment process, physiotherapists have a role in ensuring that patients who are at risk of, or who have dropped out of treatment are identified and followed up. This means putting systems in place so that when patients do not attend for follow-up visits as scheduled this is noted and there is a means of contacting them to remind them of their appointment and encourage them to attend.

V. a. Define growth and development.

Growth and development go together but at different rates.
1. Growth is the progressive increase in the size of a child or parts of a child.
2. Development is progressive acquisition of various skills (abilities), such as head support, speaking, learning, expressing the feelings and relating with other people.

b. Enlist the any five principles of growth and development.

1. Development follows a pattern.
2. Development proceeds from general to specific responses.
3. Development is a continuous process.

4. Although development is continuous process, yet the tempo of growth is not even.
5. Different aspects of growth develop at different rates.
6. Most traits are correlated in development.
7. Growth is complex. All of its aspects are closely inter-related.
8. Growth is a product of the interaction both heredity and environment.

c. Explain the factors influencing growth and development.

Factors affecting child growth and development: The rate of child growth and development varies considerably from child to child. Child growth and development rate depends in part on:

1. Heredity
2. Constitutional make up like father and mother
3. Nationality
4. Sex
5. Fetal hormones and fetal growth factors
6. Environment and climate
7. Nutritional status
8. Socioeconomical status of the family
9. Physical problems in the child
10. Illness and injury during birth
11. Infections and infestations.

OR

a. Define anorectal malformation.

Definition: This condition occurs when the rectum of the baby does not come all the way through the tissue of the bottom leaving no opening for the stool to be passed from the body. Depending on the severity of the condition, it is often classified as a low, intermediate of or a high anorectal malformation. It is also known as "imperforate anus".

Signs and symptoms: Anorectal malformations cause problems with how a child has a bowel movement. Most anorectal malformations are found before a newborn leaves the hospital. If the problem is not found in the hospital, symptoms may include:

1. Lack of stool
2. Stool coming from the vagina
3. Urine coming from the anus
4. Trouble having a bowel movement, or constipation.

b. Enlist the causes and types anorectal malformation.

Causes of anorectal malformation

1. VACTERL association (a syndrome in which there are vertebral, anal, cardiac, tracheal, esophageal, renal and limb abnormalities)
   V: Veretebral anomanlies
   A: Anal atresia
   C: Cardiovascular anomalies
   T: Tracheoesophageal fistula

E: Esophageal atresia
R: Renal and/or radial anomalies
L: Limb defects
2. Digestive system abnormalities
3. Urinary tract abnormalities
4. Abnormalities of the spine

Types of anorectal malformation

Malformations found in both males and females:
1. Imperforate anus without fistula—the anal opening is missing or in the wrong place.
2. Rectal atresia and stenosis—the anus or rectum is too small to allow stool to pass.
3. Rectoperineal fistula—the rectum connects to the perineum, an area of skin between the anus and genitals.

Malformations found in males:
1. Rectobulbar urethral fistula and rectoprostatic urethral fistula—the rectum connects directly into the urethra.
2. Rectobladder neck fistula—the rectum connects to the bottom of the bladder, where the urethra (the tube that carries urine out of the body through the genitals) begins.

Malformations found in females:
1. Rectovestibular fistula—the rectum connects to just outside of the vagina.
2. Cloaca—the vagina, rectum and urinary tract are combined into a single channel.

c. Explain in detail the nursing management of child with anorectal malformation.

Nursing consideration
1. Identification of undetected anorectal malformations.
2. A poorly developed anal dimple, a genitourinary fistula or vertebral anomalies suggest a high lesion
3. If meconium not passed within 24 hour care should be taken

Preoperative care
1. Diagnostic evaluation
2. Decompression
3. IV fluids.

Postoperative care

Goal: Prevent healing without any infection or complication.
Postoperative:
1. Keep the anal area clean—perineal care.
2. Temporary dressing and drain to manage continuous passage of stool.
3. Protective ointment, such as zinc oxide and occlusive dressing, such as hydrocolloids to decrease skin irritation from frequent.
4. Position; sidelying prone position with hips elevated or a supine position with legs suspended at a 90° angle to the trunk to prevent pressure on the perineal sutures.

5. Infant is given formula when normal peristalsis observed.
6. In the meantime NG tube for abdominal decompression and IVF.

Family support, discharge planning and home care
1. Prevent constipation
2. Encourage breastfeed
3. If cow's milk is given laxatives should be given
4. Bowel habit training, diet modification, and administration of stool softeners or fiber are important
5. Support and reassurance
6. Perineal and wound care and colostomy care
7. Observe stool pattern.

SECTION-II

VI. State wthether the following statements are *true* or *false*:
a. Apgar scoring is first done after the five minutes of birth: **TRUE**
b. Thumb sucking is psychiatric disorder: **TRUE**
c. Colostrum is the first milk of the mother: **TRUE**
d. Kangaroo mother care is used to prevent hypothermia: **TRUE**

VII. Choose the correct answer from the following:
a. The rickets is caused by deficiency of:
   i. Vitamin A   ii. Vitamin D   iii. Vitamin C   iv. Vitamin E
   Ans: ii. Vitamin D
b. Involuntary passing of urine is called as:
   i. Enuresis   ii. Encopresis   iii. Tics   iv. Nocturia
   Ans: i. Enuresis
c. Scabies in children is caused by:
   i. Fungus   ii. Mites   iii. Virus   iv. Bacteria
   Ans: ii Mites

VIII. Write shortnotes on any four of the following:

a. Management of child with patent ductus arteriosus (PDA).

Treatments for patent ductus arteriosus depend on the age of the person being treated. Options might include:
1. **Watchful waiting:** In a premature baby, a PDA often closes on its own. The doctor will monitor your baby's heart to make sure the open blood vessel is closing properly. For full-term babies, children and adults who have small PDAs that are not causing other health problems, monitoring might be all that is needed.
2. **Medications:** In a premature baby, non-steroidal anti-inflammatory drugs (NSAIDs), such as ibuprofen (Advil, Infant's Motrin, others) or indomethacin (Indocin)—might be used to help close a PDA. NSAIDs block the hormone like chemicals in the body that keep the PDA open. NSAIDs would not close a PDA in full-term babies, children or adults.
3. Surgical closure: If medications are not effective and your child's condition is severe or causing complications, surgery might be recommended. A surgeon makes a small cut between your child's ribs to reach your child's heart and repair the open duct using stitches or clips.

After the surgery, your child will remain in the hospital for several days for observation. It usually takes a few weeks for a child to fully recover from heart surgery. Occasionally, surgical closure might also be recommended for adults who have a PDA that is causing health problems. Possible risks of the surgery include hoarseness, bleeding, infection and a paralyzed diaphragm.
4. Catheter procedures: Premature babies are too small for catheter procedures. However, if your baby does not have PDA-related health problems, the doctor might recommend waiting until the baby is older to do a catheter procedure to correct the PDA. Catheter procedures can also be used to treat full-term babies, children and adults.
In a catheter procedure, a thin tube (catheter) is inserted into a blood vessel in the groin and threaded up to the heart. Through the catheter, a plug or coil is inserted to close the ductus arteriosus.

b. Care of newborn in phototherapy.

- Commence phototherapy once TSB/SBR is greater than the appropriate reference range for neonate's gestation/weight and presence of risk factors.
- Neonates should be nursed naked apart from a nappy under phototherapy and will need to be nursed in an Isolette to maintain an appropriate neutral thermal environment. (Link to:" Ward Management of a Neonate" and "Isolette use in Paediatric Wards"). In severe cases, the nappy may need to be removed and a urine bag applied to maximise skin exposure.
- Positon phototherapy units no more than 30.5 cm from the patient. neoBLUE® LED phototherapy unit can be positioned as close as 15 cm to patient. Refer to specific phototherapy units manufacturing guidelines for more details
- Expose as much of the skin surface as possible to the phototherapy light. To maximize skin exposure, dress the baby in a nappy and their protective eye covers only.
- Cover the eyes with appropriate opaque eye covers, e.g. Natus Biliband® Eye Protector (available from Butterfly ward).
- Ensure eye covers are removed 4–6 hourly for eye care during infant cares or feeding. Observe for discharge/infection/damage and document any changes.
- Daily fluid requirements should be reviewed and individualized for gestational and postnatal age.
- Maintain a strict fluid balance chart.
- Breastfeeds may need to be limited to 20 minutes if bilirubin level is high to minimize amount of time out of the lights.
- Monitor vital signs and temperature at least 4 hourly, more often if needed.
- Cover lipid lines with light resistant, reflective tape to avoid peroxidation.
- Ensure that phototherapy unit is turned off during collection of blood for TSB/SBR levels, as both conjugated and unconjugated bilirubin are photo-oxidized when exposed to white or ultraviolet light.
- Observe for signs of potential side effects.

c. Management of child with protein-energy malnutrition.

Medication
- Diet prescription in conjunction with a dietician or nutritionist.
- Appetite stimulants (e.g. megestrol acetate, mirtazapine, oxandrolone, others) may be appropriate for short-term treatment of anorexia in adults but can increase thromboembolic disease risk.

- Medications that have weight gain as a side effect (atypical antipsychotics, carbamazepine, gabapentin, corticosteroids, valproic acid, SSRIs, sulfonylureas, injectable medroxyprogesterone) may be used if indicated in patients with comorbid conditions.

General Measures
- Slowly restore and maintain fluid and electrolyte balance.
- Initiate oral iron and folate supplements (begin iron therapy ~2 weeks after initiation of dietary treatment to avoid promotion of bacterial infection).
- Administer blood transfusion in the presence of severe anemia (hemoglobin <4–6 g/dL) or symptomatic moderate anemia.
- Ensure that immunizations are up to date [protein-energy malnutrition (PEM) is not a contraindication to vaccination].

d. Pre- and postoperative nursing care of child undergoing surgery.

Preoperative care is the preparation and management of a patient prior to surgery. It includes both physical and psychological preparation.

Preoperative preparation: The period since the admission of the child to the hospital until delivery of the child to the operating room.

Target of preoperative preparation:
1. Avoid or prevent the occurrence of postoperative complications to a minimum
2. Improve postoperative outcomes
3. Reduce morbidity and mortality.

General preoperative preparation:
1. Pediatric examination + complementary examinations
2. Anesthesiology ward duration of the preoperative evaluation appropriate risk / ASA / informed consent
3. Psychological preparation - Caution: Stay in hospital can cause emotional trauma, an important psychological preparation and possibly hospitalization with parents.

General preoperative preparation fasting:
1. The last intake of food and fluids varies/in the newborn 3 hours prior to surgery
2. Premedication
3. The choice of anesthetic
4. Ensuring venous access/peripherals, CVC.

Special preoperative care: Expanding the range of examinations with respect to the current disease or associated diseases. For example, bowel preparation, and rehabilitation widen the spectrum of labor. Examination widen the spectrum of X-ray examinations.

Postoperative care
1. Continuation of beginning treatment management of pain therapy
2. Management of feeding
3. Wound care

4. Care of catheters and drains
5. Positioning and rehabilitation of patients.

Postoperative note and orders the patient should be discharged to the ward with comprehensive orders for the following:
1. Vital signs
2. Pain control
3. Rate and type of intravenous fluid
4. Urine and gastrointestinal fluid output
5. Other medications
6. Laboratory investigations.

The patient's progress should be monitored and should include at least:
1. A comment on medical and nursing observations
2. A specific comment on the wound or operation site
3. Any complications
4. Any changes made in treatment.

Aftercare: Prevention of complications:
1. Encourage early mobilization:
   a. Deep breathing and coughing
   b. Active daily exercise
   c. Joint range of motion
   d. Muscular strengthening
   e. Make walking aids, such as canes, crutches and walkers available and provide instructions for their use
2. Ensure adequate nutrition
3. Prevent skin breakdown and pressure sores:
   a. Turn the patient frequently
   b. Keep urine and feces off skin
4. Provide adequate pain control.

e. Integrated child development services programmes.

Ministry of Women and Child Development is implementing various schemes for welfare, development and protection of children.
1. Launched on 2nd October, 1975, the Integrated Child Development Services (ICDS). Scheme is one of the flagship programmes of the Government of India and represents one of the world's largest and unique programmes for early childhood care and development.
2. It is the foremost symbol of country's commitment to its children and nursing mothers, as a response to the challenge of providing preschool non-formal education on one hand and breaking the vicious cycle of malnutrition, morbidity, reduced learning capacity and mortality on the other.
3. The beneficiaries under the Scheme are children in the age group of 0-6 years, pregnant women and lactating mothers.

Objectives of the Scheme are:
1. To improve the nutritional and health status of children in the age-group 0-6 years;
2. To lay the foundation for proper psychological, physical and social development of the child;

3. To reduce the incidence of mortality, morbidity, malnutrition and school dropout;
4. To achieve effective co-ordination of policy and implementation amongst the various departments to promote child development; and
5. To enhance the capability of the mother to look after the normal health and nutritional needs of the child through proper nutrition and health education.

Services under ICDS: The ICDS Scheme offers a package of six services, viz.
1. Supplementary nutrition
2. Preschool non-formal education
3. Nutrition and health education
4. Immunization
5. Health check-up and
6. Referral services.

f. Universal immunization schedule.

Eligibility	Vaccine/s
At Birth	BCG OPV-0 Hepatitis-B
6 weeks of age	OPV-1 **Pentavalent vaccine**-1 **Rota virus**-1 (in Andhra Pradesh, Odisha, Haryana and Himachal Pradesh only at present)
10 weeks of age	OPV-2 **Pentavalent vaccine**-2 **Rota virus**-2 (in Andhra Pradesh, Odisha, Haryana and Himachal Pradesh only at present)
14 weeks of age	OPV-3 IPV **Pentavalent vaccine**-3 **Rota virus**-3 (in Andhra Pradesh, Odisha, Haryana and Himachal Pradesh only at present)
9 months of age	Measles Vitamin A—first dose
16–24 months of age	DPT–first booster OPV booster Measles—second dose Vitamin A—second dose followed by every 6 months till 5 year age, JE (in endemic districts only)
5–6 years of age	DPT second booster
10 and 16 years of age	TT

IX. Answer the following:

a. Define meningitis.

Meningitis is when the membranes that surround the brain and spinal cord (meninges) become infected. Meningitis can be caused by bacteria or viruses.
The symptoms and signs of meningitis in babies and young children include:
1. Fever
2. Refusing feeds
3. Fretfulness
4. Being difficult to wake

5. Purple–red skin rash or bruising
6. High moaning cry
7. Pale or blotchy skin.

b. Mention the causes and types of meningitis.

Bacterial meningitis: Meningitis caused by bacteria is called 'bacterial meningitis'. The organisms (germs) that cause bacterial meningitis may live in the nose and throat. People of any age can carry them without becoming ill, but they can infect others through coughing or sneezing. Meningitis caused by these bacteria is serious and requires very prompt medical attention.
Some common examples of bacterial meningitis are:
1. Haemophilus (Hib) meningitis: caused by *Haemophilus influenzae* type b
2. Meningococcal meningitis: caused by *Neisseria meningitides*
3. Pneumococcal meningitis: caused by *Streptococcus pneumoniae*.

Viral meningitis: Meningitis caused by a virus is called 'viral meningitis'. This type of meningitis is relatively common and can occasionally be serious. It can be caused by a variety of different viruses. It is often a complication of another viral illness. Some of the viruses that can cause meningitis include:
1. Enteroviruses
2. Coxsackieviruses
3. Mumps virus
4. Adenovirus.

c. Discuss the nursing and medical management of child with meningitis.

Treatment for bacterial meningitis: Early and rapid diagnosis is very important in the treatment of bacterial meningitis. Treatment may include:
1. Antibiotics (often given intravenously)
2. Hospital care
3. Anticonvulsant, cortisone and sedative medications, which may be used to treat complications.

Treatment for viral meningitis: Treatment depends on the severity of the symptoms. Treatment is the same as for any viral infection and may include supportive care such as:
1. Resting
2. Keeping warm and comfortable
3. Drinking plenty of fluids.
   a. Bed rest
   b. Increased fluid intake by mouth or IV fluids in the hospital
   c. Medicines to reduce fever and headache. Do not give aspirin or medicine that contains aspirin to a child younger than age 19 unless directed by your child's provider. Taking aspirin can put your child at risk for Reye syndrome. This is a rare but very serious disorder. It most often affects the brain and the liver.
4. Supplemental oxygen or breathing machine (respirator) if your child has trouble breathing.

X. a. Define otitis media.

Inflammation of the middle ear in which there is fluid in the middle ear accompanied by signs or symptoms of ear infection—a bulging eardrum usually accompanied by pain; or a perforated eardrum, often with drainage of purulent material (pus).

b. List down the signs and symptoms of otitis media.

Infants and children may have one or more of the following symptoms:
- Crying
- Irritability
- Sleeplessness
- Pulling on the ears
- Ear pain
- A headache
- Neck pain
- A feeling of fullness in the ear
- Fluid drainage from the ear
- A fever
- Vomiting
- Diarrhea
- Irritability
- A lack of balance
- Hearing loss.

c. Explain the management of otitis media.

The majority of AOM infections resolve without antibiotic treatment. Home treatment and pain medications are usually recommended before antibiotics are tried to avoid the overuse of antibiotics and reduce the risk of adverse reactions from antibiotics.

Treatments for AOM Include

Medication: The doctor may also prescribe eardrops for pain relief and other pain relievers. The doctor may prescribe antibiotics if your symptoms do not go away after a few days of home treatment.

Surgery: The doctor may recommend surgery if your child's infection does not respond to treatment or if your child has recurrent ear infections.

Surgery Options for AOM Include

Adenoid removal: The child's doctor may recommend that your child's adenoids be surgically removed if they are enlarged or infected and the child has recurrent ear infections.

Ear tubes: The doctor may suggest a surgical procedure to insert tiny tubes in the child's ear. The tubes allow air and fluid to drain from the middle ear.

OR

a. Define diarrhea.

A common condition that involves unusually frequent and liquid bowel movements. The opposite of constipation. There are many infectious and non-infectious causes of diarrhea. Persistent diarrhea is both uncomfortable and dangerous to the health because it can indicate an underlying infection and may mean that the body is not able to absorb some nutrients due to a problem in the bowels. Treatment includes drinking plenty of fluids to prevent dehydration and taking over-the-counter remedies. People with diarrhea that persists for more than a couple days, particularly small children or elderly people should seek medical attention.

b. Mention the causes and signs and symptoms of diarrhea.
Causes of diarrhea:
- Bacterial infection.
- Viral infection.
- Food intolerances or allergies.
- Parasites.
- Reaction to medications.
- An intestinal disease, such as inflammatory bowel disease.
- A functional bowel disorder, such as irritable bowel syndrome.

Signs and symptoms associated with diarrhea may include:
- Loose, watery stools.
- Abdominal cramps.
- Abdominal pain.
- Fever.
- Blood in the stool.
- Mucus in the stool.
- Bloating.
- Nausea.

c. Explain in detail the management of diarrhea.
Specific causes of diarrhea are treated (e.g. gluten-free diet for children with celiac disease).
General treatment focuses on hydration which can usually be done orally. IV hydration is rarely essential. [*Caution:* Antidiarrheal drugs (e.g. loperamide) are not recommended for infants and young children.]

Rehydration

Oral rehydration solution (ORS) should contain complex carbohydrate or 2% glucose and 50 to 90 mEq/L sodium. Sports drinks, sodas, juices, and similar drinks do not meet these criteria and should not be used. They generally have too little sodium and too much carbohydrate to take advantage of sodium/glucose cotransport, and the osmotic effect of the excess carbohydrate may result in additional fluid loss.

ORS is recommended by the WHO and is widely available in the US without a prescription. Premixed solutions are also available at most pharmacies and supermarkets.

2017

Pediatric Nursing

SECTION-I

I. **Give the meaning of the following:**
   a. Newborn.
   b. Weaning.
   c. Neonatal jaundice.
   d. Hernia.

II. **Fill in the blanks:**
   a. The shape of the anterior fontanelle _____
   b. The inflammation of the middle ear is known as _____
   c. Deficiency of vitamin A causes _____
   d. The route of DPT vaccine is _____

III. **Write short notes on any *four* of the following:**
   a. Advantages of breastfeeding.
   b. Immunization schedule.
   c. Principles of growth and development.
   d. Oxygen administration.

IV. **Define the following:**
   a. Define hydrocephalus.
   b. Write the causes, signs, symptoms of hydrocephalus.
   c. Explain the nursing management of child with hydrocephalus.

V. a. Define intestinal obstruction.
   b. Write the causes, signs, symptoms of intestinal obstruction.
   c. Explain the management of child with intestinal obstruction.

SECTION-II

VI. **State whether the following statements are *true* or *false*:**
   a. Worm infestation can lead to anemia in children.
   b. Hemophilia is bleeding disorder.
   c. Blephritis is a diseases associated with throat condition.
   d. Head circumference of newborn is 31-32 cm.

VII. **Choose the correct answer from the following:**
   a. Opisthotonus position is seen in:
      i. Epilepsy   ii. Typhoid   iii. Tetanus
   b. Bluish discoloration of the skin is called as:
      i. Cyanosis   ii. Erythema toxicum   iii. Acrocyanosis

c. Mental retardation is suspected in children by:
     i. Poor feeding   ii. Delayed milestone   iii. Normal milestone
VIII. **Write short notes on any *three* of the following:**
  a. Prevention measures of dengue.
  b. Importance of play.
  c. Nursing management of a child with urinary tract infection.
  d. Neonatal convulsion.
IX. **Answer the following:**
  a. Define nephrotic syndrome.
  b. Write the causes, signs and symptoms of nephrotic syndrome.
  c. Explain the nursing and medical management of child with nephrotic syndrome.
X. **Answer the following:**
  a. What is burns.
  b. Write the causes of burns.
  c. Explain nursing management of child with burns.

OR

  a. Define pneumonia.
  b. Write the causes and types of pneumonia.
  c. Write the management of child with pneumonia.

SECTION-I

I. Give the meaning of the following:

a. Newborn.

Newborn defined as birth after 28 days after delivery.

b. Weaning.

The weaning process begins the first time your baby takes food from a source other than your breast—whether it is formula from a bottle or mashed banana from a spoon. Weaning is the gradual replacement of breastfeeding with other foods and ways of nurturing.

Age	What you can offer
6 to 12 months	• Breast milk • Iron-fortified infant formula • Begin introducing solid foods
12 to 18 months	• Breast milk • Whole cow's milk (3.25%)
18 to 24 months	• Breast milk • Whole cow's milk (3.25%). • 2% milk is okay if your child is growing well and eating a variety of foods
2 to 5 years	• Breast milk • 2% milk

c. Neonatal jaundice.

Neonatal jaundice is a yellowish discoloration of the white part of the eyes and skin in a newborn baby due to high bilirubin levels. Other symptoms may include excess sleepiness or poor feeding. Complications may include seizures, cerebral palsy, or kernicterus.

Definition: Neonatal jaundice is the yellowing discoloration of the skin and sclera of a neonate, which is caused by increased levels of bilirubin in the blood. A neonate refers to an infant in the first 28 days of life.

Symptoms: Yellowing of the skin and the whites of the eyes—the main sign of infant jaundice usually appears between the second and fourth day after birth. To check for infant jaundice, press gently on your baby's forehead or nose. If the skin looks yellow where you pressed, it is likely your baby has mild jaundice. If your baby does not have jaundice, the skin color should simply look slightly lighter than its normal color for a moment.

d. Hernia.

A hernia occurs when a part of the intestine pushes through a weakness in the belly (abdominal) muscles. A soft bulge shows up under the skin where the hernia is. A hernia in the groin area is called an inguinal hernia.

If the hernia cannot be pushed back into the belly, the loop of intestine may be stuck in the weakened part of abdominal muscle. If that happens, symptoms may include:
- A full, round belly
- Vomiting
- Pain or fussiness
- Redness or a color that is not normal
- Fever.

These symptoms may look like other health problems. Make sure your child sees his or her healthcare provider for a diagnosis.

Inguinal Hernia in Children
- A hernia occurs when a part of the intestine pushes through a weakness in the belly muscles. When that happens in the groin area, it's called an inguinal hernia.
- Inguinal hernias usually occur in newborns.
- Babies born early or who have a family history of hernias are more likely to develop one.
- Inguinal hernias show up as a bulge or swelling in the groin or scrotum.
- Sometimes they can be pushed back into the belly.
- Your child needs surgery to treat an inguinal hernia.

II. Fill in the blanks:
a. The shape of the anterior fontanelle **Kite**.
b. The inflammation of the middle ear is known as **Otitis media**.
c. Deficiency of vitamin A causes **Nightblindness**.
d. The route of DPT vaccine is **IM**.

III. Write short notes on any four of the following:

a. Advantages of breastfeeding.
Breastfeeding burns extra calories, so it can help you to lose pregnancy weight faster. It releases the hormone oxytocin which helps the uterus return to its prepregnancy size and may reduce uterine bleeding after birth. Breastfeeding also lowers your risk of breast and ovarian cancer.

b. Immunization schedule.

Eligibility	Vaccine/s
At Birth	BCG OPV-0 Hepatitis-B
6 weeks of age	OPV-1 Pentavalent vaccine-1 Rota virus-1 (in Andhra Pradesh, Odisha, Haryana and Himachal Pradesh only at present)
10 weeks of age	OPV-2 Pentavalent vaccine-2 Rota virus-2 (in Andhra Pradesh, Odisha, Haryana and Himachal Pradesh only at present)
14 weeks of age	OPV-3 IPV Pentavalent vaccine-3 Rota virus-3 (in Andhra Pradesh, Odisha, Haryana and Himachal Pradesh only at present)
9 months of age	Measles Vitamin A—first dose
16–24 months of age	DPT—first booster OPV booster Measles—second dose Vitamin A—second dose followed by every 6 months till 5 year age. JE (in endemic districts only)
5–6 years of age	DPT second booster
10 and 16 years of age	TT

c. Principles of growth and development.

The process of development has been studied experimentally and otherwise. The studies and researches have highlighted certain significant facts or principles underlying this process. These are as follows:
- Development follows a pattern.
- Development proceeds from general to specific responses.
- Development is a continuous process.
- Although development is continuous process, yet the tempo of growth it not even.
- Different aspects of growth develop at different rates.
- Most traits are correlated in development.
- Growth is complex. All of its aspects are closely inter-related.
- Growth is a product of the interaction both heredity and environment.
- Each child grows in his own unique way. There are wide individual differences.

d. Oxygen administration.

Face-masks, head boxes, incubators and tents are not recommended because they waste oxygen and are potentially harmful. The recommended methods for neonates, infants and children are nasal prongs, nasal catheters and nasopharyngeal catheters.

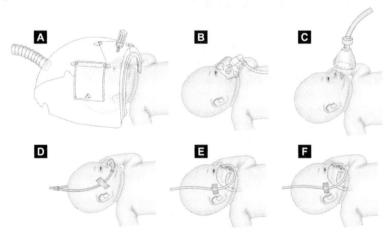

Patients with a nasopharyngeal catheter should be closely monitored, as they can develop serious complications if the catheter enters the oesophagus. Nasal prongs are the preferred oxygen delivery method in most circumstances for an optimal balance between safety, efficacy and efficiency. One of the disadvantages of nasal prongs is their cost, which is presently higher than that of catheters. This is why nasal catheters are often used in developing countries. If they are unavailable, even a cut-down nasogastric tube can suffice as a nasal catheter through which oxygen can be delivered. They are the best method for delivering oxygen to infants and children with croup or pertussis (whooping cough) to avoid provoking paroxysms of coughing.

IV. Define the following:

a. Define hydrocephalus.

Hydrocephalus is the buildup of fluid in the cavities (ventricles) deep within the brain. The excess fluid increases the size of the ventricles and puts pressure on the brain.

b. **Write the causes, signs, symptoms of hydrocephalus.**

Causes of hydrocephalus:

Obstruction: The most common problem is a partial obstruction of the normal flow of cerebrospinal fluid, either from one ventricle to another or from the ventricles to other spaces around the brain.

Poor absorption: Less common is a problem with the mechanisms that enable the blood vessels to absorb cerebrospinal fluid. This is often related to inflammation of brain tissues from disease or injury.

Overproduction: Rarely, cerebrospinal fluid is created more quickly than it can be absorbed.

Signs and symptoms: The signs and symptoms of hydrocephalus vary somewhat by age of onset.

Infants

Common signs and symptoms of hydrocephalus in infants include:

Changes in the head
- An unusually large head
- A rapid increase in the size of the head
- A bulging or tense soft spot (fontanel) on the top of the head.

Physical signs and symptoms
- Vomiting
- Sleepiness
- Irritability
- Poor feeding
- Seizures
- Eyes fixed downward (sunsetting of the eyes)
- Deficits in muscle tone and strength
- Poor responsiveness to touch
- Poor growth.

Toddlers and Older Children

Among toddlers and older children, signs and symptoms may include:

Physical signs and symptoms
- Headache
- Blurred or double vision
- Eyes fixed downward (sunsetting of eyes)
- Abnormal enlargement of a toddler's head
- Sleepiness or lethargy
- Nausea or vomiting
- Unstable balance
- Poor coordination
- Poor appetite
- Seizures
- Urinary incontinence.

Behavioral and cognitive changes
- Irritability
- Change in personality
- Decline in school performance
- Delays or problems with previously acquired skills, such as walking or talking.

Young and middle-aged adults
Common signs and symptoms in this age group include:
- Headache
- Lethargy
- Loss of coordination or balance
- Loss of bladder control or a frequent urge to urinate
- Impaired vision
- Decline in memory, concentration and other thinking skills that may affect job performance.

c. **Explain the nursing management of child with hydrocephalus.**

Nursing interventions for the newborn with hydrocephalus include:
- **Preventing injury:** At least every 2 to 4 hours, monitor the newborn's level of consciousness; check the pupils for equality and reaction; monitor the neurologic status, and observe for a shrill cry, lethargy, or irritability; measure and record the head circumference daily, and keep suction and oxygen equipment convenient at the bedside.
- **Promoting skin integrity:** After a shunting procedure, keep the newborn's head turned away from the operative site until the physician allows a change in position; reposition the newborn at least every 2 hours, as permitted; inspect the dressings over the shunt site immediately after the surgery, every hour for the first 3–4 hours, and then at least every 4 hours.
- **Preventing infection:** Closely observe for and promptly report any signs of infection; perform wound care thoroughly as ordered, and administer antibiotics as prescribed.
- **Promoting growth and development:** The newborn needs social interaction and needs to be talked to, played with, and given the opportunity for activity; and provide toys appropriate for his mental and physical capacity.
- **Reducing family anxiety:** Explain to the family the condition and the anatomy of the surgical procedure in terms they can understand; encourage them to express their anxieties and ask questions; and give accurate, nontechnical answers that are easy to understand.
- **Providing family teaching:** Demonstrate care of the shunt to the family caregivers and have them perform a return demonstration; provide them with a list of signs and symptoms that should be reported, and discuss appropriate growth and development expectations for the child, and stress realistic goals.

V. a. Define intestinal obstruction.

Bowel obstruction is a common surgical emergency for newborns. Early diagnosis and appropriate treatment usually results in positive outcomes. Delay in carrying out surgery may result in the loss of large amounts of bowel.

b. **Write the causes, signs, symptoms of intestinal obstruction.**

Causes: The most common causes of intestinal obstruction in adults are:
1. Intestinal adhesions: Bands of fibrous tissue in the abdominal cavity that can form after abdominal or pelvic surgery.
2. Colon cancer.

In children: The most common cause of intestinal obstruction is telescoping of the intestine (intussusception).

Other possible causes of intestinal obstruction include:
1. Hernias: Portions of intestine that protrude into another part of your body.
2. Inflammatory bowel diseases, such as Crohn's disease.
3. Diverticulitis: A condition in which small, bulging pouches (diverticula) in the digestive tract become inflamed or infected.
4. Twisting of the colon (volvulus).
5. Impacted feces.

Signs of bowel obstruction:

Signs of bowel obstruction can include:
1. Vomiting with or without bile stained material; never ignore bile-stained vomiting in the newborn
2. Increased gastric residuals before feedings
3. Failure to pass meconium in the first 24 hours of life
4. Abdominal distension (particularly with low level obstruction)
5. Absent or decreased bowel sounds.

c. **Explain the management of child with intestinal obstruction.**
   1. Place the infant in an incubator for close observation and temperature control.
   2. Nurse supine with the head elevated.
   3. Place an orogastric tube (8-10 FG) on low-pressure suction (or aspirate with a syringe every 60 minutes and leave on free drainage). The amount and type (for example, bile-stained, feculent) of fluid aspirated should be recorded.
   4. Place nil by mouth.
   5. Commence IV fluids. If signs of shock may need fluid resuscitation with normal saline in 10-20 mL/kg aliquots. Give maintenance fluids plus mL for mL replacement of NG aspirate with normal saline and 10 mmol KCl/500 mL.
   6. Obtain abdominal X-rays (include supine and lateral decubitus view).
   7. Note that a relatively gasless abdomen is compatible with midgut volvulus.
   8. Consult with a pediatric surgeon or PIPER neonatal to arrange transfer to an appropriate surgical center.
   9. It may be appropriate to commence antibiotics preferably after blood culture taken (discuss with the receiving unit or PIPER).
   10. Obtain blood for FBE, electrolytes, blood gas and lactate (and blood cultures if commencing antibiotics).
   11. Be aware that these infants frequently have associated problems of acidosis and shock.

SECTION-II

VI. State wthether the following statements are *true* or *false*:
a. Worm infestation can lead to anemia in children: **True**
b. Hemophilia is bleeding disorder: **True**
c. Blepharitis is a diseases associated with throat condition: **False**
d. Head circumference of newborn is 31–32 cm: **False**

VII. Choose the correct answer from the following:

a. Opisthotonus position is seen in:
   i. Epilepsy   ii. Typhoid   iii. Tetanus

   Ans: iii. Tetanus

b. Bluish discoloration of the skin is called as:
   i. Cyanosis   ii. Eerythema toxicum   iii. Acrocynosis

   Ans: i. Cyanosis

c. Mental retardation is suspected in children by:
   i. Poor feeding   ii. Delayed milestone   iii. Normal milestone

   Ans: ii. Delayed milestone

VIII. Write shortnotes on any three of the following:

a. Prevention measures of dengue.

1. Keep your house clean and tidy.
2. Do not leave stagnant water lying anywhere in or around the house. It is very dangerous as these misquotes lie on this stagnant water only, it does not matter if it is dirty or clean.
3. Spray the house with antimosquito sprays, like **Kala Hit** every day in the corners of your home to kill the hidden mosquitoes.
4. Keep your wet garbage separate and throw in a wet bin (which is kept covered)
5. In the rains, the chances of you getting infected by the dengue/mosquito are extremely high due to the level of stagnant fresh water increase; at this point all measures of safety should be used.
6. Try to wear clothes that do not leave any skin areas exposed.
7. Wear a mosquito repellent cream and carry it with you at all times.
8. Keep the doors and windows of the house closed, mostly early in the morning and during the evening.
9. Change your hand towels after a day's use.
10. Keep your wet and soggy clothes and shoes away from the dry garments. Also, try to dry the wet ones as soon as possible.
11. It is not only about our homes, we need to keep our area and city both clean. Where ever you find gutters which are not being cleaned, find some solution for it. Take it up to your local 'residence welfare association' or community head.

b. Importance of play.

1. Therapists strategically utilize play therapy to help children express what is troubling them when they do not have the verbal language to express their thoughts and feelings.
2. In play therapy, toys are like the child's words and play is the child's language.
3. Through play, therapists may help children learn more adaptive behaviors when there are emotional or social skills deficits.
4. The positive relationship that develops between therapist and child during play therapy sessions can provide a corrective emotional experience necessary for healing.
5. Play therapy may also be used to promote cognitive development and provide insight about and resolution of inner conflicts or dysfunctional thinking in the child.

c. Nursing management of a child with urinary tract infection.

Monitor vital signs for infection: Symptoms that indicate worsening infection or progression of disease include:
1. Tachycardia
2. Fever/chills
3. Elevated blood pressure.

Assess/palpate the bladder every 4 hours: Assess for bladder distention to determine if there is urinary retention.

Assess hydration status and encourage increased fluids: Increasing fluid intake will help the kidneys to flush excess waste and increase blood flow. This will also prevent dehydration with can complicate UTI.

Administer medications to treat: infection, pain, fever
1. Infection—most UTIs can be treated with common antibiotics such as nitrofurantoin, cephalexin and sulfamethoxazole/trimethoprim, depending on urine culture and sensitivity test results.
2. Pain—analgesics for urinary pain include phenazopyridine, which is a dye that helps numb the pain within the urinary tract.
3. Fever—ibuprofen or acetaminophen may be given in case of fever and chills per facility protocol.

Provide education regarding hygiene and prevention of future infections
1. Wipe from front to back when urinating and defecating to prevent bacteria being introduced to the vagina and urethra
2. Avoid scented hygiene sprays, douches and bath products to prevent infection and irritation
3. Cleanse genital area before and after sex
4. Empty bladder frequently and completely to avoid build up of toxins in the bladder
5. Drink lots of water
6. Wear cotton underwear and avoid tight fitting clothing.

Apply heating pad for comfort: Application of heat to lower back or abdomen may help relieve pain and cramping. Avoid prolonged exposure to heating pad, using only 15 minutes per session with at least 15–30 minutes in between to prevent burns.

d. Neonatal convulsion.

Neonatal seizures can be difficult to diagnose because the seizure may be short and subtle. In addition, symptoms of neonatal seizures may mimic normal movements and behaviors seen in healthy babies.

Symptoms depend on the type of seizure—subtle, clonic, tonic or myoclonic.

Symptoms of Subtle Seizures

Subtle seizures are more common among full-term babies. Symptoms of subtle seizures include:
- Random or roving eye movements, eyelid blinking or fluttering, eyes rolling up, eye opening, staring
- Sucking, smacking, chewing and protruding tongue
- Unusual bicycling or pedalling movements of the legs
- Thrashing or struggling movements
- Long pauses in breathing (apnea).

Symptoms of Clonic Seizures
Rhythmic jerking movements that may involve the muscles of the face, tongue, arms, legs or other regions of the body.

Symptoms of Tonic Seizures
- Stiffening or tightening of the muscles
- Turning the head or eyes to one side, or bending or stretching one or more arms or legs.

Symptoms of Myoclonic Seizures
Quick, single jerking motions, involving one arm or leg or the whole body.

IX. Answer the following:
a. Define nephrotic syndrome.
Nephrotic syndrome is usually caused by damage to the clusters of small blood vessels in your kidneys that filter waste and excess water from your blood. Nephrotic syndrome causes swelling (edema), particularly in the feet and ankles, and increases the risk of other health problems.

b. Write the causes, signs and symptoms of nephrotic syndrome.
Causes: Many diseases and conditions can cause glomerular damage and lead to nephrotic syndrome, including:
- **Diabetic kidney disease:** Diabetes can lead to kidney damage (diabetic nephropathy) that affects the glomeruli.
- **Minimal change disease:** This is the most common cause of nephrotic syndrome in children. Minimal change disease results in abnormal kidney function, but when the kidney tissue is examined under a microscope, it appears normal or nearly normal. The cause of the abnormal function typically can't be determined.
- **Focal segmental glomerulosclerosis:** Characterized by scattered scarring of some of the glomeruli, this condition may result from another disease or a genetic defect or occur for no known reason.
- **Membranous nephropathy:** This kidney disorder is the result of thickening membranes within the glomeruli. The exact cause of the thickening isn't known, but it's sometimes associated with other medical conditions, such as hepatitis B, malaria, lupus and cancer.
- **Systemic lupus erythematosus:** This chronic inflammatory disease can lead to serious kidney damage.
- **Amyloidosis:** This disorder occurs when substances called amyloid proteins accumulate in your organs. Amyloid buildup often affects the kidneys, damaging their filtering system.
- **Blood clot in a kidney vein:** Renal vein thrombosis, which occurs when a blood clot blocks a vein connected to the kidney, can cause nephrotic syndrome.

Symptoms: Signs and symptoms of nephrotic syndrome include:
- Severe swelling (edema), particularly around your eyes and in your ankles and feet
- Foamy urine, which may be caused by excess protein in your urine
- Weight gain due to excess fluid retention
- Fatigue
- Loss of appetite.

c. **Explain the nursing and medical management of child with nephrotic syndrome.**

Treatment for nephrotic syndrome involves treating any underlying medical condition that may be causing your nephrotic syndrome. The doctor may also recommend medications that may help control your signs and symptoms or treat complications of nephrotic syndrome. Medications may include:

- **Blood pressure medications:** Drugs called angiotensin-converting enzyme (ACE) inhibitors reduce blood pressure and also reduce the amount of protein released in urine. Medications in this category include benazepril (Lotensin), captopril and enalapril (Vasotec). Another group of drugs that works in a similar way is called angiotensin II receptor blockers (ARBs) and includes losartan (Cozaar) and valsartan (Diovan). Other medications, such as renin inhibitors, also may be used, though ACE inhibitors and ARBs are generally used first.
- **Water pills:** Water pills (diuretics) help control swelling by increasing your kidneys' fluid output. Diuretic medications typically include furosemide (Lasix). Others may include spironolactone (Aldactone) and thiazides, such as hydrochlorothiazide.
- **Cholesterol-reducing medications:** Medications called statins can help lower cholesterol levels. However, it's currently unclear whether or not cholesterol-lowering medications can specifically improve the outcomes of people with nephrotic syndrome, such as avoiding heart attacks or decreasing the risk of early death. Statins include atorvastatin (Lipitor), fluvastatin (Lescol), lovastatin (Altoprev), pravastatin (Pravachol), rosuvastatin (Crestor) and simvastatin (Zocor).
- **Blood thinners:** Medications called anticoagulants help decrease your blood's ability to clot and may be prescribed if you've had a blood clot to reduce your risk of future blood clots. Anticoagulants include heparin, warfarin (Coumadin, Jantoven), dabigatran (Pradaxa), apixaban (Eliquis) and rivaroxaban (Xarelto).
- **Immune system-suppressing medications:** Medications to control the immune system, such as corticosteroids, may decrease the inflammation that accompanies underlying conditions, such as minimal change disease, lupus and amyloidosis.

Nursing Interventions

Nursing interventions for a child with nephrotic syndrome are:
- **Monitoring fluid intake and output:** Accurately monitor and document intake and output; weigh the child at the same time every day, on the same scale in the same clothing; measure the child's abdomen daily at the level of the umbilicus.
- **Improving nutritional intake:** Offer a visually appealing and nutritious diet; consult the child and the family to learn which foods are appealing to the child; serving six small meals my help increase the child's total intake better.
- **Promoting skin integrity:** Inspect all skin surfaces regularly for breakdown; turn and position the child every 2 hours; protect skin surfaces from pressure by means of pillows and padding; protect overlapping skin surfaces from rubbing by careful placement of cotton gauze; bathe the child regularly; a sheer dusting of cornstarchma be soothing to the skin.
- **Promoting energy conservation:** Bed rest is common during the edema stage of the condition; balance the activity with rest periods and encourage the child to rest when fatigued; plan quiet, age-appropriate activities that interest the child.
- **Preventing infection:** Protect the child from anyone with an infection: staff, family, visitors, and other children; hand washing and strict medical asepsis are essential; and observe for any early signs of infection.

X. Answer the following:

a. What is burns?

Burns can be caused by flames, ultraviolet (UV) radiation, hot liquids, electricity, lightning and certain chemicals. All burns require immediate first aid treatment. Partial and full thickness burns require urgent medical attention. Full thickness burns often require skin graft surgery.

b. Write the causes of burns?

Heat burns occur by:
1. **Hot liquids (scalds):** Scalds are commonly caused by hot liquids (water, oil), steam from boiling water or heated food. Young children are mostly affected by scalds.
2. **Hot solids (contact burns):** Solid objects that are hot can cause contact burns, especially in children. Sources of burns from solid objects include ashes and coal, hot pressing irons, soldering equipment, cooking utensils (frying pans and pots), oven containers, light bulbs, and exhaust pipes.
3. **Flames:** Burns can be due to leaking gas pipe or cylinder, accidents from kerosene pressure stove, lighting of crackers during "Diwali", catching of fires in tents as pandal fires.
4. **Chemical burns:** These are accidental burns in homes (such as from toilet cleaning agents), or as acid violence attacks (throwing of acid over somebody for seeking revenge and attempts to resolve disputes of love, land or business) and work place accidents.
5. **Electrical burns:** Electrical burns are due to exposed "live" wires or short circuits. High tension wires close to homes, play areas and roads can lead to electrical burns.

Inhalational burns:
1. Inhalational burns are the result of breathing in superheated gases, steam, hot liquids or noxious products of incomplete combustion.
2. They cause thermal injury to the upper airway, irritation or chemical injury to the airways from soot, asphyxiation, and toxicity from carbon monoxide (CO) and other gases such as cyanide and accompany a skin burn in approximately 20 to 35% of cases.
3. Inhalational burns are the most common cause of death among people suffering fire-related burn.

c. Explain nursing management of child with burns.

Initial management includes assessment and maintenance of following parameters with ABCDE approach:
1. **Airway assessment and management** in case of inhalational burns (burns in closed space, deep dermal burns to face, neck, or trunk, singed nasal hair, carbon particles in oropharynx).
2. **Breathing:** Beware of inhalation and rapid airway compromise.
3. **Circulation:** Ensure fluid replacement by securing wide bore intravenous line through which Ringer lactate solution can be given rapidly. Oral fluids, such as oral rehydration solution (ORS) may be given after initial resuscitation.
4. **Disability:** Evaluation for neurological deficit or any gross disability. Compartment syndrome occurs when excessive pressure builds up inside an enclosed space in the body. The legs, arms, and abdomen are mostly affected by compartment syndrome.
5. **Exposure:** (Percentage area of burn), the whole of a patient should be examined (including the back) to get an accurate estimate of the burn area and to check for any concomitant injuries. In all cases, tetanus prophylaxis should be administered.

Wound care:
1. Adherent necrotic (dead) tissue should be cleaned.
2. After debridement, the burn should be cleansed with either 0.25% (2.5 g/L) chlorhexidine solution or 0.1% (1 g/L) cetrimide solution, or with mild water based antiseptic. (Do not use alcohol-based solutions).
3. A thin layer of antibiotic cream (silver sulfadiazine) should be applied.
4. The burn area is dressed with petroleum gauze and dry gauze thick enough to prevent seepage to the outer layers.

First aid:

Do's:
1. Stop the burning process by removing clothing, jewelry and irrigating the burns.
2. In electrical burns, put the main switch off as quickly as possible and use a wooden scale or rod wooden chair to push the victim away from electricity.
3. Extinguish flames by pouring plain water; if water is not available by applying a blanket and removing the blanket as soon as the flames are put off.
4. In chemical burns, remove or dilute the chemical agent by irrigating with large volumes of water.
5. Use cool running water to reduce the temperature of the burn.
6. Wrap the patient in a clean cloth or sheet and transport to the nearest appropriate facility for medical care.
7. Take care of fractures and probable injuries during transportation.
8. Ensure A-Airway, B-Breathing and C-Circulation before transportation to higher center.

Don'ts
1. Do not start first aid before ensuring your own safety (switch off electrical current, wear gloves for chemicals, etc.)
2. Do not apply ice because it may further damage the injured tissues.
3. Avoid prolonged cooling with water because it may cause hypothermia (low temperature).
4. Do not apply paste, oil, haldi (turmeric) or raw cotton to the burn or any other material.
5. Do not open blisters with needle or pin, until topical antimicrobials can be applied, such as by a healthcare provider.

OR

a. **Define pneumonia.**

Pneumonia is an infection that inflames the air sacs in one or both lungs. The air sacs may fill with fluid or pus (purulent material), causing cough with phlegm or pus, fever, chills, and difficulty breathing. A variety of organisms, including bacteria, viruses and fungi, can cause pneumonia.

b. **Write the causes and types of pneumonia.**

Bacteria: The most common cause of bacterial pneumonia is *Streptococcus pneumoniae*. It may affect one part (lobe) of the lung, a condition called lobar pneumonia.

Bacteria-like organisms: *Mycoplasma pneumoniae* also can cause pneumonia. It typically produces milder symptoms than do other types of pneumonia. Walking pneumonia is an informal name given to this type of pneumonia, which typically is not severe enough to require bed rest.

Fungi: This type of pneumonia is most common in people with chronic health problems or weakened immune systems, and in people who have inhaled large doses of the organisms. The fungi that cause it can be found in soil or bird droppings and vary depending upon geographic location

Viruses: Some of the viruses that cause colds and the flu can cause pneumonia. Viruses are the most common cause of pneumonia in children younger than 5 years. Viral pneumonia is usually mild. But in some cases it can become very serious.

Hospital-acquired pneumonia: Hospital-acquired pneumonia can be serious because the bacteria causing it may be more resistant to antibiotics and because the people who get it are already sick. People who are on breathing machines (ventilators), often used in intensive care units, are at higher risk of this type of pneumonia.

Health care-acquired pneumonia: Health care-acquired pneumonia is a bacterial infection that occurs in people who live in long-term care facilities or who receive care in outpatient clinics, including kidney dialysis centers. Like hospital-acquired pneumonia, health care-acquired pneumonia can be caused by bacteria that are more resistant to antibiotics.

Aspiration pneumonia: Aspiration pneumonia occurs by inhale food, drink, vomit or saliva into the lungs. Aspiration is more likely if something disturbs the normal gag reflex, such as a brain injury or swallowing problem, or excessive use of alcohol or drugs.

f. Write the management of child with pneumonia.

In many cases, the person's own immune system can deal with the infection, but antibiotics may sometimes assist recovery. Treatment depends on the age of the individual and the type of infection, but can include:

1. **Hospital admission:** For babies, young children and the elderly. Mild or moderate cases of pneumonia in people who are otherwise well can often be treated at home.
2. **Plenty of fluids:** Taken orally or intravenously
3. **Antibiotics:** To kill the infection, if bacteria are the cause
4. **Medications:** To relieve pain and reduce fever
5. **Rest:** Sitting up is better than lying dow.

2016

Pediatric Nursing

SECTION-I

I. Give the meaning of the following:
   a. Growth
   b. Pica
   c. Neonate
   d. Otitis media

II. Fill in the blanks
   a. Whooping cough is caused by _____
   b. Pathological jaundice appears within _____ hours after birth.
   c. Anterior fontanel normally closes at the age of _____ months.
   d. The period from birth to one year is called _____

III. Write short notes on any *four* of the following:
   a. Trends in pediatric nursing
   b. Neonatal hypothermia
   c. Phototherapy
   d. Assessment of newborn
   e. Physiological jaundice

IV. a. Define congenital heart diseases
   b. List the types of congenital heart disease
   c. Explain the management of a child with congenital heart disease
   Or
   a. Define pyloric stenosis
   b. List the clinical manifestations of pyloric stenosis
   c. Explain the nursing management of a child with pyloric stenosis

V. a. Define hydrocephalus
   b. List the clinical features of hydrocephalus
   c. Explain the management of a child with hydrocephalus

SECTION-II

VI. Choose the correct answer and write
   a. Circumcision is the surgical procedure performed for
      i. Wilm tumor   ii. Phimosis   iii. Exstrophy of bladder

b. Vitamin C deficiency causes:
   i. Night blindness   ii. Rickets   iii. Scurvy
c. Drug of choice for neonatal convulsion is
   i. Valporate   ii. Phenytoin   iii. Phenobarbitne

VII. State whether the following statements are *true* or *false*:
a. Blepharitis is a disease associated with throat condition
b. Decreased platelet count is termed as thrombocytopenia.
c. Lardosis is the forward curvature of the lumbar vertebrae.
d. Decreased calcium level in the blood is called as hypoglycemia

VIII. Write short notes on any *four* of the following:
a. Nursing care of a child with colostomy
b. Management of a dehydrated child
c. Restraints
d. Immunization schedule
e. Importance of play.

IX. a. Define glomerulonephritis
b. Enumeate the signs and symptoms of glomerulonephritis
c. Discuss the management of a child with glomerulonephritis

X. a. Define encephalitis
b. List the clinical manifestations of encephalitis
c. Explain the nursing management of a child with encephalitis.

SECTION-I

I. Give the meaning of the following:

a. Growth

Growth is the progressive increase in the size of a child or parts of a child. Development is progressive acquisition of various skills (abilities) such as head support, speaking, learning, expressing the feelings and relating with other people. Growth and development go together but at different rates.

Definition of growth: It is the progressive increase in the size of a child or parts of a child. **Development** is progressive acquisition of various skills (abilities) such as head support, speaking, learning, expressing the feelings and relating with other people.

Importance of assessing growth and development: The assessment of growth and development is very helpful in finding out the state of health and nutrition of a child. Continuous normal growth and development indicate a good state of health and nutrition of a child. Abnormal growth or growth failure is a symptom of disease. Hence, measurement of growth is an essential component of the physical examination.

b. Pica

Pica is a pattern of eating non-food materials, such as dirt or paper.

Causes: Pica is seen more in young children than adults. Between 10% and 32% of children ages 1–6 have these behaviors. The incidence of intentional consumption of dirt (geophagy) among children, which is a subset of children with pica behavior, is uncertain.

Pica can also occur during pregnancy. In some cases, a lack of certain nutrients, such as iron deficiency anemia and zinc deficiency, may trigger the unusual cravings. Pica may also occur in adults who crave a certain texture in their mouth.

Treatment: Treatment should first address any missing nutrients or other medical problems, such as lead poisoning. Treating pica involves behaviors, the environment, and family education. One form of treatment associates the pica behavior with negative consequences or punishment (mild aversion therapy). Then the person gets rewarded for eating normal foods. Medications may help reduce the abnormal eating behavior if pica is part of a developmental disorder, such as intellectual disability.

c. Neonate

A newborn infant, or neonate, is a child under 28 days of age. During these first 28 days of life, the child is at highest risk of dying. It is thus crucial that appropriate feeding and care are provided during this period, both to improve the child's chances of survival and to lay the foundations for a healthy life.

d. Otitis media

Otitis media is an infection of the middle section of the ear. Most of the time, it is caused by bacteria that nearly all children have in their nose and throat at one time or another. Ear infections most often develop after a viral respiratory tract infection, such as a cold or the flu. These infections can cause swelling of the mucous membranes of the nose and throat, and diminish normal host defenses, such as clearance of bacteria from the nose, increasing the amount of bacteria in the nose. Viral respiratory tract infections also can impair Eustachian tube function. Normal Eustachian tube function is important for maintaining normal pressure in the ear. Impaired Eustachian tube function changes the pressure in the middle ear (like when you are flying in an airplane). Fluid (called an effusion) may form in the middle ear and bacteria and viruses follow, resulting in inflammation in the middle ear. The increased pressure causes the eardrum to bulge, leading to the typical symptoms of fever, pain, and fussiness in young children.

Clinical manifestations: Symptoms of an ear infection in adolescents and older children may include ear aching or pain and temporary hearing loss. These symptoms usually come on suddenly. In infants and young children, symptoms of an ear infection can include:
1. Fever (temperature higher than 100.4°F or 38°C, see the table for how to measure a child's temperature)
2. Pulling on the ear
3. Fussiness or irritability
4. Decreased activity
5. Lack of appetite or difficulty, eating
6. Vomiting or diarrhea
7. Draining fluid from the outer ear (called otorrhea).

Treatment of otitis media
Treatment of an ear infection may include:
1. Antibiotics
2. Medicines to treat pain and fever
3. Observation
4. A combination of the above.

The "best" treatment depends on the child's age, history of previous infections, degree of illness, and any underlying medical problems.

II. Fill in the blanks
a. Whooping cough is caused by **DIPHTHERIA**
b. Pathological jaundice appears within **24** hours after birth.
c. Anterior fontanel normally closes at the age of **18** months.
d. The period from birth to one year is called **INFANT**

III. Write short notes on any *four* of the following:

a. Trends in pediatric nursing

Changes in the standard of care for pediatric patients are not something the medical community takes lightly. In the world of medicine, clinical care guidelines are typically developed around sound clinical research; however, there is an exception to this rule when developing clinical care guidelines for use with the pediatric patient. Although this is counterintuitive, it does make sense; there are fewer research projects involving children and, as a result, less science to support changes in clinical care guidelines.

The increasing complexity of medical and nursing techniques has created a need for special area for child care. The child care has prime importance, as the mortality and morbidity are higher in this group. Many diseases are preventable, such as nutritional deficiency. The goal of the pediatric nursing is to foster the growth and development of the children and promote an optimum state of health physically, mentally, and socially, so that they may function at the peak of their capacity.

Since most of the responses of children are influenced by the phases of growth and development, the ages of the child are the most significant factor affecting nursing activities. For example, fractured jaw is more traumatic to an infant who is in oral phase of the development than to a child of the six years of age who has already passed this phase. The separation of the family during the hospitalization will cause an anxiety in the young child and may disturb the parent–child relationship.

The nurse can minimize the psychological trauma of a hospitalization experience by helping the children to adjust to the situation rather than to repress their feelings. Play therapy has an importance in child care, by which children can play out their problems. To provide comprehensive care to children, the nurse must clearly understand the effect of illness and hospitalization experience, upon the growth and development process of children and the effect of the developmental status of the children upon their responses to therapy. The role of the pediatric nurse has been influenced by the research findings in other health disciplines of prevention and therapy, in various areas of genetics, drugs, medical, and surgical techniques. It is also influenced by the research carried out within the nursing profession itself.

The concept of assessment of children is important for providing care to patients and their families. The function of the pediatric nurse is to promote and support children in their adaptation process. The nurse must observe the children's health and illness state, their strengths and weaknesses, and effectiveness of their coping mechanism. Nursing children require a better sense of responsibility and better judgment of children's health, responses, and planning for nursing management. The nurse must have patience and emotional balance while dealing with the children and their parents, specially, in critically ill cases.

b. Neonatal hypothermia

The normal newborn continues to adapt to the extrauterine life within the first week after child birth remaining vulnerable to hypothermia. The baby remains dependent on mother for nutrition and protection. Mother is responsible for maintaining the body temperature of the baby among other functions essential for survival. Due to certain characteristics such little subcutaneous fat, low birth weight babies, exposing the baby to the cold climatic conditions increases risk of hypothermia.

Hypothermia in newborn: The newborn with a temperature of 36.0–36.4°C (96.8–97.5°F) is under cold stress (mild hypothermia). A baby with a temperature of 32.0–35.9°C (89.6–96.6°F) has moderate hypothermia, while a temperature below 32°C (89.6°F) is considered to be severe hypothermia.

Causes and risk factors: Hypothermia of the newborn is mainly due to lack of knowledge. In many hospitals incorrect care of the baby at birth is the most important factor in causing hypothermia. Delivery rooms are not warm enough and the newborn is often left wet and uncovered after delivery.

The newborn is weighed naked and washed soon after birth. The initiation of breastfeeding is frequently delayed for many hours, and the baby is kept in a nursery, apart from the mother. In many newborns, these practices will result in hypothermia.

At home, families and trained birth attendants (TBAs) may also not be aware of the importance of drying and wrapping the newborn immediately after birth. Other risk factors include asphyxia, use of anesthetic or analgesic drugs during delivery, infection or other illness of the infant and inadequate measures taken to keep the baby warm before and during transportation.

Signs of hypothermia: An early sign of hypothermia is feet that are cold to the touch. If prolonged leads to hypothermia, the baby becomes less active, suckles poorly, impaired feeding and has a weak cry. In severely hypothermic babies, the face and extremities may develop a bright red color. The baby becomes lethargic and develops slow, shallow and irregular breathing and a slow heart beat.

Low blood sugar and metabolic acidosis, generalized internal bleeding (especially in the lungs) and respiratory distress may occur. Such a level of hypothermia is very dangerous and unless urgent measures are taken, the baby will die.

Effects of hypothermia: There is no evidence that hypothermia has any beneficial effect immediately after birth; for example, cold stress is not needed at birth, as commonly believed, to initiate or stimulate breathing. Although many traditional practices are beneficial, such as heating the delivery room in cold weather, wrapping the baby and keeping it close to the mother, etc.

On the contrary, there is sample evidence that hypothermia is harmful. Prolonged hypothermia is linked to impaired growth and may make the newborn more vulnerable to infections, others are harmful, such as sprinkling the newborn with cold water to stimulate breathing, bathing the baby soon after birth, delaying breastfeeding in the belief that colostrums is harmful or useless.

Management of hypothermia: Thermal protection of the newborn is the series of measures taken at birth and during the first days of life to ensure that the baby does not become either too cold (hypothermia) and maintains a normal body temperature of 36.5–37.5°C (97.7–99.5°F).

Newborns found to be hypothermic must be rewarmed as soon as possible. It is very important to continue feeding the baby to provide calories and fluid. Breastfeeding should resume as soon as possible. If the infant is too weak to breastfeed, breast milk can be given by, spoon or cup. It is important to be aware that hypothermia can be a sign of infection. Every hypothermic newborn should therefore be assessed for infection.

Treatment: Rewarming in an incubator or under a radiant warmer: hypothermia is treated by rewarming in an incubator or under a radiant warmer. The neonate should be monitored and treated as needed for hypoglycemia, hypoxemia, and apnea. Underlying conditions, such as sepsis, drug withdrawal, or intracranial hemorrhage require specific treatment.

Prevention: Hypothermia can be prevented by immediately drying and then swaddling the neonate (including the head) in a warm blanket to prevent evaporative, conductive, and convective losses. Preterm very-low-birth-weight infants also benefit from a polyethylene occlusive wrapping at the time of delivery. A neonate exposed for resuscitation or observation should be placed under a radiant warmer to prevent radiant losses. Sick neonates should be maintained in a neutral thermal environment to minimize the metabolic rate. The proper incubator temperature varies depending on the neonate's birth weight and postnatal age, and humidity in the incubator. Alternatively, heating can be adjusted with a servomechanism set to maintain skin temperature at 36.5° C.

c. Phototherapy

Phototherapy can be used to prevent the concentration of unconjugated bilirubin in the blood from reaching levels where neurotoxicity may occur. During phototherapy the neonate's skin surface is exposed to high-intensity, light, which photochemically converts fat-soluble, unconjugated bilirubin into water-soluble bilirubin, which can be excreted in bile and urine (McFadden, 1991).

Technique
a. Bilirubin is broken down in the skin and is observed during phototherapy. Blue light is superior to white light; fluorescent tubes are remarkable as a potent source of blue light.
b. Method of phototherapy includes remove all clothing of the baby except diaper in the case of a male baby. Baby's eyes are covered with eyepad. Lights are positioned 50–75 cm from the infant. Maintain slightly more fluid intake. Phototherapy duration based on serum bilirubin

level. It is needed for 2–3 days. The observation includes body temperature, hydration status, blood levels of bilirubin as well as hemoglobin and stool examination.

d. Assessment of newborn

The purpose of the **newborn** physical examination is to **assess** the baby's transition from intrauterine line to extrauterine existence and to detect congenital malformations and actual or potential disease. The baby should be examined briefly immediately after birth.

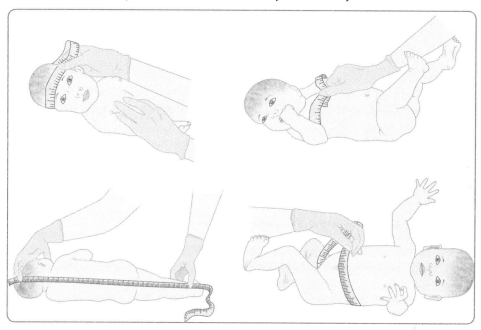

A newborn should have a thorough evaluation performed within 24 hours of birth to identify any abnormality that would alter the normal newborn course or identify a medical condition that should be addressed (e.g. anomalies, birth injuries, jaundice, or cardiopulmonary disorders).. This assessment includes review of the maternal, family, and prenatal history and a complete examination. Depending upon the length of stay, another examination should be performed within 24 hours before discharge from the hospital. Assessing the health of a newborn is very important for detecting any problems in their earliest, most treatable, stages. Listed in the directory below you will find information regarding several newborn health assessments, for which we have provided a brief overview.

Assessing Newborns Weight: A baby's birth weight is an important indicator of health. The average weight for full-term babies (born between 37 and 41 weeks gestation) is about 7 lbs (3.2 kg). In general, small babies and very large babies are more likely to have problems. Newborn babies may lose as much as 10% of their birth weight. This means that a baby weighing 7 pounds 3 ounces at birth might lose as much as 10 ounces in the first few days. Like weight, length and head circumference help your baby's healthcare provider get an idea of his or her overall health. They may also be measured using metric units, centimeters (cm) instead of inches (in). To convert inches to centimeters: 1 in = 2.54 cm.

Head circumference: The distance around the baby's head.
1. The average newborn's head measures 13 3/4 in (35 cm)
2. Generally, a newborn's head is about half the baby's body length in cm plus 10 cm. So, a baby that is 18 inches long would be 45.7 centimeters (18 x 2.54). His or her head would be about 32.9 cm or a little under 13 inches.

Length: The measurement from top of the head to the heel of one foot
1. The average newborn is about 50 cm or 19 3/4 in long.

Physical examination of the newborn: A complete physical examination is an important part of newborn care. Each body system is carefully examined for signs of health and normal function. The doctor also looks for any signs of illness or birth defects. Physical examination of a newborn often includes assessment of the following:

Vital signs
1. **Temperature:** Able to maintain stable body temperature of 97.0–98.6°F (36.1–37°C) in normal room environment.
2. **Heartbeat:** Normally 120–160 beats per minute. It may be much slower when an infant sleeps.
3. **Breathing rate:** Normally 40–60 breaths per minute.

General appearance: Physical activity, muscle tone, posture, and level of consciousness or whether or not an infant is awake and alert.

Skin: Color, texture, nails, presence of rashes.

Head and neck
1. Appearance, shape, presence of molding (shaping of the head from passage through the birth canal).
2. Fontanels (the open "soft spots" between the bones of the baby's skull).
3. Clavicles (bones across the upper chest).

Face. Eyes, ears, nose, cheeks. Presence of red reflex in the eyes

Mouth. Roof of the mouth (palate), tongue, throat

Lungs. Breath sounds, breathing pattern

Heart sounds and femoral (in the groin) pulses

Abdomen. Presence of masses or hernias

Genitals and anus. Open passage for of urine and stool and normally formed male and female genitals.

Nerves. Reflexes (for example, the Moro or startle reflex), cranial nerves (for example, eye movement), abnormal (or lack of) movements.

Arms and legs. Movement and development.

e. Physiological Jaundice

Infant jaundice is a yellow discoloration in a newborn baby's skin and eyes. Infant jaundice occurs because the baby's blood contains an excess of bilirubin, a yellow-colored pigment of red blood cells. Infant jaundice is a common condition, particularly in babies born before 38 weeks gestation (preterm babies) and some breastfed babies. Infant jaundice usually occurs because a baby's liver is not mature enough to get rid of bilirubin in the bloodstream. In some cases, an underlying disease may cause jaundice.

Clinical manifestations
1. Neonatal jaundice first becomes visible in the face and forehead. Blanching reveals the underlying color. Jaundice then gradually becomes visible on the trunk and extremities.
2. In most infants, yellow color is the only finding on physical examination. More intense jaundice may be associated with drowsiness.
3. Neurological signs (e.g. changes in muscle tone, seizures, or altered crying) require immediate attention to avoid kernicterus.
4. Hepatosplenomegaly, petechiae, and microcephaly are associated with hemolytic anemia, sepsis, and congenital infections.
5. Hepatitis (e.g., congenital rubella, CMV, toxoplasmosis) and biliary atresia cause a raised conjugated bilirubin and have a marked jaundice and pale stools and dark urine, usually presenting in the third week of life.

Causes of infant **jaundice**. Infant **jaundice** is most often **caused** by an excess of bilirubin. Bilirubin is the waste that remains after hemoglobin (the predominant protein in red blood cells) is released from the breakdown of the red blood cells that carry oxygen throughout the body. Treatment of infant jaundice often is not necessary, and most cases that need treatment respond well to noninvasive therapy. Although complications are rare, a high bilirubin level associated with severe infant jaundice or inadequately treated jaundice may cause brain damage.

IV. a. Define congenital heart diseases. b. List the types of congenital heart disease. c. Explain the management of a child with congenital heart disease

The purpose of the heart is to pump blood to the body in order to nourish it. Heart failure does not mean that the heart has stopped working, but that it just is not able to pump enough blood to meet the needs of the body. This may happen when the heart muscle itself is weaker than normal or when there is a defect in the heart that prevents blood from getting out into the circulation. When the heart does not circulate blood normally, the kidneys receive less blood and filter less fluid out of the circulation into the urine. The extrafluid in the circulation builds up in the lungs, the liver, around the eyes, and sometimes in the legs. This is called fluid "congestion" and for this reason doctors call this "congestive heart failure".

Types of congenital heart disease
1. Ventricular septal defect
2. Atrial septal defect
3. Patent ductus arteriosus
4. Coarctation of aorta
5. Transposition of great vessels
6. Tricuspid atresia
7. Truncus arteriosus
8. Fallot's tetralogy
9. Aortic stenosis
10. Pulmonic stenosis
11. Aortic or pulmonary artery dilation
12. Mitral or aortic regurgitation
13. Ebstein's anomaly
14. Dextrocardia.

Or

a. Define pyloric stenosis. b. List the clinical manifestations of pyloric stenosis. c. Explain the nursing management of a child with pyloric stenosis

Pyloric stenosis is an uncommon condition in infants that blocks food from entering the small intestine. Normally, a muscular valve (pylorus) between the stomach and small intestine holds food in the stomach until it is ready for the next stage in the digestive process. In pyloric stenosis, the pylorus muscles thicken and become abnormally large, blocking food from reaching the small intestine. Pyloric stenosis can lead to forceful vomiting, dehydration and weight loss. Babies with pyloric stenosis may seem to be hungry all the time.

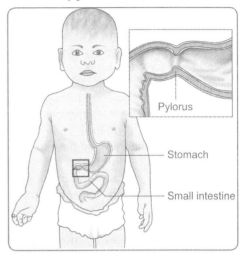

Symptoms: Signs of pyloric stenosis usually appear within three to five weeks after birth. Pyloric stenosis is rare in babies older than age 3 months.

Signs and symptoms include:
1. Vomiting after feeding. The baby may vomit forcefully, ejecting breast milk or formula up to several feet away (projectile vomiting). Vomiting might be mild at first and gradually become more severe as the pylorus opening narrows. The vomit may sometimes contain blood.
2. Persistent hunger. Babies who have pyloric stenosis often want to eat soon after vomiting.
3. Stomach contractions. You may notice wave-like contractions (peristalsis) that ripple across your baby's upper abdomen soon after feeding, but before vomiting. This is caused by stomach muscles trying to force food through the narrowed pylorus.
4. Dehydration. Your baby might cry without tears or become lethargic. You might find yourself changing fewer wet diapers or diapers that aren't as wet as you expect.
5. Changes in bowel movements. Since pyloric stenosis prevents food from reaching the intestines, babies with this condition might be constipated.
6. Weight problems. Pyloric stenosis can keep a baby from gaining weight, and sometimes can cause weight loss.

Risk factors

Risk factors for pyloric stenosis include:
1. Sex: Pyloric stenosis is seen more often in boys, especially firstborn children than in girls.
2. Race: Pyloric stenosis is more common in Caucasians of northern European ancestry, less common in African—Americans and rare in Asians.
3. Premature birth: Pyloric stenosis is more common in babies born prematurely than in full-term babies.
4. Family history: Studies found higher rates of this disorder among certain families. Pyloric stenosis develops in about 20% of male descendants and 10% of female descendants of mothers who had the condition.
5. Smoking during pregnancy: This behavior can nearly double the risk of pyloric stenosis.
6. Early antibiotic use: Babies given certain antibiotics in the first weeks of life—erythromycin to treat whooping cough, for example, have an increased risk of pyloric stenosis. In addition,

babies born to mothers who took certain antibiotics in late pregnancy also may have an increased risk of pyloric stenosis.

Bottlefeeding: Some studies suggest that bottle-feeding rather than breastfeeding can increase the risk of pyloric stenosis. Most people in these studies used formula rather than breast milk, so it is not clear whether the increased risk is related to formula or the mechanism of bottle-feeding.

Complications
Pyloric stenosis can lead to:
1. Failure to grow and develop.
2. Dehydration: Frequent vomiting can cause dehydration and a mineral (electrolyte) imbalance. Electrolytes help regulate many vital functions.
3. Stomach irritation: Repeated vomiting can irritate your baby's stomach and may cause mild bleeding.
4. Jaundice: Rarely, a substance secreted by the liver (bilirubin) can build up, causing a yellowish discoloration of the skin and eyes.

Treatment: Surgery is needed to treat pyloric stenosis. The procedure (pyloromyotomy) is often scheduled on the same day as the diagnosis. If your baby is dehydrated or has an electrolyte imbalance, he or she will have fluid replacement before surgery. In pyloromyotomy, the surgeon cuts only through the outside layer of the thickened pylorus muscle, allowing the inner lining to bulge out. This opens a channel for food to pass through to the small intestine.

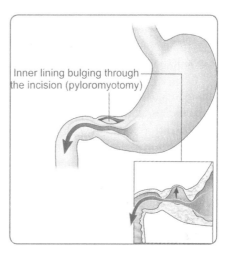

Inner lining bulging through the incision (pyloromyotomy)

Pyloromyotomy is often done using minimally invasive surgery. A slender viewing instrument (laparoscope) is inserted through a small incision near the baby's navel. Recovery from a laparoscopic procedure is usually quicker than recovery from traditional surgery, and the procedure leaves a smaller scar.

Management
1. Plot weight on growth chart and compare to previous measurements
2. Blood gas (venous or capillary): hyperchloremic hypokalaemic metabolic alkalosis is often present
3. Bloods: FBC, U/E, glucose, LFT (if jaundiced)
4. NBM
5. Abdominal ultrasound: diagnostic if pylorus is greater than 4 mm thickness and greater than 17 mm in length
6. Discuss with the surgeons
7. Regular BM monitoring 4-6 hourly via heel prick
8. Strict fluid monitoring and correct dehydration
9. NG tube on free drainage with hourly aspirations
10. Replace NG losses 'ml for ml' with 0.9% NaCl + 10 mmol KCl per 500 mL of intravenous fluid
11. Also give maintenance intravenous fluids 0.45% NaCl + 5% dextrose + 10 mmol KCl per 500 mL of fluid
12. Ensure serum bicarbonate and potassium are corrected prior to surgery

Postoperative care: Feeding is usually recommenced 4-6 hours after surgery. Vomiting may continue but should resolve within 48 hours. The main complications of the procedure are continued vomiting, infection and bowel perforation.

V. a. Define hydrocephalus, b. List the clinical features of hydrocephalus, c. Explain the management of a child with hydrocephalus

Hydrocephalus is the abnormal accumulation of cerebrospinal fluid (CSF) in the intracranial spaces. It occurs due to imbalance between production or absorption of CSF or due to obstruction of the CSF pathways. It results in the dilatation of the cerebral ventricles and enlargement of head.

Clinical manifestations

Congenital hydrocephalus starts in fetal life and presents at birth or within first few months of life. Acquired hydrocephalus develops in association with underlying cause or as its complications. Clinical manifestations depend upon age of the child, types and duration of hydrocephalus, closing of anterior fontanel or fusion of cranial sutures. The features may manifest rapidly, slowly, steadily advancing or remittent. The features include excessive enlargement of head, delayed closure of anterior fontanel, tense and bulging fontanel with open sutures. Presence of signs of increased intracranial pressure and alteration of muscle tone (spasticity) of the extremities are common presenting features. There is delayed in head holding of the infant.

Later, with gradual increase in size of the head, the child presents with protruding forehead, shiny scalp with prominent scalp veins. The eyebrows and eyelids may be drawn upwards exposing the sclera above the iris with impaired upward gaze resulting the 'sun-set' sign of eyes. The cracked-pot (Macewen's) sign may be elicited by percussion of head. Transillumination is positive. Mental functions and neurological manifestations usually vary with the causative and associated factors. The children may have normal intelligence.

Hydrocephalus occurring late in childhood may not present with large head. The features may be found as increased intracranial pressure (ICP) with papilledema, spasticity, ataxia, urinary incontinence and progressive deterioration of mental activities.

Increased ICP presents with the signs and symptoms as nausea, vomiting, restlessness, irritability, high pitched shrill cry (in infants), irregular and decreased respiration, decreased pulse, increased temperature and systolic blood pressure. Pupillary changes, tense and bulging fontanel separation of cranial sutures, increase of head circumference, papilledema, convulsions, lethargy, stupor and coma also usually present. In older children, headache, lethargy, fatigue, apathy, personality changes and visual problems are manifested.

Management

Management of hydrocephalus depends upon specific cause, associated malformations, clinical course and severity of the condition. Surgery may not be indicated, if the hydrocephalus gets spontaneous arrest. When the surgical management is not necessary, then medical management is done to reduce increased ICP by carbonic' anhydrase inhibitor, acetazolamide (Diamox) 50 mg/kg/day to reduce CSF production in slow progressive hydrocephalus. Oral glycerol and isosorbide can also be used for the same purpose.

Surgical management: It is indicated in obstructive hydrocephalus, in rapid enlargement of head, visual disturbances or in life threatening increase ICP. Ventriculostomy and choroid plexectomy have been performed with variable results. Surgical shunts are the treatment of choice at the present time.

Intracranial or extracranial shunt is done to bypass the obstruction and to divert the CSF from the ventricular system to other compartment. The most commonly performed extracranial shunt is ventriculo-peritoneal shunt (V–P shunt). Other approaches are ventriculoatrial shunt, ventriculopleural shunt or ventriculogali bladder shunt. Intrauterine surgical intervention in fetal hydrocephalus has not yet given good results.

Intracranial or extracranial shunt is done to bypass the obstruction and to divert the CSF from the ventricular system to other compartment. The most commonly performed extra- cranial shunt is ventriculoperitoneal shunt (VP shunt). Other approaches are ventriculoatrial shunt, ventriculopleural shunt or ventriculogallbladder shunt. Intrauterine surgical intervention in fetal hydrocephalus has not yet given good results.

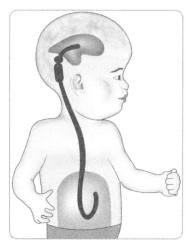

Ventriculoperitoneal shunt

Nursing management

Nursing assessment: Along with routine nursing assessment, the most important is the measurement of head circumference. The measurement should be done at the occipitofrontal circumference at largest point and approximately at some time each day and in centimeter. Other important aspects of assessment are status of fontanel, level of consciousness, pupillary response, vital signs, and pattern of respiration, signs of increased ICP, condition of the scalp, presence of pressure sore or any skin breakdown, incontinence of bladder and bowel, neurological deficits, motor activity, change in feeding behavior and signs of complications.

Nursing diagnoses: The important nursing diagnoses are:
1. Altered cerebral tissue perfusion related to increased ICP.
2. Altered nutrition, less than body requirement related to reduce oral intake and vomiting.
3. Risk for impaired skin integrity related to enlarged head.
4. Anxiety related to the abnormal condition and surgical interventions.
5. Risk for infection related to introduction of infecting organism through the shunt.
6. Risk for fluid volume deficit related to CSF drainage.
7. Ineffective family coping related to life threatening problem of infant.

Nursing interventions
1. Maintaining cerebral perfusion by assessment and management of increased ICP and assisting in/ diagnostic procedures to detect the exact pathology and administering treatment schedule as indicated.
2. Providing adequate nutrition by exclusive breastfeeding to the neonates and the infants up to 4–6 months of age. For older children, offering small frequent feeding and placing the infant or child in semi sitting position with elevation of head during and after the feeding.
3. Maintaining skin integrity by preventing pressure on the enlarged head with thinned skull and scalp. Firm- soft pillow under child's head, frequent change of position and keeping the area clean and dry are important measures. Good skin care and range of motion exercise are also essential to prevent skin breakdown.
4. Reducing parental anxiety by explanation reassurance and encouraging expressing feeling.
5. Preventing infections by aseptic technique, frequent hand washing of caregivers, maintaining general cleanliness, giving eye care and mouth care and administering antibiotics as prescribed.

6. Maintaining fluid balance by I/V fluid therapy, intake output chart, nasogastric tube feeding or oral feeding as indicated.
7. Strengthening family coping by teaching daily care of V–P shunt, as needed for the particular shunt, like pumping the shunt, positioning the child as directed (initially flat to prevent excessive CSF drainage then gradual elevation of head of child's bed to 30–45 degree) and assessing for excessive drainage of CSF (sunken fontanel, agitaion, decreased level of consciousness). Parents should also be informed about the signs of increased ICP, which indicate shunt malfunctions. Other necessary health teaching to be given to help the parents to cope with the stress situation and to provide continued home-based care with regular medical help.

SECTION-II

VI. Choose the correct answer and write

a. Circumcision is the surgical procedure performed for: **Ans: ii**
   i. Wilms tumor ii. Phimosis iii. Exstrophy of bladder
b. Vitamin-C deficiency causes: **Ans: iii**
   i. Night blindness ii. Rickets iii. Scurvy
c. Drug of choice for neonatal convulsion is: **Ans: iii**
   i. Valproate ii. Phenytoin iii. Phenobarbitone

VII. State whether the following statements are *true* or *false*

a. Blepharitis is a disease associated with throat condition: **FALSE**
b. Decreased platelet count is termed as thrombocytopenia: **TRUE**
c. Lardosis is the forward curvature of the lumbar vertebrae: **FALSE**
d. Decreased calcium level in the blood is called as hypoglycemia: **TRUE**

VIII. Write short notes on any *four* of the following:

a. Nursing care of a child with colostomy

A colostomy is a temporally or permanent opening of the colon through the abdominal wall. A placement of the colostomy will influence the nature of discharge from the colostomy. A stoma is a part of the colon brought above the abdominal wall in a colostomy.

Purpose: To provide outlet for an intestinal waste products.

Indications
1. As a lifesaving treatment for a newborn with an imperforate anus.
2. As a temporary measure to protect an anastomosis.
3. Inflammatory or obstructive processes of the lower intestinal tract.
4. Cancer of the rectum or sigmoid flexure where anastomosis is not possible.

Sites for colostomy and type of discharge
1. The ascending colostomy discharges fluid feces.
2. The colostomy near the hepatic flexure discharges semisolid feces.
3. The transverse colostomy discharges mushy feces.
4. The colostomy at the splenic flexure discharges semimushy feces.
5. The descending colostomy discharges solid feces.

Wet colostomy: A wet colostomy is that in which both urine and feces are excreted. Because of the transplantation of the ureter into the colon, this colostomy is never irrigated.

Double barrel colostomy: In double barrel colostomy, there are two openings, the proximal and distal segments of the colon. The proximal is functioning and a distal is irrigated to clean.

Postoperative care
1. Observation of a stoma and surrounding tissue is important.
   a. A stoma is deep and pink in color and moist with mucus. The stoma is soft or firm. A non-mature stoma will be friable. The peristomal skin should look healthy.
   b. The drainage characteristics and frequency should be noted. c. An abdominal distension may indicate an obstruction, and should be reported.
2. The frequency of irrigation depends on the site of the colostomy. The ascending colostomy is irrigated daily. The sigmodostomy is irrigated every two days. The first irrigation may be prescribed on the 4th - 8th postoperative day.

b. Management of a dehydrated child
Oral rehydration therapy for mild or moderate dehydration
Mild or moderate dehydration can usually be treated very effectively with oral rehydration therapy (ORT):
1. Vomiting is generally not a contraindication to ORT. If evidence of bowel obstruction, ileus or acute abdomen is noted, then intravenous rehydration is indicated.
2. Calculate fluid deficit. Physical findings consistent with mild dehydration suggest a fluid deficit of 5% of body weight in infants and 3% in children.
3. Moderate dehydration occurs with a fluid deficit of 5–10% in infants and 3–6% in children. The fluid deficit should be replaced over 4 hours.
4. The oral rehydration solution should be administered in small volumes very frequently to minimize gastric distention and reflex vomiting. Generally, 5 mL of oral rehydration solution every minute is well-tolerated. Hourly intake and output should be recorded by the caregiver. As the child becomes rehydrated, vomiting often decreases and larger fluid volumes may be used.
5. If vomiting persists, infusion of oral rehydration solution via a nasogastric tube may be temporarily used to achieve rehydration. Intravenous fluid administration (20–30 mL/ kg of isotonic sodium chloride 0.9% solution over 1–2 h) may also be used until oral rehydration is tolerated.
6. According to a Cochrane systematic review, for every 25 children treated with ORT for dehydration, one fails and requires intravenous therapy.
7. Replace ongoing losses from stools and emesis (estimate volume and replace) in addition to replacing the calculated fluid deficit.
8. An age appropriate diet may be started as soon as the child is able to tolerate oral intake.

Severe dehydration
1. Laboratory evaluation and intravenous rehydration are required. The underlying cause of the dehydration must be determined and appropriately treated.
2. Phase 1 focuses on emergency management. Severe dehydration is characterized by a state of hypovolemic shock requiring rapid treatment. Initial management includes placement of an intravenous or intraosseous line and rapid administration of 20 mL/kg of an isotonic crystalloid (e.g. lactated Ringer solution, 0.9% sodium chloride). Additional fluid boluses may be required

depending on the severity of the dehydration. The child should be frequently reassessed to determine the response to treatment.

As intravascular volume is replenished, tachycardia, capillary refill, urine output and mental status all should improve. If improvement is not observed after 60 mL/kg of fluid administration, other etiologies of shock (e.g. cardiac, anaphylactic, septic) should be considered. Hemodynamic monitoring and inotropic support may be indicated.

3. Phase 2 focuses on deficit replacement, provision of maintenance fluids and replacement of ongoing losses. Maintenance fluid requirements are equal to measured fluid losses (e.g. urine, stool) plus insensible fluid losses. Normal insensible fluid loss is approximately 400–500 mL/m^2 body surface area and may be increased by factors, such as fever and tachypnea. Alternatively, daily fluid requirements may be roughly estimated as follows:
   - Less than 10 kg = 100 mL/kg
   - 10–20 kg = 1000 + 50 mL/kg, for each kg over 10 kg
   - Greater than 20 kg = 1500 + 20 mL/kg, for each kg over 20 kg.
4. Severe dehydration by clinical examination suggests a fluid deficit of 10–15% of body weight in infants and 6–9% of body weight in older children. The daily maintenance fluid is added to the fluid deficit. In general, the recommended administration is one half of this volume administered over 8 hours and administration of the remainder over the following 16 hours. Continued losses (e.g. emesis, diarrhea) must be promptly replaced.
5. If the child is isonatremic (130–150 mEq/L), the sodium deficit incurred can generally be corrected by administering the fluid deficit plus maintenance as 5% dextrose in 0.45–0.9% sodium chloride. Potassium (20 mEq/L potassium chloride) may be added to maintenance fluid once urine output is established and serum potassium levels are within a safe range.
6. An alternative approach to the deficit therapy approach is rapid replacement therapy. With this approach, a child with severe isonatremic dehydration is administered 20–40 mL/kg of isotonic sodium chloride solution or lactated Ringer solution over 15–60 minutes. As perfusion is restored, the child improves and is able to tolerate an oral rehydration solution for the remainder of their rehydration. This approach is not appropriate for hypernatremic or hyponatremic dehydration.

c. Restraints

Mummy restraint: Used to restrain the entire body with a small blanket. Only the head is exposed.

Crib net: A net placed over the top of the crib and secured to the bed frame to keep the child from climbing or jumping out of the crib.

Papoose board: A plastic frame onto which the child can be strapped in almost any position. It is commonly used for circumcising infants. It is uncomfortable and should be used only for brief procedures, such as starting an IV.

Mitt or glove: Prevents the child from scratching or pulling on tubes.

Sleeve restraint: Tongue blades are inserted into a sleeve with long pockets and ties. The child's arm is slid into the sleeve, and straps are tied under the opposite arm. This device is used to keep a child from bending his or her arm, pulling on tubes or other devices, or disrupting a facial suture line.

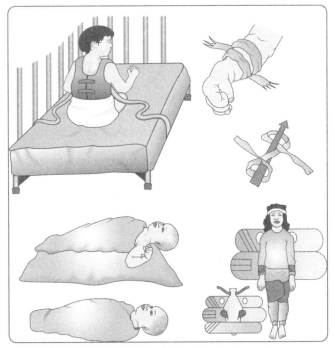
Types of restraints

Clove hitch or commercial wrist device—A Kerlix bandage or stockinette applied in a figure-8 knot, or a manufactured device, can be used to restrain one or more extremities.
1. Apply padding under the restraint.
2. Tie a knot so that device cannot become too tight.
3. Check the extremity every hour for circulation and signs of skin breakdown.
4. Remove restraints every 2 hours, and allow the child to exercise the extremity.

Arm boards: Used to protect intravenous (IV) sites.
1. Pad the board with a washcloth or small towel and fasten with tape.
   Rationale: The cloth will absorb perspiration and provide comfort. Also, the nurse can change and wash it if it becomes soiled.
2. Secure the arm board to the client's extremity after the IV is in place and secure.
   Rationale: Ensure the security of the IV even if the board needs removal.

Nursing care
1. Check the child's circulation to the arm each hour.
2. Loosen or reapply tape, as needed.
3. Document your findings.

d. Immunization schedule

Immunization schedule should be planned according to the needs of the community. It should be relevant with existing community health problems. It must be effective, feasible and acceptable by the community. Every country has its own immunization schedule. The WHO, launched global immunization program in 1974, known as Expanded Program on Immunization (EPI) to protect all children of the world against six killer diseases. In India, EPI was launched in January 1978.

The EPI is now renamed as Universal Child Immunization, as per declaration sponsored by UNICEF. In India, it is called as Universal Immunization Program (UIP) and was launched in 1985, November, for the universal coverage of immunization to the eligible population.

The Global Alliance for Vaccines and Immunization (GAVI) is worldwide coalition of organization, established h-i 1999, to reduce disparities in lifesaving vaccine access and increase global immunization coverage. GAVI is collaborative mission of Govt., NGOs, UNICEF, WHO and World Bank. The GAVI and Vaccine Fund also adopted the objective of introduction new but under used vaccines in the developing countries, where the diseases like hepatitis-B and H influenza 'B' are highly prevalent.

National Immunization Schedule as recommended by Government of India for uniform implementation throughout the country was formulated. The schedule contents the age at which the vaccines are best given and the number of doses recommended for each vaccine. The schedule also covers immunization of women during pregnancy against tetanus.

Beneficiaries	Age	Vaccine	Dose	Rout	Amount
a. Infants	• At Birth (for institutional deliveries)	• BCG • OPV	• Single • Zero dose	• Intradermal • Oral	• 0.05 mL • 2 drops
	• At 6 weeks	• BCG (if not given at birth)	• Single	• Intradermal	• 0.1 mL
		• DTP-1 • OPV-1	1st 1st	Intramuscular Oral	0.5 mL 2 drops
	• At 10 weeks	• DTP-2 • OPV-2	2nd 2nd	Intramuscular Oral	0.5 mL 2 drops
	• At 14 weels	• DTP-3 • OPV-3	3rd 3rd	Intramuscular Oral	0.5 mL 2 drops
	• At 9 months	• Measles	Single	Subcutaneous	0.5 mL
b. Children	• At 16-24 months	• DTP • OPV	Booster Booster	Intramuscular Oral	0.5 mL 2 drops
	• At 5-6 years	• DT	Single Intramuscular 0.5 mL *second dose of DT should be given after 4 weeks, if not vaccinated previoulsly with DTP		
	• At 10-16 years	• TT	Single intramuscular 0.5 mL *seocnd dose of TT should be given if not vaccinated previously		
c. Pregnant women	• Early in pregnancy • One month after	• TT-1 • TT-2	1st 2nd	Intramuscular Intramuscular	0.5 mL 0.5 mL

Note:
1. Interval between 2 doses should not be less than one month.
2. Minor cough, colds and mild fever or diarrhea are not a contraindication to vaccination.
3. In some states hepatitis 'B' vaccine is given as routine immunization.
4. Interruption of the schedule with a delay between doses not interferes with the final immunity achieved. There is no basis for the mistaken belief, that if a second or third dose in an immunization is delayed, the immunization schedule must be started all over again. So, if the child missed a dose, the whole schedule need not be repeated again.

e. Importance of Play

As children develop they will move from individual play to group play. How an older child chooses to play may depend on how they feel at the moment or a personal preference. The way most children play usually varies from day to day and situation to situation.

There are three basic forms of play:

Solitary play: Babies usually like to spend much of their time playing on their own. They are exploring all aspects of their environment from the sound of their own voice and the feel of their own body parts to those of others. They want to gaze upon, grab, suck and rattle any object that comes their way. Older children at times will also prefer to play on their own. They may spend hours making up stories with their GI Joes or Barbie Dolls. They like to build, draw, paint, invent and explore by themselves. They hopefully will also like to read and even write on their own.

Parallel play: From the age of two to about three, children move to playing alongside other children without much interaction with each other. They may be engaged in similar activities or totally different activities but they like being around others their own age. Even though it may appear that they don't care about the presence of the other children, just try separating them and you will see this contact from a far is very important to them.

Group play: By the age of three, children are ready for preschool. They are potty trained, able to communicate and socialize with others. They are able to share ideas and toys. Through interactive play they begin to learn social skills such as sharing and taking turns. They also develop the ability to collaborate on the "theme" of the play activity. The children not adults should institute play themes and structure. Adults should only intervene when children exhibit the need for coaching on social and problem solving skills. Finally, children also like to play with adults. This can be one to one or in a group. It is important that parents spend time playing with their children. It is fun. Let the kids set the pace and become a part of their world. No need to teach or preach, just enjoy the experience.

IX. a. Define glomerulonephritis.
b. Enumeate the signs and symptoms of glomerulo nephritis.
c. Discuss the management of a child with glomerulonephritis

Acute glomerulonephritis is a noninfectious renal disease found more in male children than in the female children. It is more common in the age group of 2–10 years. It is an immune complex disease, due to antigen antibody reaction following hemolytic streptococcal infection. The antibodies affect the glomerulus causing proliferation and swelling of endothelial cells obstructing the blood flow through capillaries. The amount of the glomerular infiltrate is reduced and it allows the passage of the blood cells and proteins into filtrate.

Etiology
1. Antigen antibody reaction secondary to an infection elsewhere in the body.
2. Initial infection of (upper respiratory system or skin) most frequently a beta hemolytic *Streptococcus* and other bacterias and viruses.

Pathophysiology
1. Antibodies produced to fight the invading organism also react against the glomerular tissue
2. The antigen antibody combination results in an inflammatory reaction I the kidney.

3. General vascular disturbances, including loss of capillary integrity and spasm of arterioles, are secondary to kidney changes and are responsible for much of the symptomatolgy of the disease.

Manifestation: An onset is usually, one to three weeks after the onset of infection of the upper respiratory tract or infection of the skin. Edema starts with the periorbital edema, in the morning. Urine output is decreased, with the high color urine resembling black tea or cola (due to lysis red blood cells).
1. Hypertension may be present.
2. The fever may or may not be present.
3. Children look pale, lethargic, and irritable.
4. Children may complain of a headache.
5. Gastrointestinal disturbances may occur.

Investigation
1. Urine examination for—hematuria, specific gravity, albumin, white blood cells and epithelial cells.
2. Blood examination for—urea nitrogen and creatinine, serum albumin.
3. Antistreptolysin 0 titer (ASLO).
4. Electrocardiography.

Complication
1. Hypertension
2. Hypertensive encephalopathy may occur when the diastolic blood pressure rises above 110 mm of Hg. It can cause vomiting, restlessness, convulsions, stupor, visual disturbances, or cranial nerve palsy.
3. Cardiac failure with the retention of salt and water may cause tachycardia, dyspnea, pulmonary edema, and enlargement of the heart.
4. Renal failure may occur with severe oliguria or anuria and increased blood pressure.
5. It may occur in two phases:
   – First phase: This stage of edema with oliguria may last for 5–10 days.
   – Second stage: The stage of diuresis starts with the increased output of urine and decreased edema.

Treatment
1. There is no specific treatment for acute glumerulonephritis.
2. It is self limiting and patients recover within two to three weeks.
3. Death may be due to complications.
4. Supportive treatment:
   – Antibiotics, such as, long acting penicillin may be given to treat reminent of the infection.
   – Hypotensive drugs may be prescribed to control the hypertension.
   – Magnesium sulphate may be prescribed - in the encephalopathy to reduce cerebral edema.
   – Sedatives may be required in restless patients.
5. In cardiac failure, digitalis may be prescribed.
6. In renal failure, patients may need a dialysis.

Management
1. Rest may be required for two to four weeks. Gradually, the activities may be started as the children improve.

2. The vital signs should be observed to detect early signs of complications, such as, the deviation in the pulse, may indicate cardiac failure. Headache, convulsions, and behavioral changes may be indicative of hypertensive encephalopathy.
3. Observation of the intake and output is important. An accurate recording of daily weight, edema, and appearance of the urine is necessary.
4. Nutrition should be planned according to the blood reports in the specific stage.
    a. In mild cases, salt restricted regular food may be allowed. Salty food items should be avoided. In an early phase of oliguria, the food should contain low proteins, high carbohydrates and vitamin supplement. Small, frequent feeding should be given. Fluid should be supplied according to the prescription. The parents should be explained about the accurate fluid intake.
    b. During the second phase, when the diuresis starts, the normal food with the adequate fluids, fruits can be given, as the blood reports improve.
5. Recreational facilities and play in the bed, can help divert the children's mind.

Parental advice
1. Parents should be taught about the early signs of complications and importance of early treatment.
2. Proper care of the skin and timely treatment of the skin lesions should be explained.
3. Prompt care of the respiratory problems should be insisted.
4. Parents should be instructed about the followup visits.

Nursing care
1. Maintain bed rest during the acute phase of the illness
2. Protect the child from infection
3. Provide adequate diet recommended
4. Maintain a complete record of the child's intake and output
5. Weigh the child daily
6. Record B/P at regular interval
7. Observe for signs of complication (edema, vomiting..)
8. Record appearance of urine.

X. a. Define encephalitis. b. List the clinical manifestations of encephalitis. c. Explain the nursing management of a child with encephalitis.

Encephalitis is defined as an inflammatory process of the central nervous System with dysfunction of brain. It is an acute inflammation that is caused by viral infection.

Causes
  I. **Viral:** a. RNA virus, b. DNA virus, c. Arthropod borne, d. Rabies and lymphocytic choriomeningitis, e. Dengue fever.
 II. **Nonviral:** a. Richettsia, b. Fungi, c. Protozoa, d. Bacteria.
III. **Post-infections:** Typhoid, measles, mumps, rubella, pertusis.

Pathophysiology

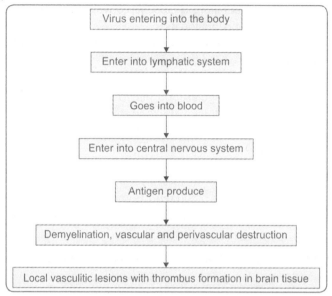

Clinical features
1. High fever
2. Headache vomiting
3. Mental confusion irritability
4. Apathy or loss of consciousness often associate with seizures
5. Sudden rise of intracranial pressure
6. Disturbance of speech
7. Neurological deficit, such as ocular palsy, hemiplegic and cerebellar syndromes, coma
8. Papilledema with brainstem dysfunction
9. Pupillary abnormalities, ptosis, sixth nerve palsy, ophthalmoplegia
10. Cheyne–Stoke breathing
11. Hyperventilation and bradycardia.

Diagnostic evaluation
1. History collection
2. Neurological examination
3. Lumbar puncture
4. CSF analysis
5. Polymerase chain reaction (PCR) on CSF
6. Stool, blood examination
7. ELISA
8. Brain biopsy
9. MRI
10. CT scan
11. EEG

Complications
1. Temporal lobe swelling which can result in compression of the brainstem.
2. Aphasia, major motor and sensory deficits.
3. Mortality and morbidity rate depend on the infectious agents, host status and other considerations.

Treatment
Symptomatic and supportive therapy
1. To reduce intracranial pressure
2. Mannitol IV -1 g/kg as a 20% solution administration should be rapid. Within 20 minutes, every 4–6 hours, not beyond 24–48 hours
4. To reduce cerebral edema e.g.: Acyclovir on suspicion of herpes
5. For treatment on suspicion of herpes, e.g. Acyclovir 10 mg /kg/dose IV every 8 hourly for 10 days.

Nursing management
1. Providing a quiet environment
2. Aspiration of nasopharyngeal secretions
3. Gavage or intravenous feeding
4. Oxygen administration
5. Oral hygiene
6. Provide skin care
7. Catheterization and enemas
8. Administration of medications
9. Parents must be helped to understand the needed of children
10. Adequate nutrition provision
11. Control the convulsions.

2015
Pediatric Nursing

SECTION-I

I. Give the meaning of the following:
   a. Hypothermia
   b. Asphyxia
   c. Toddler
   d. Weaning

II. State whether the following statement are *true* or *false*
   a. A preterm baby is born after 37 completed weeks of gestation
   b. The child starts to recognize the body parts at the age of 15 months
   c. The temporary teeth eruption starts at the age of 6 months
   d. Failure of testes to descend in the scrotum is known as hypospadias.

III. Write short notes on any three of the following:
   a. Nursing management of a child with cerebral palsy
   b. Immunization schedule
   c. Advantages of breastfeeding
   d. Principles of growth and development.

IV. a. Define pre-term baby
   b. Enumerate the causes and characteristics of pre-term baby
   c. Explain the nursing management of a pre-term baby
   Or
   a. Define PDA
   b. List the clinical manifestations of PDA
   c. Explain the nursing management of a child with PDA.

V. a. Define neonatal jaundice
   b. Explain the classification of neonatal jaundice
   c. Discuss the role of nurse in the care of a child with neonatal jaundice.

SECTION-II

VI. Choose the correct answer and write:
   a. Retinoblastoma is related to:
      i. ear   ii. Eye   iii. Nose
   b. Baby-friendly Hospital concept was launched by WHO in the year:
      i. 1997   ii. 1999   iii. 1991

c. Which vitamin deficiency is not seen in newborn:
   i. Vitamin C
   ii. Vitamin E
   iii. Vitamin K
d. The inflammation of joints is termed as:
   i. Fracture
   ii. Osteomyelitits
   iii. Arthritis

VII. State whether the following statement are *true* or *false*.
   a. Indian Red Cross Society is one of the child welfare agencies in India
   b. Infant is able to walk with support at the age of 6–8 months
   c. The 4-year-old child is not able to control bowel and bladder at nighttime

VIII. Write short notes on any *three* of the following:
   a. Nursing intervention of a child with colostomy
   b. Care of the visually handicapped child
   c. Nurses role in the administration of oxygen to children
   d. Child's reaction to hospitalization.

IX. a. Define tonsillitis
   b. List the causes, signs and symptoms of tonsillitis
   c. Explain the pre- and postoperative care of a child who undergoes tonsillitis.

X. a. Define encephalitis
   b. Enumerate the causes, signs and symptoms of encephalitis
   c. Discuss the medical and nursing management of a child with encephalitis.

SECTION-I

I. Give the meaning of the following:

a. Hypothermia
If the temperature falls below 95°F or 35°C, the condition is called hypothermia

b. Asphysia
Asphyxia neonatorum means non-establishment of satisfactory pulmonary respiration at birth. Its literal meaning is absence of pulse. It is clinically defined as failure to initiate and maintain spontaneous respiration following birth.

Clinical manifestations: Clinical features depend upon the etiology, intensity and duration of oxygen lack, plasma carbon dioxide excess and subsequent acidosis.

c. Toddler
The toddler period is usually considered from age 1–3 years, enormous changes takes place in the child and consequently, in the family. During the toddler period, the child accomplishes a wide array of developmental tasks. Promtiong toddler health and maintaining wellness involves knowledge of normal growth and development processes, an understanding of common significant milestones and the ability to anticipate deviations.

d. Weaning
Birth of a child in a family is a unique and important event in the life of a woman. There is nothing which gives the parents more happiness than a normal healthy child. To achieve this, the parents should have knowledge on feeding with clarity. Child's growth and development are rapid during the first year of life. So, it is more important that babies need extrafood along with breast milk at the right age and in sufficient amounts, to enable them to grow and stay healthy. An inclusion of semisolid foods along with Breastfeeding. Weaning excludes the formula feeding. Getting the baby accustomed to other foods from the age of fourth months along with breast milk.

Importance of weaning
1. Though breast milk is the best and safest food for an infant this can sustain the growth only for first three months and so breast milk alone cannot satisfy the growing infants on nutritional basis.
2. Storage of iron and vitamin A in liver gets used by three months and thus supplements are needed.
3. Taste buds, which at first are immature, become more sensitive to different taste.
4. In the second half of the first year, primary dentition begins as more solid diet provides a stimulus for chewing which helps new teeth to erupt.
5. Supplementary foods promote physical and cognitive growth and development.
6. Proper infant-nutrition prevents malnutrition by which infant mortality rate is reduced.

II. State whether the following statement are *true* or *false*
a. A preterm baby is born after 37 completed weeks of gestation: **FALSE**
b. The child starts to recognize the body parts at the age of 15 months: **TRUE**

c. The temporary teeth eruption starts at the age of 6 months: **TRUE**
d. Failure of testes to descend in the scrotum is known as hypospadias: **FALSE**

III. Write short notes on any *three* of the following:

a. Nursing managemt of a child with cerebral palsy

Cerebral palsy (CP) is a group of nonprogressive disorders resulting from malfunctions of the motor centers and pathways of brain. It is a noncurable and nonfatal condition due to damage of the growing brain before or during birth. It is the most common cause of crippling in children. It is severity is ranging from minor incapacitation to total handicap. Mental retardation is associated in about 25–50% of cases of CP. Other associated handicapped conditions are epilepsy, orthopedic deformities, partial or complete deafness, blindness and psychological disturbances.

Management: Management should be planned in a team approach. Coordination among team members is needed between pediatricians, pediatric surgeons, pediatric nurse specialist, physical therapist, occupational therapist, speech therapist, pediatric social worker, child psychologist, teacher, special educator, family members and parents. The holistic approach is required to achieve fullest possible functional ability and skill in keeping the child with developmental age. Management includes drug therapy, physiotherapy, and surgical corrections of deformities, occupational therapy and rehabilitation.

Drug therapy is indicated in symptomatic management for the child with CP. The commonly used drugs are diazepam for spasticity, strychnine for hypotonia, chlordiazepoxide or levodopa for athetosis, carbamazepine for dystonia, anticonvulsive for epilepsy, tranquilizers for behavioral problems and muscle relaxants to improve muscular functions.

Surgical correction may be needed for bony deformities and stabilizing the joints or relieving the contractures. Selective dorsal rhizotomy can be done to decrease spasticity. Orthopedic support can be provided by splints or orthotic devices. Physiotherapy is effective to prevent contractures, to promote relaxation of spastic muscles and for maintenance of posture. Occupational therapy can be arranged as some simple occupation (e.g. typing) so that when they grow up, they can earn something for their own. Positive application of certain repetitive movements of legs, hands and fingers can be used during occupational training which also helps to relax spastic muscles. The child should be trained in self care like feeding, dressing, bathing, brushing etc. Family support and community support are vital for socioeconomic rehabilitation of these handicapped children.

Nursing management: Nursing assessment should include the detection of ability to perform activities of daily living (ADL), developmental milestones, neurological reflexes feeding behavior, nutritional status, bladder and bowel habits, problem related to vision, hearing and language, associated health hazards or congenital anomalies, present problems, parent- child interactions, treatment compliance etc. Nursing diagnoses should be formulated accordingly to plan and to provide nursing interventions.

b. Immunization schedule

2016-VIII-D

c. Advantages of breastfeeding

1. Ideal composition. Helps in easy digestion for the baby.
2. Breast milk contains a number of protective factors. Breastfed babies are less likely to develop infections like diarrhea and respiratory infections.

3. Breast milk is readily available, usually sterile.
4. It is convenient, requiring no preparation and costs nothing.
5. It protects against allergies like asthma.
6. It has a laxative action for the baby.
7. It enhances emotional bonding between the mother and the baby.
8. Breastfeeding acts as a natural contraceptive. Chance of conception is less during lactation period.
9. Helps in involution of uterus.
10. Breastfed babies have a higher IQ and have less chance of developing hypertension, diabetes mellitus, coronary heart disease, liver disease and cancer in later life.
11. For mother, Breastfeeding reduces the risk of breast and ovarian cancer.
12. Breastfeeding saves money and time and conserves energy.
13. The family and society spend less on milk, health care and illness.

d. Principles of growth and development

1. **Development is orderly and sequential:** Development begins step and can be foreseen what will be the next from birth to one year there occurs a rapid growth, e.g. the child first learns to fall on ventral side then it starts crawling, then it sit, stands with support then without support tries to walk with support and without support.
2. **Development becomes increasingly integrated and complex:** The development abilities start from simple and gradually go to complex state. For e.g.: Before a baby learn to walk, it first crawls, then sit, stands with support, stand without support.
3. **Children are competent:** Children want them to be accepted, each child has its own ability, and they always try to achieve their needs. For example, it the child see an attractive toy in the stop somehow he would show temper tantrums to get the toy and try to possess the same. The child shows the ability in getting things done by showing the talent which is different in each child.
4. **Development involves changes:** As the development progresses the child undergoes change in all aspect, such as physical, psychological, social, spiritual, etc.
5. **Early developments is more critical than later development:** In the early stage, the child learns all skills from their parents, e.g. toilet training is not given properly, child in future will have eliminations problems like constipation.

IV. a. Define pre-term baby. b. Enumerate the causes and characteristics of preterm baby. c. Explain the nursing management of a preterm baby

In humans, preterm birth (Latin: *partus praetemporaneus* or *partus praematurus*) refers to the birth of a baby of less than 37 weeks gestational age. The cause for preterm birth is in many situations elusive and unknown; many factors appear to be associated with the development of preterm birth, making the reduction of preterm birth a challenging proposition.

Definition: Preterm labor is defined as the presence of uterine contractions of sufficient frequency and intensity to effect progressive effacement and dilation of the cervix prior to term gestation (between 20 and 37 weeks).

Causes of preterm labor
1. **Infection:** About 40–50% of all preterm labor can be traced to infection. Many women do not show classic signs of infection like fevers.

2. **Bleeding:** This does include placental abruption, where the placenta tears away from the uterine wall too early. It also includes bleeding disorders that may be genetic or acquired.
3. **Stretching of the uterus:** The stretching or overdistension of the uterus has also been linked to preterm labor and birth. This can be caused by fibroids, multiple pregnancies (twins, triplets, etc.), or even having too much amniotic fluid (polyhydramnios).
4. **Maternal factors:** Low socioeconomic status, maternal age ≤18 or ≥40 years, low prepregnancy weight, smoking, substance abuse.
5. **Maternal history:** Previous history of preterm delivery and second-trimester abortion.
6. **Uterine factors:** Uterine volume increased, uterine anomalies Trauma and Infection.

Signs and Symptoms

1. **More than 6 contractions per hour:** It is normal for the uterus to contract, or tightens, as the pregnancy progresses. Contractions that happen more than about every 10 minutes, though could be a sign of premature labor.
2. **Change in vaginal discharge:** Mother notice that there is leaking clear, watery fluid or if has any bloody discharge later weeks of pregnancy, inform the doctor know right away, mother may have preterm premature rupture of membranes (PPROM) or bloody show from early labor.
3. **Cramping:** Early labor mother may feel like the abdominal cramps (with or without diarrhea) may also be a sign of premature labor.
4. **Backache:** A low backache may be a sign of premature labor. The backache may come and go or be steady, and is usually a dullache.
5. **Pelvic pressure:** Women in premature labor may feel low-down pelvic pressure, as if the baby is pressing down on the cervix.
    a. Low back pain
    b. Suprapubic pressure
    c. Vaginal pressure
    d. Rhythmic uterine contractions
    e. Cervical dilation and effacement
    f. Possible rupture of membranes
    g. Expulsion of the cervical mucus plug
    h. Bloody show.

Warning signs.

1. Contractions every 10 minutes or more often
2. Change in vaginal discharge (leaking fluid or bleeding from your vagina)
3. Pelvic pressure–the feeling that your baby is pushing down
4. Low, dull backache
5. Cramps that feel like menstrual period pain
6. Abdominal cramps with or without diarrhea.

Factors associated with increasing rates of preterm birth

1. Increasing rates of multifetal pregnancies
2. Greater percentage of births to women of advanced maternal age
3. Increasing rates of asymptomatic infections, labor inductions, cesarean births and scheduled births
4. Advances in maternal–fetal management.

Management of Preterm Labor
Labor is judged to have started when the woman experiences regular, painful uterine contractions accompanied by either show, rupture of membranes or complete effacement of the cervix. The principles in the management of preterm labor are: (i) To prevent asphyxia, which makes the neonate more susceptible to RDS, (ii) To prevent birth trauma.

First Stage
1. The woman is put to bed to prevent early rupture of membranes.
2. Oxygen is given by mask to ensure adequate fetal oxygenation.
3. Strong sedatives or acceleration of labor is to be avoided. Epidural analgesia is the choice.
4. Progress of labor should be monitored clinically or (preferably) by electronic monitoring.
5. In case of delay or anticipating a tedious traumatic vaginal delivery, it is better to deliver by cesarean section.

Second Stage
1. The birth should be gentle and slow to avoid rapid compression and decompression of fetal head.
2. Liberal episiotomies should be done under local anesthesia, especially in primigravidae to minimize head compression.
3. Tendency to delay must be curtailed by low forceps.
4. The cord must be clamped immediately at birth to prevent the development of hypervolemia and hyperbilirubinemia.
5. To place the baby in the intensive neonatal care unit under the care of a neonatologist. Preterm fetuses before 34th week presented by breech are generally delivered by cesarean section.

Immediate Management of the Preterm Baby Following Birth
1. The cord is to be clamped quickly to prevent hypervolemia and development of hyperbilirubinemia.
2. The cord length should be about 10–12 cm in case exchange transfusion will be required due to hyperbilirubinemia.
3. The air passage should be cleared of mucus promptly and gently. The stomach contents are also to be sucked out.
4. Adequate oxygenation must be provided.
5. The baby should be wrapped in a sterile warm blanket or towel or laid in the warmer with the head slightly lowered (Temperature 36.5°–37.5°C).
6. Vitamin K 1 mg to be injected intramuscularly to prevent hemorrhagic manifestations.
7. Bathing is not appropriate for the preterm baby.
Preterm babies are functionally immature and need special care for their survival.

Or

a. Define PDA. b. List the clinical manifestations of PDA. c. Explain the nursing management of a child with PDA.

It is the persistent vascular connection between the pulmonary artery and the aorta. Functionally, the closure of ductus arteriosus (which is normally present in fetal life) occurs soon after birth. When ductus arteriosus remains patent and open after birth, the blood flows in the ductus from the aorta to the pulmonary artery due to higher pressure in the aorta. PDA is common in preterm infants who weigh less than 1.5 kg. It is the more common type in female baby and occurs approximately 11% of all CHDs.

Pathophysiology: In PDA, there is left to right shunt as blood flows from aorta (higher pressure) to pulmonary artery (lower pressure) leading to pulmonary overload. Thus oxygenated blood of systemic circulation flows back to pulmonary circulation resulting in increased vascular pressure in the pulmonary tree and volume load on left heart. In severe degree PDA, pulmonary vascular disease and pulmonary hypertension may occur.

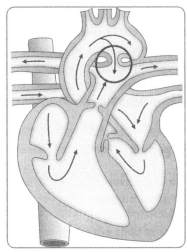

Patient ductus arteriosus

Clinical manifestations: The clinical presentations of PDA depend upon the size of ductus and its patency. Small and moderate size PDA is usually asymptomatic. Symptomatic cases manifested with tachypnea, bounding pulse and corrigan pulsation in the neck. Dyspnea and frequent respiratory infections usually found. There is increased systolic pressure and low diastolic pressure with wide pulse-pressure. Precordial pain, hoarseness of voice, feeding difficulties, slow weight gain or growth failure and CCF are common features of a child with PDA.

Diagnostic evaluation: History of illness and physical examination help in diagnostic evaluation. Auscultation of heart sound reveals continuous murmur (machinery murmur) heard at second left intercostal space or below the left clavicle or lower down, i.e. at left sternal border. There may be paradoxical spiltting of P2. Chest X-ray shows cardiomegaly and increased pulmonary vascular marking. Two-dimensional ecocardiogram with Doppler study and color flow mapping and cardiac catheterization can also be done to detect the extent of problems. ECG reveals left arterial dilation and left ventricular hypertrophy.

Management
1. **Medical management:** In symptomatic patient with PDA, indomethacin, 0.1–0.25 mg/kg/dose I/V over 30 minutes very slowly is administered, every 12–24 hours for 3 doses, for pharmacological closure of ductus arteriosus. Antiprostaglandin agents, aspirin and mefanemic acid can also be used. Supportive care is provided with rest, adequate intake of calorie for weight gain and promotion of normal growth and development with routine care. Emotional support to the parents is essential. Conservative management of CCF and other associated complications should be done with appropriate treatment.
2. **Surgical management:** Transection or ligation of patent ductus arteriosus via a lateral thoracotomy, a closed heart intervention is performed. It is done preferably between 3 and 10 years of age in asymptomatic patients and in symptomatic patients, it should be done irrespective of age and in the presence of pulmonary hypertension. The result of surgery is excellent. Preoperative and postoperative care for thoracic surgery to be provided with all precautions.

Complications: A child with PDA can have complications like CCF, infective endocarditis, pulmonary hypertension and pulmonary vascular occlusive disease. Rarely, calcification of ductus, thromboembolism, and rheumatic heart disease and Eisenmenger syndrome may develop.

V. a. Define neonatal jaundice. b. Explain the classification of neonatal jaundice. c. Discuss the role of nurse in the care of a child with neonatal jaundice.

Jaundice is the yellow discoloration of the skin caused by accumulation of excess of bilirubin in the tissues and serum. Neonatal jaundice becomes apparent at serum bilirubin concentrations of 5–7 mg/dL. Jaundiced shoulders and trunk indicates a level of 8–10 mg/dL. Jaundice of the lower body appears at 10–12 mg/dL and jaundice of the entire body at 12–15 mg/dL.

Definition: Jaundice is the yellow discoloration of the skin caused by accumulation of excess of bilirubin in the tissues and serum. Neonatal jaundice becomes apparent at serum bilirubin concentrations of 5–7 mg/dL. Jaundiced shoulders and trunk indicates a level of 8–10 mg /dL. Jaundice of the lower body appears at 10–12 mg/dL and jaundice of the entire body at 12–15 mg/dL.

Risk factors:
1. Birth trauma or evident bruising.
2. Prematurity
3. Family history of jaundiced siblings or hemolytic disease
4. Ethnic predisposition to jaundice or jaundice or inherited disease (incidence of pathological jaundice is more in Asian, African and Mediterranean male infants).
5. Delayed feeding or meconium passage.
6. Jaundice within the first 24 hours suggests hemolysis. Prolonged jaundice may indicate serious disease, such as hypothyroidism or obstructive jaundice.
7. Extent of changes in skin and sclera color.
8. Presence of lethargy, decreased eagerness to feed, vomiting, irritability, a high-pitched cry, dark urine or light stools.
9. Presence of dehydration, starvation, hypothermia, acidosis, hypoxia.

Types of jaundice

Causes of Physiological Jaundice
1. **Increased Red cell breakdown:** The newborns' red blood cells have a shorter life span (100 days in term infants and 60–80 days in preterm infants as opposed to 120 days in adults).

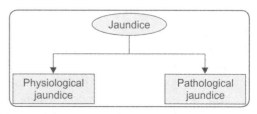

2. **Decreased albumin binding capacity:** The ability of neonates to actively transport bilirubin to the liver for conjugation is reduced because of lower albumin concentration, or decreased albumin-binding capacity. levels of unbound (free), unconjugated, fat soluble bilirubin in the blood rise as the binding sites on albumin are used up.
3. **Enzymes deficiency:** Newborn infants have low levels of uridendiphospho glucuronyl transferase (UDP-GT) enzyme activity during the first 24hours of life. UDP-GT is the major enzyme involved in bilirubin conjugation. Normal adult levels are not reached for 6–14 days.
4. **Increased Enterohepatic reabsorption:** Enterohepatic reabsorption of bilirubin is increased in neonates as they lack the normal enteric bacteria that break down bilirubin to urobilinogen

Diagnostic evaluation
1. Serum bilirubin to determine if the bilirubin is unconjugated or conjugated.
2. Direct Combs' test to detect the presence of maternal antibodies on fetal RBCs.

3. Indirect Combs' test to detect the presence of maternal antibodies in serum.
4. Hemoglobin/hematocrit estimation to assess any anemia.
5. Reticulocyte count (elevated with hemolysis when new RBC5 are being formed).
6. ABO blood group and Rheusus type for possible incompatibility.
7. Peripheral blood smear—red cell structure for abnormal cells.
8. White cell count to detect any infection.
9. Serum samples for specific immunoglobulins for the TORCH infections.
10. Glucose 6-phosphate dehydrogenase (G6PD) assay. Urine for substances, such as galactose.

Pathological jaundice: Pathological jaundice usually appears within 24 hours of birth arid is characterized by a rapid rise in serum bilirubin and prolonged jaundice. Cause of Pathological Jaundice: The underlying etiology of pathological jaundice is some interference with bilirubin production, conjugation transport and excretion.

Management: A number of treatment strategies are available to reduce bilirubin levels. These include:

Phototherapy: It can be used to prevent the concentration of unconjugated bilirubin in the blood from reaching levels where neurotoxicity may occur. During phototherapy the neonate's skin surface is exposed to high intensity light, which photochemically converts fat-soluble, unconjugated bilirubin into water soluble bilirubin, which can be excreted in bile and urine.

Exchange blood transfusions: Exchange transfusion is a lifesaving procedure in severely affected hemolytic disease of the newborn. An exchange transfusion process removes bilirubin from the body and in cases of hemolytic disease, also replaces sensitized erythrocytes with blood that is compatible with the mother's and infant's serum. Tan (1996) stated that phototherapy has largely replaced exchange transfusion when treating severe neonatal jaundice. Except in Rh incompatibility, exchange transfusion may now be seen as a second treatment of choice that is used only when phototherapy has failed. Exchange transfusion would certainly be considered when there is a risk of bilirubin toxicity or kernicterus.

Drug therapy: Drugs are used as an adjuvant therapy: (1) Phenobarbitone 2 mg/kg body weight is administered thrice daily intramuscularly for babies undergoing phototherapy. Phenobarbitone increases the glucuronyl transferase enzyme activity in the fetal and neonatal liver to conjugate the bilirubin, which hastens its clearance. (2) Antibiotics are administered for 3–5 days.

Nursing management of neonatal jaundice:
1. **Adequate feeding:** Early, frequent feeding helps newborns deal with their increased bilirubin load demand feeding ensures adequate volume of colostrums and milk in the intestine effective feeding encourages bowel colonization with normal flora and increased bowel motility, which in turn helps in production of enzymes needed for conjugation, and decreases enterohepatic reabsorption.
2. **Careful observation of newborns** will help distinguish between healthy babies with normal, physiological response (needing no active treatment) and those for whom serum bilirubin testing is required.
3. **In premature babies,** rising bilirubin level to critical level require use of phototherapy or phenobarbitone administration.

SECTION-II

VI. Choose the correct answer and write:
a. Retinoblastoma is related to: **Ans: ii**
   i. Ear   ii. Eye   iii. Nose
b. Baby-friendly hospital concept was launched by WHO in the year: **Ans: iii**
   i. 1997   ii. 1999   iii. 1991
c. Which vitamin deficiency is not seen in newborn: **Ans: i**
   i. Vitamin C   ii. Vitamin E   iii. Vitamin K
d. The inflammation of joints is termed as: **Ans: iii**
   i. Fracture   ii. Osteomyelitits   iii. Arthritis

VII. State whether the following statement are *true* or *false*
a. Indian red cross society is one of the child welfare agencies in India: **TRUE**
b. Infant is able to walk with support at the age of 6–8 months: **FALSE**
c. The 4-year-old child is not able to control bowel and bladder at night time: **FALSE**

VIII. Write short notes on any *three* of the following:

a. Nursing intervention of a child with colostomy:
2016/VIIIA

b. Care of the visually handicapped child
There are 4 levels of visual function, according to the International Classification of Diseases -10 (update and revision 2006):
1. Normal vision
2. Moderate visual impairment
3. Severe visual impairment
4. Blindness.

Moderate visual impairment combined with severe visual impairment are grouped under the term *"low vision"*: low vision taken together with blindness represents all visual impairment.

Facts about visual impairment
1. 285 million people are estimated to be visually impaired worldwide: 39 million are blind and 246 have low vision. about 90% of the world's visually impaired live in low-income settings.
2. 82% of people living with blindness are aged 50 and above.
3. Globally, uncorrected refractive errors are the main cause of moderate and severe visual impairment; cataracts remain the leading cause of blindness in middle- and low-income countries.
4. The number of people visually impaired from infectious diseases has reduced in the last 20 years according to global estimates work.
5. 80% of all visual impairment can be prevented or cured.

The causes of visual impairment
Globally the major causes of visual impairment are:
1. Uncorrected refractive errors (myopia, hyperopia or astigmatism), 43%
2. Unoperated cataract, 33%
3. Glaucoma, 2%.

People at risk: Approximately 90% of visually impaired people live in developing countries.

People aged 50 and over: about 65 % of all people who are visually impaired are aged 50 and older, while this age group comprises about 20 % of the world's population. with an increasing elderly population in many countries, more people will be at risk of visual impairment due to chronic eye diseases and aging processes.

Children below age 15: An estimated 19 million children are visually impaired. Of these, 12 million children are visually impaired due to refractive errors, a condition that could be easily diagnosed and corrected. 1.4 million are irreversibly blind for the rest of their lives and need visual rehabilitation interventions for a full psychological and personal development.

Signs of visual Impairment: Common signs that a child may have a visual impairment include the following.
1. Eyes that don't move together when following an object or a face.
2. Crossed eyes, eyes that turn out or in, eyes that flutter from side to side or up and down, or eyes that do not seem to focus.
3. Eyes that bulge, dance, or bounce in rapid rhythmic movements.
4. Pupils that are unequal in size or that appear white instead of black.
5. Repeated shutting or covering of one eye (as noticed with julian).
6. Unusual degree of clumsiness, such as frequent bumping into things or knocking things over.
7. Frequent squinting, blinking, eye-rubbing, or face crunching, especially when there's no bright light present.
8. Sitting too close to the TV or holding toys and books too close to the face.
9. Avoiding tasks and activities that require good vision.
10. If any of these symptoms are present, parents will want to have their child's eyes professionally examined. early detection and treatment are very important to the child's development.

The global response to prevent blindness: Globally, 80% of all visual impairment can be prevented or cured. Areas of progress over the last 20 years include:
1. Governments established national programs and regulations to prevent and control visual impairment.
2. Eye care services increasingly available and progressively integrated into primary and secondary health care systems, with a focus on the provision of services that are high quality, available and affordable.
3. Campaigns to educate about visual function importance and raise awareness, including school-based education, and
4. Stronger government leadership on international partnerships, with increasing engagement of the private sector.

WHO response: WHO coordinates the international efforts to reduce visual impairments? it is role is to:
1. Monitor the worldwide trends of visual impairment by country and by region.
2. Develop policies and strategies to prevent blindness appropriate for various development settings.
3. To give technical assistance to member states and partners.
4. To plan, monitor and evaluate programmes, and
5. To coordinate effective international partnerships in support of national efforts.

Vision impairment and nursing diagnoses: In assisting residents with these kinds of vision impairments, it is important to plan and also apply certain principles in order for the care to be effective. Vision loss is an hindrance in determining who might be entering the room, therefore, it is important to knock and identify one's self first before entering. This is to keep the resident informed and be able to know the person coming in. When placing the resident in a room, keep them well-versed of the surroundings and the organization of things inside, in order for the resident to visualize where he is and so he knows where to go and get the things he needs.

Nursing care for visual impairment: It is really important to pay special attention to impaired vision in nursing care plan. Some residents who still have little vision left need less attention; still the nurse should maintain the right lighting in order for them to use their available vision. When giving care or doing a procedure to the resident, explain it to them before doing it, in order to keep them aware of what is happening to them and encourage cooperation. Keep the bed in the lowest position possible, so that visually impaired residents will not have problems in going out of bed when they want to. Every person has fears of the unknown therefore explain noises that might be heard or sound different.

When feeding a resident with vision impairment describe each food and balance the pace of feeding to ensure safety and maintain appetite of the food. Give assistance while feeding, but also encourage them to be as independent as they can be. Let the residents feel the light switch before leaving the room so that they will be familiar where to locate it. When walking with the resident and assisting him, stand next to the resident but slightly be behind them in order to be cautious for possible fall of residents and be able hold them.

Use a gait belt: In order to securely hold the resident but make sure that the belt is properly placed around them. Use devices that can help improve the vision of residents, such as magnifying glass, eyeglasses and other reading devices and keep these equipments clean and in perfect condition. Any damage or loss of the devices should be reported to the nurse immediately

c. Nurses role in the administration of oxygen to children

A **nasal cannula** is a plastic tube, held in place over the victim's ears, with two small prongs that are inserted into the victim's nose. This device is used to administer oxygen to a breathing victim with minor breathing problems. Oxygen is normally delivered through a nasal cannula at a low flow rate of 1–6 LPM, giving about 25–45% oxygen. Nasal cannulas also can be used if the victim does not want a mask on his or her face. A **resuscitation mask** with an inlet valve may be used with emergency oxygen to give rescue breaths to breathing and nonbreathing victims. The recommended flow rate when using a resuscitation mask is 6–15 LPM.

A **non-rebreather mask** is an effective method for delivering high concentrations of oxygen to a breathing victim. Non-rebreather masks consist of a face mask with an attached oxygen reservoir bag and a one-way valve, which prevents the victim's exhaled air from mixing with the oxygen in the reservoir bag. Flutter valves on the side of the mask allow exhaled air to escape freely. As the victim breathes, he or she inhales oxygen from the bag.

Because young children and infants may be frightened by a mask being placed on their faces, consider a blow-by technique. The rescuer, parent or guardian should hold a non-rebreather mask approximately 2 inches from the child's or infant's face, waving it slowly side to side. This will allow the oxygen to pass over the face and be inhaled. Or the end of the tube from the tank can be placed next to or even *in* a toy/stuffed animal, and held close enough to the child's mouth/nose.

The **reservoir bag** should be sufficiently inflated (about two-thirds full) by covering the one-way valve with your thumb before placing it on the victim's face. If it begins to deflate when the victim inhales, increase the flow rate of the oxygen to refill the reservoir bag. The flow rate when using this device is 10–15 LPM.

A non-rebreather mask can deliver an oxygen concentration of 90% or more. A BVM can deliver up to 100% oxygen to a breathing or non-breathing victim when attached to emergency oxygen. Feeding a baby while in incubator.

d. Child's reaction to hospitalization

Hospitalization is the disruption of the lifestyle of children and their families. The children's reactions to the hospitalization and coping strength depend on the age, developmental stage, body image, fear, reason for hospitalization, and the previous experience about hospitalization. The change from home to hospital environment creates stress. The difference in hospital and home disturbs the child and adds to the stress, for example, environment, mealtime, toileting, feeding, bath time, and recreation. By understanding these factors, the nurse can explore the child's reaction, describe nursing care to provide safety, promote sleep and rest, manage sensory deprivation, relieve pain, give medications, and assist in other procedures.

Infants
Reactions:
1. Crankiness and irritability caused by a disruption, or change, in their normal routine.
2. Infants have an immediate reaction to pain or discomfort.
3. Infants may not be able to verbalize their feelings, but can show their feelings through their actions (withdrawing from interaction, eating or drinking less than usual, crying, sleeping more or less than usual).
4. Stranger anxiety usually begins at about 6 months of age; being separated from a caregiver can be extremely difficult for an infant in the hospital.

What you can do:
1. A favorite pacifier may provide some comfort
2. A familiar blanket
3. Soothing music

Toddlers
Reactions:
1. Fear of strangers
2. Separation anxiety
3. Toddlers often have an immediate physical response to pain and unfamiliar surroundings, such as crying.
4. A regression in established skills, for example, use of baby talk, wanting to be carried, or refusing to use the toilet.

What you can do:
1. A favorite blanket
2. A favorite stuffed animal
3. A familiar object may provide some comfort

Preschool-aged Children
Reactions:
1. Separation anxiety; fear of what might happen when a caregiver is not there.
2. Display increased magical or fantasy thinking; fear that hospitalization is a punishment or was caused by something that he or she did or did not do.
3. Fear usually regarding things that hurt, such as shots; that having a shot is a punishment.

4. Fear that an action caused the illness to occur, leading to feelings of guilt.
5. Regression of skills.

What you can do:
1. Reassure the child that nothing he did caused the illness
2. Avoid threatening tests or procedures as a punishment, this can cause a later avoidance of seeking medical care or not admitting discomfort for fear of additional pain
3. Participate in prehospital visit, when possible
4. Read books about visiting the hospital
5. Include the child in his or her care.

School-aged Children

Reactions:
1. Fear of pain; real or imagined.
2. Fear of loss of control; fear of inability to return to doing what he or she was able to do before hospitalization.
3. Fear of loss of respect; loss of respect of parents as being seen as weak or not as strong as one "should" be.
4. Fear of loss of love; fear of loss of love due to causing a disruption in the family's normal routine.
5. Fear of anesthesia; fear that if he or she goes to sleep that they may not wake up/loss of control due to anesthesia.
6. Fear of bodily injury, causing the child to question whether or not he or she will return to "normal" after the hospitalization.
7. Stress over separation from school and friends.
8. Concerns over loss of body privacy.

What you can do:
1. Encourage communication between school and child, dependent upon child's feelings and wants regarding friends' knowing private information.
2. Offer the child as much privacy as possible and as many choices as are reasonably available.
3. Read books about hospital visits.
4. Provide preparation on expected hospital experiences.
5. Include the child in his or her care.

Adolescents

Reactions:
1. Stress regarding separation from friends.
2. Fear of loss of status among group of friends.
3. Anxiety related to changes in physical appearance.
4. Anxiety related to long term illness.
5. Concern for privacy.
6. Regression can occur during uncomfortable situations.

What you can do:
1. Encourage communication between the adolescent and friends, dependent upon teen's feelings.
2. Provide accurate and honest information about their hospital experiences, this will help the teen to feel more comfortable knowing what to anticipate.
3. Encourage teens to participate in their own care.

IX. a. Define tonsillitis. b. List the causes, signs and symptoms of tonsillitis. c. Explain the pre- and postoperative care of a child who undergoes tonsillitis.

Tonsillitis is an infection of the tonsils. A sore throat is the most common of all tonsillitis symptoms. In addition, you may also have a cough, high temperature (fever), headache, feel sick, feel tired, find swallowing painful, and have swollen neck glands. The tonsils may swell and become red. Pus may appear as white spots on the tonsils. Symptoms typically get worse over 2–3 days and then gradually go, usually within a week. The picture below shows inflamed tonsils.

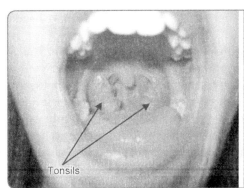 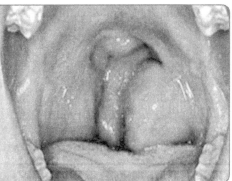

Causes

Tonsils are your first line of defense against illness, and they produce white blood cells to help the body fight infection. The tonsils combat bacteria and viruses that enter the body through the mouth, but are vulnerable to infection from these invaders themselves.

1. Tonsillitis can be caused by a virus, such as the common cold, or by a bacterial infection, such as strep throat.
2. Children come into close contact with others at school and play, exposing them to a variety of viruses and bacteria. This makes them particularly vulnerable to the germs that cause tonsillitis.

Clinical manifestations: There are many symptoms of tonsillitis, but you are unlikely to have them all. The most common include as follows:

1. A very sore throat
2. Difficulty swallowing or painful swallowing
3. A scratchy-sounding voice
4. Bad breath
5. Fever
6. Chills
7. Earaches
8. Stomach aches
9. Headaches
10. Stiff neck
11. Jaw and neck tenderness (due to swollen lymph nodes)
12. Tonsils that appear red and swollen
13. Tonsils that have white or yellow spots.

Diagnosis
Diagnosis is based on a physical examination of the throat and may include a throat culture. To take a throat culture, the doctor will gently swab the back of the throat and send the sample to a laboratory to identify the cause of the throat infection.

Management
1. **Not treating** is an option, as many tonsil infections are mild and soon get better.
2. **Have plenty to drink:** It is tempting not to drink very much if it is painful to swallow. The client may become mildly dehydrated if don't drink much, particularly if you also have a high temperature (fever). Some lack of fluid in the body (mild dehydration) can make headaches and tiredness much worse.
3. **Paracetamol or ibuprofen:** ease pain, headache, and fever. To keep symptoms to a minimum it is best to take a dose at regular intervals as recommended on the packet of medication rather than now and then. For example, take paracetamol four times a day until symptoms ease. Although either paracetamol or ibuprofen will usually help, there is some evidence to suggest that ibuprofen may be more effective than paracetamol at easing symptoms in adults. Paracetamol is usually the preferred first-line option for children, but ibuprofen can be used as an alternative. **Note**: some people with certain conditions may not be able to take ibuprofen. So, always read the packet label.
4. **Other gargles, lozenges, and sprays** that you can buy at pharmacies may help soothe a sore throat. However, they do not shorten the illness.

A mild case of tonsillitis does not necessarily require treatment, particularly if it is caused by a virus, such as a cold. Treatments for more severe cases of tonsillitis may include:

1. **Antibiotics:** Antibiotics will be prescribed to fight a bacterial infection. It is important that you complete the full course of antibiotics. The doctor may want you to schedule a follow-up visit to ensure that the medication was effective.
2. **Tonsillectomy:** Surgery to remove the tonsils is called a tonsillectomy. This was once a very common procedure. However, tonsillectomies today are only recommended for people who experience repeated tonsillitis, tonsillitis that does not respond to other treatment or tonsillitis that causes complications. Tonsillectomy, the surgical removal of masses of lymphoid tissue located in the back of the mouth, may have seemed like a childhood rite of passage for many children of previous generations. Tonsillectomy became a popular treatment for recurrent sore throats and respiratory infections as early as 1800s, and its frequency peaked in the United States in the late 1950s to the 1970s. Today, doctors are more conservative in recommending tonsillectomy.

Prevention: Tonsillitis is highly contagious. To decrease odds of getting tonsillitis, stay away from people who have active infections. Wash hands often, especially after coming into contact with someone who has a sore throat, is coughing, or is sneezing.

X. a. Define encephalitis. b. Enumerate the causes, signs and symptoms of encephalitis. c. Discuss the medical and nursing management of a child with encephalitis.

2016-X

2014
Pediatric Nursing

SECTION-I

I. Give the meaning of the following:
   a. Infant.
   b. Hernia.
   c. Daycare centers.
   d. Mongolian spots.
   e. Hyperbilirubinemia.

II. Fill in the blanks:
   a. Purulent discharge from the eyes of a newborn is known as: _____
   b. Child is able to hold head at: _____
   c. _____ is the failure of the esophagus to develop as continuous canal.

III. Write short notes on any *three* of the following:
   a. Concept of preventive pediatrics.
   b. Advantages of breastfeeding.
   c. Growth and development of a toddler.
   d. Spina bifida.

IV. a. Define hypospadiasis.
   b. Explain the surgical and nursing management of child with hypospadiasis.

   Or

   a. Define ventricular septal defect.
   b. List the clinical manifestation of VSD.
   c. Explain the nursing management of a child with VSD.

V. a. What is cleft lip and cleft palate?
   b. Write the signs and symptoms.
   c. Explain the treatment and nursing management of a child with cleft lip and cleft palate.

SECTION-II

VI. State whether the following statements are *true* or *false*:
   a. Lumbar puncture procedure is used to diagnose meningitis.
   b. The onset of disease for juvenile diabetes mellitus is before 5 years of age.
   c. Typhoid is caused by *Salmonella typhi*.

VII. Choose the correct answer and write:
   a. Scabies in children is caused by: _____
      (i. Mites, ii. Fungus, iii. Virus)
   b. Rubella can be prevented by administering: _____
      (i. MMR, ii. DPT, iii. BCG)
   c. Tetanus neonatorum is caused by: _____
      (i. *Staphylococcus*, ii. *Vibrio*, iii. *Clostridium tetani*)
   d. Mental retardation is suspected in children by: _____
      (i. Delayed milestone, ii. Poor feeding. iii. Normal milestone)

VIII. Write short notes on any *three* of the following:
   a. Oral rehydration therapy.
   b. Common worm infestation in children.
   c. Down's syndrome.
   d. Nursing management of a child with entric fever.

IX. A 10-year-old child is admitted with hemophilia:
   a. Define hemophilia.
   b. Explain the medical and nursing management.

Or

   a. Define nephritic syndrome.
   b. List the causes and signs and symptoms.
   c. Explain the nursing management of a child with nephritic syndrome.

X. a. What is otitis media?
   b. Write the signs and symptoms.
   c. Explain the treatment and management.

SECTION-I

I. Give the meaning of the following:

a. Infant
The term infant is typically applied to young children between the ages of 1 month and 12 months; however, definitions may vary between birth and 1 year of age, or even between birth and 2 years of age. A newborn is an infant who is only hours, days, or up to a few weeks old. In medical contexts, newborn or neonate (from Latin, *neonatus*, newborn) refers to an infant in the first 28 days after birth; the term applies to premature infants, postmature infants, and full term infants.

b. Hernia
It is an abnormal protrusion of an organ or a part of an organ, tissue through the structure that normally contains it. The causes of hernia are congenital, increased intra-abdominal pressure, muscle weakness (due to aging). The types are inguinal, indirect, femoral, umbilical, incision, and diaphragmatic hernia.

c. Daycare center
The scheme of Crèches/Daycare Centers extends daycare services for the children of casual, migrant, agricultural and construction laborers. Children of those women who are sick or incapacitated due to sickness or suffering from communicable diseases are covered under the scheme. This Central Sector Scheme which is being implemented through the medium of NGOs is a non-expanding scheme and is expected to be merged with the National Crèche Fund.

d. Mongolian spots
Mongolian spots are not cancerous and are not associated with disease. The markings may cover a large area of the back. Mongolian blue spots are sometimes mistaken for bruises. This can raise a question about possible child abuse. It is important to recognize that Mongolian blue spots are birthmarks, not bruises. The marking are usually: (1) Blue or blue-gray spots on the back, buttocks, base of spine, shoulders, or other body areas, (2) Flat with irregular shape and unclear edges, (3) Normal in skin texture, (4) 2–8 centimeters wide.

e. Hyperbilirubinemia
Hyperbilirubinemia is one of the most common problems encountered in term newborns. Historically, management guidelines were derived from studies on bilirubin toxicity in infants with hemolytic disease. More recent recommendations support the use of less intensive therapy in healthy term newborns with jaundice. Phototherapy should be instituted when the total serum bilirubin level is at or above 15 mg per dL (257 mol per L) in infants 25–48 hours old, 18 mg per dL (308 mol per L) in infants 49–72 hours old, and 20 mg per dL (342 mol per L) in infants older than 72 hours. Few term newborns with hyperbilirubinemia have serious underlying pathology. Jaundice is considered pathologic if it presents within the first 24 hours after birth, the total serum bilirubin level rises by more than 5 mg per dL (86 mol per L) per day or is higher than 17 mg per dL (290 mol per L), or an infant has signs and symptoms suggestive of serious illness. The management goals are to exclude pathologic causes of hyperbilirubinemia and initiate treatment to prevent bilirubin neurotoxicity.

II. Fill in the blanks:

a. Purulent discharge from the eyes of a newborn is known as: **Gonococcal conjunctivitis**
b. Child is able to hold head at: **6 months**
c. **Esophageal atresia** is the failure of the esophagus to develop as continuous canal.

III. Write short notes on any *three* of the following:

a. Concept of preventive pediatrics

Child health depends upon preventive care. Majority of the child health problems are preventable. Preventive pediatrics is a specialized area of child health comprises efforts to avert rather than cure disease and disabilities.

Preventive pediatrics has been defined as "the prevention of disease and promotion of physical, mental and social wellbeing of children with the aim of attaining a positive health". Pediatrics is largely preventive in its objectives.

Preventive pediatrics have been broadly divided into antenatal preventive pediatrics and postnatal preventive pediatrics.

Antenatal preventive pediatrics includes care of the pregnant mothers with adequate nutrition, prevention of communicable diseases, preparation of the mother for delivery, breastfeeding and mother craft training, etc. Prepregnant health status of the mother also influences the child health. Promotion of health of girl child and non-pregnant state should be emphasized as the future mother, who is soil and seed of future generation.

Postnatal preventive pediatrics includes promotion of breastfeeding, introduction of complementary feeding in appropriate age, immunization, prevention of accidents, tender loving care with emotional security, growth monitoring, periodic medical supervision and health check-up, psychological assessment, etc.

Another new concept of child healthcare is social pediatrics. The challenge of the time is to study child health in relation to community, to social values and to social policy.

Social pediatrics has been defined as "the application of the principles of social medicine to pediatrics to obtain a more complete understanding of the problems of children in order to prevent and treat disease and promote their adequate growth and development, through an organized health structure". It is concerned with the delivery of comprehensive and continuous child healthcare services and to bring these services within the reach of the total community. It also covers the various social welfare measures-local, national and international-aimed to meet the health needs of a child. To ensure adequate physical, mental and social growth of the child, total health needs should be provided as:

a. Healthy and happy parents.
b. Balanced and nutritious diet.
c. Clean, healthful house and living environments.
d. Developmental needs like play, recreation, love and affection, safety and security, recognition and companionship as emotional food.
e. Educational provisions and opportunities.

For the comprehensive services to the mothers and children, primary healthcare strategy is adopted by the healthcare delivery system. Government of India accepted a national policy for children in 1974 and implemented various health programs for preventive and social services along with curative care for the millions of children.

b. Advantages of breastfeeding

Breast milk is best for your baby, and the benefits of breastfeeding extend well beyond basic nutrition. In addition to containing all the vitamins and nutrients your baby needs in the first 6 months of life, breast milk is packed with disease-fighting substances that protect your baby from illness.

1. Research shows that breastfed infants have fewer and shorter episodes of illness.
2. Breastfeeding is the most natural and nutritious way to encourage your baby's optimal development.
3. Colostrum (the first milk) is a gentle, natural laxative that helps clear baby's intestine, decreasing the chance for jaundice to occur.
4. The superior nutrition provided by breast milk benefits your baby's IQ.
5. Breastfeeding is a gentle way for newborns to transition to the world outside the womb.
6. The skin-to-skin contact encouraged by breastfeeding offers babies greater emotional security and enhances bonding.
7. The activity of sucking at the breast enhances development of baby's oral muscles, facial bones, and aids in optimal dental development.
8. Breastfeeding appears to reduce the risk of obesity and hypertension.
9. Breastfeeding delays the onset of hereditary allergic disease, and lowers the risk of developing allergic disease.
10. Breastfeeding helps the baby's immune system mature, protecting the baby in the meantime from viral, bacteria, and parasitic infections.
11. Breastfeeding increases the effectiveness of immunizations, increasing the protection against polio, tetanus, and diphtheria vaccines.
12. Breastfeeding protects against developing chronic diseases such as: celiac disease, inflammatory bowel disease, asthma, and childhood cancers.

c. Growth and development of a toddler

The toddler period is usually considered from age 1–3 years, enormous changes takes place in the child and consequently, in the family. During the toddler period, the child accomplishes a wide array of developmental tasks. Promtiong toddler health and maintaining wellness involves knowledge of normal growth and development processes, an understanding of common significant milestones and the ability to anticipate deviations.

Physical Development

1. A child gains only about 5–6 lb (2.5 kg) and 5 inch (12 cm) a year during toddler.
2. Physical growth is slow during toddlerhood, this is because of the toddler's decline in appetite and erratic eating habits.
3. Head Circumference equals chest circumferences at 6 months to 1 year of age. At 2 years, chest circumferences are greater than of the head.
4. Toddler tend to have a prominent abdomen—a pouchy belly—because, although they are walking, their abdominal muscles are not yet strong enough to support abdominal contents as well as they will later.
5. They also have a forward curve of the spine at the sacral area (lordosis). As they walk longer, this will correct itself naturally.
6. The toddler waddles or walks with a wide stance, this stance seems to increase the lordotic curve, but it keeps the child on his or her feet.

Physiological Development

1. Brain growth continues slowly, corresponding to advancing intellectual skills and fine motor development.
2. Improved coordination and equilibrium parallels the most complete (by 2 years) myelination of the spinal cord as evidenced by refined walking, jumping and climbing.
3. Respirations slow slightly but continue to be mainly abdominal.
4. The heart rate slows from 110 to 90 bpm; blood pressure increases to about 99/64 mm Hg.
5. In the respiratory system, the lumen of vessels increases progressively, so that threat of lower respiratory infection is less.
6. Stomach capacity increases to the point that the child can eat three meals a day.
7. Stomach secretions become more acid, therefore, gastrointestinal infections also become less common.
8. Urinary and anal sphincter control becomes possible with complete myelincation of the spinal cord.
9. In the immune system, IgG and IgM antibody production become mature at 2 years of age, the passive immunity effects from intrauterine life are no longer operative.
10. The sense of hearing, smell, taste, touch and vision develop and begin to connect, since toddler utilize all fine senses to explore the world and exert autonomy and independence.
11. Bladder and bowel control is typically achieving during this time period and children are able to retain urine up to 4 hours before needing to void.

d. Spina bifida

Spina bifida is a neural tube defect—a type of birth defect of the brain, spine, or spinal cord. It happens if the spinal column of the fetus does not close completely during the first month of pregnancy. This can damage the nerves and spinal cord. Screening tests during pregnancy can check for spina bifida. Sometimes, it is discovered only after the baby is born.

During the first month of life, an embryo (developing baby) grows a structure called the neural tube that will eventually form the spine and nervous system. In cases of spina bifida, something goes wrong and the spinal column (the bone that surrounds and protects the nerves) does not fully close. Spina bifida is also known as split spine. The exact causes are unknown, but several risk factors have been identified, the most significant being a lack of folic acid before and at the very start of pregnancy.

The symptoms of spina bifida vary from person to person. Most people with spina bifida are of normal intelligence. Some people need assistive devices such as braces, crutches, or wheelchairs. They may have learning difficulties, urinary and bowel problems, or hydrocephalus, a buildup of fluid in the brain.

IV. a. Define hypospadiasis

Hypospadias is an abnormality of anterior urethral and penile development in which the urethral opening is ectopically located on the ventrum of the penis proximal to the tip of the glans penis, which, in this condition, is splayed open. The urethral opening may be located as far down as in the scrotum or perineum. The penis is more likely to have associated ventral shortening and curvature, called chordee, with more proximal urethral defects.

Hypospadias is a congenital defect that is thought to occur embryologically during urethral development, from 8–20 weeks' gestation. The external genital structures are identical in males and females until 8 weeks' gestation; the genitals develop a masculine phenotype in males primarily under the influence of testosterone. As the phallus grows, the open urethral groove extends from its base to the level of the corona. The classic theory is that the urethral folds coalesce in the midline from base to tip, forming a tubularized penile urethra and median scrotal raphe. This accounts for the posterior and middle urethra. The anterior or glanular urethra is thought to develop in a proximal direction, with an ectodermal core forming at the tip of the glans penis, which canalizes to join with the more proximal urethra at the level of the corona. The higher incidence of subcoronal hypospadias supports the vulnerable final step in this theory of development.

b. Explain the surgical and nursing management of child with hypospadiasis

Classification of hypospadias is done by the position of the urethral opening.
The types of hypospadias include:

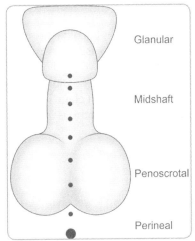

1. Distal or glanular—most common form when opening is found near the head of the penis.
2. Midshaft—when opening is found in the middle to the lower shaft of the penis.
3. Penoscrotal—when opening is on the scrotum.
4. Perineal—when opening is behind the scrotal sac. These are the most severe forms of hypospadias.

Surgical Management of Hypospadiasis

The goals of treating hypospadias are to create a straight penis by repairing any curvature (orthoplasty), to create a urethra with its meatus at the tip of the penis (urethroplasty), to re-form the glans into a more natural conical configuration (glansplasty), to achieve cosmetically acceptable penile skin coverage, and to create a normal-appearing scrotum. The resulting penis should be suitable for future sexual intercourse, should enable the patient to void while standing, and should present an acceptable cosmetic appearance.

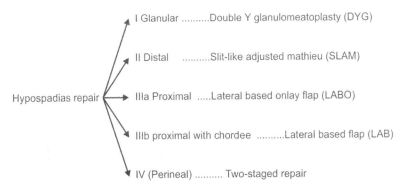

After fully assessing the penile anatomy, the shaft skin of the penis is degloved to eliminate any skin tethering, and an artificial erection is performed to rule out any curvature. Mild-to-moderate chordee may be repaired by excising any ventral fibrous tethering tissue or by plicating the dorsal tunics of the corporal bodies, compensating for any ventral-to-dorsal disproportion. More severe chordee may require grafting of the ventral corporal bodies using synthetic, animal (small intestinal subunit), cadaveric, or autologous tissues (tunica vaginalis or dermal grafts) to avoid excessive shortening of penile length. On rare occasion, the urethral plate may be tethered and transection of the plate may be required, precluding the use of native urethral tissues for urethroplasty.

The urethra may be extended using various techniques. These techniques are generally categorized as primary tubularizations, local pedicled skin flaps, tissue grafting techniques, or meatal advancement procedures.

The tubularized incised plate (TIP) repair has become the most commonly used repair for both distal and midshaft hypospadias. This technique is a primary tubularization of the urethral plate, with incision of the posterior wall of the plate, which allows it to hinge forward. This creates a greater diameter lumen than would otherwise be possible, obviating the routine use of a flap or graft to bridge a short narrow segment of urethral plate. The procedure has proved adaptable to various settings, and current surveys indicate that this is the procedure of choice for most repairs by most urologists.

Or

a. Define ventricular septal defect

VSDs - are a "hole" in the wall between the two lower chambers of the heart—the ventricles. This hole may be small, medium-sized or large, and may be single or multiple. The defect may occur in different parts of the muscular wall between the lower heart chambers, and may sometimes be found along with other heart defects.

The muscular wall between the lower heart chambers is meant to separate blood passing through each (i.e. "ventricle"). This separtion prevents unhealthy mixing of blue blood from the veins with red, oxygen-rich blood going to the arteries. When the muscular wall (i.e. septum) is incomplete or "broken", mixing occurs. In most situations, this leads to red blood passing across the defect and mixing with the blue blood on the right side of the heart. This is called a left-to-right-shunt and leads to abnormally high blood flow into the lungs. Just as in atrial septal defects (ASD), this causes frequent "chest colds" and breathing difficulty in children. When the VSD is large in a very small child, lung blood flow may be so enormous that the tiny ventricles cannot pump such a volume. This causes congestive heart failure. Heart failure in a child produces fast shallow breathing, excessive sweating, inability to feed well, irritability, constant crying, and a failure to grow at a normal pace.

b. List the clinical manifestation of VSD

Signs and symptoms of serious heart defects often appear during the first few days, weeks or months of a child's life. Ventricular septal defect symptoms in a baby may include:
1. A bluish tint to the skin, lips and fingernails (cyanosis)
2. Poor eating, failure to thrive
3. Fast breathing or breathlessness
4. Easy tiring
5. Swelling of legs, feet or abdomen
6. Rapid heart rate

Although these signs can be caused by other conditions, they may be due to a congenital heart defect.

c. Explain the nursing management of a child with VSD

The VSD, a communication allowing left-to-right shunting of blood at the ventricular level, is the most common congenital heart defect. Surgical correction is often required for large defects before the age of 12 months, and primary correction is now considered standard procedure. Small defects usually close spontaneously, and moderate defects are closely monitored for signs indicating the need for surgical intervention. Nursing care begins with child and family assessment and evaluation of the strengths and weaknesses of the family system. The child's developmental level is a major consideration in formulating interventions for his benefit.

Play therapy is a useful vehicle in relating to the child in a nonthreatening manner preoperatively and in allowing the child to work through his hospitalization postoperatively. Maintaining the physical integrity of a child just out of the operating room is a challenge. Continuing support of the family system is a significant aspect of nursing's responsibility toward child and family. Discharge planning and intervention strive to prepare the family for the transition from hospital to home both physically and emotionally.

V. a. What is cleft lip and cleft palate?

A cleft lip is a physical split or separation of the two sides of the upper lip and appears as a narrow opening or gap in the skin of the upper lip. This separation often extends beyond the base of the nose and includes the bones of the upper jaw and/or upper gum.

A cleft palate is a split or opening in the roof of the mouth. A cleft palate can involve the hard palate (the bony front portion of the roof of the mouth), and/or the soft palate (the soft back portion of the roof of the mouth).

Cleft lip and cleft palate can occur on one or both sides of the mouth. Because the lip and the palate develop separately, it is possible to have a cleft lip without a cleft palate, a cleft palate without a cleft lip, or both together.

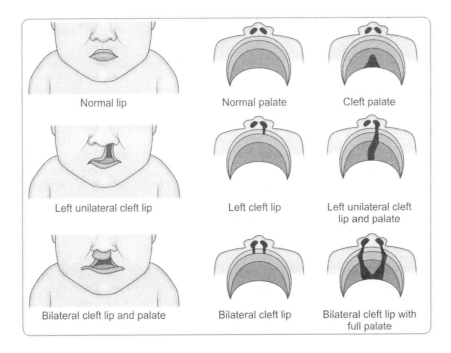

b. Write the signs and symptoms

A child may have one or more birth defects.

A cleft lip may be just a small notch in the lip. It may also be a complete split in the lip that goes all the way to the base of the nose.

A cleft palate can be on one or both sides of the roof of the mouth. It may go the full length of the palate. Other symptoms include:
1. Change in nose shape (how much the shape changes varies)
2. Poorly aligned teeth

Problems that may be present because of a cleft lip or palate are:
1. Failure to gain weight
2. Feeding problems
3. Flow of milk through nasal passages during feeding
4. Poor growth
5. Repeated ear infections
6. Speech difficulties.

c. Explain the treatment and nursing management of a child with cleft lip and cleft palate

Surgery to close the cleft lip is often done when the child is between 6 weeks and 9 months old. Surgery may be needed later in life if the problem has a big effect on the nose area. A cleft palate is usually closed within the first year of life, so that the child's speech develops normally. Sometimes, a prosthetic device is temporarily used to close the palate, so the baby can feed and grow until surgery can be done. Continued follow-up may be needed with speech therapists and orthodontists.

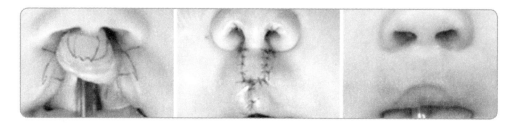

A cleft lip may require one or two surgeries depending on the extent of the repair needed. The initial surgery is usually performed by the time a baby is 3 months old.

Repair of a cleft palate often requires multiple surgeries over the course of 18 years. The first surgery to repair the palate usually occurs when the baby is between 6 and 12 months old. The initial surgery creates a functional palate, reduces the chances that fluid will develop in the middle ears, and aids in the proper development of the teeth and facial bones.

Children with a cleft palate may also need a bone graft when they are about 8 years old to fill in the upper gum line, so that it can support permanent teeth and stabilize the upper jaw. About 20% of children with a cleft palate require further surgeries to help improve their speech.

Once the permanent teeth grow in, braces are often needed to straighten the teeth.

Additional surgeries may be performed to improve the appearance of the lip and nose, close openings between the mouth and nose, help breathing, and stabilize and realign the jaw. Final repairs of the scans left by the initial surgery will probably not be performed until adolescence, when the facial structure is more fully developed.

SECTION-II

VI. State whether the following statements are *true* or *false*:
a. Lumbar puncture procedure is used to diagnose meningitis: **TRUE.**
b. The onset of disease for juvenile diabetes mellitus is before 5 years of age: **TRUE.**
c. Typhoid is caused by *Salmonella typhi*: **TRUE.**

VII. Choose the correct answer and write:
a. Scabies in children is caused by: **Fungus.** (i. Mites, ii. Fungus, iii. Virus)
b. Rubella can be prevented by administering: **MMR.** (i. MMR, ii. DPT, iii. BCG)
c. Tetanus neonatorum is caused by: **Clostridium tetani.**
   (i. *Staphylococcus*, ii. *Vibrio*, iii. *Clostridium tetani*)
d. Mental retardation is suspected in children by: **Delayed milestone.**
   (i. Delayed milestone, ii. Poor feeding. iii. Normal milestone)

VIII. Write short notes on any *three* of the following:

a. Oral rehydration therapy

Oral rehydration therapy (ORT) is a treatment response to dehydration which involves drinking water with small amounts of sugar and salt. When dehydration is severe, the therapy also includes supplemental zinc for two weeks, encouraging the dehydrated person to eat to speed recovery of normal intestinal functioning, and having family members and caretakers learn the signs of worsening dehydration. Oral rehydration salts (ORS) is a special drink that consists of a combination of dry salts. When properly mixed with safe water, the ORS drink can help rehydrate the body when a lot of fluid has been lost due to diarrhea. A child with diarrhea should never be given any tablets, antibiotics or other medicines unless these have been prescribed by a medical professional or a trained health worker. The best treatment for diarrhea is to drink lots of liquids and oral rehydration salts (ORS) properly mixed with water.

Steps in Preparing ORS
1. Purchase the required quantity of ORS. A sick infant should be given half liter of ORS drink per day, a child should be given one liter a day, and adults can consume up to two liters a day. Buy the necessary number of packets based on the calculated number of liters you'll be consuming; in most countries, ORS packets are available from health centers, pharmacies, markets and shops.
2. Put the contents of the ORS packet in a clean container. It is easiest to mix the ORS solution in a pitcher or bottle. Pour the necessary amount into your container, as per the package directions. diarrhea worse.

3. Add in your water. Slowly pour in cool or warm water to your container. Follow the measurements on the packet, so that you create the solution with the right proportion of water to solvent. Do not add ORS to milk, soup, fruit juice or soft drinks.
   Do not add sugar or other sweeteners and flavor enhancers.
4. Stir the solution. Use a spoon or whisk to mix the ORS powder into the water. After a minute or so of vigorous stirring, the solution should be completely dissolved. At this point, it is ready to be consumed.
5. Drink the ORS solution. Drink the ORS solution just like you would water or another fluid throughout the day. It is particularly important for sick children to drink enough of the solution, so as to balance their electrolytes and prevent further dehydration. Infants can be switched between breast milk and ORS solution throughout the day.

b. Common worm infestation in children

Worm infestation in children is very commonly seen in India. The common worm infestations are threadworm, round worm and hookworm. The child suffering from worms usually presents with the following symptoms.

Symptoms of worm infestations
1. The child complains of a stomach pain off and on after eating his food.
2. Lack of appetite and poor digestion.
3. Child looks weak and sick and anemic.
4. Sometimes a larger bunch of worms may block the intestinal tract and cause total constipation, abdominal distension and vomiting.
5. Itching round the anal region.

Diagnosis: The presence of infestation is diagnosed by the detection of ova (the egg of the parasite) in the stools. To avoid missing the diagnosis of worm infestation the stool samples of the child should be examined on three consecutive days.

Treating a child for worms gives us an opportunity to tell mother how to prevent the disease. Infective role of stools is to be emphasized. Washing of vegetable and roots in clean water, eating and preparing food with clean hands, water and proper excreta disposal are the most effective measures to control ascarias: periodic deworming (at 6 month interval) is no feasible for mass treatment. For enterobius infection, keeping the nails trimmed and clothes clean may prevent reinfection.

c. Down syndrome

Down syndrome (DS) or Down's syndrome, also known as trisomy 21, is a genetic disorder caused by the presence of all or part of a third copy of chromosome-21. It is typically associated with physical growth delays, characteristic facial features and mild to moderate intellectual disability. The average IQ of a young adult with Down syndrome is 50, equivalent to the mental age of an 8- or 9-year-old child, but this varies widely.

Body Shape and Size

1. Short stature (height). A child often grows slowly and is shorter than average as an adult.
2. Weak muscles (hypotonia) throughout the body. Weak belly muscles also make the stomach stick out.
3. A short, wide neck. The neck may have excess fat and skin.
4. Short, stocky arms and legs. Some children also have a wide space between the big toe and second toe.

Face Shape and Features

1. **Slanted eyes:** Tissue may also build up on the colored part of the eye (iris). But the child's vision is not affected by this buildup.
2. **A nasal bridge that looks pushed in:** The nasal bridge is the flat area between the nose and eyes.
3. **Small ears:** and they may be set low on the head.
4. **Irregularly shaped mouth and tongue:** The child's tongue may partly stick out. The roof of the mouth (palate) may be narrow and high with a downward curve.
5. **Irregular and crooked teeth:** Teeth often come in late and not in the same order that other children's teeth come in.

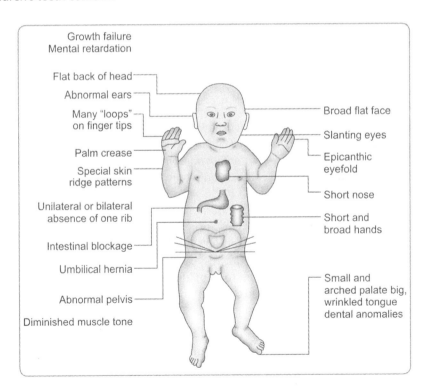

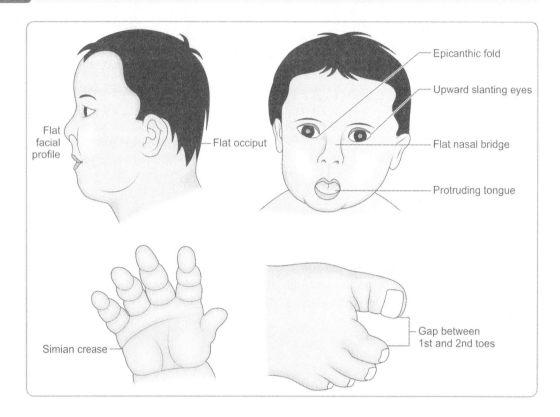

d. Nursing management of a child with entric fever

Typhoid and paratyphoid fevers—collectively known as enteric fevers—are bacterial infections. Typhoid is caused by the bacterium *Salmonella typhi*, while paratyphoid fever, which is usually a milder infection, is caused by *Salmonella enteritidis paratyphi* A, B and C. Unlike other *Salmonella* species, both *S. typhi* and *S. paratyphi* colonize only humans and can be acquired from either patients or carriers.

The diseases mainly affect those living in poorer regions of the world where sanitation and clean water are lacking. The World Health Organization (2000) estimates that typhoid fever affects 17 million people a year, causing approximately 600,000 deaths. Typhoid fever has a typical case fatality rate of 10%, but this can be reduced to as little as 1% with appropriate antimicrobial therapy. Paratyphoid fever is a similar illness but tends to be milder, with a lower case fatality rate. Effective prevention and control of imported typhoid or paratyphoid infections require an evidence-based risk assessment approach by nurses in primary care.

Primary care professionals should make every effort to:
1. Improve public understanding of the risk factors and trends of typhoid and paratyphoid infections.
2. Understand the potential threat to wider public health from typhoid and paratyphoid infections.
3. Monitor the effectiveness of prevention, including immunization against typhoid fever, by checking the health status of returning travelers.
4. Ensure that people who return after acquiring the infections from countries where they are endemic receive a high standard of primary and secondary care and have access to specialist advice when appropriate.

IX. A 10-year-old child is admitted with hemophilia.

a. Define hemophilia

Hemophilia is a bleeding problem. People with hemophilia do not bleed any faster than normal, but they can bleed for a longer time. Their blood does not have enough clotting factor. Clotting factor is a protein in blood that controls bleeding. Hemophilia is quite rare. About 1 in 10,000 people are born with it.

Types of hemophilia: The most common type of hemophilia is called hemophilia A. This means the person does not have enough clotting factor VIII (factor eight). Hemophilia B is less common. A person with hemophilia B does not have enough factor IX (factor nine). The result is the same for people with hemophilia A and B; that is, they bleed for a longer time than normal.

The signs of hemophilia A and B are the same:
1. Big bruises
2. Bleeding into muscles and joints
3. Spontaneous bleeding (sudden bleeding inside the body for no clear reason)
4. Prolonged bleeding after getting a cut, removing a tooth, or having surgery.
5. Bleeding for a long time after an accident, especially after an injury to the head.

Bleeding into a joint or muscle causes:
1. An ache or "funny feeling"
2. Swelling
3. Pain and stiffness
4. Difficulty using a joint or muscle.

b. Explain the medical and nursing management

Treatment for hemophilia today is very effective. The missing clotting factor is injected into the bloodstream using a needle. Bleeding stops when enough clotting factor reaches the spot that is bleeding. Bleeding should be treated as quickly as possible. Quick treatment will help reduce pain and damage to the joints, muscles, and organs. If bleeding is treated quickly, less blood product is needed to stop the bleeding. With an adequate quantity of treatment products and proper care, people with hemophilia can live perfectly healthy lives. Without treatment, most children with severe hemophilia will die young. An estimated 400,000 people worldwide are living with hemophilia and only 25% receive adequate treatment. The World Federation of Hemophilia is striving to close this gap.

Treatment Products

Factor concentrates are the treatment of choice for hemophilia. They can be made from human blood (called plasma-derived products) or manufactured using genetically engineered cells that carry a human factor gene (called recombinant products). Factor concentrates are made in sophisticated manufacturing facilities. All commercially prepared factor concentrates are treated to remove or inactivate blood-borne viruses.

Cryoprecipitate is derived from blood and contains a moderately high concentration of clotting factor VIII (but not IX). It is effective for joint and muscle bleeds, but is less safe from viral contamination than concentrates and is harder to store and administer. Cryoprecipitate can be made at local blood collection facilities.

In fresh frozen plasma (FFP) the red cells have been removed, leaving the blood proteins, including clotting factors VIII and IX. It is less effective than cryoprecipitate for the treatment of hemophilia A because the factor VIII is less concentrated. Large volumes of plasma must be transfused, which can lead to a complication called circulatory overload. FFP is still the only product available for treatment of hemophilia A and B in some countries.

Or

a. Define nephritic syndrome

Acute nephritic syndrome is a group of disorders affecting kidney by causing inflammation and pores in glomerulus which results in passage of red blood cells and excess proteins into the urine and restores excess fluid in the body.

b. List the causes and signs and symptoms

Acute nephritic syndrome is generally associated with immune response triggered by infection like pneumococcal, coxsackie virus or herpes zoster or other disease. The most common causes includes hemolytic uremic syndrome, Henoch-Schönlein purpura, IgA nephropathy, post-streptococcal glomerulonephritis, Abdominal abscesses, good pasture syndrome, hepatitis B or C, infective endocarditis, membranoproliferative GN I, Membranoproliferative GN II, SLE or lupus nephritis, vasculitis and few viral diseases like mononucleosis and measles.

Symptoms of Acute Nephritic Syndrome

The main symptom shown by acute nephritic syndrome patient is blood in urine (hematuria) and excess secretion of protein in urine (proteinuria). Apart from the above mentioned, a few other symptoms include:
1. Decreased or no urine (oliguria)
2. Elevated blood nitrogen (azotemia)
3. Swelling of body parts such as face, eye socket, legs, arms, hands, feet, abdomen, etc.
4. Blurred or abnormal vision
5. Cough having frothy material
6. Lack of attention
7. Confusion and drowsiness
8. Pain in muscles and joints
9. Malaise
10. Headache
11. Difficulty in breathing
12. Difficulty in movement
13. Hypertension
14. Renal insufficiency.

Prolonged condition may develop complications like chronic kidney failure, end-stage kidney disease, high blood pressure, congestive heart failure, pulmonary edema, chronic glomerulonephritis and nephrotic syndrome.

c. Explain the nursing management of a child with nephritic syndrome

The goal of treatment is to reduce inflammation in the kidney and control high blood pressure. The child may need to stay in a hospital to be diagnosed and treated. Treatment may include antibiotics or other medications or therapies.

Treatment of acute nephritic syndrome includes medication therapy and lifestyle modification which aim at reducing inflammation in the kidney and control high blood pressure.

Medication therapy may include corticosteroids or other anti-inflammatory medications, antibiotics and antihypertensive drugs prescribed by the doctor. Other supportive treatments such as regular blood tests and dialysis may be required. Home remedies include bed rest, reducing salt intake and inclusion of fluid and potassium in the diet.

Nursing intervention of nephritic syndrome
  I. Has proteinuria of more than trace:
   1. Daily morning urinalysis recorded when the urine is at its most concentrated to determine level of proteinuria. Ensure renal nurse is contacted to initiate discharge planning.
   2. Keep the morning sample in a universal container in case the doctor asks for a protein creatinine ratio (PCR) or urinary sodium (Na).
   3. A relapse is determined as $\geq 2+$ for 5 days or $\geq 3+$ for 3 days, and remission is determined as negative or trace for three consecutive days.
  II. Is prone to weight gain: Daily morning weight recorded with minimal clothing and empty bladder to determine real weight gain/loss (1liter fluid is equal to 1 kg of weight).
  III. Has edema
   1. Requires a no added salt diet (contact renal/pediatric dietician for advice) whilst edematous.
   2. Needs to be fluid restricted whilst edematous (contact renal/pediatric dietician for advice).
   3. Needs to have their lower limbs elevated when sitting to encourage vascular return.
  IV. Is at risk of hypovolemia
   1. 4 hourly (increase if concerned) blood pressure monitoring using appropriate cuff size (2/3rds of upper arm).
   2. 4 hourly (increase if concerned) heart rate.
   3. Strict fluid balance input versus output.
   4. Contact medical staff if signs of hypovolemia (tachycardia, cool peripheries, capillary refill time >2 sec). Hypotension is a late sign of hypovolemia. A urinary sodium < 10 mmol/L can confirm hypovolemia. An infusion of 4.5% human albumin 10 mL/kg over 30–60 minutes can be given if clinically shocked. An infusion of 20% human albumin 5 mL/kg over 4–6 hours along with 1–2 mg/kg IV furosemide mid infusion can be given if evidence of hypovolemia without shock.
  V. Is at risk of thrombosis: If clinical hypovolemia is suspected the child may be nursed with anti-embolism stockings.
  VI. Is at risk of infection
   1. Avoid infectious disease contacts. Nurse in a cubicle if immunocompromised.
   2. Prophylactic antibiotics (Penicillin V 125 mg if <5 years old or 250 mg >5 years old, twice daily) should be considered whilst significant proteinuria persists. This can be discontinued once in remission.
   3. Ensure skin condition is monitored daily if skin becomes red/warm/painful contact medical staff.
  VII. Is at risk pulmonary edema.
   1. 4 Hourly (increase if concerned) spot O_2 saturation levels and respiratory rate.
   2. Nurse in semi-recumbent position whilst sleeping to relieve respiratory distress and prevent fluid shifting to the lungs if grossly edematous.
  VIII. Is on steroids
   1. Ensure steroids are given with breakfast in the morning.

2. Ensure ranitidine (2 mg/kg twice a day) or omeprazole (10 or 20 mg daily) is prescribed with the steroids to prevent gastric irritation.
3. Support parents/child/carers when mood swings are present.
4. Contact renal dietician for support and education with increased appetite.

X. a. What is otitis media?

Otitis media (OM) is any inflammation of the middle ear without reference to etiology or pathogenesis. It is very common in children. There are several subtypes of OM, as follows:
1. Acute otitis media (AOM)
2. Otitis media with effusion (OME)
3. Chronic suppurative otitis media
4. Adhesive otitis media.

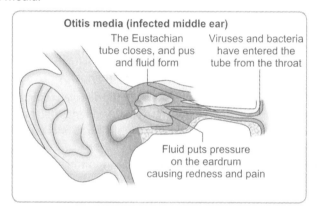

b. Write the signs and symptoms

An integral symptom of acute otitis media is ear pain; other possible symptoms include fever, and irritability (in infants). Since an acute otitis media is usually precipitated by an upper respiratory tract infection, there often are accompanying symptoms like cough and nasal discharge. Otorrhea, which is a discharge from the ear, can be caused by acute otitis externa, chronic suppurative otitis media, tympanostomy tube otorrhea, or acute otitis media with perforation. Acute otitis media (AOM) implies rapid onset of disease associated with one or more of the following symptoms: 1. Otalgia, 2. Otorrhea, 3. Headache, 4. Fever, 5. Irritability, 6. Loss of appetite, 7. Vomiting, 8. Diarrhea, Otitis media with effusion (OME) often follows an episode of AOM. Symptoms that may be indicative of OME include the following: 1. Hearing loss, 2. Tinnitus, 3. Vertigo, 4. Otalgia.

Chronic suppurative otitis media is a persistent ear infection that results in tearing or perforation of the eardrum.

Adhesive otitis media occurs when a thin retracted ear drum becomes sucked into the middle ear space and stuck.

c. Explain the treatment and management.

Treatment of an ear infection may include:
1. Antibiotics
2. Medicines to treat pain and fever

3. Observation
4. A combination of the above.

The "best" treatment depends on the child's age, history of previous infections, degree of illness, and any underlying medical problems.

Antibiotics: Antibiotics are usually given to infants who are younger than 24 months or who have high fever or infection in both ears. Children who are older than 24 months and have mild symptoms may be treated with an antibiotic or observed to see if they improve without antibiotics. Antibiotics can have side effects, such as diarrhea and rash, and overusing antibiotics can lead to more difficult to treat (resistant) bacteria. Resistance means that a particular antibiotic no longer works or that higher doses are needed next time.

Observation: In some cases, your child's doctor or nurse will recommend that you watch your child at home before starting antibiotics; this is called observation. Observation can help determine whether antibiotics are needed.

Pain management: Pain-relieving medicines, including ibuprofen (sample brand name: Motrin), acetaminophen (sample brand name: Tylenol), or ear drops that contain a numbing medicine, may be used to reduce discomfort.

Decongestants and antihistamines: Cough and cold medicines (which usually include a decongestant or antihistamine) have not been proven to speed healing or reduce complications of ear infections in children. In addition, these treatments have side effects that can be dangerous. Neither decongestants nor antihistamines are recommended for children with ear infections.

2013
Pediatric Nursing

SECTION-I

I. Give the meaning of the following:
   a. Apgar score.
   b. Hypoglycemia.
   c. Weaning.
   d. Cleft palate.

II. Fill in the blanks
   a. A tiny white papillae seen on the nose and chin of the newborn is: _____
   b. Normal respiratory rate of a newborn is: _____
   c. Temper tantrums are common among: _____
   d. In children, tumors of the kidney is termed as _____

III. Write short notes on any *three* of the following:
   a. Nursing management of neonatal convulsions.
   b. Factors affecting growth and development.
   c. Immunization schedule.
   d. Prevention of accidents in school age children.
   e. National child labor policy.

IV. a. Define preterm baby.
   b. List the characteristics of preterm baby.
   c. Explain the nursing management of a preterm baby.
                              OR
   a. Define neonatal hypoglycemia.
   b. Explain the medical and nursing management of a neonate with hypoglycemia.

SECTION-II

VI. State whether the following statements are *true* or *false*:
   a. Dysphonia is a disorder of locomotion.
   b. Deficiency of vitamin C leads to goiter.
   c. Plantar flexion of the foot in which the toes are fixed lower than the heel is talipes calcaneus.
   d. Typhoid fever is caused by *Salmonella typhi*.

VII. Fill in the blanks
   a. Whooping cough is caused by: _____
   b. Conjunctivitis is inflammation of the: _____
   c. Decreased platelet count is known as: _____

VIII. Write short notes on any *three* of the following:
   a. Care of a child after tonsillectomy.
   b. Care of a visually handicapped child.
   c. Protein-energy malnutrition.
   d. Nursing care of a child with infantile seborrheic dermatitis.
   e. Juvenile delinquency.

IX. a. What is chickenpox?
   b. List the etiology and mode of transmission of chickenpox.
   c. Explain the nursing management of a child with chickenpox.

X. a. What is urinary tract infection?
   b. List the causes.
   c. Explain the management and parental advice in the care and prevention of urinary tract infection in children.

SECTION-I

I. Give the meaning of the following:

a. Apgar score

The Apgar score is a simple assessment of how a baby is doing at birth, which helps determine whether the newborn is ready to meet the world without additional medical assistance. the practitioner will do this quick evaluation one minute and five minutes after the baby is born. This score—developed in 1952 by anesthesiologist Virginia Apgar and now used in modern hospitals worldwide—rates a baby's appearance, pulse, responsiveness, muscle activity, and breathing with a number from 0 to 2 (2 being the strongest rating). The five numbers are then totaled.

Apgar scale (evaluate @ 1 and 5 minutes postpartum)			
Sign	2	1	0
A Activity (muscle tone)	Active	Arms and legs flexed	Absent
P Pulse	>100 bpm	<100 bpm	Absent
G Grimace (reflex irritability)	Sneezes, coughs, bulls away	Grimaces	No response
A Appearance (skin color)	Normal over entire body	Normal except extremities	Cyanotic or pale all over
R Respirations	Good, crying	Slow, irregular	Absent

It is easy to remember what's being tested by thinking of the letters in the name "Apgar": Activity, pulse, grimace, appearance, and respiration. Here's how each is used to assess a baby's condition at birth:

b. Hypoglycemia

Hypoglycemia is a condition characterized by abnormally low blood glucose (blood sugar) levels, usually less than 70 mg/dL. However, it is important to talk to your health care provider about your individual blood glucose targets, and what level is too low for you. Hypoglycemia may also be referred to as an insulin reaction, or insulin shock. Hypoglycemic symptoms are important clues that you have low blood glucose. Each person's reaction to hypoglycemia is different, so it is important that you learn your own signs and symptoms when your blood glucose is low. The only sure way to know whether you are experiencing hypoglycemia is to check your blood glucose, if possible. If you are experiencing symptoms and you are unable to check your blood glucose for any reason, treat the hypoglycemia. Severe hypoglycemia has the potential to cause accidents, injuries, coma, and death. Symptoms of low blood sugar can occur suddenly. They include blurry vision, rapid heartbeat, sudden mood changes, sudden nervousness, unexplained fatigue, pale skin.

c. Weaning

Weaning your baby from the breast or the bottle starts from about 4–6 months. From about 4–6 months old, your baby needs more iron and other nutrients like vitamin D and vitamin C that milk alone cannot give. The idea of weaning is the process of gradual introduction to a wide range of 'non milk' foods so that by age of one, your baby will be joining in family meals. Weaning is a transition from breast milk or formula milk to solid foods. It is divided into the following stages: Stage 1: Babies are usually ready to start on solid foods between 4–6 months, Stage 2: 6–9 months, Stage 3: 9–12 months.

Principles of Introduction of Weaning Foods

During introduction of weaning foods following principles to be remembered:
1. Milk is the main food of infant, so additional feeds should provide extra requirements as per needs of the baby, that must be obtained from good quality food items and should be home made.
2. A small amount of new foods to be given in the beginning and gradually the amount of food to be increased during the course of a week.
3. New food to be placed over the tongue of the baby to get the taste of the food and to feel the consistency. The baby may spit the food out, but with patience the feed to be given again to get accustomed with it. A single weaning food is added at a time.
4. Additional food can be given in the daytime. Initially, it can be given once, then twice or thrice.
5. There should not be any strict rule for serving new foods, it may be modified. But the foods to be given regularly.
6. New foods should be given when the infant is hungry, but never force the child to take the feeds.
7. Observe the problems related to weaning process. The infant may have indigestion, pain in abdomen, weaning diarrhea, skin rash, specially in case of food allergy and psychological upset of the baby due to withdrawn from breast milk and sucking. The problems should be managed carefully.
8. Weaning should be started between 4–6 months of age to all children but breastfeeding to be continued up to 2 years of age or beyond.
9. Delayed weaning result in malnutrition and growth failure.

d. Cleft palate

A cleft palate is a split or opening in the roof of the mouth. A cleft palate can involve the hard palate (the bony front portion of the roof of the mouth), and/or the soft palate (the soft back portion of the roof of the mouth).

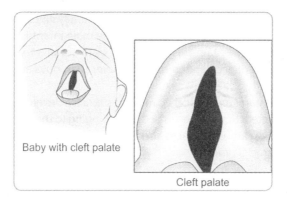

Baby with cleft palate

Cleft palate

If the cleft does not affect the palate structure of the mouth, it is referred to as cleft lip. Cleft lip is formed in the top of the lip as either a small gap or an indentation in the lip (partial or incomplete cleft) or it continues into the nose (complete cleft). Lip cleft can occur as a one sided (unilateral) or two sided (bilateral). It is due to the failure of fusion of the maxillary and medial nasal processes (formation of the primary palate).

II. Fill in the blanks

a. A tiny white papillae seen on the nose and chin of the newborn is: **Milia**
b. Normal respiratory rate of a newborn is: **45 BPM**
c. Temper tantrums are common among: **Toddler**
d. In children, tumors of the kidney is termed as: **Wilms' tumors**

III. Write short notes on any three of the following:

a. Nursing management of neonatal convulsions

A seizure is a paroxysmal behavior caused by hypersynchronous discharge of a group of neurons. Neonatal seizures are the most common overt manifestation of neurological dysfunction in the newborn. Seizures in the newborn period constitute a medical emergency. Subtle seizures are the commonest type of seizures occurring in the neonatal period. Myoclonic seizures carry the worst prognosis in terms of long-term neurodevelopment outcome. Hypoxic–ischemic encephalopathy is the most common cause of neonatal seizures. Multiple etiologies often coexist in neonates and hence it is essential to rule out common causes such as hypoglycemia, hypocalcemia, and meningitis before initiating specific therapy. A comprehensive evidence-based approach for management of neonatal seizures has been described in this protocol.

b. Factors affecting growth and development

Growth and development depend on not one but combination of many factors, all interdependent. The relatively typical pattern of growth and development is influenced by heredity and environment. Also genetic inheritance and environmental influences are two primary factors in determining a child's pattern of growth and development.

Genetic factors

1. **Heredity:** The heredity of a man and woman determines their children. Heredity decides the size and shape of the body, hence family member bear resemblance. The characteristics are transmitted through genes, which are responsible for family illness, e.g. diabetes.
2. **Sex:** Sex is determined at conception, after birth the male infant is both longer and heavier than female infant. Boys maintain this superiority until about 11 years of age. Girls mature earlier, reach the period of accelerated growth earlier than boys and are taller than boys on the average.
3. **Race:** Distinguishing characteristics called racial or subracial developed in prehistoric humans. Similar physical characteristics are seen in people belonging to the same race. As too height, tall and short examples exist among all races and subraces. Among civilized groups, intermarriage has produced mixed racial types.

Nutritional factors

1. **Poor nutrition:** Nutrition plays a vital role in the bodies susceptibility to disease because poor nutrition limits the body ability to resist infection. Poor nutrition also plays a major role in the development of chronic illnesses. Growth and development suffering from protein–energy malnutrition, anemic and vitamin deficiency states are retarded.
2. **Maternal nutrition:** intrauterine growth retardation and consequently small size of the fetus occur due to nutritional deficiency in mothers, infection and drugs used during pregnancy.

Environmental Factors

1. **Physical environment:** Environment forces act upon the individual. It is the exploding force of an individual potentially to different stimulating forces. The physical environment includes food, temperature, climate, resources, etc.
2. **Mental environment:** It includes the intellectual atmosphere of the school, the libraries, the recreation rooms, laboratories, etc.
3. **Social environment:** It includes social association the child gets from the beginning. It also includes cultural atmosphere of the society, e.g. religion, folklore, literature, art, music, social conversions and political organizations. The richer is the environment, better is the scope for developing an individual into a healthy human being.
4. **Socioeconomic level:** The child born into a family of low socioeconomic means may not receive adequate health supervision could leave a child without immunization against measles or other childhood illnesses and thus vulnerable to disease that could cause permanent neurological damage.
5. **Cultural influences:** Groups of human being create their own cultures, whereas each individual is influenced or shaped by the culture of which he or she is a part. The effects of a particular culture on a child begin before birth because of the manner in which culture views and treat the members of the pregnant women's family.
6. **Internal influences:** There is evidence that all the hormones in the body affect growth in some manner. Deficiency of growth hormone retards growth while over production results in gigantism.
7. **Characteristics of parents:** Parents with high intelligence quotient are more likely to have children with higher level of inherent intelligence.

Prenatal environment: Prenatal environment climate in which the child's develops. The influences of the intrauterine environment on the child's future development are great, particularly since the uterus shields the fetus from the full impact of external adverse condition.

Postnatal environment: An environment that provides satisfying experiences promote growth. Since growth and development are interrelated, growth in one area influences and in turn is influenced by growth in all other areas.

c. Immunization schedule

Immunization schedule should be planned according to the needs of the community. It should be relevant with existing community health problems. It must be effective, feasible and acceptable by the community. Every country has its own immunization schedule. The WHO, launched global immunization program in 1974, known as Expanded Program on Immunization (EPI) to protect all children of the world against six killer diseases. In India, EPI was launched in January 1978. The EPI is now renamed as Universal Child Immunization as per declaration sponsored by UNICEF. In India, it is called as Universal Immunization Program (UIP) and was launched in 1985, November, for the universal coverage of immunization to the eligible population. The objective of introduction new but under used vaccines in the developing countries, where the diseases like hepatitis-B and *H. influenzae* 'B' (Hib) are highly prevalent. National Immunization Schedule as recommended by Government of India for uniform implementation throughout the country was formulated. The schedule contents the age at which the vaccines are best given and the number of doses recommended for each vaccine. The schedule also covers immunization of women during pregnancy against tetanus.

Beneficiaries	Age	Vaccine	Dose	Route	Amount
(a) Infants	• At Birth (for institutional deliveries)	• BCG	• Single	Intradermal	0.05 mL
	• At 6 weeks	• BCG (it not given at birth)	• Single	Intradermal	0.1 mL
		• DTP-1	1st	Intramuscular	0.5 mL
		• OPV-1	1st	Oral	2 drops
	• At 10 weeks	• DTP-2	2nd	Intramuscular	0.5 mL
		• OPV-2	2nd	Oral	2 drops
	• At 14 weeks	• DTP-3	3rd	Intramuscular	0.5 mL
		• OPV-3	3rd	Oral	2 drops
	• At 9 months	• Measles	Single	Subcutaneous	0.5 mL
(b) Children	• At 16–24 months	• DTP	Booster	Intramuscular	0.5 mL
		• OPV	Booster	Oral	2 drops
	At 5–6 years	DTP	Single intramuscular 0.5 mL • Second dose of DT should be given after 4 weeks, if not vaccinated previously with DTP		
	At 10–16 years	TT	Single intramuscular 0.5 mL • Second dose of DT should be given if not vaccinated previously		
(c) Pregnant women	• Early in pregnancy	• TT-1	1st	Intramuscular	0.5 mL
	• One month after	• TT-2	2nd	Intramuscular	0.5 mL

d. Prevention of accidents in school age children

1. Parents must be educated regarding the dangers associated with medicines, household substances and agrochemicals. A poison label should appear on all dangerous medicines, including aspirin and paracetamol.
2. Parents must begin to teach their children at an early age the danger of touching, eating or playing with unknown objects including medicines, pesticides and insecticides, household chemicals or plants.
3. Medicines, insecticides and pesticides and other poisonous substances should be stored in locked cabinets.
4. Dyes, polishes, kerosene and other poisonous household chemicals should never be left on a low shelf or on the floor. Do not store in kitchen or bathroom.
5. Combustion devices should be adequately ventilated.
6. Inhalation of spray or fumes should be prevented during painting
7. Unnecessary toxic substances should be discarded.
8. Carefully check the label of any medicine before use. Do not put different tablets or pills in the same bottle.
9. Do not store any poisonous liquid in a beverage bottle.
10. Wear protective clothing, goggles, gloves and masks during spraying of insecticide and always spray downwind. Protective clothing should be removed and exposed skin washed thoroughly before eating anything.
11. Dispense medicine and dangerous household's chemicals in childproof, tamperproof containers.
12. Education on proper hygiene and storage of food to avoid food poisoning.
13. Workers and other persons working in industries should be trained in safe use of chemicals.

14. Industries should have complete knowledge and information in the toxicity and management of the chemicals they are using.
15. Persons having suicidal tendencies should not be given a large amount of drugs at a time and should be given adequate psychiatric follow-up and counseling.

e. National child health policy

government recognized the need to protect child labor from exploitation and from being subjected to work in hazardous conditions that endanger such children's physical and mental development, and the need to ensure the health and safety of children at the workplace. It recognized that they should be protected from excessively long working hours and from night work, that work even in non-hazardous occupations should be regulated, and all working children should be provided with sufficient weekly rest periods and holidays.

The main objective of the National Child Labor Project (NCLP) is to eliminate the prevalence of child labor in this country. The components of the running of the NCLP are:

1. Enforcement of the Child labor (Prohibition and Regulation) Act, 1986, the Factories Act, 1948, the Mines Act, 1952 and such other acts within the project area.
2. Coverage of families of child labor under the income/employment generating programs under the over aegis of antipoverty programs.
3. Formal and non-formal education for child labor in hazardous employments. Also, a stepped-up program of adult education (including non-formal education) of the parents of the working parents.
4. Setting up of special schools for child workers together with provision of vocational education/training in such special schools, supplementary nutrition, and stipend to the children taken out from the prohibited employments and health care for all the children attending at such special schools.
5. Creating awareness among the different target groups in the society through governmental and non-governmental organizations to raise their consciousness on the issue of child labor.
6. Survey of child labor in the project areas and also evaluate the progress of the project periodically.

In the year 1994, a National Authority on Elimination of Child Labor was constituted under the Chairmanship by Union Labor Minister with Secretaries of nine Departments of Government of India concerned with Child Labor. In Tamil Nadu State Authority on Child Labor was constituted under the Chairmanship of Chief Secretary. A State Monitoring Committee on Child Labor has been constituted to monitor the National Child Labor Projects in the State.

IV. a. Define preterm baby

A neonate with a birth weight of less than 2500 g irrespective of the gestational age are termed as low birth weight (LBW) baby. They include both preterm and small-for-dates (SFD) babies. These two groups have different clinical problems and prognosis. In India about 30–40% neonates are born LBW. Approximately, 80% of all neonatal deaths and 50% of infant death are related to LBW. These LBW babies are more prone to malnutrition, infections and neurodevelopment handicapped conditions. They are more vulnerable to develop hypertension, diabetes mellitus, and coronary artery disease in adult life.

High incidence of LBW babies in our country is due to higher number of babies with intrauterine growth retardation (small for dates) rather than preterm babies. It is not possible to provide special care to all LBW babies, especially in India. The baby with a birth weight of less than 2000 g is more vulnerable and need special care. About 10% of all LBW babies require admission to the special care nursery.

b. Characteristic features of preterm baby

Premature babies have a number of characteristics depending on their gestational age:
1. Skin: May be reddened. The skin may be thin so blood vessels are easily seen.
2. Lanugo: There is a lot of fine hair all over the baby's body.
3. Limbs: The limbs are thin and may be poorly flexed or floppy due to poor muscle tone.
4. Head size: Appears large in proportion to the body. The fontanelles (open spaces where skull bones join) are smooth and flat.
5. Chest: No breast tissue before 34 weeks of pregnancy.
6. Sucking ability: Weak or absent.
7. Genitals: In boys the testes may not be descended and the scrotum may be small; in girls the clitoris and labia minora may be large.
8. Soles of feet: Creases are located only in the anterior (front) of the sole, not all over, as in the term baby.

c. Explain the nursing management of a preterm baby

Hospital care of LBW infant: Ideally, the delivery of an anticipated LBW baby should be conducted in a hospital. Premature labor as well as intrauterine growth retardation is indications for referral of the pregnant mother to a well-equipped facility. This in-utero transfer of a low birth weight fetus is desirable, convenient and safe than the transport of a low weight baby after birth. Trained health professionals should conduct delivery and standard procedure of resuscitation should be followed efficiently.

The indications for hospitalization of a LBW neonate delivered at home include birth weight <1800 g, gestational age 33 weeks, neonate who is not able to take feeds from both the breasts or by katori-spoon or a sick neonate.

The principles of management of LBW neonate in the hospital are essentially the same as described for home care, viz., and temperature maintenance, providing fluids and feeds and prevention of infection.

Keeping LBW babies warm: The mother herself is a source of warmth for the baby (Cot-in baby). The room, where the baby is nursed should be kept warm (temperature between 28° and 30° C in all seasons). While in summer months no extraeffort is required to maintain this temperature, in winter months a room heater may have to be used. The baby should be clothed well. If baby does not maintain temperature, overhead radiant warmer or incubator may be used to keep the baby warm. Regular monitoring of axillary temperature by placing low reading thermometer should be carried out in all hospitalized babies. Rectal temperature is recorded only in a sick, hypothermic newborn. Normal axillary temperature is 36.5° C. In hypothermia the temperature are below 36.5° C (Cold stress <36.5° to >36.0°C, Moderate hypothermia <36.0° to >32.0°C, Severe hypothermia <32.0° C). The temperature range during which the basal metabolic rate of the baby is at minimum, oxygen utilization is least and baby thrives well is known as "thermoneutral range of temperature". For each baby, this range of temperature varies depending on gestational age, weight and postnatal age. Hypothermia can lead to hypoglycemia, bleeding diathesis, pulmonary hemorrhage, acidosis, apnea, respiratory failure, shock and even death.

Nutrition and fluids: Birth weight, gestation, presence of sickness and individual feeding effort of the baby determine the fluid and feed supplements to a baby. Ultimate goal is to meet both these requirements from direct and exclusive breastfeeds. Breast milk is the ideal feed for the low birth weight babies.

Prevention of infection: LBW babies are predisposed to serious bacterial infections. Even when treated aggressively, the mortality due to sepsis is high. Therefore, the importance of preventing sepsis cannot be overemphasized. Following measures will help prevent infections:

1. Hand washing by the health professional attending delivery and by the mother and family before handling the baby.
2. Ensuring early and exclusive breastfeeding and avoiding all prelacteal feeds. Careful attention to the hygiene of katori-spoon feeds. Dropper/bottle/nipple/cotton wicks should never be used for feeding the baby.
3. Care of the umbilical stump.
4. Avoiding unnecessary interventions such as intravenous lines and needle pricks.

OR

a. Define neonatal hypoglycemia

Blood glucose concentrations as low as 30 mg/dL are common in healthy neonates by 1–2 hours after birth; these low concentrations, seen in all mammalian newborns, usually are transient, asymptomatic, and considered to be part of normal adaptation to postnatal life. Most neonates compensate for "physiologic" hypoglycemia by producing alternative fuels including ketone bodies, which are released from fat.

1. Neonatal hypoglycemia is a common metabolic disorder and the operational threshold values of blood glucose <40 mg/dL (plasma glucose <45 mg/dL) should be used to guide management.
2. All "at risk" neonates and sick infants should be monitored for blood glucose levels. Term healthy AGA infants without any risk factors need not be monitored routinely.
3. Screening for hypoglycemia can be done by glucose reagent strips but confirmation requires laboratory estimation by either glucose oxidase or glucose electrode method. Treatment should not be delayed for confirmatory results.
4. Asymptomatic hypoglycemia can be managed with a trial of measured oral feed if blood glucose is >25 mg/dL and there is no contraindication to feeding.
5. Symptomatic hypoglycemia should be treated with a minibolus of 2 ml/kg 10% dextrose and continuous infusion of 6 mg/kg/min of 10% dextrose.
6. Refractory and prolonged hypoglycemia should be suspected and investigated if the glucose infusion requirement is >12 mg/kg/min for more than 24 hours or the hypoglycemia persists >5–7 days, respectively.
7. Babies with hypoglycemia should be followed up for neurodevelopment sequelae.

Infants in the first or second day of life may be asymptomatic or may have life-threatening central nervous system (CNS) and cardiopulmonary disturbances. Symptoms can include the following: Hypotonia, Lethargy, apathy, Poor feeding, Jitteriness, seizures, Congestive heart failure, Cyanosis, Apnea, and Hypothermia.

Clinical manifestations associated with activation of the autonomic nervous system include the following: Anxiety, tremulousness, diaphoresis, tachycardia, pallor, hunger, nausea, and vomiting.

Clinical manifestations of hypoglycorrhachia or neuroglycopenia include the following: Headache, mental confusion, staring, behavioral changes, difficulty concentrating, visual disturbances (e.g. decreased acuity, diplopia), dysarthria, seizures, ataxia, somnolence, coma, stroke (hemiplegia, aphasia), paresthesias, dizziness, amnesia, decerebrate or decorticate posturing.

b. Explain the medical and nursing management of a neonate with hypoglycemia

Hypoglycemia should be treated as soon as possible to prevent complications of neurologic damage. Early feeding of the newborn with breast milk or formula is encouraged. The mainstay of therapy for children who are alert with intact airway protection includes orange juice at 20 mL/kg.

For patients who cannot protect their airway or are unable to drink, nasogastric, intramuscular, intraosseous, or intravenous (IV) routes can be employed for the following drugs used to raise glucose levels: dextrose, glucagon, diazoxide, and octreotide. Start a 5% or 10% dextrose drip when hypoglycemia is recurrent.

Surgical exploration usually is undertaken in severely affected neonates who are unresponsive to glucose and somatostatin therapy. Near-total resection of 85–90% of the pancreas is recommended for presumed congenital hyperinsulinism, which is most commonly associated with an abnormality of beta-cell regulation throughout the pancreas. Risks include the development of diabetes.

SECTION-II

VI. State whether the following statements are *true* or *false*

a. Dysphonia is a disorder of locomotion: **TRUE.**
b. Deficiency of vitamin C leads to goiter: **FALSE.**
c. Plantar flexion of the foot in which the toes are fixed lower than the heel is talpes calcaneus: **TRUE.**
d. Typhoid fever is caused by *Salmonella typhi*: **TRUE.**

VII. Fill in the blanks

a. Whooping cough is caused by: **Bordetella pertussis**
b. Conjunctivitis is inflammation of the: **Conjunctiva**
c. Decreased platelet count is known as: **Thrombocytopenia**

VIII. Write short notes on any *three* of the following:

a. Care of a child after tonsillectomy

A tonsillectomy is surgery to remove the child's tonsils. Tonsils are 2 large lumps of tissue in the back of the child's throat. Adenoids are small lumps of tissue on top of the throat. Tonsils and adenoids both fight infection. The child may need his tonsils removed to improve breathing and asthma, and to reduce throat, sinus, and ear infections. His adenoids may be taken out at the same time if they are large or infected.

1. A tonsillectomy with or without an adenoidectomy is a painful and uncomfortable procedure. Your child's throat can be sore for 10–14 days after the operation.
2. 5–6 days after the operation the pain may get worse as the white membrane over the healing area contracts.
3. There is much less discomfort after an adenoidectomy alone.
4. The child may have referred pain to the ear for 7–10 days following an adenotonsillectomy.
5. White areas over the throat where the tonsils were removed is seen; this does not mean infection and will resolve within the first 2–3 weeks after surgery.
6. Bad breath is common during healing.
7. There can be some blood-stained saliva, nasal discharge or bleeding after the operation. Sucking ice can help this, but if there is a larger amount of fresh blood (more than 1–2 teaspoonful) or if the bleeding continues for more than 5 minutes, dial 111 and ask for emergency medical help.
8. Some children's voices can be slightly different after the operation but soon return to normal after 3 or 4 weeks.

9. Some children experience a change in their sense of taste after the operation but this usually only lasts for a few weeks.

b. Care of a visually handicapped child

Visual impairment (or vision impairment) is vision loss (of a person) to such a degree as to qualify as an additional support need through a significant limitation of visual capability resulting from either disease, trauma, or congenital or degenerative conditions that cannot be corrected by conventional means, such as refractive correction or medication.

Maslow's five-stage hierarchy of needs model offers a means of raising awareness of the care requirements of both young and older patients with visual impairment. Using the model has highlighted the challenges involved when planning and managing their care. Meeting individual needs through effectively managed care may help to make a difference to patients with visual impairment. Effective communication is instrumental in achieving this, and remains the single most important aspect of nursing practice.

Nurses who have a knowledge and understanding of ocular pathology and the nature of visual impairment may be able to provide the effective communication and care management skills required to meet the special needs of patients who have visual impairment, their families and significant others.

c. Protein–energy malnutrition

Protein–energy malnutrition (PEM) is the term given to a group of clinical conditions which occur due to inadequate protein and calorie intake, especially in children. PEM is also referred to as protein-calorie malnutrition. It develops in children and adults whose consumption of protein and energy (measured by calories) is insufficient to satisfy the body's nutritional needs. While pure protein deficiency can occur when a person's diet provides enough energy but lacks the protein minimum, in most cases the deficiency will be dual. PEM may also occur in persons who are unable to absorb vital nutrients or convert them to energy essential for healthy tissue formation and organ function.

Causes of protein–energy malnutrition

1. When PEM is purely due to dietary deficiency, it is termed as the primary type. This begins at the fetal stage and continues into infancy and childhood. Nearly 25% of the pediatric hospital beds in India are occupied by children suffering from malnutrition and around 80% of hospitalized children are malnourished to some extent. Hence, this contributes to the infant mortality ratio in a big way.
2. Secondary malnutrition arises due to a serious illness like tuberculosis, cancer or inability of the body to absorb nutrients, e.g. in bowel disease like ulcerative colitis, metabolic syndromes and long standing gastroenteritis.
3. Dietary factors contributing to PEM are inadequate breastfeeding by the mother due to inability of mother's body to make milk due to inadequate nutrition, stopping breastfeeding early in case of working mothers and inadequate supplementation of other foods, ignorance of weaning and weaning foods, inverted or cracked nipples in mother causing difficulty in breastfeeding. Another important reason is nipple confusion when the baby is switched from breast to the artificial nipple and bottle. Formula milk may not be well tolerated leading to diarrhea.
4. Problems in the mother, such as mental or psychiatric illnesses, postnatal depression (severe cases), poor maternal health like anemia and having too many children in quick succession

or having twins may lead to the mother producing not enough milk to meet the demand of the infants.
5. Traditional methods which are harmful to the baby may be practiced in villages and rural areas, such as not offering colostrum (the fluid that comes out of the nipple in the first few hours after delivery) which is very healthy and boosts the baby's immune system and withholding breast milk when the baby has diarrhea. Even in remote areas, health professions should conduct antenatal classes for mothers-to-be and educated them.
6. All kinds of infections in the baby, such as oral ulcers, gastroenteritis, food poisoning, diarrhea and serious conditions, such as congenital heart or kidney disease may cause inability to suckle which causes malnutrition. Thus, infection and malnutrition is a vicious cycle as one contributes to the other.
7. Low socioeconomic status of the people coupled with the desire to have more children (especially boys) is the social malady that many uneducated people suffer from.

d. Nursing care of a child with infantile seborrheic dermatitis

Seborrheic dermatitis is a skin condition in which the skin becomes red and inflamed before developing scaly flakes of white, gray, or yellow skin. This condition is most common on areas of the body where sweat glands are abundant, such as the scalp and groin, and it can also appear in the folds of the skin, in areas such as the neck and armpits. This condition is not harmful, but it can be unsightly, and many people choose to seek treatment for it for this reason.

When a patient presents with a condition which looks like seborrheic dermatitis, the doctor may decide to take a scraping to examine it under the microscope. This can reveal clues to other skin conditions which might be causing the outbreak. If the samples do not provide additional information, the doctor may proceed with treatment for seborrheic dermatitis and recommend a follow up visit to confirm that the diagnosis was correct.

Infantile seborrheic dermatitis: This starts as red scaly patches present on the scalp and on the flexures of the body. The scales are greasy and are on the scalp and on the other areas of the body. It starts at the age of three to four months and generally clears up spontaneously in three to six weeks. Secondary bacterial or candidal infections may occur. The use of alkali soap may cause an irritation.

Treatment: Simple corticosteroid cream with antibiotics or hydroxyquinoline may be prescribed.

e. Juvenile delinquency

Juvenile delinquency is the broad-based term given to juveniles who commit crimes. Juveniles are defined as those people who have not reached adulthood or the age of majority. What defines adulthood or the age of majority in a court system may be predetermined by law, especially for minor crimes. Major crimes may force the courts to decide to try a juvenile as an adult, a very important distinction, since sentencing can then mean not just spending adolescence, but a lifetime in prison. Delinquency can be defined as the committing of those things considered crimes by the state, although delinquent can also mean abandoned. Thus, juvenile delinquency can cover anything from small crime—a student who cuts school repeatedly is delinquent—to very serious crimes like felony theft and murder. When a child, anyone under the age of majority, commits a crime, most frequently they are tried and sentenced through a court system separate from that which tries adults. There are also confinement centers, in other words, prisons, specifically designed for children who commit serious crimes. These are often called juvenile detention centers.

IX. a. What is chickenpox?

Chickenpox is a viral infection in which a person develops extremely itchy blisters all over the body. It used to be one of the classic childhood diseases. However, it has become much less common since the introduction of the chickenpox vaccine. Most children with chickenpox have the following symptoms before the rash appears: fever, headache, stomach ache.

The chickenpox rash occurs about 10–21 days after coming into contact with someone who had the disease. The average child develops 250–500 small, itchy, fluid-filled blisters over red spots on the skin.

1. The blisters are usually first seen on the face, middle of the body, or scalp.
2. After a day or two, the blisters become cloudy and then scab. Meanwhile, new blisters form in groups. They often appear in the mouth, in the vagina, and on the eyelids.
3. Children with skin problems, such as eczema, may get thousands of blisters. Most pox will not leave scars unless they become infected with bacteria from scratching.

Some children who have had the vaccine will still develop a mild case of chickenpox. They usually recover much more quickly and have only a few pox (fewer than 30). These cases are often harder to diagnose. However, these children can still spread chickenpox to others.

b. List the etiology and mode of transmission of chickenpox

Chickenpox is caused by the varicella-zoster virus, a member of the herpes virus family. The same virus also causes herpes zoster (shingles) in adults.

Chickenpox can be spread very easily to others. You may get chickenpox from touching the fluids from a chickenpox blister, or if someone with the disease coughs or sneezes near you. Even those with mild illness may be contagious.

A person with chickenpox becomes contagious 1–2 days before their blisters appear. They remain contagious until all the blisters have crusted over.

Most cases of chickenpox occur in children younger than 10 years. The disease is usually mild, although serious complications sometimes occur. Adults and older children usually get sicker than younger children.

Children whose mothers have had chickenpox or have received the chickenpox vaccine are not very likely to catch it before they are 1 year old. If they do catch chickenpox, they often have mild cases. This is because antibodies from their mothers' blood help protect them. Children under 1-year-old whose mothers have not had chickenpox or the vaccine can get severe chickenpox.

Severe chickenpox symptoms are more common in children whose immune system does not work well because of an illness or medicines, such as chemotherapy and steroids.

c. Explain the nursing management of a child with chickenpox

Treatment involves keeping the person as comfortable as possible. Here are things to try:
1. Avoid scratching or rubbing the itchy areas. Keep fingernails short to avoid damaging the skin from scratching.
2. Wear cool, light, loose bedclothes. Avoid wearing rough clothing, particularly wool, over an itchy area.
3. Take lukewarm baths using little soap and rinse thoroughly. Try a skin-soothing oatmeal or cornstarch bath.
4. Apply a soothing moisturizer after bathing to soften and cool the skin.
5. Avoid prolonged exposure to excessive heat and humidity.
6. Try over-the-counter oral antihistamines, such as diphenhydramine (Benadryl), but be aware of possible side effects such as drowsiness.
7. Try over-the-counter hydrocortisone cream on itchy areas.

Medications that fight the chickenpox virus are available but not given to everyone. To work well, the medicine usually must be started within the first 24 hours of the rash.
1. Antiviral medication is not usually prescribe to otherwise healthy children who do not have severe symptoms. Adults and teens, who are at risk for more severe symptoms, may benefit from antiviral medication if it is given early.
2. Antiviral medication may be very important in those who have skin conditions (such as eczema or recent sunburn), lung conditions (such as asthma), or who have recently taken steroids.
3. Some doctors also give antiviral medicines to people in the same household who also develop chickenpox, because they will usually develop more severe symptoms.

Do not give aspirin or ibuprofen to someone who may have chickenpox. Use of aspirin has been associated with a serious condition called Reye's syndrome. Ibuprofen has been associated with more severe secondary infections. Acetaminophen (Tylenol) may be used.

A child with chickenpox should not return to school or play with other children until all chickenpox sores have crusted over or dried out. Adults should follow this same rule when considering when to return to work or be around others.

X. a. What is urinary tract infection?

Urinary tract infections (UTI) are the presence of infective agents (usually bacteria) that exists anywhere between the renal cortex and the urethral meatus. It is sometimes difficult to determine the exact location of the infections. It may cause irreversible renal damage, especially in association with urinary tract anomalies and vesicoureteric reflux (VUR). The most common causative organism is *E. coli*. Other organisms are *Streptococcus*, *Staphylococcus*, *Pseudomonas*, etc. The most common route of entry is the ascending infections from the urethra or may be hematogenous spread. This infection is more common in girls.

The contributing causes of UTI are urinary stasis, congenital anomalies or obstruction of urinary tract (PUJ, bladder-neck obstruction, PUV), VUR, poor perineal hygiene, short female urethra, urinary catheterization, or instrumentation, local inflammation, chronic constipation or infection anywhere in the body.

Pathophysiology: Most commonly UTI are found in lower urinary tract. It may occur as cystitis or pyelonephritis. Inflammation results in urinary retention and stasis. Backflow of urine (reflux) into the kidney may occur though ureter. Inflamed part become edematous, thickened and fibrosed. Ureter and renal pelvis may be dilated. If left untreated, kidney may become small and tissue may be destroyed resulting disturbances of renal functions.

Clinical manifestations: The onset of symptoms may be abrupt or gradual, even the condition may have no symptoms. The patient usually have moderate to high fever with chills, rigors, convulsions, anorexia, malaise, irritability and vomiting. Urinary symptoms may be found as frequency and urgency, dysuria, dribbling and bed wetting. Urine may be foul-smelling. The child may complain abdominal or flank or suprapubic pain. It may present as acute abdomen. Neonates with UTI may have lethargy, diarrhea, jaundice, poor weight gain and features of sepsis.

Diagnosis: The diagnosis of UTI is confirmed by urine culture and urine analysis (routine and microscopic) by clean catch or sterile urine specimen. Associated congenital anomalies or obstructive uropathies should be detected by USG, MCU, IVP, renal scan, etc. Blood examination shows increased TLC and ESR with decreased Hb%.

X. b. Causes of urinary tract infection?

Urine is normally sterile, which means it doesn't contain any bacteria, fungus or viruses. To infect the urinary system, a micro-organism usually has to enter through the urethra or, rarely, from the bloodstream. The most common culprit is a bacterium common to the digestive tract called *Escherichia coli (E. coli)*. It is usually spread to the urethra from the anus. Other micro-organisms, such as *Mycoplasma* and *Chlamydia*, can cause urethritis in both men and women. These micro-organisms are sexually transmitted so, when these infections are detected, both partners need medical treatment to avoid re-infection.

Risk factors for developing UTIs: Some people are at greater risk than others of developing UTIs. These include:

Women—sexually active women are vulnerable, in part because the urethra is only 4 cm long and bacteria have only this short distance to travel from the outside to the inside of the bladder.

People with urinary catheters—such as the critically ill, who can't empty their own bladder.

People with diabetes—changes to the immune system make a person with diabetes more vulnerable to infection.

Men with prostate problems—such as an enlarged prostate gland that can cause the bladder to only partially empty.

Babies—especially those born with physical problems (congenital abnormalities) of the urinary system.

c. Explain the management and parental advice in the care and prevention of urinary tract infection in children

Management of UTI is mainly done with antibiotic therapy. Specific symptomatic and supportive treatment is essential. Associated congenital anomalies should be detected early for prompt management.

The antibiotic therapy is given with combination of ampicillin and gentamicin or amikacin for 7–10 days. Other antibiotics also can be used, i.e. ceftriaxone, cefotaxime, etc.

Supportive measures include management of fever by rest, tepid sponge and/or antipyretics, with large amount of fluid intake. Improvement of personal hygiene (perineal hygiene) is important preventive measure. Frequent emptying of bladder should be encouraged to prevent stasis of urine. Repeat urine culture to be done to discontinue the treatment. The UTI may be complicated with recurrent infections, renal damage and severe VUR.

Antibiotic therapy for UTIs is based upon the sensitivity profile obtained from the urine-culture results. Cystitis (infection limited to the bladder) should respond quickly to routine oral antibiotics. Pyelonephritis may need hospitalization for intravenous administration of antibiotics along with fluid therapy if the patient is experiencing associated vomiting and dehydration. Oral antibiotic therapy, however, may be appropriate if these complications are not present.

Preventive Measures

1. **Hygiene:** Wipe females from front to back during diaper changes or after using the toilet in older girls. With uncircumcised males, mild and gentle traction of the foreskin helps expose the urethral opening. Most boys are able to fully retract the foreskin by 4 years of age.
2. **Complete bladder emptying:** Some toilet-trained children are in hurry to leave the bathroom. Encourage "double voiding" (urinating immediately after finishing the first void). Children should be encouraged to urinate approximately every two to three hours. Some children ignore the sensation of a full bladder in the desire to continue to play.
3. **Avoid the "4 C's":** **C**arbonated drinks, high amounts of **c**itrus, **c**affeine (sodas), and **c**hocolate. Some kidney specialists are not as adamant about this option.

2012
Pediatric Nursing

SECTION-I

I. Give the meaning of the following:
  a. Meningocele
  b. Hypospadias
  c. Leukemia
  d. Atrial septal defect (ASD)
  e. Exstrophy of bladder

II. Fill in the blanks:
  a. Whooping cough is caused by: _____
  b. Decreased calcium in the blood causes: _____
  c. Inflammation of middle ear is known as: _____

III. Write short notes on any *three* of the following:
  a. Trends in pediatric nursing.
  b. Guidance to parents on toddler care.
  c. Care of a child with hemolytic disorder.
  d. Welfare of delinquent and destitute children.

IV. a. What is dengue fever?
  b. List the types of dengue fever.
  c. Briefly explain the medical and nursing management of a child with dengue fever.

V. a. What is cleft lip and cleft palate?
  b. Explain surgical treatment and management of a child with cleft lip and cleft palate.

SECTION-II

VI. Choose the correct answer and write:
  a. Normal head circumference of newborn is: _____
    (i. 31–33 cm, ii. 33–35 cm, iii. 35–40 cm)
  b. Chickenpox is caused by: _____
    (i. Varicella zoster, ii. Myxovirus, iii. Itch mite)
  c. The most common cause of abdominal pain in children is: _____
    (i. Dysentery, ii. Worm colic, iii. Appendicitis)

VII. State whether the following statements are *true* or *false*:
  a. Spina bifida is one of the most uncommon anomalies in children.
  b. Cerebral palsy is the most frequent permanent disability of childhood.

c. Phototherapy is a treatment for intrauterine growth retardation.
   d. Pleural effusion is the collection of fluid in pleural space.

VIII. **Write short notes on any *three* of the following:**
   a. Ascariasis.
   b. Child reaction to hospitalization.
   c. Medical and nursing management of a child with HIV infection.
   d. Management of a child with rheumatic fever.

IX. a. What is diarrhea?
   b. List the causes and clinical features of diarrhea.
   c. Write the complications and nursing management of a child with diarrhea.

X. a. Define osteomyelitis.
   b. List the signs and symptoms of osteomyelitis.
   c. Explain the nursing management of a child suffering from osteomyelitis.

SECTION-I

I. Give the meaning of the following:

a. Meningocele

Meningocele is a form of spina bifida, a relatively common birth defect. This congenital condition affects the meninges, or the membranes surrounding the spinal cord. There is an abnormal opening in the back through which the meninges bulge through, forming a sac. Meningocele is typically less severe than other forms of spina bifida, and patients are usually able to function well. Nearly all patients with this birth defect will need a type of surgery called a meningocele repair in order to prevent further damage.

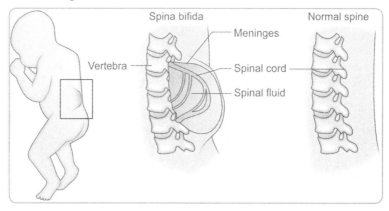

A meningocele repair will usually be required within 24–48 hours of the child's birth, which will typically occur via cesarean section to prevent the area from becoming more damaged. The promptness of this surgery is essential to prevent infections in the opening of the back. While this procedure cannot fix the defects, it will prevent the nerves and spinal cord from becoming damaged as the child grows.

b. Hypospadias

Hypospadias is the congenital abnormal urethal opening on the ventral aspect (under surface) of the penis. It is one of the commonest malformations of male children.

Undescended testes or inguinal hernia or upper urinary tract anomalies may be associated with hypospadias. It may found in females as urethal opening in the vagina with dribbling of urine.

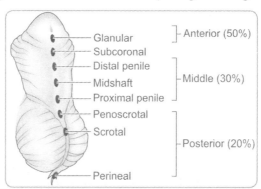

c. Leukemia

Leukemia is the cancer of blood forming tissue. It is the common form of childhood cancer. It is more common between the ages of two to live years.

Leukemia is a proliferation of immature white blood cells in the blood-forming tissues. The cells count of mature cells is decreased and the count of immature cells is increased. It depresses the bone marrow production. Effects of proliferating cells in leukemia are anemia due to decreased erythrocytes, infections from neutropenia and bleeding from decreased platelets.

Classification: Acute lymphoid leukemia and acute myeloid leukemia.

Acute lymphoid leukemia: This includes lymphocytic leukemia, lymphatic leukemia and lymphoblastic leukemia.

Acute myelogenous leukemia: This includes granulocytic leukemia, myelocytic leukemia, monoblastic leukemia, and monomyeloblastic leukemia.

d. Atrial septal defect (ASD)

All infants have a small opening in their atria right after birth, called a foramen ovale. Sometimes, as the fetal heart forms, lower pressure in the right heart causes the left atrium to send more blood through the foramen ovale, creating a larger than usual hole. While the normal foramen ovale closes shortly after the baby is born, this larger hole may not close and is termed an atrial septal defect.

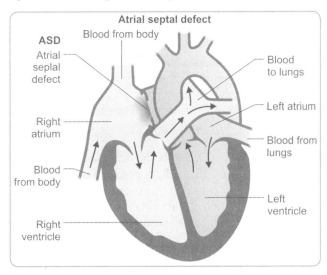

An atrial septal defect is classified by the position of the hole in the septum, as well as by size. When the hole is in the middle of the septum, it is called a sinus venosus defect. A hole in the lower part of the septum is termed an ostium primum, and one at the top of the septum is an ostium secundum.

e. Exstrophy of bladder

Bladder exstrophy (also known as Ectopia vesicae) is a congenital anomaly in which part of the urinary bladder is present outside the body. It is rare, occurring once every 10,000–50,000 live births with a 2:1 male: female ratio. The diagnosis involves a spectrum of anomalies of the lower abdominal wall, bladder, anterior bony pelvis, and external genitalia. It occurs due to failure of the abdominal wall to close during fetal development and results in protrusion of the anterior bladder wall through the lower abdominal wall. Treatment is with surgical correction of the defect, but patients can still have long-term issues with urinary tract infections and urinary incontinence.

II. Fill in the blanks

a. Whooping cough is caused by: **Bordetella pertussis**
b. Decreased calcium in the blood caused by: **Chronic kidney diseases**
c. Inflammation of middle ear is known as: **Otitis media**

III. Write short notes on any *three* of the following:

a. Trends in pediatric nursing

The increasing complexity of medical and nursing techniques has created a need for special area for child care. The child care has prime importance, as the mortality and morbidity are higher in this group. Many diseases are preventable, such as nutritional deficiency. The goal of the pediatric nursing is to foster the growth and development of the children and promote an optimum state of health physically, mentally, and socially, so that they may function at the peak of their capacity.

Since most of the responses of children are influenced by the phases of growth and development, the ages of the child are the most significant factor affecting nursing activities. For example, fractured jaw is more traumatic to an infant who is in oral phase of the development than to a child of the six years of age who has already passed this phase. The separation of the family during the hospitalization will cause an anxiety in the young child and may disturb the parent–child relationship.

The nurse can minimize the psychological trauma of a hospitalization experience by helping the children to adjust to the situation rather than to repress their feelings. Play therapy has an importance in child care, by which children can play out their problems. To provide comprehensive care to children, the nurse must clearly understand the effect of illness and hospitalization experience, upon the growth and development process of children and the effect of the developmental status of the children upon their responses to therapy. The role of the pediatric nurse has been influenced by the research findings in other health disciplines of prevention and therapy, in various areas of genetics, drugs, medical, and surgical techniques. It is also influenced by the research carried out within the nursing profession itself.

The concept of assessment of children is important for providing care to patients and their families. The function of the pediatric nurse is to promote and support children in their adaptation process. The nurse must observe the children's health and illness state, their strengths and weaknesses, and effectiveness of their coping mechanism. Nursing children require a better sense of responsibility and better judgment of children's health), responses, and planning for nursing management. The nurse must have patience and emotional balance while dealing with the children and their parents, specially, in critically ill cases.

b. Guidance to parents on toddler care

1. Parents must be educated regarding the dangers associated with medicines, household substances and agrochemicals. A poison label should appear on all dangerous medicines, including aspirin and paracetamol.
2. Parents must begin to teach their children at an early age the danger of touching, eating or playing with unknown objects including medicines, pesticides and insecticides, household chemicals or plants.

3. Medicines, insecticides and pesticides and other poisonous substances should be stored in locked cabinets.
4. Dyes, polishes, kerosene and other poisonous household chemicals should never be left on a low shelf or on the floor. Do not store in kitchen or bathroom.
5. Combustion devices should be adequately ventilated.
6. Inhalation of spray or fumes should be prevented during painting or application of insecticides.
7. Unnecessary toxic substances should be discarded.
8. Carefully check the label of any medicine before use. Do not put different tablets or pills in the same bottle.
9. Do not store any poisonous liquid in a beverage bottle.
10. Wear protective clothing, goggles, gloves and masks during spraying of insecticide and always spray downwind. Protective clothing should be removed and exposed skin washed thoroughly before eating anything.
11. Dispense medicine and dangerous household's chemicals in childproof, tamperproof containers.
12. Education on proper hygiene and storage of food to avoid food poisoning.
13. Workers and other persons working in industries should be trained in safe use of chemicals.
14. Industries should have complete knowledge and information in the toxicity and management of the chemicals they are using.
15. Persons having suicidal tendencies should not be given a large amount of drugs at a time and should be given adequate psychiatric follow-up and counseling.

c. Care of a child with hemolytic disorders

Hemolytic disease of the newborn (HDN), also called erythroblastosis fetalis, is a blood disorder that occurs when the blood types of a mother and baby are incompatible. The following are the most common symptoms of hemolytic disease of the newborn. However, each baby may experience symptoms differently.

During pregnancy symptoms may include:
1. With amniocentesis, the amniotic fluid may have a yellow coloring and contain bilirubin.
2. Ultrasound of the fetus shows enlarged liver, spleen, or heart and fluid buildup in the fetus's abdomen, around the lungs, or in the scalp.

After birth, symptoms may include:
1. A pale coloring may be evident, due to anemia.
2. Jaundice, or yellow coloring of amniotic fluid, umbilical cord, skin, and eyes may be present. The baby may not look yellow immediately after birth, but jaundice can develop quickly, usually within 24–36 hours.
3. The newborn may have an enlarged liver and spleen.
4. Babies with hydrops fetalis have severe edema (swelling) of the entire body and are extremely pale. They often have difficulty breathing.

During pregnancy, treatment for HDN may include:
1. Intrauterine blood transfusion of red blood cells into the baby's circulation. This is done by placing a needle through the mother's uterus and into the abdominal cavity of the fetus or directly into the vein in the umbilical cord. It may be necessary to give a sedative medication to keep the baby from moving. Intrauterine transfusions may need to be repeated.

2. Early delivery if the fetus develops complications. If the fetus has mature lungs, labor and delivery may be induced to prevent worsening of HDN.

After birth, treatment may include:
1. Blood transfusions (for severe anemia)
2. Intravenous fluids (for low blood pressure)
3. Help for respiratory distress using oxygen, surfactant, or a mechanical breathing machine
4. Exchange transfusion to replace the baby's damaged blood with fresh blood. The exchange transfusion helps increase the red blood cell count and lower the levels of bilirubin. An exchange transfusion is done by alternating giving and withdrawing blood in small amounts through a vein or artery. Exchange transfusions may need to be repeated if the bilirubin levels remain high.
5. Intravenous immunoglobin (IVIG). IVIG is a solution made from blood plasma that contains antibodies to help the baby's immune system. IVIG may help reduce the breakdown of red blood cells and lower bilirubin levels.

d. Welfare of delinquent and destitute children

One of the major objectives of the society is to explore the unidentified areas through research work where the child can be helped and to place before the government for future action plan.

Aims and objectives of the society
1. To coordinate activities and help in the development of child welfare movement specially delinquent and destitute children and children of other backward classes.
2. To organize public opinion to secure progressive legislation, its better enforcement of child welfare mainly in the state of Delhi.
3. To provide medical aid and relief to the needy children including the establishment maintenance and support of institutions of medical aid and relief.
4. Awarding scholarship, grant or monetary aid and assistance to deserving children for the purpose of undertaking, prosecuting and encouraging research work in any branch of education, technology, medical science, agricultural science, commercial accountancy, business management or any branch or branches of applied sciences or higher learning.
5. To provide grants in aids of any kind for the benefit of deserving indigent and needy children.
6. To organize conferences, seminars and exhibitions to promote the interests of children.
7. To maintain a library of books and publications.
8. To promote and encourage cultural activity among the children.
9. To foaster and encourage friendly, brotherly feelings, better understandings, cooperation and to develop unity, among the children.
10. To distribute free books food and clothing to the poor and needy children.
11. To act as representative between the official and non-official agencies and organizations, at the local district and state level.
12. To initiate action for promoting child welfare services in slum areas, re-settlement colonies, etc. for meeting their needs, by setting up essential relief projects.

IV. a. What is dengue fever?
   b. List the types of dengue fever
   c. Briefly explain the medical and nursing management of a child with dengue fever

Dengue fever is one of the most important emerging diseases of the tropical and subtropical regions, affecting urban and periurban areas.

Dengue fever is a self limiting disease and represents the majority of cases of dengue infection. These infections may be asymptomatic or may lead to: (a) "Classical" dengue fever or; (b) Dengue hemorrhagic fever without shock or; (c) Dengue hemorrhagic fever with shock.

Pathogenesis

1. Agent factors—it is caused by an RNA virus that has 4 subtypes infecting humans. A prevalence of *Aedes aegypti* and *Aedes albopictus* together with the circulation of dengue fever.
2. Host factors—it is estimated that each year 50 million infections occur with 500,000 cases of dengue hemorrhagic fever and at least 12,000 deaths, mainly among children, although fatalities could be twice as high.
3. Environmental factors—the increase of dengue and DHF is due to uncontrolled population growth and urbanization without appropriate water management, to the global spread of dengue via travel and trade and to erosion of vector control program.
4. Mode of transmission—dengue fever transmitted by *Aedes agape*.
5. Incubation period—about 8–10 days commonly (5–6 days).

Clinical Manifestations

1. Classical dengue fever—it also called "breakbone fever". The onset is sudden with chills and high fever, intense headache, muscle and joint pains which prevent all movements.
2. Within 24 hours retro-orbital pain, particularly on eye movement or eye pressure and photophobia develops. Some common symptoms include extreme weakness anorexia, constipation, altered taste sensation, colicky pain and abdominal tenderness, dragging in inguinal region, sore throat and general depression. Fever is usually between 39°C and 40°C.
3. The rash is accompanied by similar but milder symptoms. The rash may be diffuse flushing, mottling or fleeting pin point eruptions on the face, neck and chest during the first half of the febrile period and a conspicuous rash that may be maculopapular or scarlatiniform on 3rd or 4th day.

Dengue Hemorrhagic Fever

1. Dengue hemorrhagic fever is a severe form of dengue fever, caused by infection with more than one dengue virus.
2. The incubation period of four to six days, the illness commonly begins abruptly with high fever, accompanied by discomfort, tenderness at the right costal margin and generalized abdominal pain are common.
3. Occasionally, the temperature may be 40–41°C and febrile convulsions may occur particularly in infants.

Dengue Shock Syndrome

Shock—manifested by rapid and weak pulse with narrowing of the pulse pressure (20 mm Hg or less) or hypotension with the presence of cold, clammy skin and restlessness.

Grading the Severity of DHF
1. Grade I—Fever and only hemorrhagic manifestations.
2. Grade II—Spontaneous bleeding usually in the form of skin.
3. Grade III—Circulatory failure leads to shock.
4. Grade IV—Profound shock with undetectable blood pressure and pulse.

Diagnostic Tests
1. Thrombocytopenia (100,000/mm^3 or less) and
2. Hemoconcentration: Hematocrit increased by 20% or more of baseline value.
3. The above mentioned two clinical criteria plus thrombocytopenia and hemoconcentration or a rising hematocrit are sufficient to establish a clinical diagnosis of DHF.

Management
1. Management of dengue fever is symptomatic and supportive—bed rest, antipyretics or sponging, oral fluids and electrolyte therapy is recommended for patients with excessive sweating, vomiting or diarrhea.
2. The fluid replacement should be the minimum volume that is sufficient to maintain effective circulation during the period of leakage.
3. Management of shock is a medical emergency that requires prompt and vigorous volume replacement therapy. Colloidal fluid is indicated incases with massive leakage and to whom a large volume of crystalloid fluid has been given.

Complications: There is also electrolyte (sodium) and acid–base disturbances. It must be considered that there is a high potential for developing disseminated intravascular clotting (DIC) and that stagnant anemia blood will promote or enhance DIC, which may lead to severe hemorrhage or irreversible shock.

Preventive and Control Measures
1. Mosquito control—the principle can be controlled by individual and community action, using anti-adult and antilarval measures.
2. Isolation under nets during the first few days, individual protection against mosquitoes.

V. a. What is cleft lip and cleft palate?
b. Explain surgical treatment and management of a child with cleft lip and cleft palate

See question no. V of GNM paper-2-2014.

SECTION-II

VI. Choose the correct answer and write:
a. Normal head circumference of newborn is: **31–33 cm:**
   (i) 31–33 cm, (ii) 33–35 cm, (iii) 35–40 cm
b. Chickenpox is caused by: **Vericella zoster:**
   (i) Vericella zoster, (ii) Myxovirus, (iii) Itch mite
c. Commonest cause of abdominal pain in children is: **Worm colic:**
   (i) Dysentery, (ii) Worm colic, (iii) Appendicitis

VII. State whether the following statements are *true* or *false*

a. Spina bifida is one of the most uncommon anomalies in children: **FALSE**.
b. Cerebral palsy is the most frequent permanent disability of childhood: **TRUE**.
c. Phototherapy is a treatment for intrauterine growth retardation: **FALSE**.
d. Pleural effusion is the collection of fluid in pleural space: **TRUE**.

VIII. Write short notes on any *three* of the following:

a. Ascariasis

Ascaris lumbricoides is a nematode, mostly known as roundworm. it is most common helminthic infestation. It lives in the lumen of small intestine. The adult female roundworm measures 20–40 cm and the male 12–30 cm in length. Each female round worm produces 2,40,000 eggs per day. The eggs are excreted in the feces and in the external environment they become infective in favorable conditions. On ingestion of mature egg by the human host (definitive host), it hatches out in the duodenum to release larvae. The larvae penetrate the intestinal wall and are carried to liver then to the lungs through bloodstream. In the lungs they break through the alveolar walls and migrate into the bronchioles, then coughed up through the trachea and reswallowed to reach the small intestine, where they become mature into adult worms in 60–80 days. The life span of an adult roundworm is between 6 and 12 months and maximum 1.5–2 years.

b. Child reaction to hospitalization

Infants

1. Crankiness and irritability caused by a disruption, or change, in their normal routine.
2. Infants have an immediate reaction to pain or discomfort.
3. Infants may not be able to verbalize their feelings, but can show their feelings through their actions (withdrawing from interaction, eating or drinking less than usual, crying, sleeping more or less than usual).
4. Stranger anxiety usually begins at about 6 months of age; being separated from a caregiver can be extremely difficult for an infant in the hospital.

Toddlers

1. Fear of strangers.
2. Separation anxiety.
3. Toddlers often have an immediate physical response to pain and unfamiliar surroundings, such as crying.
4. A regression in established skills, for example, use of baby talk, wanting to be carried, or refusing to use the toilet.

Preschool-aged Children

1. Separation anxiety; fear of what might happen when a caregiver is not there.
2. Display increased magical or fantasy thinking; fear that hospitalization is a punishment or was caused by something that he or she did or did not do.
3. Fear usually regarding things that hurt, such as shots; that having a shot is a punishment.
4. Fear that an action caused the illness to occur, leading to feelings of guilt.
5. Regression of skills.

School-aged Children
1. Fear of pain; real or imagined.
2. Fear of loss of control; fear of inability to return to doing what he or she was able to do before hospitalization.
3. Fear of loss of respect; loss of respect of parents as being seen as weak or not as strong as one "should" be.
4. Fear of loss of love; fear of loss of love due to causing a disruption in the family's normal routine.
5. Fear of anesthesia; fear that if he or she goes to sleep that they may not wake up/loss of control due to anesthesia.
6. Fear of bodily injury, causing the child to question whether or not he or she will return to "normal" after the hospitalization.
7. Stress over separation from school and friends.
8. Concerns over loss of body privacy.

Adolescents
1. Stress regarding separation from friends.
2. Fear of loss of status among group of friends.
3. Anxiety related to changes in physical appearance.
4. Anxiety related to long-term illness.
5. Concern for privacy.
6. Regression can occur during uncomfortable situations.

c. Medical and nursing management of child with HIV infection

ART is the mainstay in human immunodeficiency virus (HIV) treatment. Appropriate antiretroviral therapy (ART) and treatment of specific infections and malignancies are critical in treating patients who are HIV positive. Intervening early may prevent damage to the immune system and potentially retard dissemination of infection. Combination ART is recommended for all infants, children, and adolescents who meet treatment criteria.

Reduction in the mortality rate associated with perinatally acquired HIV-1 over the past 10 years is a result of improved ART. However, only triple combination ART appears to significantly reduce the relative hazard ratio of death, as compared with no treatment.

The inadequacy of merely reducing the viral load has been realized in recent years. Quick suppression of the viral load with highly active ART (HAART) substantially slows viral replication and prevents resistant mutations.

Medical Management of HIV-Infected Children
The following are the 2010 goals for treating pediatric patients with HIV infection, from the Panel on Antiretroviral Therapy and Medical Management of HIV-Infected Children:
1. Reducing HIV-related mortality and morbidity.
2. Restoring and/or preserving immune function.
3. Maximally and durably suppressing viral replication.
4. Minimizing drug-related toxicity.
5. Maintaining normal physical growth and neurocognitive development.
6. Improving quality of life.

The following are several important factors to consider in making treatment decisions about when to initiate antiretroviral therapy:
1. Severity of HIV disease.
2. Risk of disease progression.
3. Laboratory assessments (e.g. $CD4^+$ count, plasma HIV RNA levels).
4. Availability of appropriate and palatable drug formulations.
5. Adverse effects of the antiretroviral medications.
6. Effect of initial treatment regimen choice on later therapeutic options.
7. Presence of comorbidities that may affect drug choices.

Potential antiretroviral drug interactions with required concomitant medications.
Ability of the child and caregiver to adhere to treatment regimen.

As the disease progresses, wasting is noted, with weight loss and growth retardation in children. Low protein stores can be countered by increasing the intake of amino acids, specifically threonine and methionine.

Address abnormalities in psychological and neurologic development, due, in part, to the tropism of the virus for CNS tissue in children who are HIV positive. Social, economic, and psychological factors impair the ability of many HIV-infected children and their parents to attend regular clinic appointments. This problem can be challenging and may require substantial use of social and child protective services on a regular basis. Psychosocial support is extremely important. Failure to provide such services can result in a lack of compliance with medications and appointments.

d. Management of a child with rheumatic fever

Rheumatic fever is a serious immune disease that affects different areas of the body, including the joints, heart, skin, nervous system, and brain. Rheumatic fever may develop after a serious infection with *Streptococcus* bacteria, especially strep throat. Family history of the disease also plays an important part in who gets rheumatic fever and who does not. While rheumatic fever is more frequent in children under 15 years old, it can occur at any age if a serious case of strep throat is left untreated treated inadequately for more than 20 days.

Rheumatic fever (RF) is a systemic illness that may occur following group A beta hemolytic streptococcal (GABHS) pharyngitis in children. Rheumatic fever and its most serious complication, rheumatic heart disease (RHD), are believed to result from an autoimmune response; however, the exact pathogenesis remains unclear. Studies in the 1950s during an epidemic on a military base demonstrated 3% incidence of rheumatic fever in adults with streptococcal pharyngitis not treated with antibiotics.

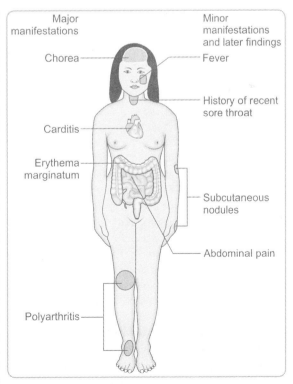

Treatment of rheumatic fever

Name of medicine	Age	Dose	When to take
Penicillin V or G (by mouth)	up to 3 years over 3 (includes adults)	125 mg 250 mg	4 times a day for 10 days
OR Benzathine penicillin (by injection)	up to 3 years over 3 (includes adults)	600,000 units 1,200,000 units	Single injection (Give one-half in each buttock)
OR Procaine penicillin (by injection)	up to 3 years over 3 (includes adults)	600,000 units 1,200,000 units	Inject one-half into each buttock muscle once a day for 10 days
For persons allergic so penicillin give: Erythromycin (by mouth)	up to 3 years over 3 (includes adults)	125 mg 250 mg	4 times a day for 10 days

NOTE: Whenever possible, it is safer to give children medicine by mouth than by injection

While there is no cure for rheumatic fever, the disease can be effectively treated with a dual approach, which includes antibiotics, such as penicillin, to cure any remainders of the streptococcal infection, and no steroidal anti-inflammatory medication to reduce inflammation and ease the bothersome symptoms. Bed rest is also a common prescription for patients. Patients who have been diagnosed with rheumatic fever usually must take antibiotics throughout life to prevent recurrences. If left untreated, rheumatic fever can result in serious complications, including scarring of the heart's valves and even congestive heart failure. Rheumatic fever has also been known to affect the brain and cause loss of coordination. Since no definite treatments exist for rheumatic fever, prevention is essential. Treating throat infections with antibiotics is the easiest way to avoid later complications.

IX. a. What is diarrhea?

Diarrhea diseases rank among the top three causes of childhood death in the developing countries. On an average a child suffers from about 12 episodes of diarrhea, 4 such episodes occurring during the very first year of life. Existence of malnutrition makes the child very much vulnerable to diarrheal diseases.

Diarrhea is defined as the passage of loose, liquid or watery stools, more than three times per day. The recent change in consistency and character of stool rather than number of stools is more important. Especially in children one large amount watery motion may constitute diarrhea. 'Acute diarrhea' is an attack of loose motion with sudden onset which usually lasts 3–7 days but may last up to 10–14 days. it is caused by an infection of the large intestine, but maybe associated with infection of gastric mucosa and small intestine. The term 'acute gastroenteritis' (AGE) is most frequently used to describe acute diarrhea.

Chronic diarrhea is termed when the loose motion is occurring for 3 weeks or more. It is usually related to underlying organic diseases with or without malabsorption.

Diarrhea with watery stools and visible blood in the stools is called as dysentery. Persistent diarrhea refers to the episodes of acute diarrhea that last for 2 weeks or more and may be due to infective origin.

b. List the causes and clinical features of diarrhea

Epidemiology: Diarrhea is a major public health problem in India, among children below the age of 5 years. About one-third of total hospitalized children are due to diarrheal diseases and 17% of all deaths in indoor pediatric patients are related to this condition. The morbidity rate in terms of diarrhea episodes per year per child under the age of 5 years is about 1.7. Diarrheal diseases cause a heavy economic burden on health services.

Agent factors: Diarrhea is mostly infectious. A large numbers of organism are responsible for acute diarrhea. The infectious agents causing diarrhea with enteric infection include the followings:
1. **Viruses:** Rotavirus, adenovirus, enterovirus, Norwalk group viruses, measles virus, etc.
2. **Bacteria:** *Campylobacter jejuni, Euclid, Shigella, Salmonella, Cholera vibrio, Vibrio parahemolyticus,* etc.
3. **Parasites:** *Cryptospo ridium, H. nana,* malaria, etc.
4. **Fungi:** *Candida albicans.*

Diarrhea may occur due to spread of infection by parenteral route from other infections like pneumonia, tonsillitis, upper respiratory infections, otitis media, urinary tract infection, etc. Other important causes of diarrhea are related to dietary or nutritional factors, e.g. over feeding, under feeding or malnutrition, food allergy and food poisoning. Some drugs (antibiotics) also can cause diarrhea.

Noninfectious causes of diarrhea are congenital anomalies of GI tract, malabsorption syndrome, inflammatory bowel disease, immunodeficiency conditions, inappropriate use of laxative and purgatives, emotional stress and excitement.

Types of Diarrhea

Secretory diarrhea: It is caused by external or internal secretagogue (cholera toxin, lactase deficiency). It has tendency to be watery, voluminous and persistent, even if no oral feeding is allowed. There is decrease absorption and increased secretion.

Osmotic diarrhea: It is due to ingestion of poorly absorbed solute (alcohol, sorbitol) or maldigestion or a small bowel defect. It tends to be watery and acidic with reducing substances.

Motility diarrhea: It is associated with increased or delayed motility of the bowel. There is decreased transit time or stasis of bacteria leading to overgrowth.

Clinical manifestations: The clinical presentations of diarrheal diseases may vary with severity, specific cause and type of onset. Dehydration is the important life-threatening feature which is usually associated with diarrhea. It should be assessed accurately for the appropriate management. Diarrhea stools are usually loose or watery in consistency. It may be greenish or yellowish-green in color with offensive smell. It may contain mucus, pus or blood and may expel with force, preceded by abdominal pain. Frequency of stools varies from 2–20 per day or more.

The child may have low-grade fever, thirst, anorexia with intermittent vomiting and abdominal distention. Behavioral changes like irritability, restlessness, weakness, lethargy, sleepiness, delirium, stupor and flaccidity are usually present. Physical changes like loss of weight, poor skin turgor, dry mucus membranes, dry lips, pallor, sunken eyes, and depressed fontanelles are also usually found. The vital signs are changed as low blood pressure, tachycardia, rapid respiration, cold limbs and collapse. There is decreased or absent urinary output. Convulsions and loss of consciousness may also present in some children with diarrheal diseases.

Complication: Dehydration, abdominal distension, acute renal failure, peripheral circulatory failure, thrombophlebitis, convulsions, intussusception, bronchopneumonia and malnutrition.

c. Write the complications and nursing management of a child with diarrhea

Supportive Care
1. Fluid and electrolyte balance should be maintained. The amount and type of fluid depends on the severity of diarrhea.

a. In mild diarrhea with few loose stools, small amount (about 300 mL) of oral rehydration solution may be given every hour.
b. In moderate diarrhea, with several loose stools and 10% weight with dehydration, clear fluid intake should be encouraged.

   The amount of oral rehydration solution is increased up to 200 mL/kg/day. A nasogastric drip may be started as it may help to prevent gastrocolic reflex. The care should be taken to prevent circulatory overload.

   If children have no nausea, vomiting or abdominal distension, they should be encouraged to drink oral electrolyte solution: Sodium chloride 3.5 g, sodium bicarbonate 2.5 g, potassium chloride 1.5 g, glucose 20 g, water 1000 mL.
c. In severe dehydration with more than 10% weight loss, intravenous fluids are necessary. The fluids may be administered at 225 mL/kg/day. Fifty percent of the calculated fluids should be given by a fast drip, over a period of six hours. Twenty five percent in the next four hours and remaining amount over the rest of the day.
2. Specific antibiotics are prescribed for *E. coli*, *Shigella* and *Salmonella*.
3. Sedatives may be prescribed only to the children with the severe restlessness, to control the pain and cramps.
4. Adsorbents, such as kaolin and pectin may decrease the frequency of evacuation, may not reduce the fluid loss but mask the volume loss.

Management

1. Children should be isolated to prevent the spread of infection. The excreta should be disinfected and disposed. The contamination should be prevented.
2. If children have no vomiting and are conscious, they should be encouraged to take oral fluids, such as buttermilk, coconut water, skimmed milk, weak tea, and apple juice. In case of severe dehydration, when intravenous fluids are necessary. The rate of the fluid intake should be monitored carefully, as prescribed. In the beginning, the fluid is given at faster and then the rate is gradually decreased. A care of the intravenous infusion site is important to prevent the infiltration, infection, or thrombosis.
3. Observation is required, for the signs of complication, by monitoring vital signs, skin changes, and behavior changes of the patient.
4. Assessment of the characteristics of diarrhea and recording of the number, amount, and consistency of stools. Any vomiting and cramps should be noted.
5. Care of the skin at the perineum and buttocks is important because the stools have chemicals that affect the skin around the anal region, causing irritation, redness, and excoriation. The diaper should be changed immediately after each soiling. The cleaning and dying after each soiling and application of a cream or zinc paste can prevent skin irritation.
6. Comforting the patient is essential. Dry, clean, and comfortable linen should be provided.
7. The close contact and affection can be provided by holding the children whenever necessary. The diversional measures, such as toys suitable for the age and developmental level of children can be used.
8. General hygienic care should be provided.
9. Nutritional status should be monitored. During the diarrhea, if children are on intravenous fluids or in severe diarrhea where nutritional balance cannot be met, they may develop malnutrition. Therefore, as soon as vomiting stops, oral feeding should be started which are easily digestible such as soft cooked rice, banana, curds, and buttermilk.

10. Once loose motions are controlled, high calories and high protein diet should be given to make up the weight loss.

Parental advice

1. The parents should be supported especially when their children can not have anything by mouth and when they are on intravenous fluids.
2. The parents should be explained about the following precautions related to feeding:
   a. To follow the cleanliness while preparing feeds and feeding the children.
   b. The importance of hand washing before handling the food and after cleaning 'the patient. Need for boiling of the vessels used for feeding and preventing contamination is required especially for the infant. Use of boiled and cooled water for drinking should be emphasized.
3. Parents should be explained about the early signs of diarrhea and dehydration.
4. The parents should be explained about the use of oral rehydration fluids, in the early stage of diarrhea.

X. a. Define osteomyelitis.
b. List the signs and symptoms of osteomyelitis.
c. Explain the nursing management of a child suffering from osteomyelitis.

Definition: Osteomyelitis is an infection of the bone. It is commonly caused by an infection, usually bacterial in nature, which starts in another part of the body and spreads by the blood. It can be acute, i.e. it has a rapid onset, or chronic, i.e. it is persistent and long-lasting.

Causes: This infection can be caused by a complication somewhere else in the body like pneumonia or a urinary tract infection. The most common bacteria that causes, it is *Staphylococcus aureus*. This infection is then carried through the body in the blood, also known as sepsis, a whole body or systemic inflammatory condition, or bacteremia, a condition where there is bacteria present in the blood. It can also be caused by a trauma, typically where there is a break in the skin. Chronic open wounds, such as diabetic ulcers, can also open up a path for the bacteria to spread to the bone.

Typically, osteomyelitis is found in the feet, vertebrae or spine, and in the pelvis in adults. Children usually experience this infection in the long bones, such as the femer or thigh bone. People with certain other health problems, such as diabetes, sickle cell disease immune system compromise and the elderly in general are at a higher risk.

Clinical manifestations: Osteomyelitis symptoms can include local inflammation, warmth and redness of the area, pain in the bone, fever with or without malaise and nausea. Malaise is a general feeling of discomfort. The victim can also experience things such as chills, excessive sweating, low back pain or generalized swelling of the ankles, feet and legs.

Diagnosis: Diagnosis of osteomyelitis is made through a general physical examination where pain, swelling and redness can be detected. Blood tests, bone scans, MRIs, and bone lesion biopsies are also helpful diagnostic tools. In some cases, a needle aspiration is necessary. This is where the infected fluids causing swelling are drawn out from the area.

Management: The typical course of treatment for osteomyelitis is antibiotics to destroy the bacteria. In severe cases, surgery may be needed if the infection is resistant to antibiotics to remove the dead bone tissue. Surgery is then followed by a six-week course of antibiotics. In most cases, if treated, osteomyelitis can be successfully solved. But if it becomes chronic, the abscesses, or pus-filled pockets in the bone, can inhibit blood flow to the bone and spread the infection. Chronic osteomyelitis sufferers occasionally need more drastic measures, such as amputations, to avoid further spread of the bacteria.

2011
Pediatric Nursing

SECTION-I

I. Give the meaning of the following:
   a. Juvenile delinquency.
   b. Omphalocele.
   c. Apgar score.
   d. Neonatal mortality rate.
   e. Hernia.

II. Fill in the blanks
   a. Deficiency of vitamin D causes _____ in children.
   b. Normal length of a newborn is: _____
   c. Depressed fontanelle is the sign of: _____

III. Write short notes on any *four* of the following:
   a. Tetralogy of Fallot.
   b. The battered child syndrome.
   c. Nursing management of a child with cerebral palsy.
   d. Phototherapy.
   e. Growth and development of toddler.

IV. Differentiate between the following:
   a. Hypospadias and epispadias.
   b. Meningocele and meningomyelocele.

V. A child is admitted with history of cleft lip and cleft palate, explain
   a. Surgical treatment.
   b. Preoperative and postoperative nursing management.

SECTION-II

VI. Choose the correct answer
   a. Opisthotonus position is seen in: _____
      (i) Measles, (ii) Tetanus, (iii) Typhoid
   b. State with the lowest infant mortality rate is: _____
      (i.) Kerala, (ii) Goa, (iii) Madhya Pradesh
   c. The traction which is used to treat upper extremity is: _____
      (i) Russel traction, (ii) Dunlop traction, (iii) Ninety-ninety traction.

VII. State whether following statements are *true* or *false*:
   a. Hemophilia is due to deficiency of plasma factor VIII.
   b. The disease caused by Klebs Loeffler bacillus is called pertussis.
   c. Emphysema is the condition of the pus in the pleural cavity.
   d. Cryptorchidism is failure of testes to descend into the scrotum.

VIII. Write short notes on any three of the following:
   a. Juvenile diabetes mellitus.
   b. Worm infestations.
   c. Administration of oxygen for infants and children.

IX. Ramu aged about 8 years is suffering from acute glomerulonephritis
   a. Explain acute glomerulonephritis.
   b. Enumerate the clinical manifestations and treatment of acute glomerulonephritis.
   c. Explain the nursing management of glomerulonephritis.

OR

   a. Define convulsion.
   b. List the causes of convulsion.
   c. Explain the management of a child with convulsion during and after attack.

X. Seema aged 6 years is admitted to pediatric ward with the diagnosis of rheumatic fever
   a. Define rheumatic fever.
   b. List the causes of rheumatic fever.
   c. Explain the medical and nursing management of rheumatic fever.

SECTION-I

I. Give the meaning of the following:

a. Juvenile delinquency

Delinquency is a kind of abnormality. When an individual deviates from the course of normal social life, his behavior is called "delinquency". When a juvenile, below an age specified under a statute exhibits behavior which may prove to be dangerous to society and/or to him he may be called a 'Juvenile delinquent'. Each state has its own precise definition of the age range covered by the word 'juvenile'.

Juvenile delinquents are those offenders including boys and girls who are normally under 16 years of age. A juvenile delinquent is a young person incorrigible, or habitually disobedient. Acts of delinquency may include (i) running away from home without the permission of parents, (ii) habitual truancy beyond the control of parents, (iii) spending time idly beyond limits, (iv) use of vulgar languages, (v) wandering about rail-roads, streets, market places, (vi) visiting gambling centers, (vii) committing sexual offences, (viii) shop-lifting, (ix) stealing, etc. Juveniles may do such activities singly or through a gang.

b. Omphalocele

An omphalocele technically is a malformation or a birth defect in the wall of the abdomen, often along the area of the umbilical cord. It generally is characterized by the protrusion of internal abdominal organs outside the umbilicus and is covered by a thin transparent membrane. Some parts or most parts of the intestines, stomach, spleen, and liver can be seen through this thin covering depending on the size of the opening.

On the sixth week of fetal life, the intestines generally develop and tend to protrude out of the abdomen and grow longer. By the end of the tenth week, they usually return inside the abdominal cavity, technically followed by closure of the abdominal wall. Failure of this process sometimes happens during the development of the fetus, often resulting in the formation of an omphalocele. There are some studies that point to inherited genetic disorders as possible causes of omphalocele.

During the second and third trimesters of pregnancy, an omphalocele technically can be detected by ultrasound if present in the fetus. It often is advised by a physician to evaluate the fetus further for any presence of other abnormalities. Down syndrome, Turner syndrome, and Beckwith-Wiedemann syndrome, among many others, often are found in children born with omphaloceles. Repair procedures often are decided before the birth of the affected child, depending mostly on the size of the defect as seen in an ultrasound.

c. Apgar score

(See Questions No. I-a of GNM Paper-2-2013)

d. Neonatal mortality rate

The ratio of the number of deaths in the first 28 days of life to the number of live births occurring in the same population during the same period of time.

$$\text{Neonatal mortality rate} = \frac{\text{Number of neonatal deaths}}{\text{Number of live births in the same year and areas}} \times 1{,}000 \text{ births}$$

e. Hernia
(See Question No I-b of GNM Paper-2-2014)

II. Fill in the blanks
a. Deficiency of vitamin D causes **Rickets** in children.
b. Normal length of a newborn is: **45–50 cm.**
c. Depressed forntanelle is the sign of: **Diarrhea.**

III. Write short notes on any *four* of the following:

a. Tetralogy of Fallot

Tetralogy of Fallot (TOF) is the most common cyanotic congenital heart disease. It accounts for 6–10% of all CHDs. This condition is characterized by the combinations of four defects (i) pulmonary stenosis, (ii) ventricular septal defect, (iii) overriding or dextroposition of the aorta, and (iv) right ventricular hypertrophy.

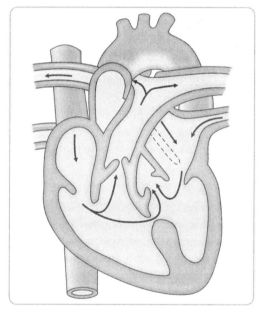

Pathophysiology: Due to structural defects, there is right to left heart shunt causing cyanosis. The most vital abnormalities are pulmonary stenosis and VSD (generally perimembraneous variety). Obstruction of blood flow from the right ventricle due to pulmonary valve stenosis results in shunting of deoxygenated blood through the VSD into the left ventricle, then to the aorta causes cyanosis. Degree of cyanosis depends upon the degree of right ventricular outflow tract obstruction and the size of the VSD. Outflow obstruction can also occur due to infundibular hypertrophy and supravalvular stenosis. Right ventricular hypertrophy develops due to the obstruction. Finally, the condition is complicated by persistent arterial unsaturation, poor pulmonary vascularity, polycythemia to compensate cyanosis and increased blood viscosity resulting thrombophlebitis and formation of emboli. Minimum right to left shunt in small obstruction causes mild form of TOF and termed as pink or acyanotic tetralogy of Fallot.

b. The battered child syndrome

the battered child syndrome, a clinical condition in young children who have received serious physical abuse, is a frequent cause of permanent injury or death. The syndrome should be considered in any child exhibiting evidence of fracture of any bone, subdural hematoma, failure to thrive, soft tissue swellings or skin bruising, in any child who dies suddenly, or where the degree and type of injury is at variance with the history given regarding the occurrence of the trauma. Psychiatric factors are probably of prime importance in the pathogenesis of the disorder, but knowledge of these factors is limited. Physicians have a duty and responsibility to the child to require a full evaluation of the problem and to guarantee that no expected repetition of trauma will be permitted to occur.

c. Nursing management of child with cerebral palsy

Cerebral palsy (CP) is a group of nonprogressive disorders resulting from malfunctions of the motor centers and pathways of brain. It is a noncurable and nonfatal condition due to damage of the growing brain before or during birth. It is most common cause of crippling in children. Its severity is ranging from minor incapacitation to total handicap. Mental retardation is associated in about 25–50% of cases of CP. Other associated handicapped conditions are epilepsy, orthopedic deformities, partial or complete deafness, blindness and psychological disturbances.

Nursing management: Nursing assessment should include the detection of ability to perform activities of daily living (ADL), developmental milestones, neurological reflexes feeding behavior, nutritional status, bladder and bowel habits, problem related to vision, hearing and language, associated health hazards or congenital anomalies, present problems, parent-child interactions, treatment compliance, etc. Nursing diagnoses should be formulated accordingly to plan and to provide nursing interventions.

d. Phototherapy

Phototherapy is a form of medical treatment in which some form of light is used to address a medical issue. Babies born with jaundice are also treated with phototherapy. Jaundice in newborns is caused by a buildup of a pigment called bilirubin. Phototherapy helps the body convert the bilirubin into a form which can be urinated or excreted, allowing the baby's skin to return to a more usual color. Treatment for babies is usually conducted in a hospital immediately after birth, with staff keeping an eye on the baby to make sure that he or she is not struggling with other medical problems.

e. Growth and development of toddler

(See Question No. III-c of GNM Paper-2-2014)

IV. Differentiate between the following:

a. Hypospadias and epispadias

Hypospadias is a congenital defect, primarily of males, in which the urethra opens on the underside (ventrum) of the penis. It is one of the most common congenital abnormalities in the United States, occurring in about one of every 125 live male births. The corresponding defect in females is an opening of the urethra into the vagina and is rare.

Epispadias (also called bladder exstrophy) is a congenital defect of males in which the urethra opens on the upper surface (dorsum) of the penis. The corresponding defect in females is a fissure in the upper wall of the urethra and is quite rare.

b. Meningocele and meningomyelocele

A **meningocele** is sessile, sometimes pedunculated and of variable size. It is covered by full-thickness skin, which occasionally may be thin and translucent. It transilluminates brilliantly with no evidence of neural tissue or strands. An impulse on coughing or crying is apparent. There is no neurological deficit.

In a meningomyelocele, transillumination is positive and neural tissue may be demonstrable within the sac. It is usually not reducible, though a crying impulse and cross fluctuation with the open fontanel may be elicited. The sac is usually in communication with the subarachnoid space, but may also be multiloculated and divided into non-communicating compartments by fibrous or fibrolipomatous septa. The amount of neural tissue in the sac varies from case to case. A few strands of ectopic nerve fibers to the spinal cord or a part of the cauda equina may be found in the sac. The neural tissue is closely adherent to the fundus with only flimsy adhesions to the neck. Rarely such a meningomyelocele may be associated with angiomatous, cartilaginous or lipomatous tissue.

V. A child is admitted with history of cleft lip and cleft palate, explain:

a. Surgical treatment,
b. Preoperative and postoperative nursing management.
See Question No. V-c of GNM Paper-2-2014.

SECTION-II

VI. Choose the correct answer:

a. Opisthotonus position is seen in: **Tetanus**
   (i) Measles, (ii) Tetanus, (iii) Typhoid
b. State with the lowest infant mortality rate is: **Goa**
   (i) Kerala, (ii) Goa, (iii) Madhya Pradesh
c. The traction which is used to treat upper extremity is: **Dunlop traction**
   (i) Russell traction, (ii) Dunlop traction, (iii) Ninety-ninety traction.

VII. State whether following statements are *true* or *false*:

a. Hemophilia is due to deficiency of plasma factor VIII: **FALSE**
b. The disease caused by Klebs Loeffler bacillus is called pertussis: **FALSE**
c. Emphysema is the condition of the pus in the pleural cavity: **TRUE**
d. Cryptorchidism is failure of testes to descend into the scrotum: **TRUE**

VIII. Write short notes on any *three* of the following:

a. Juvenile diabetes mellitus

Type 1 diabetes can occur at any age. It is most often diagnosed in children, adolescents, or young adults. Insulin is a hormone produced in the pancreas by special cells, called beta cells. The pancreas is behind the stomach. Insulin is needed to move blood sugar (glucose) into cells. There, it is stored and later used for energy. In type 1 diabetes, beta cells produce little or no insulin.

Without enough insulin, glucose builds up in the bloodstream instead of going into the cells. The body is unable to use this glucose for energy. This leads to the symptoms of type 1 diabetes. The exact cause of type 1 diabetes is unknown. Most likely, it is an autoimmune disorder. This is a condition that occurs when the immune system mistakenly attacks and destroys healthy body tissue. With type 1 diabetes, an infection or another trigger causes the body to mistakenly attack the cells in the pancreas that make insulin. Type 1 diabetes can be passed down through families. When sugar builds up in the blood instead of going into cells, the body's cells starve for nutrients and other systems in the body must provide energy for many important bodily functions. As a result, high blood sugar develops and can cause:

1. **Dehydration.** The buildup of sugar in the blood can cause an increase in urination (to try to clear the sugar from the body). When the kidneys lose the glucose through the urine, a large amount of water is also lost, causing dehydration.
2. **Weight loss.** The loss of sugar in the urine means a loss of calories which provide energy and therefore many people with high sugars lose weight (Dehydration also contributes to weight loss).
3. **Diabetic ketoacidosis (DKA).** Without insulin and because the cells are starved of energy, the body breaks down fat cells. Products of this fat breakdown include acidic chemicals called ketones that can be used for energy. Levels of these ketones begin to build up in the blood, causing an increased acidity. The liver continues to release the sugar it stores to help out. Since the body cannot use these sugars without insulin, more sugars piles into the blood stream. The combination of high excess sugars, dehydration, and acid build up is known as "ketoacidosis" and can be life-threatening if not treated immediately.
4. **Damage to the body.** Over time, the high sugar levels in the blood may damage the nerves and small blood vessels of the eyes, kidneys, and heart and predispose a person to atherosclerosis (hardening) of the large arteries that can cause heart attack and stroke.

b. Worm infestations

Worm infestations is a helminthic infection of the upper intestine, is chronic and debilitating. The disease's major sign is anemia.

Pathogenesis

1. **Agent factors:** Adult worms live in the small intestine, mainly jejunum where they attach themselves to the villi. Man is the only important reservoir of human hookworm infection. Feces containing the ova of hookworms. However, the immediate source of infection is the soil contaminated with infected larvae.
2. **Host factors:** All ages and both sexes are susceptible to infection, in endemic areas, the highest incidence is found in the age group 15–25 years. It is an occupational disease of the farming community.
3. **Environmental factors:** The soil must be suitable for the eggs and larvae, a temperature 24°–32°C is considered favorable for the survival.
4. **Mode of transmission:** Hook worm enters the body usually feet, by penetrating the skin. Ancylostoma may also be acquired by the oral route by direct ingestion of infective larvae via contaminated fruits and vegetables. Transmission may take place in the warmer and wet seasons.
5. **Incubation period:** After entry of infection, 6 weeks are required for feces to have ova or eggs in it. Symptoms may appear after few weeks, months or even years, depending on the intensity of the infection.

Clinical Features
1. The patient may report that he recently walked barefoot in an area with contaminated soil. The earliest symptom findings are irritation and pruritus at the entry site.
2. When the larvae reach the lungs, the patient may complain of sore throat and cough, possibly productive of bloody sputum.
3. When intestinal infection occurs, he may report fatigue, nausea, weight loss, dizziness, uncontrolled diarrhea, black tarry stool. Fever occurs when larvae migrate through the lungs.
4. Inspection may reveal edema and an erythematous papulovesicular rash at an entry site. Auscultation of the chest may reveal crackles as larvae migrate through the lungs.

Complications
1. Identification of hookworm ova in a stool smear confirms the diagnosis. Anemia suggests severe chronic infection.
2. In an infected patient, blood studies show:
   a. Hemoglobin level of 5–9 g/dL (in a severe case)
   b. White blood cell count as high as 47,000/mm^3
   c. Eosinophil count of 500–700 /mm^3.

Management: Mebendazole or pyrantel pamoate is prescribed for hookworm infection. The patient also needs an iron rich diet or iron supplementations to prevent or correct anemia.

Preventive Measures
1. People should have habit of wearing chappals, shoes or boots and should not go out barefooted.
2. Provision for proper disposal of human excreta is necessary to prevent pollution of soil and water.
3. Provision of adequate latrines and urinals should be made to avoid in discriminated defecation and teach proper use of latrines to the public.
4. Vegetables and fruits must be washed properly before eating. Special care is required when these are taken raw.
5. Educate people about the spread, dangers and prevention of the disease.

c. Administration of oxygen for infants and children

Oxygen is used as a drug to change the concentration of inspired air in the conditions of deficiency of oxygen. It is one of the most common procedures carried out in the management of children with respiratory diseases and other illnesses. The young children are unable to express their breathing discomfort. The pediatric nurse should have knowledge, good observation skill and ability for assessment of need for oxygen therapy.

Purpose of Oxygen Therapy

Oxygen is administered to achieve satisfactory level of PaO_2, range between 60 and 80 or 90 mm Hg. It is used as temporary measures to relieve hypoxemia and hypoxia, but does not replace definite treatment of underlying cause of these conditions.

The general purposes of oxygen therapy are:
1. To correct hypoxemia and hypoxia.
2. To increase oxygen tension of blood plasma.
3. To restore the oxyhemoglobin in red blood cells.
4. To maintain the ability of body cells to carry on normal metabolic functions.

Assessment of Need for Oxygen Therapy

Oxygen administration is indicated in numbers of medical and surgical conditions.

The need for oxygen is assessed by the followings:
1. Observing symptoms of respiratory distress and hypoxia, i.e. inadequate breathing pattern, labored respiration, dysrhythmias, cyanosis, change of activity like restlessness, lethargic and unresponsiveness, change in level of consciousness, hypothermia, etc.
2. Analysis of arterial blood gases (ABGs) for PaO_2, $PaCO_2$ pH, HCO_3, etc.
3. Pulse oximetry.
4. Measuring of inspired O_2 concentration (FiO_2).

Methods of Oxygen Administration

It depends upon age and condition of the child, cause of hypoxia, required concentration of oxygen and ventilator assistance, available facilities, etc. Oxygen therapy can be given continuous or intermittent. It can be dispensed from a cylinder, piped-in-system, liquid oxygen reservoir or oxygen concentrator. It should be administered in higher concentration than is present in air (21%). Usually, it is given in 40–60% concentration but sometimes 100% can also be given.

Oxygen can be administered by following methods:
1. **Non-invasive method:** by (a) oxygen mask which can be simple face mask, venturi mask or partial rebreathing mask, (b) oxygen hood or face tent, (c) oxygen tent or canopy and (d) Isolette incubator or other closed incubator.
2. **Invasive method:** by (a) orotracheal or nasotracheal or tracheostomy route and (b) nasopharyngeal catheter or nasal cannula or nasal prong.

Complications of Oxygen Therapy

Prolonged exposure to high concentrations of oxygen may result in constriction of cerebral blood vessels leading to irreversible brain damage and constriction of retinal blood vessels causing retinopthy of prematurity or retrolental fibroplasia. Pulmonary complications are pulmonary congestion, bronchiolar edema, bronchopulmonary dysplasia (in neonates), respiratory depression, necrotizing bronchiolitis, etc. Long-term complications due to oxygen toxicity are chronic pulmonary diseases, seizure disorders and epilepsy.

Safety Precautions during Administration of Oxygen

1. Oxygen acts as a drug: It must be prescribed and administered in specific dose in terms of rate, concentration and duration.
2. Humidifier and regulator must be used.

IX. **Ramu aged about 8 years is suffering from acute glomerulonephritis:**
   a. Explain acute glomerulonephritis
   b. Enumerate the clinical manifestations and treatment of acute glomerulonephritis
   c. Explain the nursing management of glomerulonephritis

Acute glomerulonephritis is a noninfectious renal disease found more in male children than in the female children. It is more common in the age group of 2–10 years. It is an immune complex disease, due to antigen antibody reaction following hemolytic streptococcal infection. The antibodies affect the glomerulus causing proliferation and swelling of endothelial cells obstructing the blood flow through capillaries. The amount of the glomerular filtrate is reduced and it allows the passage of the blood cells and proteins into filtrate.

Manifestation

1. An onset is usually, one to three weeks after the onset of infection of the upper respiratory tract or infection of the skin.
2. Edema starts with the periorbital edema, in the morning.
3. Urine output is decreased, with the high color urine resembling black tea or cola (due to lysis red blood cells).
4. Hypertension may be present.
5. The fever may or may not be present.
6. Children look pale, lethargic, and irritable.
7. Children may complain of a headache.
8. Gastrointestinal disturbances may occur.

Investigation

1. Urine examination for: Hematuria, specific gravity, albumin, white blood cells and epithelial cells.
2. Blood examination for: Urea nitrogen and creatinin, serum albumin.
3. Anti-streptolysin O titer (ASLO).
4. Electrocardiography.

Complication

1. **Hypertension:** Hypertensive encephalopathy may occur when the diastolic blood pressure rises above 110 mm of Hg. It can cause vomiting, restlessness, convulsions, stupor, visual disturbances, or cranial nerve palsy.
2. **Cardiac failure** with the retention of salt and water may cause tachycardia, dyspnea, pulmonary edema, and enlargement of the heart.
3. **Renal failure** may occur with severe oliguria or anuria and increased blood pressure. It may occur in two phases:

    First phase: This stage of edema with oliguria may last for 5–10 days.

    Second stage: The stage of diuresis starts with the increased output of urine and decreased edema.

Treatment

1. There is no specific treatment for acute glumerulonephritis.
2. It is self limiting and patients recover within 2–3 weeks.
3. Death may be due to complications.

Supportive Treatment

1. Antibiotics, such as, long-acting penicillin may be given to treat reminent of the infection.
2. Hypotensive drugs may be prescribed to control the hypertension.
3. Magnesium sulfate may be prescribed in the encephalopathy to reduce cerebral edema.
4. Sedatives may be required in restless patients.
5. In cardiac failure, digitalis may be prescribed.
6. In renal failure, patients may need a dialysis.

Management

1. Rest may be required for two to four weeks. Gradually, the activities may be started as the children improve.
2. The vital signs should be observed to detect early sign of complications, such as, the deviation in the pulse, may indicate cardiac failure. Headache, convulsions, and behavioral changes may be indicative of hypertensive encephalopathy.
3. Observation of the intake and output is important. An accurate recording of daily weight, edema, and appearance of the urine is necessary.
4. Nutrition should be planned according to the blood reports in the specific stage.
   a. In mild cases, salt restricted regular food may be allowed. Salty food items should be avoided. In an early phase of oliguria, the food should contain low proteins, high carbohydrates and vitamin supplement. Small, frequent feeding should be given. Fluid should be supplied according to the prescription. The parents should be explained about the accurate fluid intake.
   b. During the second phase, when the diuresis starts, the normal food with the adequate fluids, fruits can be given, as the blood reports improve.
5. Recreational facilities and play in the bed, can help divert the children's mind.

Parental advice

1. Parents should be taught about the early signs of complications and importance of early treatment.
2. Proper care of the skin and timely treatment of the skin lesions should be explained.
3. Prompt care of the respiratory problems should be insisted.
4. Parents should be instructed about the follow up visits.

OR

a. Define convulsion
b. List the causes of convulsion
c. Explain the management of a child with convulsion during and after attack

Convulsions, also sometimes called seizures, are a medical condition in which a person's body appears to shake in an uncontrollable manner. When a person experiences them, his or her muscles quickly contract and relax repeatedly. This is what causes the appearance of rapid shaking movements. Convulsions are when a person's body shakes rapidly and uncontrollably. During convulsions, the person's muscles contract and relax repeatedly. The term "convulsion" is often used interchangeably with "seizure," although there are many types of seizures, some of which have subtle or mild symptoms instead of convulsions. Seizures of all types are caused by disorganized and sudden electrical activity in the brain.

When a person experiences convulsions, he or she may suddenly fall or experience uncontrollable muscle spasms. He or she may also begin to drool or froth from the mouth, start snorting and grunting, and stop breathing for a period of time. Other symptoms include briefly blacking out, feelings of confusion, unusual eye movement, loss of bowel or bladder control, and clenching of the teeth. The person may also act in an unusual manner, such as laughing for no reason, suddenly becoming angry, or picking at his or her clothes.

Causes: Convulsions are caused by a variety of factors, including epilepsy, fever, low blood sugar, meningitis, stroke, uremia (from kidney failure), head or brain injury and withdrawal from sedatives.

Clinical Manifestations

The signs of seizures in children can include confusion, hallucinations, motor impairment, behavioral changes, a blank stare, repetitive gestures, odd physical sensations and impaired communication. Not all of these symptoms are generally present during a child's seizure and, in some instances, the signs of seizures in children go unnoticed as a child will appear to behave normally despite a neurological dysfunction. Symptoms also differ according to the types of seizures that affect children.

There are more than 20 different types of seizures and most are developed in early childhood. Seizures are characterized by abnormal electrical discharges in the brain. Depending on where these discharges occur, the signs of seizures in children will differ. For instance, focal seizures, which occur on a single side of the brain, do not interrupt a child's consciousness, but may cause minor to severe muscle spasms. During a focal seizure, a child may be completely alert and able to communicate.

Symptoms of seizures in children are sometimes unrecognized. This is particularly true in instances where symptoms, such as a blank stare or minor confusion, only last for a few seconds. Other signs of seizures in children, such as reports of a peculiar taste or smell, may be overlooked or even assumed to be due to some other explanation. Sometimes mild signs of seizures in children tend to occur during a child's sleep and are, therefore, often easily missed by adults. Although a child may appear to function as she or he normally would, in some types of seizures brief disturbances in the brain lasting from a few seconds to several minutes may be taking place.

Management

In the highly stressed setting of this type of medical emergency, a familiar standardized protocol of recommended management saves time, prevents errors and facilitates care. Although the outcome is mainly determined by its cause, the duration of CSE is very important. A timely approach may be more important than the exact individual pharmacological interventions. Particular local expertise or resource limitations may provide legitimate reasons to adapt or adjust the recommended protocol. For individual children, who are known to respond well to specific medications, a more tailored approach may be more appropriate.

The objectives for the acute management of CSE are as follows:
1. Maintenance of adequate airway, breathing and circulation (ABCs).
2. Termination of the seizure and prevention of recurrence.
3. Diagnosis and initial therapy of life-threatening causes of CSE (e.g. hypoglycemia, meningitis and cerebral space-occupying lesions).
4. Arrangement of appropriate referral for ongoing care or transport to a secondary or tertiary care center.
5. Management of refractory status epilepticus (RSE).

X. Seema aged 6 years is admitted to pediatric ward with the diagnosis of rheumatic fever:
a. Define rheumatic fever
b. List the causes of rheumatic fever
c. Explain the medical and nursing management of rheumatic fever

See Question No. VIII-d of GNM Paper-2-2012

2010 (August)
Pediatric Nursing

SECTION-I

I. Give the meaning of the following:
  a. Mid-day meal.
  b. Hernia.
  c. Clubfoot.
  d. Gynecomastia.
  e. Hyperglycemia.

II. Fill in the blanks with suitable answers:
  a. Normal Apgar score of a newborn is: _____
  b. Startle reflex can be elicited by: _____
  c. The comfortable position for a 4-year-old child with cyanotic spell is: _____

III. Write short notes on any three of the following:
  a. Day care centers.
  b. Care of the child with marasmus.
  c. Concept of preventive pediatrics.
  d. Care of child with hydrocephalus.
  e. Growth and development during infancy.

IV. a. What is congenital heart disease?
  b. Write the types.
  c. Explain the clinical manifestation and management of a child with patent ductus arteriosus.

V. a. Define low birth weight baby.
  b. Explain the management of low birth weight baby.

Or

Baby Niranjan is admitted for hypospadiasis
  a. Define hypospadiasis.
  b. Write the signs and symptoms of hypospadiasis.
  c. Explain the surgical and nursing management of a child with hypospadiasis.

SECTION-II

VI. State whether the following statements are *true* or *false*
  a. Immunization is contraindicated if the child has febrile condition.
  b. Oral thrush is caused by *Candida albicans*.
  c. BCG vaccine is administered to prevent chickenpox.
  d. Planter flexion of the foot in which the toes are fixed lower than the heel is talipes calcaneus.

VII. Choose the correct answer and write
a. Which assessment finding is documented in case of an infant with Hirschsprung's diseases: _____
(i. Diarrhea, ii. Projectile vomiting, iii. Regurgitation of feed, iv. Foul smelling ribbon like stools)
b. Whooping cough is caused by: _____
(i. Vericella zoster, ii. Paramyxovirus, iii. Bordetella pertussis, iv. Enterovirus)
c. While administering oral liquid iron supplement to a child the nurse instructs the mother to: _____
(i. Administer iron throw straw, ii. Administer iron at meal time, iii. Add iron to formula for easy administration, iv. Mix iron with cereal)

VIII. Write short notes on any *three* of the following:
a. Prevention of home accident in toddlers.
b. Use of play as nursing intervention.
c. Respiratory distress syndrome.
d. Oral rehydration therapy.

IX.
a. What is bronchial asthma?
b. List the causative factors and clinical features.
c. Write in detail the medical and nursing management of an 8-year-old child with bronchial asthma.

X.
a. What is poliomyelitis?
b. Write the causes and signs and symptoms.
c. Explain the preventive measures and management of a child with polio attack.

SECTION-I

I. Give the meaning of the following:

a. Mid-day meal

Mid-day meal program has an important role in providing balanced diet to school children. This is an effect taken by government of India. Since 1960 to provide at least one nutritious meal and diet supplements to children in primary and middle schools. It was first organized in 1957 in Tamil Nadu successfully. In this one third of the child's daily requirement can be fulfilled. CARE, UNICEF and many international, governmental voluntary agencies give their contribution in this. The primary objective of mid-day meal program is to improve the nutritional status of children and imparting nutritional education and to ensure universal primary education.

b. Hernia

It is an abnormal protrusion of an organ or a part of an organ, tissue through the structure that normally contains it. The causes of hernia are congenital, increased intra-abdominal pressure, muscle weakness (due to aging). The types are inguinal, indirect, femoral, umbilical, incision, and diaphragmatic hernia.

c. Club foot

Congenital club foot (talipes equinovarus) is a deformity consists on an inversion of the forefoot and its downward displacement at the ankle.

d. Gynecomastia

Gynecomastia is enlargement of the gland tissue of the male breast. During infancy, puberty, and in middle-aged to older men, gynecomastia can be common. Gynecomastia must be distinguished from pseudogynecomastia or lipomastia, which refers to the presence of fat deposits in the breast area of obese men. True gynecomastia results from growth of the glandular, or breast tissue, which is present in very small amounts in men. Gynecomastia is the male breast. Gynecomastia results from an imbalance in hormone levels in which levels of estrogen (female hormones) are increased relative to levels of androgens (male-hormones). Gynecomastia that occurs in normally-growing infant and pubertal boys that resolves on its own with time is known as physiologic gynecomastia.

e. Hyperglycemia

Hyperglycemia is a condition that increased blood glucose level. The normal blood sugar level is 80–100 mg/dL.

II. Fill in the blanks with suitable answers:

a. Normal Apgar score of a newborn is: **7–10.**
b. Startle reflex can be elicited by: **Clapping the hands.**
c. The comfortable position for a 4-year-old child with cyanotic spell is: **Fowler's position.**

III. Write short notes on any *three* of the following:

a. Daycare centers
Crèches/Day care centers: The Scheme of Crèches/Day care centers extends day care services for the children of casual, migrant, agricultural and construction laborers. Children of those women who are sick or incapacitated due to sickness or suffering from communicable diseases are covered under the scheme. This Central Sector Scheme which is being implemented through the medium of NGOs is a non-expanding scheme and is expected to be merged with the National Crèche Fund.

b. Care of the child with marasmus
Nutritional marasmus: This is caused by severe deficiency of proteins and calories in the diet. The important features of growth retardation and severe wasting of muscle and loss of subcutaneous fat. The skin is dry and atrophic. Eye lesions due to vitamin A deficiency and anemia may also be present.

Sl. No.	Features	Marasmus	Kwashiorkor
	Clinical	Always present	
1.	Muscle wasting	Obsious	Hidden by edema and fat
2.	Edema	None	Present in lower legs, face, lower arms
3.	Fat wasting	Loss of subcutaneous fat	Fat often retained but not firm
4.	Weight for height	Very low	Weight may be less than 60% of standard
5.	Mental changes	Quiet	Irritable

Treatment: The main principles of treatment are (a) to ensure an acceptable and readily digestible diet (liquid diet initially for a week) rich in proteins, calories and supplying all other dietary essentials in required amounts and (b) treatment of any bacterial and parasitic infections present. The diet is usually contains of skim milk powder (reconstituted), sugar, cooked cereals and banana. Fat is introduced in the diet from the 2nd week of treatment. The daily calorie intake should be 140–150 kcal/kg and protein intake 3–5 g/kg body weight. Vitamin A deficiency is corrected by the administration of the required amounts of synthetic vitamin A.

Prevention and control: The PEM like any other disease can be prevented and controlled by comprehensive approach involving primary level secondary level and tertiary level preventive measures. Primary preventive measures include health promotion and specific protection. The secondary and tertiary level preventive measures include early diagnosis treatment and rehabilitation.

c. Concept of preventive pediatrics
Child health depends upon preventive care. Majority of the child health problems are preventable. Preventive pediatrics is a specialized area of child health comprises efforts to avert rather than cure disease and disabilities.

Preventive pediatrics has been defined as "the prevention of disease and promotion of physical, mental and social wellbeing of children with the aim of attaining a positive health". Pediatrics is largely preventive in its objectives.

Preventive pediatrics have been broadly divided into antenatal preventive pediatrics and postnatal preventive pediatrics.

Antenatal preventive pediatrics includes care of the pregnant mothers with adequate nutrition, prevention of communicable diseases, preparation of the mother for delivery, breastfeeding and mother craft training, etc. Prepregnant health status of the mother also influences the child health. Promotion of health of girl child and nonpregnant state should be emphasized as the future mother, who is soil and seed of future generation.

Postnatal preventive pediatrics includes promotion of breastfeeding, introduction of complementary feeding in appropriate age, immunization, prevention of accidents, tender loving care with emotional security, growth monitoring, periodic medical supervision and health check-up, psychological assessment, etc.

Another new concept of child health care is social pediatrics: The challenge of the time is to study child health in relation to community, to social values and to social policy. Social pediatrics has been defined as "the application of the principles of social medicine to pediatrics to obtain a more complete understanding of the problems of children in order to prevent and treat disease and promote their adequate growth and development, through an organized health structure". It is concerned with the delivery of comprehensive and continuous child health care services and to bring these services within the reach of the total community. It also covers the various social welfare measures—local, national and international—aimed to meet the health needs of a child.

To ensure adequate physical, mental and social growth of the child, total health needs should be provided as:
a. Healthy and happy parents.
b. Balanced and nutritious diet.
c. Clean, healthful house and living environments.
d. Developmental needs like play, recreation, love and affection, safety and security, recognition and companionship as emotional food.
d. Educational provisions and opportunities.

For the comprehensive services to the mothers and children, primary health care strategy is adopted by the health care delivery system. Government of India accepted a national policy for children in 1974 and implemented various health programs for preventive and social services along with curative care for the millions of children.

d. Care of child with hydrocephalus

Hydrocephalus is a condition of imbalance between the production of cerebrospinal fluid and its absorption over the surface of the brain into the circulatory system. Cerebrospinal fluid is formed in the choroid plexuses of the ventricles of the brain, 50–100 ml/day. The large portion of the cerebrospinal fluid is reabsorbed through the arachnoid villi but the sinuses vein, brain substance and dura matter also participates in the absorption. Hydrocephalus is characterized by an abnormal increase in cerebrospinal fluid volume within the intracranial cavity and by the enlargement of the young child's head. Due to increased amount of cerebrospinal fluid and intracranial pressure, ventricles become dilated and brain substance is compressed against the bony cranium. It is common in the age groups from birth to 2 years.

Causes
1. Excessive secretion of cerebrospinal fluid due to chronic plexuses papillon class or tumor.
2. Noncommunication of the cerebrospinal fluid due to blockage of the circulation in the ventricle, which prevents the escape of cerebrospinal; fluid in to subarachnoid space.
3. There may be a blocked circulation of cerebrospinal fluid in the extraventricular space.

Manifestations

1. Anterior fontanel is tense, bulging, enlarged and nonpulsatile. Scalp veins may be prominent and dilated on city.
2. A large skull with separated skull sutures may be seen up to three years of age.
3. Eyes have setting sun sign, eyes cannot gaze upward due to increase of thin orbital roof.
4. Difficulty in sucking and feeding.
5. Shrill, high pitch cry, restlessness, and irritability.
6. Alteration of vital signs, such as increased blood pressure, decreased pulse and respiration
7. Vomiting, seizures, squint, mental deficiency, and spastic paralysis may develop.
8. If hydrocephalus is allowed to progress, development of lower brain functions are disrupted.

Investigation

1. X-ray shows widening of the fontanel and sutures.
2. Transliteration of infant's head allows visualization of fluid collection.
3. Percussion of the human skull may produce a typical 'Cracked pot' sound (Macewen's sign).
4. In ventriculography, abnormalities are visualized in the ventricular system of the subarachnoid space.
5. Pneumoencephalography may show the dilated ventricles and the extent of the brain damage and the location of the obstruction.
6. Ophthalmoscopy may show papilledema.
7. Computerized Axial Tomography (CAT) provides computer analysis of X-ray transmission data.

Treatment: Installation of shunting device is the surgical treatment. Surgically, ventriculoperitoneal and ventriculoatrial drainage shunt can be made. This shunt contains a one way valve mechanism that directs flow on one direction and prevents reflux. This helps to reduce the volume, thus, the pressure of the cerebrospinal fluid within the ventricles is reduced.

Ventriculoperitoneal shunt (VP shunt): VP shunt directs cerebrospinal fluid from lateral ventricles or the spinal subarachoid space to the preritoneal cavity. In VP shunt, the tube is passed from lateral ventricles through an occipital burr hole subcutaneously through the posterior aspect of the neck and paraspinal region to the peritoneal cavity through a small incision in the right lower quadrant.

Ventriculoatrial shunts (VA shunt): VA shunt is passed from the dilated ventricle through a burr hole in the partial region of the skull. It is then passed under the skull behind the ear into a vein down to a point where it discharges into the right atrium and superior vena cava. The tube is passed at the point through a one-way pressure sensitive system. The valve or valves close to prevent reflux of blood into the ventricles and open as ventricular pressure rises, allowing the fluid pass from the ventricles into bloodstream.

Management

Preoperative care

1. The head circumference should be measured daily.
2. The vital signs should be watched to detect increased intracranial tension.
3. The adequate nutritious food should be provided. The children should be fed in semisitting position. After every feeding, the children should be placed on their right side with the elevated head to prevent aspiration.
4. Pressure sores should be prevented by taking care of the skin and changing the position every two hours.

5. Contracture of the joints can be prevented by physiotherapy.
6. While turning these children, the head and the body should be rotated together to prevent a strain on the neck. A firm pillow may be kept under the head and shoulder, for further support while lifting the child.
7. The eye care should be given if eyes cannot be closed.
8. The parents should be provided with the necessary support and explained about the need of the love and affection for their children.

Postoperative care

1. The vital signs should be checked and recorded every hour or frequently till the children are recovered from anesthesia.
2. The body temperature should be maintained within the normal limits, especially for the infants.
3. The mucous and secretions should be removed from the nose and the air passage, to help the respiration.
4. Nasogastric free drainage can prevent aspiration.
5. Oral hygiene should be maintained by taking care of the mouth to prevent dryness and infection.
6. To allow proper flow of the cerebrospinal fluid through the shunt, the shunt should be pumped and children should be positioned as ordered by the surgeon. To pump the shunt, the valve should be compressed carefully, for the specified number of times, at regular intervals.
7. A special care should be taken to prevent the sore at the site of the valve.
8. Avoid positioning the child on the area of the valve or the incisional area, until the incision is healed.
9. Fluid, electrolytes and nutritional balance should be maintained.

Oral feeding can be started as the children get recovered. Gradually the feeding can be increased and encourage high protein diet.

Complications

1. Increased intracranial tension occurs, if the shunt malfunctions.
2. Dehydration should be suspected, if the fontanel is suckered, output is decreased or the dryness is observed around the shunt.

Parental advice: The parents should be explained about the specific precautions to be taken while giving care to the children at home. For example, the care of the shunt, symptoms of increased intracranial tension, and follow up.

e. Growth and development during infancy

Infancy is traditionally designed as the period from 1 month to 1 year of age. This year is one of rapid growth and development, with the infant tripling birth weight and increasing length by 50%. During this period, the baby's senses sharpen and with the process of attachment to primary care givers, from his or her first social relationships. Infants are seen at healthcare facilities for health maintenance at least 6 months during the first year.

Physical Growth

I. Weight
1. As a rule, most infant double their weight at 4–6 months, they triple it by 1 year.
2. During the first 6 months, infants typically average a weight gain of 2 lb per month.
3. During second 6 months, weight gain is approximately 1 lb per month.

4. The average 1 year old male weight 10 kg (22 lb), the average female weight 9.5 kgs (21 lb).

II. Height
1. The infant increases in height during the first year by 50% or grows from the average birth length of 20 inch to about 30 inch (50.8–76.2 cm).
2. Height, like weight is best assessment if it is plotted on a standard growth chart.

III. Head circumference
1. Head circumference increase rapidly during the infant period, reflecting rapid brain growth.
2. By the end of the first year, the brain has already reached two thirds of its adult size.

IV. Body proportion
1. Body proportion changes during the first year from that of a newborn to a more typical infant appearance.
2. The mandible becomes more prominent as bone grows.
3. The circumference of. the chest is generally less than that of the head at birth by about 2 cm. It is even with the head circumference in some infants as early as 6 months and in most by 12 months.
4. The abdomen remains protuberant until the child has been walking well.

V. Body systems
1. In the cardiovascular system, heart rate slows from 120–160 bpm to 100–120 bpm by the end of the first year.
2. Respiratory rate of the infant slows from 30–60 breaths/min to 20–30 breaths/min by the end of the first year.
3. At birth, the gastrointestinal tract is immature in its ability to digest food and mechanically move it along. These functions mature gradually during the infant year.
4. The immune system becomes functional by at least 2 months of age, the infant is able to produce both IgC and IgM antibodies by 1 year of age.
5. Ability to adjust to cold is mature by age 6 months.
6. Kidney, liver and endocrine glands remains immature and not as efficient at eliminating body wastes as in the adult.

VI. Teeth
1. The first baby tooth usually erupts at age 6 months, followed by a new one monthly.
2. Teething pattern can vary greatly among children.

IV. a. What is congenital heart disease?
  b. Write the types
  c. Explain the Clinical manifestation and management of a child with patent ductus arteriosus

Congenital heart disease (CHD) is the structural malformations of the heart or great vessels, present at birth. It is the most common congenital malformations. The exact number of prevalence is not known.

Etiology: The exact cause of CHD is unknown in about 90% of cases. Heredity and consanguinous marriage are important etiological factors. Genetic disorders and chromosomal aberrations (trisomy —21, Turner's syndrome) are also known to predispose congenital heart disease. Other associated factors responsible for CHD include fetal and maternal teratogenic infections (rubella), teratogenic drug (thalidomide) intake, alcohol intake by the mother and irradiation in first trimester of pregnancy, maternal IDDM, high altitude, fetal hypoxia, birth asphyxia, etc.

Classification of CHD: CHD can be grouped into three categories:
A. *Acyanotic CHD:* There is increased pulmonary blood flow due to left to right shunt. It includes:
  a. Ventricular septal defect (VSD).
  b. Atrial septal defect (ASD).

c. Patent ductus arteriosus (PDA).
   d. Atrioventricular canal (AVC).
B. Cyanotic CHD:
   a. Tetralogy of Fallot (TOF).
   b. Tricuspid atresia (TA).
   c. Transposition of great arteries (TGA).
   d. Truncus arteriosus.
   e. Hypoplastic left heart syndrome.
   f. Total anomalous pulmonary venous return.
   g. Eisenmenger's syndrome or complex.
C. Obstructive lesions
   a. Coarctation of aorta.
   b. Aortic value stenosis.
   c. Pulmonary valve stenosis.
   d. Congenital mitral stenosis.

Patent ductus arteriosus: Patent ductus arteriosus allows shunting oxygenated blood directly into the systemic circulation by bypassing the lungs which do not oxygenate during fetal life. Soon after birth, the ductus arteriosus gets closed because of arteriosus gets closed, as a result of constriction of smooth muscles in its vessel walls. When it remains open, it results in patent ductus arteriosus. As pulmonary resistance falls, the pulmonary artery pressure drops and the blood with higher pressure from aorta is shunted from aorta to the pulmonary artery.

Thus, part of the blood is recirculated through the lungs.

Clinical Manifestations
1. Murmur is heard at the middle to the upper left sternal border.
2. Pulse pressure is increased.
3. Enlargement of left atrium, left ventricle, and right ventricle. If the volume overload of left ventricle occurs, it causes pulmonary.

Diagnosis
1. PDA murmur is heard.
2. X- ray shows that left side of the heart and right ventricle are enlarged.
3. Echocardiogram to find out increased left atrial and aortic ratio.

Treatment: Surgical correction by division and ligation of patent vessels. In asymptomatic children, generally, the repair is done at one to two years of age.

In serious neonates, sometimes indomethacin is used for closure.

V. a. Define low birth weight baby
b. Explain the management of low birth weight baby

A neonate with a birth weight of less than 2500 g irrespective of the gestational age are termed as low birth weight (LBW) baby. They include both preterm and small-for-dates (SFD) babies. These two groups have different clinical problems and prognosis. In India, about 30–40 percent neonates are born LBW. Approximately, 80% of all neonatal deaths and 50% of infant death are related to LBW. These LBW babies are more prone to malnutrition, infections and neurodevelopment handicapped conditions. They are more vulnerable to develop hypertension, diabetes mellitus, and coronary artery disease in adult life.

High incidence of LBW babies in our country are due to higher number of babies with intrauterine growth retardation (small for dates) rather than preterm babies. It is not possible to provide special care to all LBW babies, especially in India. The baby with a birth weight of less than 2000 g is more vulnerable and need special care. About 10 percent of all LBW babies require admission to the special care nursery.

Prevention of LBW babies: Prevention and reduction in incidence of LBW babies is the most important strategy to reduce perinatal and infant mortality rates and improve the quality of life among those who survive. Causes of preterm birth and SFD babies should be eliminated to fulfill the objectives.

Hospital care of LBW infant: Ideally, the delivery of an anticipated LBW baby should be conducted in a hospital. Premature labor as well as intrauterine growth retardation is indications for referral of the pregnant mother to a well-equipped facility. This in-utero transfer of a low birth weight fetus is desirable, convenient and safe than the transport of a low weight baby after birth. Trained health professionals should conduct delivery and standard procedure of resuscitation should be followed efficiently.

The indications for hospitalization of a LBW neonate delivered at home include birth weight <1800 g, gestational age <33 weeks, neonate who is not able to take feeds from both the breasts or by katori-spoon or a sick neonate.

The principles of management of LBW neonate in the hospital are essentially the same as described for home care, viz. temperature maintenance, providing fluids and feeds and prevention of infection.

Keeping LBW babies warm: The mother herself is a source of warmth for the baby (Cot-in baby). The room, where the baby is nursed should be kept warm (temperature between 28°–30°C in all seasons). While in summer months no extraeffort is required to maintain this temperature, in winter months a room heater may have to be used. The baby should be clothed well. If baby does not maintain temperature, overhead radiant warmer or incubator may be used to keep the baby warm. Regular monitoring of axillary temperature by placing low reading thermometer should be carried out in all hospitalized babies. Rectal temperature is recorded only in a sick, hypothermic newborn. Normal axillary temperature is 36.5°C. In hypothermia the temperature are below 36.5°C (cold stress <36.5°C to >36.0°C, moderate hypothermia <36.0°C to >3 2.0°C, severe hypothermia <32.0°C). The temperature range during which the basal metabolic rate of the baby is at minimum, oxygen utilization is least and baby thrives well is known as "thermoneutral range of temperature". For each baby, this range of temperature varies depending on gestational age, weight and postnatal age. Hypothermia can lead to hypoglycemia, bleeding diathesis, pulmonary hemorrhage, acidosis, apnea, respiratory failure, shock and even death.

Nutrition and fluids: Birth weight, gestation, presence of sickness and individual feeding effort of the baby determine the fluid and feed supplements to a baby. Ultimate goal is to meet both these requirements from direct and exclusive breastfeeds. Breast milk is the ideal feed for the low birth weight babies.

Prevention of Infection: LBW babies are predisposed to serious bacterial infections. Even when treated aggressively, the mortality due to sepsis is high. Therefore, the importance of preventing sepsis cannot be overemphasized.

Following measures will help prevent infections:

1. Hand washing by the health professional attending delivery and by the mother and family before handling the baby.

2. Ensuring early and exclusive breastfeeding and avoiding all prelacteal feeds. Careful attention to the hygiene of katori-spoon feeds. Dropper/bottle/nipple/cotton wicks should never be used for feeding the baby.
3. Care of the umbilical stump.
4. Avoiding unnecessary interventions such as intravenous lines and needle pricks.

If the LBW baby is not sick, the vaccination schedule is the same as for the normal babies. Hence, BCG and OPV should be given at the earliest. A sick LBW baby, however, should receive these vaccines only on recovery.

Or

Baby Niranjan is admitted for hypospadiasis:
a. Define hypospadiasis
b. Write the signs and symptoms of hypospadiasis
c. Explain the surgical and nursing management of a child with hypospadiasis

Hypospadias is the congenital abnormal urethral opening on the ventral aspect (under surface) of the penis. It is one of the most common malformations of male children. Undescended testes or inguinal hernia or upper urinary tract anomalies may be associated with hypospadias. It may found in females as urethal opening in the vagina with dribbling of urine.

Classification

Hypospadias can be classified depending upon the site of the urethral meatus.
1. **Anterior hypospadias** (65–70%). It may be found as glandular or coronal or on distal penile shaft.
2. **Middle (10–15%) penile shaft hypospadias.**
3. **Posterior hypospadias** (20%). It may be found on proximal penile shaft or as penoscrotal, scrotal or perineal type.

Problems Related to Hypospadias

A child with hypospadias may have following problems:
1. Presence of painful downward curvature of the penis during erection as chordee.
2. Due to chordee, there is deflected stream of urine and the child wets his thigh during urination.
3. Inability to void urine while standing, in case of penoscrotal, scrotal and perineal hypospadias. It also may found with the penis in the normal elevated position.
4. If appropriate management is not done or left untreated, the condition, in later life, interferes during sexual intercourse with difficulty in penetration due to the presence of chordee. Severe forms of hypospadias interfere with reproductive ability as the sperms are deposited outside the vagina due to proximal situation of meatus.
5. There can be meatal stenosis, fistula, urethral stricture or stenosis or diverticulum.

Management: Management of hypospadias is done by surgical reconstruction to obtain straight penis at erection, to form urethral tube and urethral meatus at the tip of glans penis. Meatotomy is done at any age after birth. Chordee correction and advancement of prepuce can be done at the age of 2–3 years. Urethroplasty is done 3–4 months after chordee correction. The surgical repair should be completed before admission to the school. Operation can be performed as multistage or single stage repair.

SECTION-II

VI. State whether the following statements are *true* or *false*.

a. Immunization is contraindicated if the child has febrile condition: **TRUE**
b. Oral thrush is caused by *Candida albicans*: **TRUE**
c. BCG vaccine is administered to prevent chickenpox: **FALSE**
d. Plantar flexion of the foot in which the toes are fixed lower than the heel is talipes calcaneus: **FALSE**

VII. Choose the correct answer and write.

a. Which assessment finding is documented in case of an infant with Hirschsprung's diseases: **Foul smelling ribbon like stools**.
   (i. Diarrhea, ii. Projectile vomiting, iii. Regurgitation of feed, iv. Foul smelling ribbon like stools)
b. Whooping cough is caused by: **Bordetella pertussis**.
   (i. *Vericella zoster*, ii. Paramyxo virus, iii. *Bordetella pertussis*, iv. Enterovirus)
c. While administering oral liquid iron supplement to a child the nurse instructs the mother to: **Administer iron at meal time.**
   (i. Administer iron throw straw, ii. Administer iron at mealtime, iii. Add iron to formula for easy administration, iv. Mix iron with cereal)

VIII. Write short notes on any three of the following:

a. Prevention of home accident in toddler

World Health Organization defines accident as an event which is independent of human will power, caused by an external force, acts rapidly and results in bodily or mental damage. If death occurs at once or within a week after the accident, it is termed as fatal accident. Death is considered as due to an accident, if it occurs more than a week and less than a month after the accident. Death is stated to be due to sequel of an accident, if it occurs one year or more after the accident.

Education and Persuasion Strategy

1. Parents must be educated regarding the dangers associated with medicines, household substances and agrochemicals. A poison label should appear on all dangerous medicines, including aspirin and paracetamol.
2. Parents must begin to teach their children at an early age the danger of touching, eating or playing with unknown objects including medicines, pesticides and insecticides, household chemicals or plants.
3. Medicines, insecticides and pesticides and other poisonous substances should be stored in locked cabinets.
4. Dyes, polishes, kerosene and other poisonous household chemicals should never be left on a low shelf or on the floor. Do not store in kitchen or bathroom.
5. Combustion devices should be adequately ventilated.
6. Inhalation of spray or fumes should be prevented during painting or application of insecticides.
7. Unnecessary toxic substances should be discarded.
8. Carefully check the label of any medicine before use. Do not put different tablets or pills in the same bottle.
9. Do not store any poisonous liquid in a beverage bottle.

10. Wear protective clothing, goggles, gloves and masks during spraying of insecticide and always spray downwind. Protective clothing should be removed and exposed skin washed thoroughly before eating anything.
11. Dispense medicine and dangerous household's chemicals in childproof, tamperproof containers.
12. Education on proper hygiene and storage of food to avoid food poisoning.
13. Workers and other persons working in industries should be trained in safe use of chemicals.
14. Industries should have complete knowledge and information in the toxicity and management of the chemicals they are using.
15. Persons having suicidal tendencies should not be given a large amount of drugs at a time and should be given adequate psychiatric follow-up and counseling.

b. Use of play as nursing intervention

Play is an essential element to the development of a normal, well-adjusted personality in all means, i.e. physically, emotionally, mentally, socially and morally through a single type of activity; the child will learn how to adjust in the life and provides a valuable learning experience.

1. It is an important tool for socialization, the child tries to learn to understand and communicates with others, enjoys their company and establishes an effective interpersonal relationship through which, child learns to assume responsibilities.
2. Child learns social adjustment pattern, play will teach the children adult roles including sex role behavior.
3. Play activities help the children to develop muscular coordination, communication skills and senses are exercised; it encourages exploration of physical nature of the world, provides release of surplus energy.
4. Helps in maintaining the body weight through outdoor games.
5. Increases the endurance of the child.
6. Fulfills the needs and desires of children by participant and leadership role.
7. Acts like a stimulant for creative activities through painting, drawing, clay dolls, puppets; provides an expressive outlet for creative ideas and interests; enhances development of special talents and skills.
8. Self-awareness: Encourages regulation of own behavior; allows for testing of own abilities; provides for comparison of own abilities with those of others and learns how own behavior affects others.
9. Therapeutic values: Means of outlet for pent up release of energy to relieve emotional tensions, conflicts and worries; allows for expression of emotions and release of unacceptable impulses in a socially acceptable fashion; encourages experimentation and testing of fearful situation in a safe manner; facilitates nonverbal and indirect verbal communication of needs, fears and desires.
10. Develops more definite and realistic concepts of themselves by developing insight into the situations; provides multiple sources of learning, exploration and manipulation of shapes, sizes, texture and colors, experiences with numbers, spatial relationships and abstract concepts; it provides opportunity to practice and expand language skills.
11. Helps children to understand the world in which they live and to distinguish reality and fantasy.

Makes the Child to Learn the Problem-solving Approach

1. Learns the moral standards, values, procedures and appropriate roles by following the rules, regulations of the specific game; encourages interaction and development of positive attitudes towards others pattern, reinforces approved behavior.

2. Desirable personality traits will be acquired, e.g. cooperation, truthful, generous and pleasantness, etc.
3. Increases attention, concentration and ability in task oriented activities, thus the child learns to control the emotions.
4. Child learns the spatial relationships for abstract thinking.
5. The child learns to understand the concept, cause and effect, learn to think and solve the problem.
6. Develops honesty, sportsmanship and compassion.
7. Speech and language: Listening to others and family members; saying sounds and words, expressing wants and needs while playing. Speaking increases language ability, improves verbal and non-verbal communication, e.g. speech, gestures.
8. As the child grows the amount of time spends for play decreases or narrowed and they pursue in other interests and spend their leisure time with those interests.
9. Play establishes and maintains emotional balance; enables the child to develop characters such as self-control, self-reliance, patience, perseverance, skills and neuromuscular coordination.

c. Respiratory distress syndrome

Respiratory distress syndrome (RDS) or hyaline membrane disease (HMD): It is caused by deficient surfactant in the lungs and thus seen more often in premature babies. The baby has difficulty in initiating normal respiration. After birth, the child is tachypneic. This is accompanied by chest retractions, nasal flaring and expiratory grunting. Later, cyanosis may appear. X-ray reveals a whiteout lung (ground glass appearance). Shake test can be done on the gastric aspirate to determine lung maturity. Mix 0.5 mL of gastric aspirate with 0.5 mL of absolute alcohol in a test-tube and shake for 15 seconds. Formation of bubbles indicates adequate surfactant and less chances of HMD.

Treatment: Prolongation of pregnancy with bed rest and/or drugs that inhibit premature labor, as well as the induction of pulmonary surfactant with antenatal steroid administration play an important role in reducing the incidence of respiratory distress syndrome. Postnatal treatment consists of surfactant replacement therapy and supportive therapy. These babies need respiratory support, intensive monitoring, and IV fluids. Collapse of the alveoli may be prevented by application of CPAP (continuous positive airway pressure) by nasal prongs or endotracheal tube. CPAP can be delivered through a ventilator. Start with a minimum pressure of 4–6 cm water.

d. Oral rehydration rherapy

Oral rehydration therapy (ORT) is the giving of fluid by mouth to prevent and or correct the dehydration that is a result of diarrhea.

Purpose
1. To prevent dehydration.
2. To prevent morbidity and mortality due to acute diarrheal diseases.

The Formula for ORS
The formula for ORS recommended by WHO and UNICEF contains:
1. 3.5 g sodium chloride.
2. 2.9 g trisodium citrate dihydrate (or 2.5 g sodium bicarbonate).

3. 1.5 g potassium chloride.
4. 20 g glucose (anhydrous).

The above ingredients are dissolved in one liter of clean water.

Equipments needed

1. Take one liter of boiled and cooled drinking water.
2. Clean glass of 200 mL capacity.
3. A clean vessel to mix the solution.
4. A clean spoon to mix the solution and feed the child.

Procedure

1. Pour one liter of clean water into a clean vessel.
2. Open a packet of ORS and pour all the contents into the vessel.
3. Stir with a clean spoon till it completely dissolves.
4. Take some solution in a clean glass.
5. Feed the child frequently with small doses of the solution.

Action of ORT

1. Oral rehydration therapy does not stop the diarrhea, but it replaces the lost fluids and essential salts, thus preventing or treating dehydration and reducing the danger.
2. The glucose contained in ORS solution enables the intestine to absorb the fluid and the salts more effectively. ORT alone is an effective treatment for 90–95% of patients suffering from acute watery diarrhea regardless of cause.

General Instructions

1. Oral rehydration therapy is the cheap, simple and effective way to treat dehydration caused by diarrhea.
2. ORT is safe and can be used to treat anyone suffering from diarrhea, without having to make a detailed diagnosis before the solution is given.
3. Children must always treat immediately because they become dehydrated more quickly.

IX. a. What is bronchial asthma?
    b. List the causative factors and clinical features
    c. Write in detail the medical and nursing management of an 8-year-old child with bronchial asthma

It is a syndrome in which repeated attack of breathlessness and wheezing occurs due to irreversible narrowing of airway.

Pathophysiology: When the person is exposed to an allergen or antigen, a large amount of antibody, i.e. IgE is produced and this antigen attacks to the mast cells which are found in the lungs, as a result mast cell products (cell mediators) are released such as histamine, bradykinin, leukotrinase, prostagladin and slow reactive activating substance of anaphylaxis. The release of these mediators from the lung tissue affects the smooth muscle and glands of the airway causing bronchospasm, or bronchoconstriction, mucus plugging, vascular congestion, and narrowing of the vessels.

Clinical Manifestations

1. Wheezing.
2. Non-productive cough.
3. Dyspnea.
4. Chest tightness.
5. Prolonged expansion, i.e. is 1:3 or 1:4 (normal inspiratory-expiratory ratio is 1:2).
6. Restlessness.
7. Increased anxiety.
8. Increased pulse and respiratory rate.

Nursing Management

I. Impair gas exchange related to brochoconstriction and mucosal edema
1. Provide comfortable position that is Fowler's position.
2. Auscultate breath sounds every 1–2 hours.
3. Assess blood pressure, heart rate, respiratory rate and level of consciousness every 15 minutes until stable and then every 2–4 hours.
4. Administer bronchodilators as prescribed.
5. Administer oxygen as prescribed.

II. Ineffective airway clearance related to increased thick mucus secretions and fatigue
1. Cough and deep-breath adequately to expectorate secretions.
2. Demonstrate skill in conserving energy while attempting to clear airway.
3. Provide chest physiotherapy or postural drainage.
4. Give steam inhalation as per requirement.
5. Encourage to take more warm fluid/ liquid intake.
6. Administer bronchodilator or steroid therapy as prescribed.

III. Anxiety related to inability to breath and interference with activities
1. Verbalize fears related to breathing problems.
2. Encourage to express his fears and concerns about his illness and answer his questions honestly.
3. Encourage him to identify and comply with care measures and activities that promote relaxation.
4. Demonstrate measures to decrease anxiety during an attack.
5. Reassure during as asthma attack and stay with him.
6. Place in semi-Fowler's position and encourage diaphragmatic breathing.

IV. High risk for infection related to decrease pulmonary function, ineffective airway clearance and possible steroid therapy
1. If effective sputum is mucopurulent, obtain sputum for culture and sensitivity and also Gram's stain.
2. Administer antibiotics as prescribed.
3. Monitor TPR every 4th hourly.
4. Monitor all respiratory treatments that are administered.
5. Provide deep breathing and coughing exercises.

V. Knowledge deficit related to health maintenance.
Teaching needs to be given to the child parents:
1. Teach the family members about diaphragmatic and pursed lip breathing.
2. Teach the parents how to use an oral or turbo-inhaler.

3. Show the patient how to breath deeply.
4. Instruct him to coup up secretions accumulated overnight and to allow time for medications to work.
5. Emphasize consistency of medications for maximum benefits, even though he is feeling well.
6. Instruct to drink plenty of oral fluids to help loosen secretions and maintain hydration.
7. Tell to eat well-balanced diet to prevent respiratory infection and fatigue.
8. Teach him to avoid substances that trigger an attack.
9. Encourage the patient to take light nutritious and well balanced diet and not full stomach meal particularly at night because it causes discomfort in breathing.
10. Avoid foods and place, which is allergic to the patient if occupation induces allergy, change of occupation is needed.
11. Advise to carry bronchodilators and to take whenever he gets an attack of wheezing.

X. a. **What is poliomyelitis?**
   b. **Write the causes and signs and symptoms**
   c. **Explain the preventive measures and management of a child with polio attack**

Definition

Poliomyelitis also called polio and infantile paralysis. In poliomyelitis, there will be inflammation of the grey matter of the spinal cord.

1. Poliomyelitis is an acute communicable disease caused by the poliovirus. Most patients present with minor illness (fever, malaise, headache, sore throat and vomiting) but a few develop aseptic meningitis and paralytic illness.
2. Poliomyelitis is an acute systemic disease caused by an RNA virus, which replicates mainly in the gastrointestinal tract. In some cases, the virus may reach the CNS and damage anterior horn cells of the spinal cord and occasionally the medulla and motor cortex.

Pathogenesis

1. **Agent:** It is caused by poliomyelitis virus, i.e. type I-Brunhilde type, type II-lansing type and type III- Leon type. The virus is resistant and stable, remaining viable for months outside the body.
2. **Reservoir of infection:** Man is the only known reservoir of infection. Most infections are subclinical. It is the mild and sub-clinical infection that play a dominant role in the spread of infection.
3. **Source of infection:** The virus is found in the feces and oropharyngeal secretions of an infected person.
4. **Host factor:** In India, about 50% of cases are reported in infancy. The most vulnerable age is between 6 months and 3 years.
5. **Environmental factors:** Approximately 60% of cases recorded in India were during June to September. The environmental sources of infection are contaminated water, food and flies.
6. **Mode of transmission:** Fecal–oral route is the main route of spread in developing countries. The infection may spread directly through contaminated fingers where hygiene is poor or indirectly through contaminated water, milk, foods, flies and articles of daily use. Droplet infection — this may occur in the acute phase of disease when the virus occurs in the throat.
7. **Incubation period:** Usually 7–14 days.

Clinical Features

1. **Prodormal stage:** *Respiratory*—coryza, sore throat or cough. *GIT*— vomiting, diarrhea and constipation. *Constitutional*—fever, headache, drowsiness, restlessness, irritability and sweating.
2. **Pre-paralytic stage:** Fever, pain and stiffness in the neck. Headache, nausea, hyperesthesia, nuchal and spinal rigidity, muscle fasciculation and micturition disturbances.
3. **Paralytic stage:** Usually develops between 2nd and 5th days after onset of signs of involvement of nervous system. Paralysis usually begins within 1–5 days after onset of illness. Distribution of paralysis usually patchy, may produce monoplegia, paraplegia, and quadriplegia. Lower limbs more commonly affected.
4. **Convalescence:** Initial paralysis usually diminishes to some extent after a period of two or more weeks and improvement may continue for several months. When the chronic stage is reached six months to a year after initial infection, no further spontaneous improvement can be expected.

Clinical Types of Poliomyelitis

1. **Abortive poliomyelitis:** Presumptive diagnosis during epidemic. Brief influenza like illness with one or more of the following symptoms malaise, anorexia, nausea, vomiting, headache, sore throat constipation and localized abdominal pain. Fever seldom more than 103°F coryza and cough uncommon.
2. **Nonparalytic poliomyelitis:** Subjective symptoms as in abortive type but headache, nausea, vomiting more intense and soreness and stiffness of posterior muscles of neck, trunk and limbs. Fleeting paralysis of flaccid type usually asymmetrical and scattered in distribution though more severe in one extremity. Legs most frequently involved. Respiratory paralysis may result from involvement of diaphragm and intercostals muscles.

Bulbar form: Muscles supplied by bulbar nuclei involved alone or with spinal musculature. Facial, palatal and sometimes pharyngeal paralysis causes change in voice, difficulty in swallowing, nasal regurgitation and choking when attempting to drink.

Diagnostic findings: Isolation of the poliovirus from throat washings early in the disease and from stools throughout the disease confirms the diagnosis. If the patient has a central nervous system infection, cerebrospinal fluid cultures may aid diagnosis. Coxsackievirus serum antibody titters four

Management of Poliomyelitis

Preparalytic Stage

1. **Rest in Bed:** On a firm mattress with as little disturbance of patient as possible. A padded foot board serves to protect the legs from pressure of bed-clothes and keep ankles flexed at 90°.
2. **Sedation:** With barbiturate if required.
3. **Heat:** In form of moist (but not wet) packs of value in relieving muscle soreness or spasm.

Paralytic Stage

1. **Splints;** Paralysis of muscles which results in stretching or malposition may require application of removable splints.
2. **Maintenance** of fluid intake, vitamins.
3. **Physiotherapy:** When muscle tenderness has subsided gentle massage, together with active and passive movements for purpose of relaxing the muscles and preventing contracture.

4. **Catheterization:** May be necessary for few days.
5. **Enemas;** given if abdominal muscles are weak.

Paralysis of Respiratory Muscles

1. Patient should be watched for signs of respiratory embarrassment and as soon as these have become apparent, placed in artificial respirator immediately.
2. A patient will require assistance with his respiration if normal acts like speaking make him breathless, if cough is ineffective, if he cannot count to 20 after deep inspiration, if chest excursions are feeble or he cannot push out his upper abdomen.
3. Tracheotomy may be needed when air passages are occluded by mucus or spasm of laryngeal muscles or may be done as a routine procedure. IV fluids, penicillin or other antibiotic to prevent pulmonary complications. Use of respirator should be continued in bulbar cases until respiratory centers have continued in bulbar cases until respiratory centers have recovered.

Convalescent stage: Physiotherapy muscles re-education application of appropriate corrective appliances and orthopedic surgery. Rehabilitation of the severely paralyzed patient.

Preventive Measures of Poliomyelitis

1. **Active immunization:** Two types of polio vaccine are used (a) Salk inactivated polio vaccine (IPV) administered by injection, (b) Sabin oral live attenuated vaccine (OPV). It is the recommended vaccine in most countries.
2. **Passive immunization:** With 5–15 mL according to age of child of gamma globulin. Some measures of protection are afforded for 6 weeks. Indications—Newborn in hospital are exposed to infection, unimmunized children in hospital ward in which a case of poliomyelitis develops.

Complications of Poliomyelitis

1. Possible complications include respiratory failure, pulmonary edema. Pulmonary embolism, urinary tract infection, urolithiasis, atelectasis, pneumonia, or pulmonale, soft tissue and skeletal deformities and paralytic ileus.
2. In polio survivors latents poliomyelitis can lead to muscle spasticity and weakness 20–30 years after initial infection. Delayed poliomyelitis also can affect respiratory muscles leading to hypoxemia.

Nursing Interventions

1. Observe for signs of paralysis and other neurological damage, which can occur rapidly. Maintain a patient airway and look for respiratory weakness and difficulty swallowing.
2. Frequently check blood pressure, especially if the patient has bulbar poliomyelitis. This form of the disease can cause hypertension or shock.
3. Watch for signs of stool impaction caused by dehydration and intestinal inactivity. To prevent this, give enough fluids to ensure an adequate daily urine output of low specific gravity (1.5–2 L/day for adults).
4. To prevent pressure ulcers, provide skin care, reposition bladder weakness or transient bladder paralysis with urine retention.
5. Provide emotional support to the patient and family members. Long-term support and encouragement is essential for maximum rehabilitation.

2010 (February)
Pediatric Nursing

SECTION-I

I. Give the meaning of the following:
   a. Preventive pediatrics.
   b. Daycare centers.
   c. Reproductive health.
   d. Polycystic kidney.
   e. Pyloric stenosis.

II. State whether the following statements are *true* or *false*:
   a. Talipes equinovarus is also known as clubbed fingers.
   b. Hermaphroditism is a condition in which both ovarian and testicular tissue exists in the same individual.
   c. The evaluation of Apgar score was introduced by Virginia Anderson in 1972.

III. Write short notes on any three of the following:
   a. Weaning and complementary feeding.
   b. Factors influencing growth and development.
   c. Role of parents in sex education of child.
   d. Management of a child with cerebral palsy.

IV. a. Explain the physical and neurological assessment of a newborn.
   b. Write the management of a preterm baby.

V. Baby Suma is admitted and diagnosed as having tetralogy of Fallot:
   a. Write the clinical manifestation and diagnosis.
   b. Explain the management of a child with tetralogy of Fallot.

SECTION-II

VI. Fill up the blanks:
   a. Ascariasis is caused by: _____
   b. Phototherapy is used in case of: _____
   c. Lobar pneumonia affects the: _____
   d. Wilms' tumor is the tumor of the: _____

VII. State whether the following statements are *true* or *false*:
   a. Tetanus is caused by *Clostridium tetani*.
   b. Acute sinusitis is a condition in which there is inflammation of the oral mucous membrane.
   c. Meningitis is a condition in which there is infection of the muscle.

VIII. Write short notes on any *three* of the following:
   a. Care of a child in oxygen tent.
   b. Management of a child with thalassemia.
   c. Management of a child with chronic glomerulonephritis.
   d. Juvenile diabetes mellitus.

IX. Mr Nandi aged 10 years admitted and diagnosed as acute appendicitis:
   a. Define appendicitis.
   b. Write the signs and symptoms.
   c. Explain the pre and postoperative care of Mr Nandi.

X. Explain the management of an 8-year-girl with hearing impairment.

SECTION-I

I. Give the meaning of the following:

a. Preventive pediatrics
Child health depends upon preventive care. Preventive pediatrics is a specialized branch in child health. It has subdivisions of antenatal preventive pediatrics and postnatal preventive pediatrics.

b. Daycare centers
It is a special program in which the special care given to preschool children. Most of the day care programs incorporate a daily schedule of quite play, outdoor activities, group games and projects, creative or educational play and snack and rest periods.

c. Reproductive health
It is the ability to reproduce and regulate their fertility, women are able to go through pregnancy and child birth safely, the outcome of pregnancies is successful in terms of maternal and infant survival and well-being and couples are able to have sexual relations free of fear of pregnancy and of contracting diseases.

d. Polycystic kidney
It is an abnormal condition in which the kidney is enlarged and contains many cysts. There are three forms of the diseases: (1) Childhood polycystic disease (CPD), (2) Adult polycystic disease (APD), (3) Congenital polycystic diseases (CPD).

e. Pyloric stenosis
It is an obstruction at the pyloric sphincter caused by a hypertrophy of the circular muscles. It is occur soon after birth. It is generally recognized 3 weeks after birth.

II. State whether the following statements are *true* or *false*:
a. Talipes equinovarus is also known as clubbed fingers: **FALSE**
b. Hermaphroditism is a condition in which both ovarian and testicular tissue exists in the same individual: **TRUE**
c. The evaluation of Apgar score was introduced by Virginia Anderson in 1972: **FALSE**

III. Write short notes on any *three* of the following:

a. Weaning and complementary feeding
Breastfeeding alone is adequate and sufficient to maintain optimum growth and development of an infant up to the age for 4–6 months. It is, therefore, necessary to introduce more concentrated energy riched nutritional supplements by this age. Infants also required iron containing food supplements after this age to prevent iron deficiency anemia.

Weaning or complementary feeding is the process of gradual and progressive transfer of the baby from the breastfeeding to the usual family diet. During this process, the infant gets accustomed to foods other than mother's milk. Weaning does not mean discontinuity of breastfeeding. Weaning foods are given in addition of breastfeed when the amount of breastfeeding is inadequate.

Qualities of Complementary Foods

The weaning foods should be:
1. Liquid at starting then semisolid and solid foods to be introduced gradually.
2. Clean, fresh and hygienic, so that no infections can occur.
3. Easy to prepare at home with the available food items and not costly.
4. Easily digestible, easily acceptable and palatable for the infants.
5. High in energy density and low in bulk viscosity and contains all nutrients necessary for the baby.
6. Based on cultural practices and traditional beliefs.
7. Well-balanced, nourishing and suitable for the infant.

Principles of Introduction of Weaning Foods

During introduction of weaning foods following principles to be remembered:
1. Milk is the main food of infant, so additional feeds should provide extra-requirements as per needs of the baby, that must be obtained from good quality food items and should be home made.
2. A small amount of new foods to be given in the beginning and gradually the amount of food to be increased during the course of a week.
3. New food to be placed over the tongue of the baby to get the taste of the food and to feel the consistency. The baby may spit the food out, but with patience the feed to be given again to get accustomed with it. A single weaning food is added at a time.
4. Additional food can be given in the daytime. Initially it can be given once, then twice or thrice.
5. There should not be any strict rule for serving new foods, it may be modified. But the foods to be given regularly.
6. New foods should be given when the infant is hungry, but never force the child to take the feeds.
7. Observe the problems related to weaning process. The infant may have indigestion, pain in abdomen, weaning diarrhea, skin rash, especially in case of food allergy and psychological upset of the baby due to withdrawn from breast milk and sucking. The problems should be managed carefully.
8. Weaning should be started between 4–6 months of age to all children but breastfeeding to be continued up to 2 years of age or beyond.
9. Delayed weaning result in malnutrition and growth failure.

Complementary Feeding at Different Age

4–6 months: Weaning to be initiated with fruit juices, especially the grape juice, which is low in sorbitol. Within one or two weeks new foods to be introduced with suji, biscuit soaked in milk, vegetable soup, mashed banana, mashed and boiled potato, etc. Each food should be given with one or two teaspoons at first for 3–6 times per day. Foods should not be over diluted. Within 3–4 weeks amounts to be increased to half a cup. Breastfeeding must be continued.

6–9 months: Food items to be given in this period include soft mixture of rice and dal, khichri, pulses, mashed and boiled potato, bread or roti soaked in milk or dal, mashed fruits like banana, mango, papaya, stewed apple, etc. Egg yolk can be given from 6–7 months onwards. Curd and khir can be introduced from 7–8 months onwards. By the age of 6–9 months the infant can enjoy to bite biscuits, piece of carrot and cucumber. The infant can have these foods 5–6 times per day and amount of food to be increased gradually. Breastfeeding should be continued.

9–12 months: More variety of household foods can be added. New food items like fish, meat, and chicken can be introduced during this period. The infant can eat everything cooked at home but spices and condiments to be avoided. Feeds need not to be mashed but should be soft and well-cooked. Breastfeeding to be continued.

12–18 months: The child can take all food cooked in the family and needs half amount of mother's diet. Number of feeds can be 4–5 times or according to the child's need. Breastfeeding to be continued, especially at night.

The weaning period is most crucial period in child development. The appropriate weaning practices are an important aspect of child rearing and significant approach of preventive pediatrics towards healthy children.

b. Factors influencing growth and development

Growth and development depend on not one but combination of many factors, all interdependent. The relatively typical pattern of growth and development is influenced by heredity and environment. Also genetic inheritance and environmental influences are two primary factors in determining a child's pattern of growth and development.

Genetic Factors

1. **Heredity:** The heredity of a man and women determines their children. Heredity decides the size and shape of the body, hence family member bear resemblance. The characteristics are transmitted through genes, which are responsible for family illness, e.g. diabetes.
2. **Sex:** Sex is determined at conception, after birth the male infant is both longer and heavier than female infant. Boys maintain this superiority until about 11 years of age. Girls mature earlier, reach the period of accelerated growth earlier than boys and are taller than boys on the average.
3. **Race:** Distinguishing characteristics called racial or subracial developed in prehistoric humans. Similar physical characteristics are seen in people belonging to the same race. As too height, tall and short examples exist among all races and subraces. Among civilized groups, intermarriage has produced mixed racial types.

Nutritional Factors

1. **Poor nutrition:** Nutrition plays a vital role in the bodies susceptibility to disease because poor nutrition limits the body ability to resist infection. Poor nutrition also plays a major role in the development of chronic illnesses. Growth and development suffering from protein-energy malnutrition, anemic and vitamin deficiency states are retarded.
2. **Maternal nutrition:** Intrauterine growth retardation and consequently small size of the fetus occur due to nutritional deficiency in mothers, infection and drugs used during pregnancy.

Environmental Factors

1. **Physical environment:** Environment forces act upon the individual. It is the exploding force of an individual potentially to different stimulating forces. The physical environment includes food, temperature, climate, resources, etc.
2. **Mental environment:** It includes the intellectual atmosphere of the school, the libraries, the recreation rooms, laboratories, etc.

3. **Social environment:** It includes social association the child gets from the beginning. It also includes cultural atmosphere of the society, e.g. religion, folklore, literature, art, music, social conversions and political organizations. The rich is the environment, better is the scope for developing an individual into a healthy human being.
4. **Socioeconomic level:** The child born into a family of low socioeconomic means may not receive adequate health supervision could leave a child without immunization against measles or other childhood illnesses and thus vulnerable to disease that could cause permanent neurological damage.
5. **Cultural influences:** Groups of human being create their own cultures, whereas each individual is influenced or shaped by the culture of which he or she is a part. The effects of a particular culture on a child begin before birth because of the manner in which culture views and treat the members of the pregnant women's family.
6. **Internal influences:** There is evidence that all the hormones in the body affect growth in some manner. Deficiency of growth hormone retards growth while over production results in gigantism.
7. **Characteristics of parents:** Parents with high intelligence quotient are more likely to have children with higher level of inherent intelligence.

Prenatal environment: Prenatal environment climate in which the child's develops. The influences of the intrauterine environment on the child's future development are great, particularly since the uterus shields the fetus from the full impact of external adverse condition.

Postnatal environment: An environment that provides satisfying experiences promote growth. Since growth and development are interrelated, growth in one area influences and in turn is influenced by growth in all other areas.

c. Role of parents in sex education of child

Sexuality during the school years: Between 8 and 11 years, children begin to perceive sex roles in a near adult—fashion. Questions about one's sexuality continue, and the ultimate goal of all education about sexuality is the ability of the individual to merge biologic impulses with a satisfying family life. School-age children will continue, as they did during the preschool period, to ask questions concerning reproduction, but the questions will be more specific. While the 5-year old may say "Daddy put the seed in" as a way of explaining birth, the 7 or 8 year old may want an explanation about how daddy did it. Such questioning depends upon alertness, the ability of the child to articulate, and the permissiveness of the parents.

Boys and girls should be informed about the reproductive cycle and their respective roles as they approach puberty. Both female and male sexual changes should be discussed by caring, informed parents.

Usually if a daughter has not asked about menses by the age of 10 years, the parent should gently introduce the topic. Her questions should be answered fully and completely. Techniques of self-care during menstruation can be explained and the girl given some choice in the technique to be used. Fathers should explore the menstrual cycle with their sons. Mothers also should share their feelings with their sons.

d. Management of child with cerebral palsy

Cerebral palsy (CP) is a group of nonprogressive disorders resulting from malfunctions of the motor centers and pathways of brain. It is a noncurable and nonfatal condition due to damage of the growing brain before or during birth. It is commonest cause of crippling in children. Its severity is ranging from minor incapacitation to total handicap. Mental retardation is associated in about 25–50% of cases of CP.

Other associated handicapped conditions are epilepsy, orthopedic deformities, partial or complete deafness, blindness and psychological disturbances.

Management: Management should be planned in a team approach. Coordination among team members is needed between pediatricians, pediatric surgeons, pediatric nurse specialist, physical therapist, occupational therapist, speech therapist, pediatric social worker, child psychologist, teacher, special educator, family members and parents. The holistic approach is required to achieve fullest possible functional ability and skill in keeping the child with developmental age. Management includes drug therapy, physiotherapy, and surgical corrections of deformities, occupational therapy and rehabilitation.

Drug therapy is indicated in symptomatic management for the child with CP. The commonly used drugs are—diazepam for spasticity, strychnine for hypotonia, chlordiazepoxide or levodopa for athetosis, carbamazepine for dystonia, anticonvulsive for epilepsy, tranquilizers for behavioral problems and muscle relaxants to improve muscular functions.

Surgical correction may be needed for bony deformities and stabilizing the joints or relieving the contractures. Selective dorsal rhizotomy can be done to decrease spasticity. Orthopedic support can be provided by splints or orthotic devices. Physiotherapy is effective to prevent contractures, to promote relaxation of spastic muscles and for maintenance of posture. Occupational therapy can be arranged as some simple occupation (e.g. typing), so that when they grow up, they can earn something for their own. Positive application of certain repetitive movements of legs, hands and fingers can be used during occupational training which also helps to relax spastic muscles. The child should be trained in self care like feeding, dressing, bathing, brushing, etc. Family support and community support are vital for socio-economic rehabilitation of these handicapped children.

Nursing management: Nursing assessment should include the detection of ability to perform activities of daily living (ADL), developmental milestones, neurological reflexes feeding behavior, nutritional status, bladder and bowel habits, problem related to vision, hearing and language, associated health hazards or congenital anomalies, present problems, parent–child interactions, treatment compliance, etc. Nursing diagnoses should be formulated accordingly to plan and to provide nursing interventions.

IV. a. Explain the physical and neurological assessment of a newborn.
b. Write the management of a preterm baby.

Physical assessment: The order of assessment can be planned to the individual neonate. The cardiac and abdominal parts are examined when the neonate is quiet. The observation of the nose and mouth may be done with the neonate crying or very active.

General appearance: The infant lies with extremities flexed. The activity may be increased with the stimuli. The infant may have a loud lusty cry with irritability or sluggishness should be noted and reported.

Measurement of the size: The size of the head, length, and weight is measured and compared with the growth chart based on gestational age. The disproportion in any parameter can be identified. Any significant disproportion may be a sign of the potential problem.

Head circumference: After birth, molding of the skull may give inaccurate measurement of the head circumference. Therefore, the measurement should be repeated 48 hours after the birth. It is 33–35 cm. It is 2–3 cm larger than the chest circumference. The head circumference may be unusually large in a hydrocephalus, and significantly small in a macrocephalus or premature closure of sutures (craniostenosis).

Chest circumference: Chest circumference is about 30.5–33 cm. It may be smaller in case of malnutrition and preterm neonate. The thorax is barrel shaped. The breathing is quiet and mainly with the diaphragm (the abdomen rises and falls with the breath).

Length (head to heal): On average the neonate's length is 45–50 cm.

Body weight: The body weight of the neonate should be measured immediately after the birth. It is on an average 2.5–3 kg. The neonatal loss the body weight about 10% within the first 4–5 days after the birth. The birth weight is regained by 10th day after the birth. Accurate weight measurement is necessary as it is the base line for evaluation of the progress.

Body temperature: Many nurseries practice axillary temperature. The normal temperature ranges between 35.5 °C and 37.5 °C. Some nurseries practice rectal temperature. The normal rectal temperature is 37°C.

Heart rate: It may vary according to the phase of reactivity. Also it may increase when the neonate cries. It should be auscultated with the stethoscope when the neonate is calm. Apical beat normally ranges from 120–140/min.

Respiratory rate: The respiratory rate normally ranges between 30 and 60 per minute, when the neonate is calm. It may be irregular in the initial hours but comes to normal rhythm within a few hours.

Blood pressure: The normal systolic pressure may be 70 mm of mercury, at the age of first few days. By the end of two weeks, the systolic blood pressure may be 84 mm of mercury.

Posture: In full-term babies, generalized flexion is seen. The extremities and neck are flexed. The feet are dorsiflexed. Any deviation from the flexion may be tested with care. Erb's palsy may result in the extension of an arm and flexion in the other parts of the body. Frank breech shows extended legs.

Activity: The normal neonate is alert and active. This can be observed as his response to stimulus of loud noise, presence of Moro's reflex. The degree of alertness should be observed. The baby may be irritable or drowsy with neurological disturbances,

Skin: The neonate's skin is soft, smooth and puffy. At birth, the skin is covered with a grayish white cheese like substance called vernix caseosa. Vernix caseosa has insulating and bacteriostatic power.

Head: Newborn's skull consists of bones that do not close completely, so the shape of the skull is easily moulded by the passage through the birth canal. At the junction of the suture lines, the fontanels can be palpated. The anterior fontanelle bounded by the parietal and frontal bone is diamond shaped. It is 2.5 cm Long and 4 cm wide. The posterior fontanel, bounded by the occipital and parietal bones, is triangular shaped. The anterior fontanel is assessed with the infant relaxed and in an upright position. Lie is normally soft and pulsates with each heartbeat. The fontanel will feel fuller when the infant is lying down and will bulge slightly when the infant coughs. The widely spaced sutures and bulging fontanel may suggest increased intracranial pressure, seen in the hydrocephalus, infections of the nervous system or bleeding in the central nervous system. Depressed fontanelle may indicate dehydration. The nurse must observe for caput succedaneum and cephathematoma.

Face: The newborn's face is observed for asymmetry, position, proportion of facial sutures and any signs of malformation. Unusual facies, including unusual shape and position of the eyes, tilt to the nose, shape of the mouth, and size of the jaw may suggest possible inherited or congenital disorder.

Eye: An awake quiet newborn will usually open the eyes readily. Size and position of the eyes should be noted. The distance between the inner canthi should be 2 cm. Neonates' pupils are generally round and of equal size and they react to the light. The neonate does not form tears. Any abnormal eye discharge should be notified. The eyes should be examined for edema, hemorrhage or inflammation.

Ear: The ear cartilage in the term infant is sufficiently formed that the ear retains its shape. Malformed or low-set ears may be associated with other abnormalities. Startle reflex on loud noise indicates the audibility.

Nose: The neonate is a nasal breather. If the neonate is breathing quietly with the mouth closed and is pink, it can be assumed that the nose is functioning. Just after the birth, sneezing is common to remove the secretions from airway. Nasal flaring indicates respiratory distress.

Mouth: The mouth and throat can be examined when the neonate is crying or yawning. It should be observed for existing structures. Normally the lips and palate are intact. Whitish plaques adhering to the mucosa may indicate infection by *Candida albicans*.

Neck: Newborns' neck is short and with folds. It is in a full range of motion. It should be checked for abnormal masses.

Chest: The thorax of the neonate is a barrel shaped. The breast may be engorged and have milky discharge because of the stimulation by the maternal hormones. This resolves gradually and requires no treatment. Parents should be explained about it. Neonates should breathe quietly mainly with the diaphragm. The abdomen rises and falls at each breathe.

Abdomen: The abdomen should not be distended or scaphoid. It should appear flat. Bowel sounds must be present. On palpation it should feel soft. The liver edge can be normally palpated from one to three centimeters below the coastal margin. The spleen tip is palpated on the left. There should be no masses or enlargement of the kidneys. The umbilical cord should contain two arteries and one vein.

Stools: The stools are unformed but not watery. The color is golden yellow. The reaction of the stool is acid. When cows' milk is fed, the stools are passed less frequently, it is firmer, and has yellow color. The reaction of the stools is alkaline or neutral. The odor is noticeable.

Genitalia: In female neonates, the labia and clitoris must be inspected carefully. In normal newborns, the labia minora are covered by the labia majora. The urethral opening is situated behind the clitoris. Hymenal tag may be visible from the posterior opening of a vagina. Vaginal Bloody discharge may be noticed during the first week due to abrupt decrease of maternal hormones. This is called pseudomenstruation. In male neonates, the penis should be inspected for location of the urethral opening. It is usually at the tip. The prepuce is normally not retractable and should not be forcefully retracted. Smegma, a white cheesy substance is accumulated around the glans penis under the foreskin. The scrotum is dark pigmented with rougae. The testes are generally descended in the scrotum at birth. An absence of testes in the scrotum may be seen in premature babies, in the ectopic testes or in sexual abnormalities.

Back and spine: The shape of the back is slightly rounded. An abnormal depression in the spine may indicate spina bifida.

Extremities: Extremities are inspected for symmetry, range of motion, and any malformation or injury. The reflexes and muscle tone are assessed. When the attempt is made to extend any extremity the neonate resists and when released, the extremity will return to its previous flexed position.

Neurological status: Assessment of neurological status is very important. In the neonates, neurological mechanisms are immature both anatomically and physiological which result in disturbance of temperature regulation, uncoordinated movements and lack of control over musculature.

Examination of muscle tone, head control and reflexes are essential aspects. Two types of reflexes are present in the neonates, i.e. protective reflex (blinking, coughing, sneezing and gagging) and primitive reflex (rooting, sucking, Moro, or startle, tonic neck, stepping and palmer grasp).

Neurological assessment: Neurological assessment in general includes observation of posture, neonate's reflexes, muscle tone, head control, and movements. The nervous system develops in orderly consistent patterns related to the age right from the conception. That is why assessment of neurological development and reflexes helps in determining the gestational age of the neonate. For example, the term newborn has stronger muscle flexion than muscle extensor, whereas preterm has an extended posture. There are many reflexes seen in the neonate that disappear after maturity of nervous system.

Reflexes of the Neonate

1. **Rooting:** When the cheek is touched along the side of the mouth, the neonate will turn his head to that side.
2. **Sucking:** The neonate sucks when its mouth comes in contact with a nipple, or may occur as a part of a rooting response.
3. **Gag reflex:** Stimulation of posterior pharynx by food, suction or while passing tube causes the neonate to gag.
4. **Extrusion:** When tongue is touched or depressed the neonate resists by forcing it outward.
5. **Yawning:** It is spontaneous response to decreased oxygen level by increasing inspired air.
6. **Grasp reflex:** Touching palm or sole of feet near the base of digits causes flexion of hands and toes.
7. **Moro's reflex:** Moro's reflex can be elicited by holding the neonate in a supine position, with the trunk just above the table and then suddenly allowing the neonate drop backwards on the level of the table. Sudden jarring or sudden lack of support causes sudden extension and abduction of extremities, fanning of fingers and then bringing the arms together in the midline (in an "embrace"). This may be accompanied by crying, extension of head and trunk.
8. **Startle reflex:** A sudden loud noise causes abduction of the arms with flexion of elbows, hands remain clenched.
9. **Tonic neck reflex:** The asymmetrical tonic neck reflex is elicited by placing the neonate in the supine position and turning the head.

V. Baby Suma is admitted and diagnosed as having tetralogy of Fallot.
a. Write the clinical manifestation and diagnosis
b. Explain the management of a child with tetralogy of Fallot

Tetralogy of Fallot (TOF) is the most common cyanotic congenital heart disease. It accounts for 6–10% of all CHDs. This condition is characterized by the combinations of four defects (1) pulmonary stenosis (2) ventricular septal defect (3) overriding or dextroposition of the aorta and (4) right ventricular hypertrophy.

Pathophysiology: Due to structural defects, there is right to left heart shunt causing cyanosis. The most vital abnormalities are pulmonary stenosis and VSD (generally perimembraneous variety). Obstruction of blood flow from the right ventricle due to pulmonary valve stenosis results in shunting of deoxygenated blood through the VSD into the left ventricle, then to the aorta causes cyanosis. Degree of cyanosis depends upon the degree of right ventricular outflow tract obstruction and the size of the VSD. Outflow obstruction can also occur due to infundibular hypertrophy and

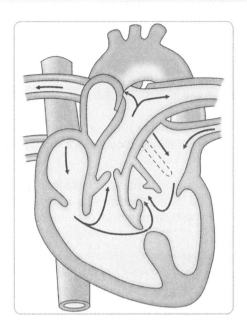

supravalvular stenosis. Right ventricular hypertrophy develops due to the obstruction. Finally, the condition is complicated by persistent arterial unsaturation, poor pulmonary vascularity, polycythemia to compensate cyanosis and increased blood viscosity resulting thrombophlebitis and formation of emboli. Minimum right to left shunt in small obstruction causes mild form of TOF and termed as pink or acyanotic tetralogy of Fallot.

Clinical manifestations: Clinical features of TOF depend upon size of VSD and degree of right ventricular outflow obstruction. Blue baby or cyanosis of lips and nail beds with dyspnea is found initially with crying and exertion in neonates especially when the ductus arteriosus begins to close.

As the infant grows, other presenting features are observed, i.e. hypoxic-anoxic or blue (hypercyanotic) spells, which occur due to cerebral anoxia. The spell consists of irritability, dyspnea, and cyanosis, flacidity with or without unconsciousness. The spell is also termed as Tet-spell, and found in the morning soon after awakening, during or after feeding and painful procedures. The child feels comfortable in squatting posture or in lying down position. Slow weight gain and mental slowness are found. By the age of two years, the child usually develops clubbing. CCF is unusual in infants and children suffering from TOF.

Diagnostic evaluation: Details history of illness and thorough clinical examination are important diagnostic approach. Auscultation of soft or harsh systolic ejection murmur heard best at the upper left sternal border in third space. P2 is usually single. Chest X-ray shows poorly vascularized lung fields, a small boot-shaped heart (due to RVH) and cancavity of the pulmonary artery segment. There may be right aortic arch.

ECG shows right axis deviation and RVH. Two-dimensional echocardiogram and cardiac catheterization help to detect structural abnormalities, degree of obstruction and coronary artery pattern.

Management

A. Medical management: The child with TOF should be managed for cyanosis, hypoxic spells and other associated complications. Oxygen therapy, correction of dehydration, anemia, antibiotic therapy, supportive nursing care and continuous monitoring of child's condition are very important measures.

Hypoxic spells should be managed by placing the baby in knee-chest position, sedatives, oral propranolol therapy, I/V fluid, treatment of acidosis, oxygen therapy and administration of I/V vasopressors (phenylephrine, methoxamine). Oxygen therapy during the spells has limited value. Planning for surgical correction of defects should be done as soon as the child starts having spells. Parents should be taught about the immediate care at home during the spells and necessary medical help.

Neonates with severe TOF, may be benefited from prostaglandin E1 (IV) which causes dilatation of the ductus and allows adequate pulmonary blood flow. It should be administered immediately on diagnosis of cyanotic CHD.

B. Surgical management: Surgical interventions can be planned as palliative surgery or definitive correction in one stage repair. One stage repair may be contraindicated in abnormal coronary artery distribution, multiple VSDs, hypoplastic branch of pulmonary arteries and small infant with less than 2.5 kg body weight.

SECTION-II

VI. Fill up the blanks

a. Ascariasis is caused by: **Lumbricoides**
b. Phototherapy is used in case of: **Hyperbilirubinemia**
c. Lobar pneumonia affects the: **Lobes of the lung**
d. Wilms' tumor is the tumor of the: **Kidney**

VII. State whether the following statements are *true* or *false*:

a. Tetanus is caused by *Clostridium tetani*: **TRUE**
b. Acute sinusitis is a condition in which there is inflammation of the oral mucous membrane: **FALSE**
c. Meningitis is a condition in which there is infection of the muscle: **FALSE**

VIII. Write short notes on any *three* of the following:

a. Care of child In oxygen tent

Oxygen is used as a drug to change the concentration of inspired air in the conditions of deficiency of oxygen. It is one of the most common procedures carried out in the management of children with respiratory diseases and other illnesses. The young children are unable to express their breathing discomfort. The pediatric nurse should have knowledge, good observation skill and ability for assessment of need for oxygen therapy.

Purpose of Oxygen Therapy

Oxygen is administered to achieve satisfactory level of PaO_2, range between 60 and 80 or 90 mm Hg. It is used as temporary measures to relieve hypoxemia and hypoxia, but does not replace definite treatment of underlying cause of these conditions.

The general purposes of oxygen therapy are:
1. To correct hypoxemia and hypoxia.
2. To increase oxygen tension of blood plasma.
3. To restore the oxyhemoglobin in red blood cells.
4. To maintain the ability of body cells to carry on normal metabolic functions.

Assessment of Need for Oxygen Therapy—Oxygen administration is indicated in numbers of medical and surgical conditions. The need for oxygen is assessed by the followings:
1. Observing symptoms of respiratory distress and hypoxia, i.e. inadequate breathing pattern, labored respiration, dysrhythmias, cyanosis, change of activity like restlessness, lethargic and unresponsiveness, change in level of consciousness, hypothermia, etc.
2. Analysis of arterial blood gases (ABGs) for PaO_2, $PaCO_2$, pH, HCO_3, etc.
3. Pulse oximetry.
4. Measuring of inspired O_2 concentration (FiO_2).

Methods of Oxygen Administration

It depends upon age and condition of the child, cause of hypoxia, required concentration of oxygen and ventilatory assistance, available facilities, etc. Oxygen therapy can be given continuous or intermittent. It can be dispensed from a cylinder, piped-in-system, liquid oxygen reservoir or oxygen concentrator. It should be administered in higher concentration than is present in air (21%). Usually, it is given in 40–60% concentration but sometimes 100% can also be given.

Oxygen can be administered by following methods:
1. **Noninvasive method:** by (a) Oxygen mask which can be simple face mask, venturi mask or partial rebreathing mask, (b) Oxygen hood or face tent,(c) Oxygent tent or canopy and (d) Isolette incubator or other closed incubator.
2. **Invasive method:** by (a) Orotracheal or nasotracheal or tracheostomy route and (b) nasopharyngeal catheter or nasal canula or nasal prong.

Complications of oxygen therapy: Prolonged exposure to high concentrations of oxygen may result in constriction of cerebral blood vessels leading to irreversible brain damage and constriction of retinal blood vessels causing retinopathy of prematurity or retrolental fibroplasia. Pulmonary complications are pulmonary congestion, bronchiolar edema, bronchopulmonary dysplasia (in neonates), respiratory depression, necrotizing bronchiolitis, etc. Long-term complications due to oxygen toxicity are chronic pulmonary diseases, seizure disorders and epilepsy.

Safety Precautions during Administration of Oxygen
1. Oxygen acts as a drug—it must be prescribed and administered in specific dose in terms of rate, concentration and duration.
2. Humidifier and regulator must be used.

b. Management of a child with thalassemia

Thalassemia is a chronic congenital hemolytic anemia in which red blood cells have abnormal hemoglobin. In this condition, synthesis of beta polypeptides is deficient. This causes chronic microcytic hypochromic anemia. There is more production of fetal hemoglobin. Large number of immature and defective hemoglobin damages red blood cells and increases hemolyis. Thalassemia is classified as thalassemia minor and thalassemia major. Thalassemia minor is caused when genes responsible for the disease are of heterogeneous traits. These children have no symptoms of anemia. Sometimes, the spleen gets enlarged. Thalassemia major is caused by homogeneous traits of genes. They have severe anemia.

Manifestation
1. Anemia.
2. Fever.
3. Poor feeding.
4. Enlarged spleen.
5. Hemosiderosis (bronze skin).
6. Hemochromatosis (fibrosis causing destruction of tissue).
7. Chronic effect results in skeletal changes, cardiac enlargement. Myocardial changes, splenomegaly and destruction of pancreas.

Investigation
1. Blood examination to detect changes in red blood cells, such as, hypochronic, microcytic, anisocytosis, or poikilocytosis.
2. Hemoglobin level.
3. X-ray of bones to detect widening.

Treatment
1. Frequent blood transfusions are required to maintain the level of hemoglobin above 6 g per 100 mL.
2. Use of iron chelating agent (deferoxamine) helps to excrete the excessive iron stored through the kidney.
3. Splenectomy may be done to decrease discomfort and promote normal growth.
4. Folic acid may be prescribed to prevent its deficiency.

Management
1. Circulating capacity can be increased by blood transfusions which will increases hemoglobin level and prevent hypoxia.
2. Observation during the transfusion and checking for the reaction to the blood is necessary.
3. Prevention of the infection can be done by avoiding contact with infection and prophylactic antibiotics according to the doctor's prescription.
4. Fracture prone activities should be avoided, because the bones have lost their strength.
5. Children should be helped to cope up with the effects of the disease.
6. Children's feelings should be explored and they should be provided with the support.
7. Emphasis should be on the quiet activities.
8. Maintenance of good hygiene will help to prevent infection.
9. Encouragement for interactions with peers will help in diversional effect.

Parental advice
1. Parental support can be provided by exploring their feelings and explaining the care of the children.
2. The children may be referred to social and supportive agencies as advisable.
3. Parents may be referred to the genetic counseling to prevent occurrence in the consequitive children.

c. Management of a child with chronic glomerulonephritis

Acute glomerulonephritis is a noninfectious renal disease found more in male children than in the female children. It is more common in the age group of 2–10 years. It is an immune complex disease, due to antigen antibody reaction following hemolytic streptococcal infection. The antibodies affect the glomerulus causing proliferation and swelling of endothelial cells obstructing the blood flow through capillaries. The amount of the glomerular filtrate is reduced and it allows the passage of the blood cells and proteins into filtrate.

Manifestation: An onset is usually, one to three weeks after the onset of infection of the upper respiratory tract or infection of the skin.
1. Edema starts with the periorbital edema, in the morning.
2. Urine output is decreased, with the high color urine resembling black tea or cola (due to lysis red blood cells).
3. Hypertension may be present
4. The fever may or may not be present
5. Children look pale, lethargic, and irritable.
6. Children may complain of a headache.
7. Gastrointestinal disturbances may occur.

Investigation
1. Urine examination for: Hematuria, specific gravity, albumin, white blood cells and epithelial cells.
2. Blood examination for: Urea nitrogen and creatinine, serum albumin.
3. Antistreptolysin O titer (ASLO).
4. Electrocardiography.

Complication
1. Hypertension.
2. Hypertensive encephalopathy may occur when the diastolic blood pressure rises above 110 mm of Hg. It can cause vomiting, restlessness, convulsions, stupor, visual disturbances, or cranial nerve palsy.
3. Cardiac failure with the retention of salt and water may cause tachycardia, dyspnea, pulmonary edema, and enlargement of the heart.
4. Renal failure may occur with severe oliguria or anuria and increased blood pressure; it may occur in two phases.
5. First phase: This stage of edema with oliguria may last for 5–10 days.
6. Second stage: The stage of diuresis starts with the increased output of urine and decreased edema.

Treatment
1. There is no specific treatment for acute glumerulonephritis.
2. It is self limiting and patients recover within 2–3 weeks.
3. Death may be due to complications.

Supportive Treatment
1. Antibiotics, such as, long-acting penicillin may be given to treat reminent of the infection.
2. Hypotensive drugs may be prescribed to control the hypertension.
3. Magnesium sulfate may be prescribed in the encephalopathy to reduce cerebral edema.
4. Sedatives may be required in restless patients.
5. In cardiac failure, digitalis may be prescribed.
6. In renal failure, patients may need a dialysis.

Management

1. Rest may be required for two to four weeks. Gradually, the activities may be started as the children improve.
2. The vital signs should be observed to detect early sign of complications, such as, the deviation in the pulse, may indicate cardiac failure. Headache, convulsions, and behavioral changes may be indicative of hypertensive encephalopathy.
3. Observation of the intake and output is important. An accurate recording of daily weight, edema, and appearance of the urine is necessary.
4. Nutrition should be planned according to the blood reports in the specific stage.
    a. In mild cases, salt restricted regular food may be allowed. Salty food items should be avoided. In an early phase of oliguria, the food should contain low proteins, high carbohydrates and vitamin supplement. Small, frequent feeding should be given. Fluid should be supplied according to the prescription. The parents should be explained about the accurate fluid intake.
    b. During the second phase, when the diuresis starts, the normal food with the adequate fluids, fruits can be given, as the blood reports improve.
5. Recreational facilities and play in the bed, can help divert the children's mind.

Parental Advice

1. Parents should be taught about the early signs of complications and importance of early treatment.
2. Proper care of the skin and timely treatment of the skin lesions should be explained.
3. Prompt care of the respiratory problems should be insisted.
4. Parents should be instructed about the follow up visits.

d. Juvenile diabetes mellitus

Diabetes mellitus is a hereditary disorder associated with derangement in carbohydrate, protein, and fat metabolism, leading to high serum levels of glucose and presence of glucose in the urine. Predisposing factors include deficiency of insulin, heredity, obesity, and correlated endocrine factors. In juvenile diabetes melitus, onset occurs before 15 years of age. A pancreas produces inadequate insulin. The proper oxidation of glucose does not occur. Proteins and fats are oxidized in abnormal rates. Hyperglycemia results from deficient oxidation of glucose.

Manifestation

1. Rapid onset.
2. Major symptoms include polyuria, polydypsia, polyphagia, loss of weight, and tiredness.
3. Minor symptoms include skin and urinary infections and dry skin.
4. Diabetes acidosis. Precomatose state includes the symptoms such as, drowsiness, dry skin, red lips, tachypnea, nausea, and abdominal pain.
5. Comatose state includes the symptoms such as, extreme hyperapnea (Kussmaul's breathing), rapid and weak pulse, decreased blood pressure, decreased body temperature, sunken eyes, and a rigid abdomen.
6. Circulatory collapse and renal failure may occur as a result of acidosis and dehydration.

Complication

1. Stunting of growth.
2. Gangrene.

3. Cataract.
4. Diabetic nephropathy.

Treatment
1. Intravenous sodium bicarbonate and potassium may be administered as prescribed.
2. Insulin should be available, if patient suddenly becomes hypoglycemic. Soluble insulin is administered intravenously. The dose of insulin depends on the degree of ketosis and glucose level in the blood.

Management
1. The common causes of acidosis should be remembered such as untreated diabetes, inadequate insulin, failure to follow diet, and chronic and repeated infection.
2. In case of coma, principles of the nursing management of an unconscious patient should be followed. In addition, following care is required.
3. Maintenance of intravenous therapy:
   a. Intravenous sodium bicarbonate and potassium supplement may be required to administer.
   b. Intravenous glucose may be required, if a patient becomes suddenly hypogycemic.
   c. A soluble insulin, such as regular insulin should be ready for intravenous administration if required.

   The dose of insulin depends on the level of ketosis and glucose level of the blood. The urine examination of glucose and acetones is necessary.
4. Nasogastric intubation may be required to relieve abdominal detention and prevent vomiting. Oral feeding is started when patient recovers from acidosis and becomes alert. The food is started with low fat liquid diet. Lost potassium can be replaced by giving fruit juices, coffee, and milk.

   The diet should be adequate for the child's normal growth and development; and sufficient to satisfy the appetite. A prescribed diet is decided on the child's symptoms, family, and cultural habits.

   A diet is distributed throughout the day to accommodate varying peak actions of insulin.
5. Insulin is administered to maintain the balance of the blood glucose level. The knowledge of type and effect of insulin is necessary. The dose and type of insulin is decided by the results of diabetic neuropathy reaction testing of urine for sugar and acetone.

   Insulin should be administered by rotating sites. It should be administered subcutaneously to prevent local skin reaction and to promote absorption.

   Extrabottles of insulin should be stored in the refrigerator.
6. Encourage exercises within the normal limits which help to reduce blood glucose. Prevent infections by maintaining hygiene, daily bath and skin care.

Parental Advice
1. Explain the parents and child about the immediate care of the wound, care of foot, dental checkup and dental care.
2. Parents and child should be taught the administration of insulin in the correct dose by correct method.
3. The diet of the child should be explained
4. The urine examination should be taught because; it has to be done at home.

IX. Mr Nandi aged 10 years admitted and diagnosed as acute appendicitis:
   a. Define appendicitis.
   b. Write the signs and symptoms.
   c. Explain the pre and postoperative care of Mr Nandi.

Appendicitis is the inflammation of the vermiform appendix caused by the obstruction of the intestinal lumen. It may occur due to fecalith, infection, stricture, foreign body or tumor. It is common surgical emergency in childhood and usually found in age group of 5–15 years.

Pathophysiology
Obstruction of the intestinal lumen results in edema, infection and ischemia. Collection of secretion inside the lumen leads to distension and pressure on the intramural blood vessels. Inflammation leads to ulceration and gangrene. Necrosis and perforation usually occur due to intraluminal tension. Ruptured appendix followed by peritonitis may develop following inflammatory changes.

Clinical Manifestations
Initially the child presents with classical triad symptoms of periumbilical pain followed by vomiting and fever. The pain usually starts in epigastrium and colicky in nature. Later, within 2–12 hours pain shifts and localizes at right lower quadrant or McBumey's point in right iliac fossa and increases in intensity.

There may be some variations of site of pain depending upon the position of the appendix. In retrocecal appendix, pain may radiate to the right flank which may be mistaken as ureteric colic. In pelvic appendix, pain may radiate to lower abdomen. In appendicular perforation, pain becomes generalized. In peritonitis, the pain usually present over whole of the lower abdomen.

Other presenting features are anorexia, nausea and constipation. Diarrhea may occur occasionally. Rebound tenderness and involuntary guarding with generalized abdominal rigidity are found during abdominal examination. Positive Psoas sign and Rovsing's sign are suggestive of appendicitis.

Complications: The appendicitis can be complicated with ruptured appendix, intestinal perforation, paralytic ileus, peritonitis, pelvic abscess and subphrenic abscess.

Diagnosis: The diagnosis of acute appendicitis is done on the basis of detailed history and thorough clinical examination. Other investigative methods are useful in case of any doubt.
1. Urine examination to be done to exclude urinary problems.
2. Blood examination shows moderate leukocytosis.
3. Abdominal X-ray helps identify the presence of fecalith or perforation or intestinal obstruction.
4. USG abdomen helps in the diagnosis of ruptured appendix or abscess formation.

Management
The treatment of acute appendicitis is mainly appendectomy and necessary symptomatic and supportive management. There is no role of conservative management, as the chance of perforation and peritonitis are very high in children.

Appendicular mass should be treated with I/V antibiotics, fluid therapy and analgesics. Interval appendectomy is done if the mass undergoes resolution. Otherwise immediate exploration is indicated when fever and appendicular mass persist with increased abdominal pain.

Nursing interventions should emphasize on the basic preoperative and postoperative care including special attention on pain management and prevention of infections. Parents should be involved in care of the child. Emotional support to the child and parents is important in relation to surgery. Instructions and necessary information's should be given regarding continuation of care after discharge with special attention of operative area and follow-up.

X. Explain the management of an 8-year-girl with hearing impairment.

Hearing is important for the development of speech and verbal communication. Impairment of hearing may be congenital or acquired. It may be temporary or permanent, organic or inorganic and peripheral or central in origin. Hearing deficit can be mild, moderate, severe or profound. It is one of the common handicapped conditions in children. It is found about 9–15% among Indian school children.

Common causes of Hearing Impairment

1. **Genetic:** familial deafness, chromosomal abnormalities like trisomy 21, Pierre–Rubin syndrome, Alport's syndrome, Hunter–Hurler syndrome and congenital craniofacial anomalies.
2. **Intrauterine infections:** Rubella, CMV, syphilis, toxoplasma, chickenpox,
3. **Teratogenic exposure during pregnancy:** Drug therapy with quinine, streptomycin, thalidomide and irradiation.
4. **Infection in postnatal period:** Meningitis, encephalitis, mumps, measles, chickenpox, recurrent and supportive otitis media.
5. **Mechanical obstruction** of external auditory canal by wax and foreign body.
6. **Brain damage,** cerebral palsy, mental retardation, LBW baby (below 1500 g), severe respiratory depression, birth asphyxia, prolonged (more than 5 days) mechanical ventilation, birth injury.
7. **Toxic:** Neonatal hyperbilirubinemia.
8. **Ototoxic drug therapy:** Streptomycin, gentamicin, neomycin, chloroquine, loop diuretics.
9. **Endocrinal:** Cretinism.
10. **Injury:** Direct injury of ear, head injury, indirect injury by explosion (cracker, fireworks), constant exposure to loud noise.
11. Nutritional-malnutrition, vitamin 'B' complex deficiency.

Classification of hearing impairment: In a quiet environment, the healthy child can hear tones between 0 and 25 decibel ranges. Hearing impairment is described as follows:
1. Slight hearing impairment—15–25 decibels.
2. Mild hearing impairment—25–40 decibels.
3. Moderate hearing impairment—40–65 decibels.
4. Severe hearing impairment—65–95 decibels.
5. Profound hearing impairment—95 or more decibels.

Types

Hearing deficits can be classified as follows:

Conductive hearing deficit: It is dysfunction of sound transmission or conduction of sound wave through the external ear and middle ear. Any process interfering with sound transmission through ear canal, ear drum or ossicles may result in conductive hearing loss. It is common type of hearing deficit. The most common cause of conductive deafness is otitis media with effusion. Other causes are impacted wax. Foreign body, tympanic perforation, cholesteatoma, otosclerosis, etc. Several congenital syndromes may also be associated with conductive hearing deficit, e.g. Aperts syndrome, Crouzon's, syndrome, etc.

Sensorineural hearing deficit: This condition is cause by damage or lesions of the cochlea (organ of Corti), auditory nerve or central auditary pathways. It is usually an acquired problem due to meningitis, perinatal CNS infection, birth asphyxia, neonatal hyperbilirubinemia, ototoxic drug effect and loud noise. This condition may be congenital due to genetic or nongenetic causes. Genetic causes are associated with Alport's syndrome, Jervell's syndrome, etc. Nongenetic causes are LBW baby, prematurity, neonatal sepsis, etc. These problems damage the auditary nerve and hair cells in the cochlea, thus prevent transmission of sound impulses to the brain for interpretation resulting in sensorineural hearing deficit.

Mixed type: It includes both conductive and sensorineural hearing deficit.

Hearing deficit can also be classified as central or peripheral hearing deficit. It may also be due to psychogenic factor. Central hearing deficit indicates auditory deficit originating along central auditory nervous system from the proximal 8th nerve to cortex due to convulsive disorders, tumors, demyelinating disease, etc. Peripheral hearing deficit indicates dysfunction in the sound transmission through the external or middle ear as also its conversion into neural activity at the inner ear and the 8th nerve. It may be conductive, sensorineural or mixed type.

Consequence of hearing impairment: Children with hearing impairment may not complain that they cannot hear well. Only about 6% of the hearing impaired children have profound hearing loss. The rest have some hearing ability. But even mild or unilateral hearing deficit has detrimental effect on development and performance of the child. Consequences of hearing impairment may be found as poor or lack of response to sounds, delayed or poor speech development, poor attention span, poor academic performance, behavior problems in home and school, speaking loudly, listening radio and television at a loud volume, inadequate social and emotional development.

Diagnostic Evaluation

1. Assessment of developmental milestones, especially language development and personal social behavior along with response to sound help in suspicion of hearing impairment. Otoscopic examination to be done along with physical examination and history collection related to the condition for the suspected cases.
2. Hearing tests
   a. Using tuning fork-Weber test, Rinne test and Schwabach test are done in school children to detect the types of hearing deficit. These tests are not fully reliable. Before testing with these techniques, wax from ear canal to be removed.
   b. An ordinary test using wrist watch can be useful to detect the hearing deficit.
3. Audiometry to be done to confirm the diagnosis and the type of deficit. This test should be done through play and behavior assessment, when the child can cooperate and follow the instructions. The result is recorded in the form of audiogram. Pure tone audiometry is usually possible in children above 5 years of age.
4. Tympanometry may be performed to detect mobility of the tympanic membrane.
5. Labyrinthine test to be performed to detect vestibular functions in older children and adolescence. it is simple, inexpensive and accurate diagnostic test indicating presence or absence of labyrinthine response.
6. Auditory brainstem response (ABR) or otoacoustic emissions (OAE) test should be done to detect hearing impairment for all neonates with risk factors for hearing loss.

Management: Early detection and prompt treatment of ear diseases by medical and surgical interventions are important, aspect of management. Treatment of infections by antibiotic therapy removal of cerumen or toxic agent and management the specific cause should be done effectively. Surgical interventions may be required especially in conductive problems as myringotomy, tympanoplasty, tympanostomy tube insertion, stapedectomy and insertion of graft or prosthesis, adenotonsilectomy, cochlear implant, etc. Supportive and rehabilitative management are provided with hearing aids, speech therapy, lip reading, sign language, deaf education, etc. Cochlear implants are indicated in profound sensorineural deafness, which is unresponsive to 3–6 month's trial with powerful hearing aids.

COMMUNITY HEALTH NURSING

2019
Community Health Nursing

SECTION-I

I. **Give the meaning of the following:**
   a. Health records.
   b. Community health nursing.
   c. Geriatric nursing.
   d. Rehabilitation nursing.

II. **State whether the following is *true* or *false*:**
   a. Inhalation of silica dust causes silicosis.
   b. Corporation in urban areas have a population of above 2 lakhs.
   c. The road to health card is important tool for monitoring growth of under five children.
   d. 11th five-year plan was started in the year of 2005.

III. **Write short notes on any *three* of the following:**
   a. Government health insurance scheme.
   b. Recommendations of Mudaliar committee.
   c. Indigenous system of medicine.
   d. Environmental sanitation.
   e. Central health administration.

IV. **Answer the following:**
   a. What is occupational nursing?
   b. List down the occupational diseases.
   c. Explain the role of community health nurse in industrial health nursing.

V. a. Define primary health care.
   b. List down the elements of primary health care.
   c. Explain the role of community health nurse.

SECTION-II

VI. **Fill in the blanks:**
   a. Scientific study of human population is: _____
   b. One tribal sub centre covers a population of: _____
   c. Mid-day meal programme was established in the year of: _____
   d. United nations international childrens emergency fund (UNICEF) headquarters is in: _____

VII. Choose the correct answer from the following:
   a. Oral pills contains small amount of: _____
      i. Estrogens and progesterones   ii. Norplant   iii. Oxytoxin   iv. Progesterone
   b. The registration of deaths are done within: _____
      i. 7 days   ii. 14 days   iii. 21 days   iv. 28 days
   c. MTP Act came into force in: _____
      i. 1971   ii. 1975   iii. 1980   iv. 1970

VIII. Write the short notes on any *three* of the following:
   a. National Urban Health Mission (NUHM).
   b. Village health guides.
   c. National health agencies.
   d. Intrauterine contraceptive devices.

IX. Answer the following:
   a. Define vital statistics.
   b. Explain the sources and uses of vital statistics.

X. a. What is expanded programmes of immunization?
   b. Explain the role of community health nurse in pulse polio programme.

SECTION-I

I. Give the meaning of the following:

a. Health records.

A health record is a confidential compilation of pertinent facts of an individual's health history, including all past and present medical conditions, illnesses and treatments, with emphasis on the specific events affecting the patient during the current episode of care. The information documented in the health record is created by all healthcare professionals providing care and is used for continuity of care.

b. Community health nursing.

Community health nursing is the synthesis of nursing and public health practice applied to promote and protect the health of population. It combines all the basic elements of professional, clinical nursing with public health and community practice.

c. Geriatric nursing. (2016-I-b)

d. Rehabilitation nursing.

Rehabilitation nursing defined as diagnosis and treatment of human responses of individuals and groups to actual or potential health problems with the characteristics of altered functional ability and altered life-style

II. State whether the following are *true* or *false*:

a. Inhalation of silica dust causes silicosis: **TRUE**
b. Corporation in urban areas have a population of above 2 lakhs: **FALSE**
c. The road to health card is important tool for monitoring growth of under five children: **TRUE**
d. 11th five-year plan was started in the year of 2005: **TURE**

III. Write short notes on any *three* of the following:

a. Government health insurance scheme.

National Health Insurance Schemes are the health insurance programs initiated by the National government. To make health insurance accessible to the poor and destitute, our government has launched some health insurance schemes such as Rashtriya Swasthya Bima Yojana, Central Government Health Scheme, Employment State Insurance Scheme, Universal Health Insurance Scheme, Aam Aadmi Bima Yojana, and Janashree Bima Yojana among others.

Let's check out the benefits offered by these schemes in detail:
1. **Rashtriya Swasthya Bima Yojana (RSBY):** Ministry of Labour and Employment, Government of India launched this National Health Insurance Scheme for families who are below the poverty line. The aim is to offer health insurance coverage to BPL families in an economical manner. Under RSBY, the government has fixed the hospitalization cover limit at ₹ 30,000. The government has also fixed the hospital package rates.

    Pre-existing illnesses are also covered without any age limit criterion. 5 family members including self, three dependents, and spouse can be covered. The registration fee for the recipients is only thirty rupees and the premium is paid by the government to the insurance company.

2. **Employment State Insurance Scheme:**
   a. Employees' State Insurance Scheme (ESIS) is a Government's scheme and is customized insurance that provides socio-economic security to workers and their dependents.
   b. Apart from full medical cover for self and dependents, the beneficiaries can also avail cash benefits if there is any health emergency, permanent and temporary disabilities, death due to occupation hazard, employment injury, etc.
   c. Employment State insurance Scheme is valid for non-seasonal factory employees. But the factory should have more than 10 employees.
   d. The Scheme is also applicable to hotels, shops, cinemas, restaurants, newspaper establishments and road-motor transport enterprises employing more than 20 people.
   e. Employment State Insurance Scheme is implemented area-wise in all the States apart from Sikkim, Manipur, Mizoram, Arunachal Pradesh, and Union Territories.
3. **Central Government Health Scheme:** CGHS or the Central Government Health Scheme offers all-inclusive health care services to the Central government employees. It includes the pensioners as well as their dependents who are living in specific cities. It was started in 1954 by the Central Government. The healthcare services are offered through Wellness Centres (CGHS Dispensaries/ Allopathic, Yoga/Ayurveda, Siddha, Unani, and Homeopathic Centres). The Major Components of this Scheme are:
   a. Dispensary services
   b. Domiciliary care
   c. Consultation with a specialist at hospital, polyclinic and dispensary
   d. Medical tests including ECG, X-Ray and laboratory tests
   e. Hospitalization cover
   f. Medicines requirements
   g. Health education.
4. **Aam Admi Bima Yojana:** Aam Admi Bima Yojana or AABY scheme was commenced on October 02, 2007 for rural, landless households. The National Health Insurance Scheme covers the earning member of a household between the age group of 10 and 59 years. Compensation provided is as follows:
   a. Compensation of ₹ 30,000 in case of natural death
   b. Compensation of ₹ 75,000 in case of accidental death, partial or permanent disabilities (loss of 2 limbs or 2 eyes)
   c. Compensation of ₹ 37,500 in case of partial permanent disabilities resulting from an accident (one limb or an eye)
5. **Universal Health Insurance Scheme:** UHIS scheme is being implemented by four public insurers to provide health insurance coverage to poor families. In this scheme, the sum assured limit is up to ₹ 30,000 on family floater basis for hospitalization expenses. Accidental death cover offered to the policyholder is 25,000 rupees. Compensation of ₹ 50 is provided on a daily basis, if there is a loss of income.
   In the case of an individual the premium subsidy is now increased to ₹ 200 from ₹100, for 5 members, it has been increased to ₹ 300 and for seven members, it has been increased to ₹ 400 with the same benefits.
6. **Janashree Bima Yojana:** Janashree Bima Yojana or JBY scheme was launched by the Government of India in August 2000. People between the age group of 18 and 59 years (members of the specific 45 professional groups) can get covered under JBY scheme.

7. **Ayushman Bharat-National Health Protection Mission:** Ayushman Bharat, a National Health Protection Scheme, will offer cover to more than 10 Crore vulnerable and poor families offering coverage up to Rs. 5 Lakh per family every year for tertiary and secondary care hospitalization. This scheme aims at subsuming the schemes that are in progress and are sponsored by the Central Government such as Senior Citizen Health Insurance Scheme (SCHIS) along with Rashtriya Swasthya Bima Yojana (RSYB).

b. Recommendations of Mudaliar committee. (2014-III-e)
c. Indigenous system of medicine. (2014-III-c)
d. Environmental sanitation.

Environmental sanitation encompasses the control of environmental factors that are connected to disease transmission. Subsets of this category are solid waste management, water and wastewater treatment, industrial waste treatment and noise and pollution control. Sanitation generally refers to the provision of facilities and services for the safe disposal of human urine and feces. The word 'sanitation' also refers to the maintenance of hygienic conditions, through services such as garbage collection and wastewater disposal.

These are environmental factors which impact on the infectious agents and transmission of disease. These include:
1. Disposal of human excreta
2. Sewage
3. Household waste and other waste likely to contain infectious agents
4. Water drainage
5. Domestic water supply
6. Housing

Sanitation practices: These are various hygienic practices of the communities, basic knowledge, skills and human behaviors as well as social and cultural factors concerning health, life-styles and environmental awareness. These include:
1. Personal hygiene (washing, dressing, eating, etc)
2. Household cleanliness (kitchen, bathroom cleanliness, etc)
3. Community cleanliness (waste collection, common places, etc)

Environmental sanitation strongly depends on social and cultural practices and beliefs and these have to be considered when planning interventions.

To allow for transmission of infectious agents they have to be present in the immediate human environment, exposure has to take place, and transmission has to occur by uptake of the agents through unsafe practices. To interrupt the transmission, environmental sanitation can act on reducing exposure to infectious agents by limiting contact to wastes or polluted media, and by changing hygiene and socio-cultural practices.

e. Central health administration. (2011-I-a)

IV. **Answer the following:**
a. **What is occupational nursing?**

Occupational health nursing is a specialty nursing practice that provides for and delivers health and safety programs and services to workers, worker populations, and community groups.

b. List down the occupational diseases. (2015-IV-b)
c. Explain the role of community health nurse in industrial health nursing. (2015-IV-c)

V. a. Define primary health care. (2015-V-a)
b. List down the elements of primary health care. (2015-V-b)
c. Explain the role of community health nurse. (2015-V-c)

SECTION-II

VI. Fill in the blanks:
   a. Scientific study of human population is: **Demography**
   b. One tribal sub centre covers a population of: **5,000**
   c. Mid-day meal programme was established in the year of: **1995**
   d. United nations international children's emergency fund (UNICEF) headquarters is in: **Geneva**.

VII. Choose the correct answer from the following:
a. Oral pills contains small amount of:
   i. Estrogens and progesterones   ii. Norplant   iii. Oxytoxin   iv. Progesterone
   Ans: i. Estrogens and progestrones
b. The registration of deaths are done within:
   i. 7 days   ii. 14 days   iii. 21 days   iv. 28 days
   Ans: iii. 21 days
c. MTP act came into force in:
   i. 1971   ii. 1975   iii. 1980   iv. 1970
   Ans: i. 1971

VIII. Write the short notes on any three of the following:
a. **National Urban Health Mission (NUHM):**

The National Urban Health Mission (NUHM) as a sub-mission of National Health Mission (NHM) has been approved by the Cabinet on 1st May 2013. NUHM envisages to meet health care needs of the urban population with the focus on urban poor, by making available to them essential primary health care services and reducing their out of pocket expenses for treatment. This will be achieved by strengthening the existing health care service delivery system, targeting the people living in slums and converging with various schemes relating to wider determinants of health like drinking water, sanitation, school education, etc. implemented by the Ministries of Urban Development, Housing and Urban Poverty Alleviation, Human Resource Development and Women and Child Development.

NUHM Goals

1. Need based city specific urban health care system to meet the diverse health care needs of the urban poor and other vulnerable sections.

2. Institutional mechanism and management systems to meet the health-related challenges of a rapidly growing urban population.
3. Partnership with community and local bodies for a more proactive involvement in planning, implementation, and monitoring of health activities.
4. Availability of resources for providing essential primary health care to urban poor.
5. Partnerships with NGOs, for profit and not for profit health service providers and other stakeholders.

b. Village health guides. (2014-III-a)
c. National health agencies.

In the developing nation's non-governmental organizations have played an important role in promoting health. Often governments in developing countries are constrained from specific activities by political and economic limitations. Non-governmental agencies, because they are not subject to these constraints, often play a key role in disease intervention and promotion of health.

National Agencies

Working in the field of MCH: Family Planning Association of India, Indian Council of Child Welfare and Kasturba Memorial Fund.

Working for specific disease problem: Hind Kushta Nivaran Sangh, Indian Cancer Society etc. Working for general health care: Indian Red Cross Society, Central Social Welfare and all India Women's and Conference.

Professional bodies: INC, IMA, IDA, TNAI, etc.

International NGO/PVO: Multilateral Organizations: receive found from multiple governments and nongovernmental sources and support developmental effort of governments and organization in less-developed nations of the world. Examples are WHO, UNICEF, World Bank, UNFPA, ILO, UNDP, FAO.

Bilateral single government agency: That provides aid to lesser developed countries. They usually deal directly with other government, e.g. are USAID, DANIDA, Colombo plan, SIDA.

Non-governmental: They include humanitarian (philanthropic agencies) and professional organizations concerned with global health. These are not under government sponsorships or control, e.g. International Red Cross, Rockefeller foundation, ford foundation, CARE, etc.

d. Intrauterine contraceptive devices:

An intrauterine device (IUD), also known as intrauterine contraceptive device (IUCD or ICD) or coil is a small, often T-shaped birth control device that is inserted into a woman's uterus to prevent pregnancy. IUDs are one form of long-acting reversible birth control (LARC).

There are two types of IUDs:
1. Copper IUD—contains copper, a type of metal
2. Hormonal IUD—contains the hormone progestogen (Mirena or Jaydess).

Advantages:
1. Long acting—it lasts for up to 10 years
2. Reversible—you can choose to have it taken out at any time. After that, you will be able to get pregnant again
3. 99% effective—it works very well

4. Does not affect breastfeeding
4. Does not get in the way of sex
5. The copper IUD does not contain any hormones
6. The copper IUD can also be used as emergency contraception
7. The hormonal IUD has a very small amount of hormones and most people have no side effects from this
8. The Mirena (a hormonal IUD) can help with period bleeding and pain, and most will have light bleeding or no periods at all.

Studies show that IUDs do not cause pimples, headaches, sore breasts, nausea, mood changes, loss of sex drive or weight gain. There is no evidence of an extra risk of cancer.

Disadvantages: Some people feel pain, cramps or dizziness when the IUD is put in or taken out.

Risks from having an IUD put in:
1. There is a small risk of infection (about 1%) when an IUD is put in
2. There is a very small risk of damage to the uterus (about 1 in 1,000 people)
3. A copper IUD might give you more bleeding and cramping during your period, but this usually gets better over time
4. The copper IUD can cause an allergic reaction, but this is very rare
5. The hormonal IUD might give you irregular or light bleeding
6. The IUD can sometimes come out by itself (about 5% of all IUDs). You can check the strings are still in the right place at any time.

IX. Answer the following:
a. Define vital statistics. (2010-IX-a)
b. Explain the sources and uses of vital statistics. (2010-IX-b)

X. a. What is expanded programmes of immunization. (2015-X-a)
b. Explain the role of community health nurse in pulse polio programme. (2015-X-b)

2018
Community Health Nursing

SECTION-I

I. Give the meaning of the following:
   a. Voluntary health agency.
   b. Immunization.
   c. Village health guide.
   d. Population explosion.

II. State wthether the following statements are *true* or *false*:
   a. 12th five-year plan was started in the year 1990.
   b. Farmer's lung is caused by inhalation of grain dust.
   c. School health services are started 1st at Baroda city.
   d. Subcenters covers 10,000 population.

III. Write short notes on any *three* of the following:
   a. Functions of primary health care.
   b. Components of school health services.
   c. Janani Suraksha Yojana.
   d. ESIA scheme and its benefits.

IV. a. Write the organization of directorate general of health services.
   b. Explain the functions of directorate general of health services.

V. a. List the various national health problems in India.
   b. Explain the role of nurse in prevention of nutritional problems.

SECTION-II

VI. Fill in the blanks:
   a. Vitamin A prophylaxis is given to children to prevent _____
   b. Permanent family planning method for men is _____
   c. Pulse polio programme was started in the year _____
   d. Headquarters of WHO is situated at _____

VII. Choose the correct answer from the following:
   a. The drug given for treatment of tuberculosis is:
      i. Rifampicin   ii. Chloroquinine   iii. Calcium
   b. For the better absorption iron and folic acid tablets should be taken with:
      i. Milk   ii. Citrous fruits   iii Calcium
   c. In India CARE began its operation in:
      i. 1960   ii. 1950   iii. 1970

VIII. Write short notes on any *three* of the following:
   a. Integrated child development services.
   b. Indian red cross society.
   c. Functions of heath worker female.
   d. Intrauterine devices.
IX. a. Define vital health statistics.
   b. List the sources of vital health statistics.
   c. Explain the uses of vital health statistics.
X. a. Mention the different national health programmes.
   b. Explain the iodine deficiency disease control programme.

Community Health Nursing: 2018

SECTION-I

I. **Give the meaning of the following:**
   a. **Voluntary health agency:** Voluntary health agency is a non-profit, non-governmental agency, governed by lay or professional individuals and organized on a national, state, or local level, whose primary purpose is health related.
   b. **Immunization:** Immunization is the process whereby a person is made immune or resistant to an infectious disease, typically by the administration of a vaccine. Vaccines stimulate the body's own immune system to protect the person against subsequent infection or disease.
   c. **Village health guide:** Village Health Guides Scheme was designed to provide simple promotive, preventive, and curative services to the rural population.
   d. **Population explosion:** Population explosion refers to great and sudden increase in the number of people through natural means within a short period of time.

II. **State wthether the following statements are *true* or *false*:**
   a. 12th five year plan was started in the year 1990: **FALSE**
   b. Farmer's lung is caused by inhalation of grain dust: **TRUE**
   c. School health services are started 1st at Baroda city: **TRUE**
   d. Sub-centers cover 10,000 populations: **FALSE**

III. **Write short notes on any three of the following:**

a. Functions of primary health care. (2013-IV-b)

b. Components of school health services. (2013-V-b)

c. Janani Suraksha Yojana.

1. Janani Suraksha Yojana (JSY) is a safe motherhood intervention under the National Health Mission.
2. It is being implemented with the objective of reducing maternal and neonatal mortality by promoting institutional delivery among poor pregnant women.
3. The scheme, launched on 12 April 2005 by the Hon'ble Prime Minister, is under implementation in all states and Union Territories (UTs), with a special focus on Low Performing States (LPS).
4. JSY is a centrally sponsored scheme, which integrates cash assistance with delivery and post-delivery care.
5. The Yojana has identified Accredited Social Health Activist (ASHA) as an effective link between the government and pregnant women.

Important features: The scheme focuses on poor pregnant woman with a special dispensation for states that have low institutional delivery rates, namely, the states of Uttar Pradesh, Uttarakhand, Bihar, Jharkhand, Madhya Pradesh, Chhattisgarh, Assam, Rajasthan, Odisha, and Jammu and Kashmir. While these states have been named Low Performing States (LPS), the remaining states have been named High Performing States (HPS).

d. ESI scheme and its benefits.

The Employee State Insurance Corporation Scheme provides members financial protection in case of an untimely health-related eventuality. The scheme offers medical benefits, disability benefits, maternity benefits, unemployment allowance, etc.

Benefits:
1. **Medical benefits:** The Employee State Insurance Corporation takes care of an individual's medical expenses by providing reasonable medical care. This cover comes into effect from day one of the individual's employment.
2. **Disability benefit:** In case an employee is disabled, ESIC ensures that the employee is paid their monthly wages for the period of the injury in case of a temporary disablement or for the remainder of the employee's life in case of a permanent disablement.
3. **Maternity benefit:** ESIC helps an employee welcome their baby to a household which has been showered with benefits. ESIC provides a total of 100% of the average daily wages for a period of 26 weeks from the time of going into labor and 6 weeks in case of a miscarriage. 12 weeks of pay is provided in the case of an adoption.
4. **Sickness benefit:** ESIC ensures that there is a flow of cash coming into the employee's household during medical leave. 70% of the average daily wages of an employee is paid during medical leave for a maximum period of 91 days in two successive benefit periods.
5. **Unemployment allowance:** ESI provides a monthly cash allowance for a maximum period of 24 months in case of permanent invalidity due to a non-employment injury or due to involuntary loss of employment.
6. **Dependent's benefit:** In case the employee meets with an untimely death due to an injury at the place of employment, ESIC will provide monthly payments apportioned among the surviving dependents.

Other benefits that are offered with ESI are:
1. Confinement expenses
2. Funeral expenses
3. Physical rehabilitation
4. Vocational training
5. Skill upgradation training under Rajiv Gandhi Shramik Kalyan Yojana (RGSKY).

IV. a. Write the organization of directorate general of health Services.

The directorate general of health services (DGHS) is the principal advisor to the Union government in both medical and public matters. The DGHS is headed by Director General (DG) who renders technical advice on all medical and public health matters and is involved in the implementation and monitoring of various health scheme. The DG is assisted by a team of Additional Director General of health services (ADGHS), Deputy Director General (DDG), Assistant Deputy Director General (ADDG) and large number of other administrative staff in hierarchy.

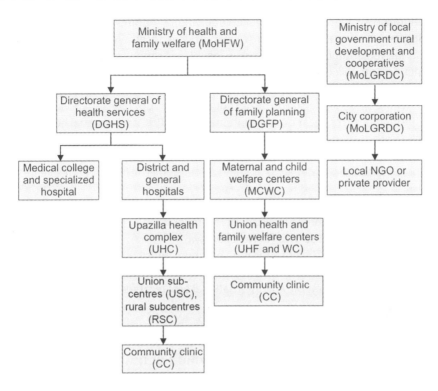

b. Explain the functions of directorate general of health services.

1. Providing educational support to all national health programmes including primary health care (PHC).
2. Providing consultative services and technical guidance to the Director General of Health Services in planning educational aspects of various health programs.
3. Planning, implementing and evaluating the health education aspects of various health programs.
4. Developing health education human resources by providing health education training to professional health educators as well as to personnel of other health and related departments and agencies.
5. Incorporating health education components in the training programmes of all categories of health personnel working in various national health programs.
6. Integrating health education components in the teaching programs of Medical and Nursing Colleges, Paramedical institutes, Teachers Training Colleges, Primary Training Institutes, Institutes of Mass Media and Journalism, etc.
7. Assisting in planning and implementation of the school health education program.
8. Planning and implementing the hospital and clinic health education program.
9. Designing and developing educational messages on different health issues.
10. Producing and disseminating different kinds of educational materials for various health programs.
11. Planning and developing mass health education programs through radio, television and newspaper.
12. Procuring and supplying health education materials and equipment.
13. Liaising and coordinating with development partners and NGOs in the promotion and implementation of health education activities.

14. Monitoring and evaluating national health education programs.
15. Providing technical guidance and advisory services to different health managers in the planning, implementation and evaluation of health education components of their programs.
16. Coordinating and collaborating with international agencies and organizations to promote health education programs.
17. Providing professional leadership in health education in support of all national health programs and promoting health education as an integral part of PHC and national health programs.
18. Conducting orientation in health education for program managers and health administrators, and arrange training courses for health personnel and faculty of teaching institutes.
19. Developing educational materials for training as well as for use in community health education programs.
20. Conducting field studies and research on sociocultural beliefs that affect health behaviors.
21. Planning the human, material and financial resources needed for the effective functioning of national health education services in the country.
22. Monitoring and evaluating health education programs and activities at division, district, upazila and union levels.
23. Coordinating and collaborating with international organizations promoting health education programs.

V. a. List the various national health problems in India. (2011-IX-a)
   b. Explain the role of nurse in prevention of nutritional problems.

Nurses are often the ones who spend the most time with the patient. Therefore, their understanding of nutrition is critical.

Proper nutrition plays a big role in disease prevention, recovery from illness and ongoing good health. A healthy diet will help you look and feel good as well. Since nurses are the main point of contact with patients, they must understand the importance of nutrition basics and be able to explain the facts about healthy food choices to their patients. Nutrition classes provide the information necessary to sort the fact from fiction about healthy eating and pass that knowledge on to their patients. Not only must nurses be able to explain the ins and outs of a healthy diet, they must also lead by example.

Education is also essential in preparing healthcare professionals to provide nutritional care appropriately. An understanding of the basic principles of nutritional science is the foundation for which healthcare professionals can help improve patient health outcomes.

SECTION-II

VI. Fill in the blanks:
a. Vitamin A prophylaxis is given to children to prevent _____
b. Permanent family planning method for men is _____
c. Pulse polio programme was started in the year _____
d. Headquarters of WHO is situated at _____

VII. Choose the correct answer from the following:
a. The drug given for treatment of tuberculosis is:
   i. Rifampicin   ii. Chloroquinine   iii. Calcium
   Ans: i. Rifampicin

b. For the better absorption iron and folic acid tablets should be taken with:
   i. Milk ii. Citrous fruits iii. Calcium
   Ans: ii. Citrus fruits
c. In India CARE began its operation in:
   i. 1960 ii. 1950 iii. 1970
   Ans: ii 1950

VIII. Write short notes on any three of the following:
a. Integrated child development services.

Integrated Child Development Services (ICDS) scheme is world's largest community based program. The scheme is targeted at children upto the age of 6 years, pregnant and lactating mothers and women 16–44 years of age. The scheme is aimed to improve the health, nutrition and education (KAP) of the target community. Launched on 2 October 1975, the scheme has completed 25 years of its operational age. The article describes in brief, the organization, achievements and drawbacks of this national program. It also suggests various thrust areas for its betterment and further improvement.

The main objectives of the scheme are:
1. Improvement in the health and nutritional status of children 0–6 years and pregnant and lactating mothers.
2. Reduction in the incidence of their mortality and school drop out.
3. Provision of a firm foundation for proper psychological, physical and social development of the child.
4. Enhancement of the maternal education and capacity to look after her own health and nutrition and that of her family.
5. Effective co-ordination of the policy and implementation among various departments and programs aimed to promote child development.

Beneficiaries

The beneficiaries are:
1. Children 0–6 years of age
2. Pregnant and lactating mothers
3. Women 15–44 year of age
4. Since 1991 adolescent girls upto the age of 18 years for non-formal education and training on health and nutrition.

Services: The program provides a package of services facilities like:
1. Complementary nutrition
2. Vitamin A
3. Iron and folic acid tablets
4. Immunization
5. Health check up
6. Treatment of minor ailments
7. Referral services
8. Non-formal education on health and nutrition to women
9. Preschool education to children 3–6 year old and
10. Convergence of other supportive services like water, sanitation, etc.

b. Indian red cross society.

During the First World War in 1914, India had no organization for relief services to the affected soldiers, except a branch of the St John Ambulance Association and by a Joint Committee of the British Red Cross. Later, a branch of the same Committee was started to undertake the much needed relief services in collaboration with the St John Ambulance Association in aid of the soldiers as well as civilian sufferers of the horrors of that Great War. A bill to constitute the Indian Red Cross Society, Independent of the British Red Cross, was introduced in the Indian Legislative Council on 3rd March 1920 by Sir Claude Hill, member of the Viceroy's Executive Council who was also Chairman of the Joint war Committee in India. The bill was passed on 17th March 1920 and became Act XV of 1920 with the assent of the Governor General on the 20th March 1920.

Seven Fundamental Principles of Red Cross

1. **Humanity:** The International Red Cross and Red Crescent Movement, born of a desire to bring assistance without discrimination to the wounded on the battlefield, endeavors, in its international and national capacity, to prevent and alleviate human suffering wherever it may be found. Its purpose is to protect life and health and to ensure respect for the human being. It promotes mutual understanding, friendship, cooperation and lasting peace amongst all peoples.
2. **Impartiality:** It makes no discrimination as to nationally, race, religious beliefs, class or political opinions. It endeavors to relieve the suffering of individuals, being solely by their needs, and to give priority to the most urgent cases of distress.
3. **Neutrality:** In orders to enjoy the confidence of all, the Movement may not take sides in hostilities or engage in controversies of a political, racial, religious or ideological nature.
4. **Independence:** The Movement is independent. The National Societies, while auxiliaries in the humanitarian services of their governments and subject to the laws of their respective countries, must always maintain their autonomy so that they may be able at all times to act in accordance with the principles of the Movement.
5. **Voluntary service:** It is voluntary relief movement not prompted in any manner by desire for gain.
6. **Unity:** There can be only one Red Cross Or Red Crescent in any one country. It must be open to all. It must carry on its humanitarian work throughout its territory.
7. **Universality:** The International Red Cross and Red Crescent Movement, in which all societies have equal status and share equal responsibilities and duties in helping each other, is worldwide.

c. Functions of health worker female.

A health worker (Female) is to cover a population of 3,000 in tribal areas and 5,000 in non-tribal areas. She will make a visit to each family once a fortnight according to fixed calendar of visit. She will carry out the following function:
1. She will register pregnant women three months of pregnancy onwards.
2. She will maintain a register enumerating all children 0-5 in her area by systematic house visits.
3. Categories the eligible couples according to the number of children and age of mothers.

Care at home:
1. She will provide care to pregnant women especially registered mothers throughout the pregnancy.

2. To give advice on nutrition to expectant and nursing mothers and responsible for storage, preparation and distribution of food to the expectant and nursing mothers under supplementary feeding.
3. Distribute iron and folic acid tablets to pregnant and nursing mothers, children and family planning adopters and vitamin 'A' solution to children at twice a year from 6 months to 60 months of age.
4. Immunise pregnant mothers with tetanus toxoid. Immunise infants with DPT, Polio and measles as per Schedule.
5. Refer cases of abnormal/high risk pregnancy and cases with medical and gynecological problems to Primary Health Centre/Hospital.
6. Conduct deliveries as per the norms prescribed in her areas.
7. Supervise deliveries conducted by Dais and guide them replenish the stock of basic drugs and dressings to Dais.
8. Refer cases of difficult Labor and newborn with abnormalities and help them to get institutional care and provide follow-up care to patient's referral to or discharged from hospital.
9. Provide at least three post-delivery visits for each delivery cases and render advice regarding feeding of the newborn.
10. Spread the message of family planning to the couples. Motivate them for family planning individuals and in groups.
11. Distribute conventional contraceptives to the couples, provide facilities and help to prospective adaptors in getting family planning services, if necessary, by accompanying or arranging Dias to accompany them to hospital.
12. Provide follow-up services to family planning adaptors, identify side effects give treatment on the spot for side effects and minor complaints and refer these cased that need attention by physicians to the Primary Health Center/Hospital.
13. Assess the growth and development of the infant and child by taking birth weight of the newborn and monthly weight of children up to 5 years of age and maintain these in the "Health Cards".
14. Do DPT and Polio and measles immunization to all the newborn infants in her area up to one year of age or till the Primary immunizations are completed and assist the Health Supervisors (Female) in the immunization program and in carrying out campaign approach activities. She will administer vitamin 'A' concentrate to all the children upto one year.
15. She will ensure effective sterilisation.
16. She will ensure the cold chain requirements for preservation of vaccine.
17. Provide treatment for minor ailments, provide first aid in case of emergencies and refer cases beyond her competency to Primary Health Centre or nearest hospital.
18. Notify notifiable diseases, which she comes across during her visits to Male Multipurpose Health Worker and the Medical Officer, Primary Health Center.
19. Record and report births and deaths occurring in her area to the local Births and Deaths Registrar and to the supervisors.
20. Test Urine for a albumen and sugar and Hemoglobin test during her home visits to the pregnant mothers.
21. Identify the case that require help for medical termination of pregnancy, provide information on the availability.

Care in clinic:
1. Arrange and help medical Officer and Health Supervisor (Female) in conducting MCH, and Family Planning Clinics at the Sub-Centers.
2. Educate mothers individually and in groups in better family health including MCH, and Family Planning Nutrition. Immunisation, Hygiene and Minor ailments.

Care in the community:
1. She will identify women leaders and help the Health Supervisor (Female) and participate in the training of Women.
2. Set up women Depot holders for Nirodh distribution and help the Health Supervisor (Female) in training them.
3. Participate in Women Welfare meetings and utilize such gatherings for educating the women family welfare programme.
4. Utilise satisfied customers, Village leaders, Dais and others for promoting Health, Nutrition, Family Welfare Programme.
5. She will attend to treatment to treatment of minor ailments and render immediate first aid as per the standing instructions issued form time to time.
6. She will arrange for Oral Rehydration in the case of diarrhea cases.

d. Intrauterine devices (IUD).

An intrauterine device (IUD), also known as intrauterine contraceptive device (IUCD or ICD) or coil is a small, often T-shaped birth control device that is inserted into a woman's uterus to prevent pregnancy. IUDs are one **form** of long-acting reversible birth control (LARC).

There are two types of IUDs:
1. Copper IUD: Contains copper, a type of metal
2. Hormonal IUD: Contains the hormone progestogen (Mirena or Jaydess)

Advantages
1. It protects against pregnancy for 5 or 10 years, depending on the type
2. Once an IUD is fitted, it works straight away.
3. Most women can use it.
4. There are no hormonal side effects, such as acne, headaches or breast tenderness.
5. It does not interrupt sex.
6. It is safe to use an IUD if you are breastfeeding.
7. It is possible to get pregnant as soon as the IUD is removed.
8. It is not affected by other medicines.

Disadvantages:
1. The periods may become heavier, longer or more painful, though this may improve after a few months.
2. It does not protect against STIs, so you may need to use condoms as well.
3. If you get an infection when you have an IUD fitted, it could lead to a pelvic infection if not treated.

4. Most women who stop using an IUD do so because of vaginal bleeding and pain, although these side effects are uncommon.

IX. a. Define vital health statistics.

Vital statistics, also known as vital events or vital records, are an important source of demographic data. They explain statistically such events as births, deaths, marriages, divorces, etc. According to NB Ryder, they "provide cumulative summaries for successive time periods of population movements like birth, death, migration, marriage and marital dissolution as well as demographic and other relevant characteristics of the individuals involved in these events."

b. List the sources of vital health statistics.

1. **Civil registration system:** It is defined as the continuous permanent and compulsory recording of the occurrence of vital events like live births, deaths, fetal deaths, marriages, divorces, as well as annulments, judicial separation, adoption.
2. **National sample survey:** The data collected from the census are not very reliable and available only once in 10 years. In absence of reliable data from the civil registration system (SRS), the need for reliable statistics at national and state levels is being met through sample surveys launched from time to time.
3. **Sample registration system:** In this system, there is continous enumeration of births and deaths in a sample of villages/urban blocks by a resident part-time enumerator and then an independent six monthly retrospective survey by a full time supervisor.

Health surveys: A few important sources for demographic data have emerged. These are National Family Health Surveys (NFHS) and the District Levels Household Surveys (DLHS) conducted for evaluation of reproductive and child health programmes. NFHS provide estimates of fertility, child mortality and a no. of fertility, child mortality and a no. of health parameters relating to infants and children at state level.

c. Explain the uses of vital health statistics.

Vital statistics are of much importance for the people and nation.
1. **For the individual:** Vital statistics are of much use for an individual. A birth certificate issued by the registering authority is an important document which records the date, time, place and parentage of the person. It establishes his identity as the citizen of the country.
2. **Legal use:** Vital statistics are legally very useful. Certificates relating to birth, death, marriage, divorce, etc. have legal importance. For instance, a death certificate is an important legal document for the settlement of property of the deceased person, the claim of his/her insurance policy, etc.
3. **Health and family planning programs:** Vital statistics relating to births and deaths can be used in health and family planning programs of the government. The causes of deaths, and the mortality rates of different categories help in assessing the health condition of the people.
4. **Study of social conditions:** Vital statistics like birth and death rates, divorce rate, widow remarriage, widowhood, etc. throw light on the social conditions of a society, as also its customs and traditions.
5. **For administrators and planners:** Data provided by vital statistics relating to trend and growth of population in the various age groups and on the whole, help planners and administrators to plan and formulate policies for public health, education, housing, transport and communications, food supplies, etc.

6. **For the Nation:** Vital statistics are of much importance for the nation. They help in analyzing the population trends at any given point of time. They try to fill the gap between two censuses. They relate to the composition, size, distribution and growth of population.

X. a. Mention the different national health programmes.

1. **National Vector Borne Disease Control Programme:** Launched in 2003-04 by merging National anti-malaria control programme, National Filaria Control Programme and Kala-azar Control programmes. Japanese B Encephalitis and Dengue/DHF have also been included in this Program Directorate of NAMP is the nodal agency for prevention and control of major Vector Borne Diseases List of Vector Borne Diseases Control Programme Legislations:
   a. National Anti-malaria Programme
   b. Kala-azar Control Programme
   c. National Filaria Control Programme
   d. Japenese Encephilitis Control Programme
   e. Dengue and Dengue Hemorrhagic fever.
2. **Revised National Tuberculosis Control Programme:** The National TB Control Programme was started in 1962 with the aim to detect cases earliest and treat them. In the district, the programme is implemented through the District Tuberculosis Centre (DTC) and the Primary Health Institutions. The District Tuberculosis Programme (DTP) is supported by the state level organization for the coordination and supervision of the programme. The Revised National Tuberculosis Control Programme (RNTCP), based on the Directly Observed Treatment, Short Course (DOTS) strategy, began as a pilot project in 1993 and was launched as a national programme in 1997 but rapid RNTCP expansion began in late 1998. The nation-wide coverage was achieved in 2006.
3. **National Leprosy Eradication Programme:** The National Leprosy Eradication Programme is a centrally sponsored Health Scheme of the Ministry of Health and Family Welfare, Govt. of India. The Programme is headed by the Deputy Director of Health Services (Leprosy) under the administrative control of the Directorate General Health Services, Govt. of India. While the NLEP strategies and plans are formulated centrally, the programme is implemented by the States/UTs. The Programmes also supported as Partners by the World Health Organization, The International Federation of Anti-leprosy Associations (ILEP) and few other Non-Govt. Organizations.
4. **National AIDS control programme:** The National AIDS Control Programme (NACP), launched in 1992, is being implemented as a comprehensive programme for prevention and control of HIV/ AIDS in India. Over time, the focus has shifted from raising awareness to behavior change, from a national response to a more decentralized response and to increasing involvement of NGOs and networks of People living with HIV (PLHIV).
5. **Janani Suraksha Yojana:** Janani Suraksha Yojana (JSY) is a safe motherhood intervention under the National Rural Health Mission (NHM). It is being implemented with the objective of reducing maternal and infant mortality by promoting institutional delivery among pregnant women. The scheme is under implementation in all states and Union Territories (UTs), with a special focus on Low Performing States (LPS).
6. **Janani Shishu Suraksha Karyakaram:** Government of India has launched the Janani Shishu Suraksha Karyakaram (JSSK) on 1st June, 2011. The scheme is to benefit pregnant women who access Government health facilities for their delivery. Moreover it will motivate those who still

choose to deliver at their homes to opt for institutional deliveries. All the States and UTs have initiated implementation of the scheme.
7. **Mission Indradhanush:** Mission Indradhanush was launched by the Ministry of Health and Family Welfare, Government of India on December 25, 2014. Between 2009-2013 immunization coverage has increased from 61% to 65%, indicating only 1% increase in coverage every year. To accelerate the process of immunization by covering 5% and more children every year, Indradhanush mission has been adopted to achieve target of full coverage by 2020.
8. **Pradhan Mantri Swasthya Suraksha Yojana (PMSSY):** It aims at correcting the imbalances in the availability of affordable healthcare facilities in the different parts of the country in general, and augmenting facilities for quality medical education in the under-served States in particular. The scheme was approved in March 2006.
9. **National Ayush Mission (NAM):** Department of AYUSH, Ministry of Health and Family Welfare, Government of India has launched National AYUSH Mission (NAM) during 12th Plan for implementing through States/UTs. The basic objective of NAM is to promote AYUSH medical systems through cost effective AYUSH services, strengthening of educational systems, facilitate the enforcement of quality control of Ayurveda, Yoga and Naturopathy, Unani, Siddha and Homoeopathy (AYUSH).
10. **National Viral Hepatitis Surveillance Programme:** Viral hepatitis is an inflammation of the liver caused by one of the five hepatitis viruses, referred to as types A, B, C, D and E. The Government of India through the National Centre for Disease Control is implementing the National Viral Hepatitis Surveillance Programme.
11. **National Programme for the Health Care for the Elderly:** The National Programme for the Health Care for the Elderly (NPHCE) is an articulation of the International and national commitments of the Government as envisaged under the UN Convention on the Rights of Persons with Disabilities (UNCRPD), National Policy on Older Persons (NPOP) adopted by the Government of India in 1999 & Section 20 of "The Maintenance and Welfare of Parents and Senior Citizens Act, 2007" dealing with provisions for medical care of Senior Citizen.
12. **National tobacoo control programme:** The Government of India has enacted the national tobacco-control legislation namely, "The Cigarettes and other Tobacco Products (Prohibition of Advertisement and Regulation of Trade and Commerce, Production, Supply and Distribution) Act, 2003" in May, 2003. India also ratified the WHO-Framework Convention on Tobacco Control (WHO-FCTC) in February 2004.

b. Explain the iodine deficiency disease control programme.

Realizing the magnitude of the problem, the Government of India launched a 100 per cent centrally assisted National Goitre Control Programme (NGCP) in 1962. In August, 1992 the National Goitre Control Programme (NGCP) was renamed as National Iodine Deficiency Disorders Control Programme (NIDDCP) with a view of wide spectrum of Iodine Deficiency Disorders like mental and physical retardation, deaf mutisim, cretinism, stillbirths, abortions etc. The programme is being implemented in all the States/UTs for entire population.

Goal:
1. To bring the prevalence of IDD to below 5% in the country
2. To ensure 100% consumption of adequately iodated salt (15 ppm) at the household level.

Objectives:
1. Surveys to assess the magnitude of Iodine Deficiency Disorders in the districts.
2. Supply of iodated salt in place of common salt.
3. Resurveys to assess iodine deficiency disorders and the impact of iodated salt after every 5 years in the districts.
4. Laboratory monitoring of iodated salt and urinary iodine excretion.
5. Health education and publicity.

Policy: On the recommendations of Central Council of Health in 1984, the Government took a policy decision to Iodate the entire edible salt in the country by 1992. The programme started in April, 1986 in a phased manner. To date, the annual production of iodated salt in our country is 65 lakh metric tones per annum.

2017
Community Health Nursing

SECTION-I

I. Give the meaning of the following:
   a. Records.
   b. DPT vaccine.
   c. Community health nursing.
   d. Primary health care.

II. State whether the following statements are *true* or *false*:
   a. Sex ratio is defined as the number of females per 1000 males.
   b. Government of India launched a national AIDS control programme in 1990.
   c. The recent census in India was conducted in the year 2010.
   d. Objective of the MCH is only to take care of children.

III. Write short notes on any three of the following:
   a. Panchayat raj.
   b. Shrivastav committee.
   c. Voluntary health agencies in India.
   d. Geriatric nursing.

IV. Answer the following:
   a. Classify the occupational hazard.
   b. Explain the role of nurse in industrial nursing.

V. a. Define health.
   b. Explain the delivery of health services at the central level.

SECTION-II

VI. Choose the correct answer from the following:
   a. BCG vaccine is given through _____ site.
      i. Intradermal   ii. Subcutaneous   iii. Intramuscular
   b. _____ is commonly used for taking weight of children under 1 year of age.
      i. Weighing scale   ii. Infant weighing scale   iii. Salter spring hanging scale
   c. World AIDS Day is celebrated on _____
      i. 23rd June   ii. 1st December   iii. 4th August

VII. Fill in the blanks:
   a. The theme of world health day in 2017 was _____
   b. A female health worker is expected to cover a population of _____
   c. National TB control programme was launched in the year _____
   d. _____ is celebrated on May 12th.

VIII. Write short notes on any *three* of the following:
  a. Temporary family planning methods.
  b. Sources of vital statistics.
  c. National malaria eradication programme.
  d. Small family norm.

IX. a. Define demography.
  b. List the sources of demography.
  c. Explain the demographic cycle.

X. a. Define health team.
  b. List the members of health team.
  c. Explain the roles of health assistant male and female in community.

Community Health Nursing: 2017

SECTION-I

I. **Give the meaning of the following:**
   a. **Records:** Records are facts and figures, arranged in a logical order, that a new worker may be able to maintain continuity if service to individual's families and communities.
   b. **DPT Vaccine:** DPT is a class of combination vaccines against three infectious diseases in humans—diphtheria, pertussis (whooping cough), and tetanus. The vaccine components include diphtheria and tetanus toxoids and killed whole cells of the bacterium that causes pertussis.
   c. **Community Health Nursing:** Community health nursing is concerned with the people who are sick as well as the healthy, young and old, male and female. Community health and community health nursing draw knowledge and practices from other disciplines such as medicine, surgery, pediatrics, obstetrics, gynecology, dentistry, health education and vital statistics.
   d. **Primary Health Care:** It is a essential health care based on practical, scientifically sound and socially accepted methods and technology, made universally acceptable to individuals and families in the community involving their full participation and at a cost that the community and country can afford to maintain at every stage of their development

II. **State whether the following statements are *true* or *false*:**
   a. Sex ratio is defined as the number of females per 1000 males: **FALSE**
   b. Government of India launched a national AIDS control programme in 1990: **FALSE**
   c. The recent census in India was conducted in the year 2010: **FALSE**
   d. Objective of the MCH is only to take care of children: **FALSE**

III. **Write short notes on any *three* of the following:**

a. **Panchayat raj.**

Parallel to this official structure of administration, there are institutions of local self government in rural areas. This refers to Panchayat raj system. This system is introduced since 1957 strengthen the administration at the gross root level.

Panchayat raj is a 3 tire structure of the rural local self government. It is a complex system, which represents the local inhabitants, possessing a range or degree of autonomy. The Panchayati Raj institutions are accepted as agencies public welfare. All development programmes are channeled through these bodies.

Panchayat raj institutions strengthen democracy at its root and ensure more effective and better participation of the people in the government. It is a three tire structure.

Panchayati raj at village level:
1. **The primary unit** or local government is the 'village' and the primary institution of local government is the 'village panchayat'. Panchayats has been in existence in India from Vedic age. They continued to exist till 1800 AD, when they were ruined and remained so until revived in 1948.
2. **Villages** throughout the country are to be served by the panchayats for panchayats have a defined role in planning and implementing the programmes in village.
3. **Grama sabha:** It is the assembly of all adult men and women of the village. The body meets at least twice in a year and discusses important issues and considers proposals for taxation; discuss the annual programme and elects members of gram panchayat.

4. **Gram panchayat:** It is executive organ of the Gram Sabha and an agency for planning and development at the village level. It consists of 15-30 elected members; it covers a population of 2000 to 5000. Every panchayat has an elected president (Sarpanch/Mukhiya/Sabhapati), a vice president and Panchayat secretary. The Panchayat secretary has been given powers to function for wide areas, such as maintenance of sanitation and public health, socioeconomic development of the villages, etc.
5. **Nyaya panchayt:** It is composed of 5 members from the panchayat. It tries to solve the dispute between the panchayat. It tries to solve the dispute between the two parties/individuals over certain matters on mutual consent.

b. Shrivastav committee.

The committee recommendations are:
1. Step should be taken to create bands of paraprofessional or semiprofessional health workers from the community itself to provide simple, protective preventive and curative services which are needed by the community.
2. Health workers should be trained and equipped to give simple specified remedies for day-to-day illness.
3. The primary health center should provide with an additional doctor and a nurse to look after the maternal and child health services.
4. Development of a "Referral services complex" by establishing proper linkage between PHC and higher level referral services.
5. Establishment of medical and health education commission for planning and implementing the referrals needed in health and medical education on the lines of the university grants commission.

c. Voluntary health agencies in India.

Voluntary health agencies: They have long history of involvement in the promotion of human welfare and well being. These agencies are helping to create condtions to the promotion and maintenance of health and prevention illness.

Types:
1. Indian Red Cross
2. Hind Kusht Nivaran Sangh
3. Indian Council of Child Welfare
4. Bharat Sevak Samaj
5. Central Social Welfare board
6. The Kasturba Memorial Fund
7. The All India Women's Conference
8. The All India Blind Relief societies

Functions of voluntary Health Agencies:
1. Creating a sense of responsibility through direct involvement.
2. Channelise human resources.
3. Effective policy formation through interpretation of public opinion.
4. Participation of beneficiaries.
5. Flexibility and experimentation.
6. Initiative and leadership.
7. Supplements the efforts of Government.

8. Help in efficient programme implementation.
9. Advancing health legislation.

d. Geriatric nursing.

Geriatric nurses are often employed at healthcare facilities such as hospitals and clinics. They also work in residential care facilities, like nursing homes and retirement communities. Some geriatric nurses also work in home healthcare, traveling to patients' homes to care for them there. As a geriatric nurse, you will be required to perform a number of duties
1. Measuring and recording vital signs;
2. Administering medications;
3. Exercising and massaging patients;
4. Watching for signs of elder abuse;
5. Transporting patients to doctor's visits and other appointments; and
6. Helping patients with their daily needs, such as bathing, dressing, and using the bathroom.

IV. Answer the following:

a. Classify the occupational hazard.

A **hazard** is anything with the potential to cause harm. **Risk** is the probability of a negative outcome from exposure to a hazard. A substance is defined as **hazardous** if it has one or more of the following characteristics: flammable, corrosive, toxic, or reactive. Also, substances are defined as **hazardous** if they are specifically listed by regulation. For example, OSHA, EPA, and DOT publish lists of materials deemed hazardous. In our discipline of occupational health and safety, the six primary **hazard categories** are:
1. Physical hazards
2. Chemical hazards
3. Biological hazards
4. Radiological hazards
5. Ergonomic hazards
6. Behavioral hazards

Category 1: Urgent public health hazard—conditions that pose a serious risk to the public's health as the result of short-term exposures to hazardous substances.

Category 2: Public health hazard—conditions that pose a public health hazard as the result of long-term exposures to hazardous substances.

Category 3: Indeterminate public health hazard—conditions for which no conclusions about public health hazard can be made because data are lacking.

Category 4: No apparent public health hazard—conditions where human exposure to contaminated media is occurring or has occurred in the past, but the exposure is below a level of health hazard.

Category 5: No Public health hazard—conditions for which data indicate no current or past exposure or no potential for exposure, and therefore no health hazard.

b. Explain the role of nurse in industrial nursing.

Industrial nursing requires specialized knowledge and skill which means they need proper additional training. Occupational health is the additional training. Occupational health is the entirely preventive medicine. The chief objective of occupational health is the safety of workers in all occupations from injuries and diseases and to improve their health status.

Components of occupational health nursing:
1. To carry out significant, positive health programs
2. To provide therapeutic service for the workers.
3. To establish meaningful interpersonal relationship between herself and the workers to indetify problems and workout solutions together.
4. To ensure that her nursing activities are compatible with the management policy and the healthcare system.

Beneficiaries of occupational health nursing:
1. **Individual-labors/employee:** Occupational health nurse has to provide health care to skilled – unskilled, trained, untrained, new or old, all types of works. The occupational untrained nurse has her primary responsibility towards workers to promote, protect and preserve their health.
2. **Employee's group:** Occupational health nurse has responsibility towards her employees to protect the company from adverse effects of work process and hazardous substances on workers.
3. **Managerial personnel:** The community health nurse has to give feedback regarding the health of workers. This includes informing the health limits of worker related to work, giving information regarding health hazards and helping the management to identify the health problem of the workers.
4. **The company:** The company gets direct or indirect benefit from the occupational health nurse.

Functions of occupational health nurse:
1. Assistance in general administration, maintenance and arrangements of health facilities in the plant.
2. Emergency and primary treatment of accidents and illness based on standing orders from physicians.
3. Arranging follow up treatments, where indicated, including health supervision of employees returning to work after illness.
4. Assistance in general preventive health measures in the plant.
5. Health education and counselling for employees.
6. Assistance in supervision of factory hygiene and accident prevention.
7. Advice on specific health question to management and workers.
8. Maintenance of records and statistics.
9. Cooperation with and referral of workers to general community agencies for help as and when necessary.
10. Participation in a health surveillance programme that includes the assessment and recording of the health status of employees.
11. Participation in the environmental control programme the aims to work related.
12. Counseling and crisis intervention for those individuals experiencing work related problems and health promotion through specific health education and screening programs.

V. a. Define health.

WHO has defined health as a "State of complete physical, mental, social, spiritual well-being, and not merely absence of disease or infirmity." The concept of positive wholeness or completeness is emphasized and health is seen as more than a physical state. An individual's health is never static and is always in a dynamic equilibrium with his environment.

b. Explain the delivery of health services at the central level.

The organization at the national level consists of the Union Ministry of Health and Family Welfare. The Ministry has three departments, viz. Department of Health and Family Welfare, Department of Ayurveda, Yoga-Naturopathy, Unani, Sidha and Homeopathy (AYUSH) and Department of Health Research. Each of these departments is headed by respective secretaries to Govt of India. The department of Health and Family Welfare is supported by a technical wing, the Directorate General of Health Services, headed by Director General of Health Services (DGHS).

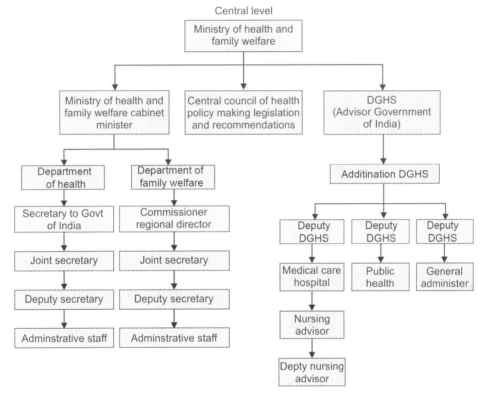

Functions of DGHS:
1. International health relations and quarantine
2. Control of drug standards
3. Medical store department
4. Postgraduate training
5. Medical education (4 colleges)
6. Medical research
7. Central government health scheme
8. National health education bureau
9. Health statistics
10. National medical library

SECTION-II

VI. Choose the correct answer from the following:
a. BCG vaccine is given through _____ site.
   i. Intradermal   ii. Subcutaneous   iii. Intramuscular
   Ans: i. Intradermal
b. _____ is commonly used for taking weight of children under 1 year of age.
   i. Weighing scale   ii. Infant weighing scale   iii. Salter spring hanging scale
   Ans: iii. Salter spring hanging scale
c. World AIDS Day is celebrated on _____
   i. 23rd June   ii. 1st December   iii. 4th August
   Ans: ii. 1st December

VII. Fill in the blanks:
a. The theme of world health day in 2017 was **Depression**.
b. A female health worker is expected to cover a population of **5000**.
c. National TB control programme was launched in the year **1997**.
d. **International Nurses Day** is celebrated on May 12th.

VIII. Write short notes on any three of the following:

a. Temporary family planning methods.
The temporary methods for family planning and contraception are enlisted as below:
1. Condoms
2. Oral pills
3. Emergency contraception
4. Injections
5. Implants
6. Intrauterine contraceptive device (IUCD).

b. Sources of vital statistics.
1. **Civil registration system:** It is defined as the continous permanent and compulsory recording of the occurrence of vital events like live births, deaths, fetal deaths, marriages, divorces, as well as annulments, judicial separation, adoption.
2. **National sample survey:** The data collected from the census are not very reliable and available only once in 10 years. In absence of reliable data from the civil registration system(SRS), the need for reliable statistics at national and state levels is being met through sample surveys launched from time to time.
3. **Sample registtration system:** In this system, there is continuous enumeration of births and deaths in a sample of villages/urban blocks by a resident part-time enumerator and then an independent six monthly retrospective survey by a full time supervisor.
   Health surveys: A few important sources for demographic data have emerged. These are National Family Health Surveys (NFHS) and the District Levels Household Surveys (DLHS) conducted for evaluation of reproductive and child health programs. NFHS provide estimates of fertility, child mortality and a no. of fertility, child mortality and a no. of health parameters relating to infants and children at state level.

c. National malaria eradication programme.

1. In the 1950's malaria was India's number one health problem. The national government launched National malaria control programme in 1953 to reduce the incidence of malaria in the country.
2. The initial success against malaria was spectacular. From 75 million cases in 1952, the incidence of malaria was brought down to 2 million in 1958.
3. In 1958 the National malaria control programme was converted into National Malaria Eradication programme.
4. The initial success against malaria by National Malaria control programme had been commendable and the incidence of malaria was brought down. Encouraged by these results and coupled with the fear that the insect (vector) might develop resistance to insecticides the programme was upgraded to National Malaria Eradication programme.
5. In 1968, the programme was reviewed; Kerala achieved complete eradication of this disease in 1965-66. In 1976 the incidence of malaria rose to 6.4 million cases with 59 deaths.
6. In view of this, Government of India reviewed and total situation with the help of expert committee and a revised strategy was recommended.

New Strategies:

1. Active surveillance for early detection of cases with fever and prompt treatment to them chloroquine.
2. To use anti-larval measures, spraying of insecticides other than DDT when DDT has shown resistance to mosquito vectors.
3. Provision of mobile teams with health inspectors and 2 spraying squads with necessary equipment. It was recommended that one mobile team for every 10 PHC's in hypoendemic areas and one for every 5 PHC's in hyperendemic areas.
4. The community health nurses have an important role in promoting this operations and participating in case findings treatment, health education and the promotion of adequate environmental sanitation in the urban and rural areas.

d. Small family norm.

The national target is to achieve a family size of 2.3 children by 2000 AD. All the efforts are being made through mass communication that the concept of "small family norms" is accepted adopted and woven into lifestyle of the people. The family size plays a very important role in the health and welfare of not only the individual, family and community but also of the nation as a whole because it affects the population growth rate.

Effects of family size:

1. **Basic human needs:** Food clothing, shelter, basic education and primary health are basic needs of human. If the family size is small, the perception share will be more.
2. **Economical needs:** Income, savings and resources may not be sufficient to meet if the family size is large. Low savings income and large family size will not help in further development.
3. **Food and nutrition:** The larger the family size will not be able to meet the nutritive requirements of the members of family.
4. **Socioeconomic:** Large family size result in migration of rural people to urban areas in search for employment resulting in urban slums and associated socioeconomic problems.
5. **Larger family size:** Has shown higher morbidity and mortality among mothers and children.
6. **Education:** It is hard for the large family to give proper education to their children.

Hazards of large family:
1. Increased maternal mortality and morbidity.
2. Increased child mortality and morbidity.
3. Increased congenital problems due to late pregnancies.
4. Unemployment, illiteracy and poverty.
5. Increased psychosocial problems.
6. Increased disease and disabilities.

Factors involve small family:
1. Sociocultural background of the society.
2. Socioeconomic aspects of the family.
3. Health center and health workers involvement and participation.
4. Family health services or programmes effectiveness.
5. Education background of the individual and family members.
6. Effective contraceptive delivery services.
7. Health education and mass media participation.
8. Legal issues by governmental sectors by maintaining proper records and reports.
9. Statistical system of particular area.
10. Periodical evaluation and revision of policies and procedures.

Barriers of small family norms:
1. Religious issues.
2. Family beliefs.
3. Customs tradition and values in the family.
4. Illiteracy.

IX. a. Define demography.

Demography is the scientific study of human population such as changes in population size, the composition of the population and distribution of population in space. It also deals with five "demographic process" namely fertility, mortality, marriage, migration and social mobility.

b. List the sources of demography.

Census: The word census originated from the Latin word censere which means to assess or to rate. The first census of India was conducted in 1872, hence the census of 1881 is considered as the first systematic census of India. Census 2001 is the 14th census the 6th census, of independent India and the first of 21st century.

Vital registration: It is a process of recording vital events that occur in a population from time to time, the events registered related to births, deaths and marriage. Vital registration helps in planning, implementation and evaluation of community health services/programs.

Institutional records: The records are routinely maintained by various categories of hospitals and healthcare institutions, operating at various levels, have limited public health relevance.

c. Explain the demographic cycle.

The demographic cycle, or population cycle, refers to the evolution over time of the population profile of a country, region or other defined geographical area. A population cycle theory has been postulated in terms of the socioeconomic history of industrialized countries.

1. **High stationary stage:** This characteristic by crude birth rate and high crude death rate with a negligible demographic gap between two.
2. **Early expanding stage:** This characterized by a crude birth rate that continues to remain high and a crude death rate that starts declining.
3. **Late expanding stage:** This characterized by a crude birth rate that continues to fall and crude birth rate that starts declining.
4. **Low stationary stage:** This characterized by a low crude birth rate and a low crude death rate with a negligible demographic gap.
5. **Declining stage:** This characterized by a low crude birth rate and a low crude death rate with a negligible demographic gap.

X. a. Define health team.

Healthcare is a team effort. Each healthcare provider is like a member of the team with a special role. Some team members are doctors or technicians who help diagnose disease. Others are experts who treat disease or care for patients' physical and emotional needs.

b. List the members of health team.

1. Doctors
2. Physician assistants
3. Nurses
4. Pharmacists
5. Dentists
6. Technologists and technicians
7. Therapists and rehabilitation specialists
8. Emotional, social and spiritual support providers
9. Administrative and support staff
10. Community health workers and patient navigators.

c. Explain the roles of health assistant male and female in community.

Female

1. ***Supervision and Guidance***
   - Supervise and guide the Health Worker Female, Dias/MSS Depot Holders in delivery of healthcare services to the community.
   - Strengthen the knowledge and clinical skills of the Health Workers Female.
   - Help the Health Worker Female in improving her skills of working in the community.
   - Help and guide the Health Worker Female in planning and organizing her program of act conduct EC survey, assess community need and prepare subcenter plan.
   - When posted at PHCs she will help MOI/c, PHC in organizing MCH Clinics and any other act she will be responsible to supervise field work of ANM, help implementation of National Programmes.

- Visit each subcenter at least once in two week on a fixed day to observe and guide the Worker Female in her day-to-day activities. A tentative tour programme has to be approved Incharge PHC, after completion of journey; she will submit the tour dairy.
- Assess fortnightly the progress of work of the Health Workers Female and submit an assessment report to the Medical Officer of the Primary Health Center.
- Carry out supervisory home visits in the area of the Health Workers Female with respect to duties under various National Health Programmes.
- Attend monthly meetings of the Panchayats and help the Panchayat to review work of MPW and female.
- She will supervise antimalaria activities, water sampling and purification at SC level.

2. **Team Work**
    - Help the workers to work as part of the health team
    - Coordinate her activities with those of the Health Assistant male and other health per including Dias and other voluntary workers.
    - Coordinate the health activities in her area with the activities of workers of other departments, e.g. ICDS, ayurved education.PRIs,revenue department.
    - Conduct regular staff meetings with Health Workers in coordination with assistant male at SHC.
    - Attend staff meeting at the Primary Health Center.
    - Assist the Medical officer of the PHC in implementation of nation health programs.
    - Practice as a member of the health team in mass camps and campaigns in health programs.
    - Help Health Workers in identification of unreached area and plan outreach activities.
    - Help the MO in organizing the school health program.

3. **Supplies, Equipment and Maintenance of Subcenter**
    - In collaboration with the Health Assistant Male, check at regular intervals the stores available at the sub-center and help in the procurement of supplies and equipment.
    - Check that the drugs at the sub-center are properly stored and that the equipment is well maintained.
    - She will ensure that all the medicines and used before their expiry.
    - Ensure that the Health Workers Female maintains her general kit, midwifery kit and Dai kit in proper way.
    - Ensure that the subcenter is kept clean and its properly maintained.

4. **Records and Reports**
    - Scrutinize maintenance of records by Health Worker Female and guide her in their proper maintenance.
    - Maintain the prescribed records and prepare the necessary reports.
    - Review reports received from the Health Workers Female, consolidate them and submit monthly reports to the Medical Officer of the Primary Health Center.
    - Provide feedback to health Worker Female on performance of subcenter.
    - She will review registration of births and deaths done by the health workers.
    - She will review each maternal and infant death in her area.
    - She will conduct preliminary investigations of all cases and death due to VDP.

5. **Training**
    - Organize and conduct training for Dais with the assistance of the Health Worker Female.

- Assist the Medical Officer of the Primary Health Center in conducting training programs for various categories of health personnel and NGOs.
- She will support and guide the ANMS/MPW (Female) for the skills of IUD insertion to untrained ANMS/MPW female required in delivering RCH services.

6. **Reproductive and Child Health**
    - Conduct weekly or biweekly RCH clinic at each sub-center with assistant of the health worker (female) and Dais as per the visit schedule.
    - Respond to calls from the Health Worker Female/Male, Jan Mangal, NGOs, MSS, AWW and trained Dais and rendered the necessary help.
    - Conduct deliveries when required at PHC level and provide domiciliary midwifery services.
    - Initiate steps to promote institutional delivery.
    - Identify and refer risk cases to FRU after counseling.
    - Help in organizing transport services for high risk cases refer to FRU.
    - To educate about adolescent health, sex education and give knowledge of reproductive organs and hazards of pregnancy in early age group.
    - Preventive methods of early pregnancy, RTI and STI.
    - Supervise the work of ANM in context of ARI/Diarrhea.

7. **Family Planning and Medical Termination of Pregnancy**
    - She will ensure through spot checking that Health Worker Female maintain up-to-date eligible couples registers all the time.
    - Conduct fortnightly family planning clinics (along with the RCH Clinics) at each subcenter with the assistance of the Health Worker Female.
    - Personally motivate non-acceptors for family planning. She will help Health Worker Female in counseling couples with expressed unmet needs, who have not accepted contraceptive services.
    - Provide information on the availability of services for medical termination of pregnancy and for sterilization.
    - Counsel and refer cases of unwanted pregnancy and seeking MTP services to PHC or designated MTP center.
    - Guide the Health Worker Female in establishing female depot holders for the distribution of conventional contraceptives and trained the depot holders with the assistance of the Health Workers Female.
    - Provide IUD services, its follow-up on consistence basis.
    - Assist MO, PHC in organization of Family Planning Camps and drive.
    - Identify cases of RTI/STI and refer them to PHC for management.
    - To give knowledge about PNDT act to health workers and community.

8. **Nutrition**
    - Ensure that all cases of malnutrition among infants and young children (zero to five years) are given the necessary treatment, advice and refer serious cases to the Primary Health Center.
    - Ensure that iron-folic acid and vitamin A are distributed to the beneficiaries as prescribed.
    - Educate the expectant mothers regarding breast-feeding.
    - On Health day they should help ANM to check the health status of children and advice accordingly.
    - Advice the parents for deworming the children of malnourished and anemic.

9. **Immunization Programs**
   - Supervise the immunization of all pregnant women and children (zero to five years).
   - She will also guide the Health Worker Female to procure supplies, organize immunization camps, and provide guidance for maintaining cold chain, storage of vaccine, immunization and health education.
   - She will supervise PPI / AFP surveillance activities in her area.
10. Primary Medical Care Ensure treatment for minor ailments, provide ORS and first aids for accidents and emergencies and refer cases beyond her competence to the PHC or nearest hospital as and where required.

Male

1. **Supervision and Guidance**
   - Supervise and guide the Health Worker male in the delivery of health care services to the community.
   - Strengthen the knowledge and clinical skills of the Health Workers male.
   - Help the Health Worker male in improving his skills of working in the community.
   - Help and guide the Health Worker male in planning and organizing his program of activities.
   - Visit each Health Worker Male at least once in 2 weeks on a fixed day to observe and guide him in his day-to-day activities. A tentative tour program has to be approved by MO In-charge, after completion of journey he will submit tour dairy to MO In-charge.
   - Assess monthly progress of work of the Health Workers male and submit an assessment report to the Medical Officer of the Primary Health Center with 25% physical verification of work done.
   - Carry out supervisory home visits in the area of the Health Workers male
   - Attend monthly meetings of the Panchayats and help the Panchayat to review work of MPW and female.

2. **Team Work Help the Help Workers to Work as Part of the Health team.**
   - Coordinate his activities with those of the Health Assistant Female and other health personnel including Jan Mangal volunteers Dais. MSS, AWW and Depot holders.
   - Coordinate the health activities in his area with the activities of workers of other departments and agencies.
   - Conduct staff meetings fortnightly with the Health Workers in coordination with the Health Assistant Female at one of the subcenters by rotation.
   - Attend staff meeting at the Primary Health Center.
   - Assist the Medical officer of the Primary Health Center in the Organization of the different health services/camps, FW, RCH, Health Mela and campaigns in health programs.
   - Assist the Medical officer of the Primary Health Center in conducting training programs for various categories of health personal.
   - Participate in CNA in preparation of subcenter and PHC annual action plan.
   - **Supplies and equipment:** In collaboration with the Health Assistant Female, check at regular intervals the stores available at the sub-center and ensure timely and logistic placement of indent and procure the supplies and equipment well in time.
   - Check that the drugs at the subcenter are properly stored and timely costumed (before expiry); that the equipment are well maintained and routinely used.
   - Ensure that the Health Workers male maintains his kit in the proper way.

Nutrition
1. Ensure that all cases of malnutrition among infants and young children (zero to five years) are given the necessary treatment, advice and refer serious cases to the Primary Health Center. Establish linkage with ICDS program.
2. Ensure that Iron–folic acid and vitamin A are distributed to the beneficiaries as prescribed.
3. Advice the parents for deworm the child if suffering with malnourished and anemia.
4. **Control of blindness:** All cases of blindness including suspected cases of cataract will be referred to concerned specialist. He will also keep records of such cases.

Vital Events
1. Collect and compile the monthly report of birth and death occurring in his area and submit them to the medical officer primary health center.
2. Educate the community regarding the need for registration of vital events. (Birth and Deaths) Primary Medical Care.
   Ensure that treatment for minor ailments is provided first aid for Accidents and refer cases beyond his competence to the Primary Health center or nearest hospital.
   Attend the cases referred by the health workers and refer cases beyond his competence to the Primary Health center or nearest hospital.

Health Education
1. Carry out educational activities for control of communicable diseases, environmental sanitation, RCH, Family Planning, nutrition, immunization, HIV/AIDS, personal hygienic and other National Health Programs
2. Arrange group meetings with leaders and involve them in spreading the message for various health programs.
3. Organise and conduct training of community leaders with the assistance of the Health team.

School Health
1. Impart knowledge about adolescent health.
2. Assist medical officers in school health programs.

Note: In PHCs where there is no HA (Male), these functions will be carried out by LHV(HA) Female.

2016
Community Health Nursing

SECTION-I

I. **Give the meaning of the following:**
   a. Eligible couple
   b. Geriatric nursing
   c. Infant
   d. Maternal mortality rate.

II. **State whether the following statements are *true* or *false***
   a. Karthar Singh Committee is otherwise known as Multipurpose Health worker committee.
   b. Colostrum is harmful to the newborn baby.
   c. Notification or reporting is the first step in the control of communicable disease.
   d. The objective of the under-five clinic is to take care of children below 5 years.

III. **Write short notes on any *three* of the following:**
   a. Postnatal care
   b. Determinants of health
   c. Antenatal diet
   d. Levels of health care

IV. a. What is school health services?
   b. List the objectives of school health services
   c. Discuss the role of nurse in school health services

V. a. Name the Health Committees in India
   b. Explain the role of nurse in school health services

SECTION-II

VI. **State whether the following statements are *true* or *false***
   a. Birth and death rates are important components of population
   b. Education is a crucial element in economic and social development
   c. BCG vaccine is given to prevent malaria.

VII. **Fill in the blanks**
   a. The World Aids Day is celebrated on _____
   b. PHC in hilly and tribal area covers the population of _____
   c. Dengue fever is caused by the bite of _____
   d. Montaux test is to diagnose_____

VIII. Write short notes on any of *three* of the following:
   a. Function of female health assistant
   b. Blindness control progress
   c. Temporary family planning methods
   d. Infertility

IX. a. What is National Malaria Control Program?
   b. Discuss the role of nurse in National Malaria Control Program.

X. a. Define vital statistics
   b. Explain briefly the concept and sources of vital statistics.
   c. Enumerate the uses of vital health statistics.

SECTION-I

I. Give the meaning of the following:

a. Eligible couple

An eligible couple refers to a currently married couple wherein the wife is in the reproductive age, which is generally assumed to lie between the ages of 15–45 years. There will be at least 150–180 such couples per 1000 populations in India. These couples are in need of family planning services. About 20% of eligible couples are found in the age group 15–24 years. On an average 2.5 million couples are joining the reproductive group every year. The eligible couple register is a basic document for organizing family planning work.

b. Geriatric nursing

Gerontological nursing is the specialty of nursing pertaining to older adults. Gerontological nurses work in collaboration with older adults, their families, and communities to support healthy aging, maximum functioning, and quality of life. Gerontological nursing is important to meet the health needs of an aging population. Due to longer life expectancy and declining fertility rates, the proportion of the population that is considered old is increasing. Between 2000 and 2050, the number of people in the world who are over age 60 is predicted increase from 605 million to 2 billion. The proportion of older adults is already high and continuing to increase in more developed countries.

c. Infant

Infancy is traditionally designed as the period from 1 month to 1 year of age. This year is one of rapid growth and development, with the infant tripling birth weight and increasing length by 50%. During this period the baby's senses sharpen and with the process of attachment to primary care givers, from his or her first social relationships. Infants are seen at health care facilities for health maintenance at least six months during the first year.

d. Maternal mortality rate

Maternal death is the death of a woman while pregnant or within 42 days of termination of pregnancy, irrespective of the duration and site of the pregnancy, from any cause related to or aggravated by the pregnancy or its management but not from accidental or incidental causes. To facilitate the identification of maternal deaths in circumstances in which cause of death attribution is inadequate, a new category has been introduced: Pregnancy-related death is defined as the death of a woman while pregnant or within 42 days of termination of pregnancy, irrespective of the cause of death.

II. State whether the following statements are *true* or *false*

a. Karthar Singh Committee is otherwise known as Multipurpose Health worker committee: **TRUE**
b. Colostrum is harmful to the newborn baby: **FALSE**
c. Notification or reporting is the first step in the control of communicable disease: **TRUE**
d. The objective of the under-five clinic is to take care of children below 5 years: **TRUE**

III. Write short notes on any *three* of the following:

a. Postnatal care

Care of the mother after delivery is known as postnatal or postpartal care or puerperium. Puerperium is a 6 week period following birth in which the reproductive organs undergo physical and physiological changes a process called involution.

Objectives of Postpartum Care

1. To prevent complications of postpartum period.
2. To provide care for the rapid restoration of the mother to optimum health.
3. To provide family planning services.
4. To check adequacy of breastfeeding.
5. To provide basic health education to mother/family.

Postnatal examination: Examining postnatal mother to rule out any fever, tachycardia, laceration, and erosion of cervix, rectocele, cystocele, displacement of uterus and inflammatory swellings in the abdomen, examining the neonates to rule out birth injuries, congenital defects and low-birth weight.

Postnatal assessment: Assessing weight changes of the neonates and the nature and extent of birth injuries and congenital defects. Assessing the temperature and pulse rate of the mothers.

Postnatal care and attention: Provide for the care of the perineum, care of the breast, prevention of infection, early ambulation, immunization and psychological support to mothers. Also provided for prevention of infection and care of the cord stump of newborns. Postnatal education and counseling includes breastfeeding, dietary intake, danger signals and family planning.

Complications of Postnatal Period

1. **Puerperal sepsis:** This is infection of the genital tract within 3 weeks after delivery. This is accompanied by rise in temperature and pulse rate, foul smelling locia, pain and tenderness in lower abdomen etc. this can be prevented by attention to asepsis before and after delivery.
2. **Thrombophlebitis:** This is an infection of the vein of the legs, frequently associated with varicose vein. The leg may become tender, pale and swollen.
3. **Secondary hemorrhage:** Bleeding from vagina anytime from 6 hours after delivery to the end of the puerperium (6 weeks) is called secondary hemorrhage and may be due to retained placenta or membranes.
4. **Others:** Urinary tract infection and mastitis, etc.

Role of Nurse in Postnatal Care

1. Care during postpartum period to the mother- enquire and observe her condition generally and with reference to sleep, diet, after the pain subsides. Check vital signs, inspect perineum for discharge and inspect breast and nipples.
2. Care of newborn is an interwoven activity along with the care to mother. It involves taking body temperature, checking skin, color, eyes, bowel movements, urination, watching the cry, checking the sleeping and feeding.

b. Determinants of health

Environmental determinants: Environment has the direct impact on the health of individual, family or community. Internal or external and physical, biological and psychosocial components of environment influence the mental, social, spiritual and physical well-being of individuals, Environmental pollution has become a global threat. We must find the ways to reduce and manage the pollution as well as waste. It is worth mentioning that Florence Nightingale had also given importance to environmental factors in the maintenance of the health and care of the sick. Air, water, noise, radiation, housing, waste-management etc. all affect the health status and quality of life.

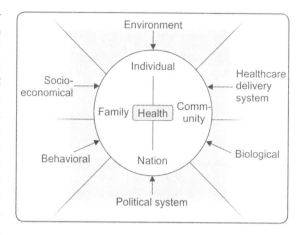

Political system: Political system has a great effect on the social climate in which we live. Political influences have the power and authority to regulate much of our surroundings in that, health care is also included. Implementation of any health program cannot be conducted properly without the strong political will. In our country health is a subject of concurrent list, so there is a need of coordination between the union and state governments in the health-related matters.

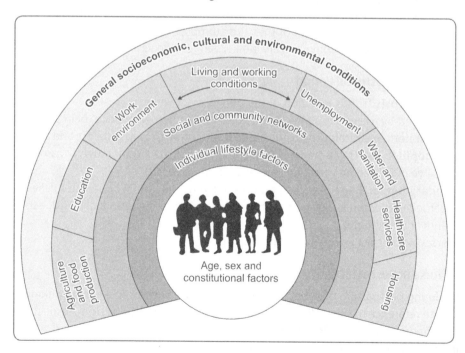

Behavioral determinants: Health is the mirror of a person's lifestyle because faulty and ill habits have the adverse effect on the health of the individual. It is an established fact that culture and ethnic heritage shape much of our lifestyle including the health care.

Socioeconomic determinants: Socioeconomic conditions have the major impact on the health status of any country. Education, economy, occupational opportunities, housing, nutritional level, per capita income, etc. determine the healthcare system and health resources.

Healthcare delivery system determinants: The healthcare delivery system plays a great role in the field of health. This is considered as a disease-oriented system, but in our country which has the second largest population in the world, providing health care services at the grassroots level is a difficult task. Besides the above-mentioned determinants women's issue, aging population, agriculture, social welfare, rural development, urban improvement, etc. also have a major impact on the health of the nation, its families and individuals.

c. Antenatal diet

During pregnancy, there should be an increase in all nutrients to meet the physiologic demands of maternal changes and fetal growth. The amount of increase in essential nutrients for each woman depends on a number of factors, such as

1. The general nutritional status before pregnancy.
2. Current health status, age and parity.
3. Time interval between pregnancies.
4. Height, weight and activity level.

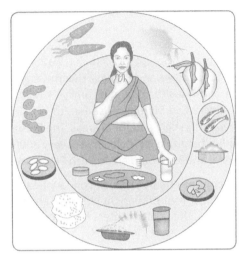

Adolescents who are pregnant before the cessation of their own growth do not have the physiologic maturity to withstand the additional stresses of pregnancy. They need greater nutritional requirements then do adults.

Calorie increase: Calorie requirements must be increased between 10 and 15% during pregnancy to meet the increased energy demands of the women's body and the development of the fetus. The total energy cost during pregnancy is approximately 80,000 calories. Therefore, an increase of about 300 calories (kcal) per day is needed during pregnancy. A well balanced diet consisting of about 2500 calories a day will meet the nutritional demands of pregnancy.

   I. **Protein:** Protein should be increased from 45 to 50 g per day in the nonpregnant women to 60 g per day for the pregnant women. For adolescent pregnancy, the protein requirement is 1.5 g per kilogram of body weight. Protein is needed to provide additional amino acids.
   1. To support rapid fetal and placental growth
   2. Growth of the breasts and uterus
   3. Expansion of maternal blood volume and
   4. To meet the demands of labour, birth and lactation.

   Sources of complete proteins: Milk, cheese and eggs, meet, fish, poultry, grains, legumes and nuts. Vegetable proteins can be combined with complete proteins, (or) two vegetable proteins that complement each other's amino acid deficiencies can be eaten together to make a complete protein.
   Example: Milk and cereal. Rice with beans.

   II. **Carbohydrates and fats:** The role of carbohydrate and fats during pregnancy are to contribute to the total calorie intake required for maternal and fetal growth.
   Sources of carbohydrates and fat: Fruits, whole grains cereal, milk and bread. Fats are found in butter, cheese, oil and nuts.

Vitamins: Vitamin intake should be maintained or increased during pregnancy and lactation. This intake should be obtained through a well-balanced diet. The role of vitamins in the diet is to maintain the normal cell structure and function and to support the growth of new tissues. The fat-soluble vitamins A, D, E and K are stored in the liver in moderate amount. They are absorbed along with the dietary fats eaten.

d. Levels of health care

Primary health care: Primary healthcare denotes the first level of contact between individuals and families with the health system. According to Alma Atta Declaration of 1978, Primary Health care was to serve the community it served; it included care for mother and child which included family planning, immunization, prevention of locally endemic diseases, treatment of common diseases or injuries, provision of essential facilities, health education, provision of food and nutrition and adequate supply of safe drinking water. In India, Primary Healthcare is provided through a network of Sub centers and Primary Health Centers in rural areas, whereas in urban areas, it is provided through Health posts and Family Welfare Centers. The Sub centre consists of one Auxiliary Nurse Midwife and Multipurpose Health worker and serves a population of 5000 in plains and 3000 persons in hilly and tribal areas. The Primary Health Centre (PHC), staffed by Medical Officer and other paramedical staff serves every 30000 population in the plains and 20,000 persons in hilly, tribal and backward areas. Each PHC is to supervise 6 Sub centers.

Secondary healthcare: Secondary health care refers to a second tier of health system, in which patients from primary health care are referred to specialists in higher hospitals for treatment. In India, the health centers for secondary health care include District hospitals and Community Health Centre at block level.

Tertiary healthcare: Tertiary health care refers to a third level of health system, in which specialized consultative care is provided usually on referral from primary and secondary medical care. Specialized intensive care units, advanced diagnostic support services and specialized medical personnel on the key features of tertiary health care. In India, under public health system, tertiary care service is provided by medical colleges and advanced medical research institutes.

IV. a. What is school health services? b. List the objectives of school health services. c. Discuss the role of nurse in school health services.

a. The School Health Program is defined as "the school procedures that contribute to the maintenance and improvement of the health of pupils and school personnel including health services healthful living and health education". Childhood is the age of learning and it is the time when a child start developing practices and attitude towards health. It is very important to target the children for oral health awareness and demonstration of correct methods for oral hygiene.

b. List the objectives of School Health Services

1. Developing schools in India as 'Health Promoting Schools'.
2. Implementing Comprehensive School Health Programme (CHSP) in schools.
3. Promotion of research and development in the field of school health and student well-being.
4. Creation of awareness among school children about healthy living.
5. Enhancement of the skills of school teachers in handling health and developmental problems among children.

6. To promote life skill education and personal development in schools.
7. To provide guidance for the establishment and maintenance of Health Clubs in schools.
8. Provision of Preventive Health Services to Schools.
9. To identify and correct psychosocial problems among school children, including substance abuse.
10. To provide counseling and guidance services to children with special problems.
11. To develop and distribute health education materials and media to schools.
12. Promotion of Educational Research.
13. To cooperate with governments and health agencies in the formulation, implementation and evaluation of school health policies and programs.
14. To set up and run establishments/institutions, that may help in furthering the objectives.
15. To bring out newsletters, pamphlets and other informational materials, that may help in furthering the objectives.
16. To formulate and implement any other activity as may be necessary or is conducive to the attainment of the above objectives.

c. Discuss the role of nurse in school health services

I. Provide health assessments.
1. Obtains a health and developmental history.
2. Screens and evaluates findings for deficits in vision, hearing, scoliosis, growth, etc.
3. Observes the child for development and health patterns in making a nursing assessment and nursing diagnosis.
4. Identifies health findings, which do not fall within the normal range.
5. Assists with physical examinations when conducted in the school.

II. Develops and implements a health plan.
1. Interprets the health status of pupils to school personnel.
2. Initiates referrals to parents, school personnel and community health resources for intervention, remediation, and follow through.
3. Provides ongoing health information to pupils, parents, school personnel and health agencies.

d. Recommends and helps to implement modifications of school programs to meet students' health needs

e. Utilizes existing health resources to provide appropriate care of pupils
3. Maintains, evaluates, and interprets cumulative health data to accommodate individual needs of students.
4. Participates as the health specialist on the child education evaluation team to develop the health individualized educational plan (IEP)
5. Plans and implements school health management protocols for the child with chronic health problems, including the administration of medication.
6. Participates in home visits to assess the family's needs as related to the child's health.
7. Develops procedures and provides for crises intervention for acute illness, injury and emotional disturbances.

8. Promotes and assists in the control of communicable diseases through preventive immunization programs, early detection, surveillance and reporting of contagious diseases.
9. Recommends provisions for a school environment conducive to learning.
10. Provides information on health.
    a. Provides health information to assist students and families in making health-related decisions.
    b. Participates in health education directly and indirectly for the improvement of health by teaching per sons to become more assertive health consumers and to assume greater responsibility for their own health.
    c. Provides information to adolescents concerning health problems in order to encourage responsible decision-making practices.
    d. Serves as a resource person to the classroom teacher and administrator in health instruction and as a member of the health curriculum development committees.
11. Coordinates school and community health activities and serves as a liaison person between the home, school, and community.
12. Acts as a resource person in promoting health careers.
13. Engages in research and evaluation of school health services to act as a change agent for school health programs and school nursing practices.
14. Assists in the formation of health policies, goals and objectives for the school unit.

III. Administration

1. Is responsible for maintaining and updating cumulative health records.
2. Helps develop/revise school health policies, procedures and standing orders.
3. Prepares the budget for school health supplies.
4. Reviews, revises and implements emergency policies, including in-service health and safety programs for personnel.
5. Prepares first aid kits for each building.
6. Organizes, instructs, and supervises school health volunteers or assistants.
7. Reports regularly in writing to the principal and superintendent on school health activities.
8. Prepares statistical reports for the Department of Educational and Cultural Services and Department of Human Services for the superintendent's signature as required.
9. Implements the school medication policy and procedure.

IV. Coordination

1. Interprets school health services to school personnel.
2. Plans, implements, and supervises school health screening programs in accordance with state and district r requirements and recommendations. Provides follow-up services when indicated.
3. Interprets appraisal findings, and helps students and parents accept responsibility for diagnosis and treatment.
4. Serves as a health liaison between school, home, and the community. Makes home visits as needed.
5. Encourages parents to maintain current immunization protection as recommended by the Department of Human Services.
6. Participates in the health aspects of kindergarten preregistration.
7. Helps school personnel recognize departures from appropriate behavior and growth patterns; helps students and staff adjust student programs when necessary to accommodate health needs of students.

8. Serves as a resource person to school personnel. Participates selectively in classroom instruction under the supervision of the teacher.

V. a. Name the health committees in India. b. Explain briefly the Bhore Committee Report?

Various committees of experts have been appointed by the government from time to time to render advice about different health problems. The reports of these committees have formed an important basis of health planning in India. The goal of National Health Planning in India is to attain Health for All by the year 2000.

1. Bhore Committee (1946)
2. Mudaliar Committee (1962)
3. Chadah Committee (1963)
4. Mukherjee Committee (1965)
5. Mukherjee Committee (1966)
6. Jungalwalla Committee (1967)
7. Kartar Singh Committee (1973)
8. Shrivastav Committee (1975)
9. Bajaj Committee Health Report (1986)
10. Krishnan Committee Health Report (1992)
11. High Power Committee Recommendations.

Bhore Committee (1946)

In 1943, the Government of India appointed a Committee as the Bhore Committee for the health survey and development committee with Sir, Joseph Bhore as Chairman. Its aim was to survey the existing position regarding the health conditions and health organization in the committee which had among its members some of the pioneers of the health, met regularly for 2 years and submitted its famous report in 1946 which runs into 4 volumes. This committee, known as the Health Survey and Development Committee, was appointed in 1943 with Sir Joseph Bhore as its Chairman. It laid emphasis on integration of curative and preventive medicine at all levels. It made comprehensive recommendations for remodelling of health services in India. The report, submitted in 1946, had some important recommendations like:

1. Integration of preventive and curative services of all administrative levels.
2. Development of Primary Health Centres in 2 stages:
    a. Short-term measure – one primary health centre as suggested for a population of 40,000. Each PHC was to be manned by 2 doctors, one nurse, four public health nurses, four midwives, four trained dais, two sanitary inspectors, two health assistants, one pharmacist and fifteen other class IV employees. Secondary health centre was also envisaged to provide support to PHC, and to coordinate and supervise their functioning.
    b. A long-term programme (also called the 3 million plan) of setting up primary health units with 75 – bedded hospitals for each 10,000 to 20,000 population and secondary units with 650 – bedded hospital, again regionalized around district hospitals with 2500 beds.
3. Major changes in medical education which includes 3-month training in preventive and social medicine to prepare "social physicians".

Important Recommendations

1. **Nutrition of the people:** They pointed out the main defects of the average Indian diet results from the insufficiency of proteins, mineral salts and vitamins. They also recommend special measures to increase the production of food rich in proteins. Also prevention of food adulteration and improvement of the quality of the food.
2. **Health education:** Bhore committee suggested that health education to school children on hygiene should begin at the earliest. The doctors, nurses, midwife and in fact every health worker will discharge his or her duties and by educating the persons with whom they deal with regard to prevention of disease and the promotion of positive health.
3. **Physical examination:** Committee stated that there is great dearth of suitable and qualified teachers for imparting instructions in this subject. Also physical training program for the community with emphasis on national games and exercises.
4. **Health services for mothers and children:** At the head quarters of each primary unit and in place where 30 bed hospitals are located the service for mothers and children should be available.
5. **Health services of the school children:** The school teachers who have to carry or certain health duties require careful training and continuous supervision. They have to conduct health education programs. In each primary unit, the male medical officer should take charge of the school health services.
6. **Occupational heath including industrial health:** The Committee recommended that the industrial health organization should form an integral part of the provincial health department and government.
7. **Health services for certain important diseases:** Bhore Committee studied the existing legal and administrative provisions to deal with communicable diseases and suggested certain measures for controlling communicable diseases.
8. **Environmental hygiene:** An essential part of the campaign for promoting public health was to improve man's physical environment. The Committee's main recommendations were improvement in village and town planning.
9. **Vital statistics:** The Committee recommended administrative organization at the center, organization at provincial head quarters and district organization. Another recommendation is provision of training facilities for statistics.
10. **Professional education:** The main objective of the Committee during his period was the provision of adequate and suitably trained staff to enable the plan of health work effectively.
11. **Drug and medical requisites:** they recommended our universities should undertake research with a view to produce life saving drugs in this country.

SECTION-II

VI. State whether the following statements are *true* or *false*

a. Birth and death rates are important components of population: **TRUE**
b. Education is a crucial element in economic and social development: **TRUE**
c. BCG vaccine is given to prevent Malaria: **FALSE**

VII. Fill in the blanks
a. The World Aids Day is celebrated on **1ST DEC**
b. PHC in hilly and tribal area covers the population of **3000**
c. Dengue fever is caused by the bite of **AEDES MOSQUITO**
d. Montaux test is to diagnoses: **TUBERCULOSIS**

III. Write short notes on any *three* of the following:
a. Functions of female health assistant
The Female Health Assistant will cover a population of 5000/3000. She should reside in the subcentre area, location of the sub-centre itself being her headquarter. She will perform 16 days field visit in a month, i.e. 4 days per week, the Saturday being the weekly meeting/diary day and another day duly earmarked being the subcenter clinic day. The following are the job functions:

I. Registration
She will:
1. Register pregnant women from 3 months onwards, married woman in the reproductive period and children through systematic home-visits and at clinics.
2. Maintain basic information regarding villages, house and population, etc. with the help of her male counterpart.
3. Maintain maternity record, register of antenatal cases, eligible couple register and children register up to date.
4. Categories the eligible couples according to the number of children and age of mothers.

II. Care at Home
1. Provide care to pregnant mothers especially the registered ones throughout the entire period of pregnancy.
2. Give advice on nutrition to expectant and lactating mothers.
3. Distribute iron-folic acid tabs to pregnant and lactating mothers and children as well as to the family planning adopters, and vitamin A in oil to the children up to 6 years of age.
4. Immunize pregnant mother with tetanus toxoid and with others to the children as per immunization schedule.
5. Conduct home deliveries whenever required in normal labor cases.
6. Prefer cases of abnormal pregnancy, difficult labour, at risk babies, cases with medical and gynecological problems and help them get institutional care properly.
7. Provide postdelivery visits for each delivery case and follow up care to the patients recovered and discharged from hospital.
8. Maintain close liaison with local trained *dais* and extend help when called for, supervise the deliveries conducted by the *dais* and forward the list of deliveries thus conducted recommending claims of payment thereafter to the concerned PHC as per rules.
9. Promote cases of sterilization and IUD through spread of small family norms to the eligible couples and arrange facilities of service to the willing acceptors.
10. Distribute conventional contraceptive to the couples during home visit as well as through the *dais* and *anganwadi* workers.

11. Take active part in the special sterilization camps when held in PHC/other areas.
12. Get herself trained in BCG technique by the local BCG technician meant for the purpose and cover the area with BCG vaccination with the help of the technician and male Health Assistant.
13. Provide follow up services to FP adopters, identify side-effects and minor compliant, if any, and refer those cases to the nearest PHC/hospital when required.
14. Detect cases of 8 target diseases under EPI and any abnormal episode within her area and arrange containment measures promptly.
15. Provide first aid and preliminary treatments of common ailments and refer cases beyond her competence to the nearest PHC/hospital.
16. Arrange testing of urine for albumin and sugar, and blood for hemoglobin of pregnant women.
17. Collect blood smears from at least suspected malaria cases and administer presumptive treatment.
18. Identify cases that require help for medical termination of pregnancy (MTP) provide information on the availability of services and refer them to the nearest approved institution.
19. Educate the female folks regarding maintenance of health and nutrition of pregnant and lactating mothers and children, importance of immunization, births and deaths registration, prompt reporting of any disease, use of safe drinking water and maintenance of personal hygiene and environmental sanitation and use of ORS in gastrointestinal diseases. She will also motivate mother to accept the health facilities including the nutrition programmes provided by the SC and PHC/SHC.
20. Enquire and record births and deaths occurring in her area and report them to the local registrar.

III Care at Clinic

1. Arrange and perform MCH clinics at subcenter once a week with the help of the concerned male health assistant.
2. Conduct urine examinations and estimate hemoglobin of the pregnant mothers.
3. Conduct IUD insertion of the willing mothers at SC
4. Conduct feeding programme at SC, if it is there.
5. Take help of the Vol. Female attendant attached to her SC.
6. Conduct other activities of the SC including immunization, prophylaxis, MCH, health and nutrition education, and preliminary treatment of common ailments.
7. Impart continuing education to the *anganwadi* workers under ICDS project and help and supervise the activities of the said workers.
8. Assess growth and development of the infants and take suitable action as called for.

IV Care in the Community

1. Identify women leaders and help the HS(F) and SWO in conducting training of those leaders.
2. Set up depot holders for Nirodh distribution and help HS(F) in training them in this.
3. Participate in Mahila Mandal Meetings and educate women in family welfare.
4. Utilize satisfied customers, village leaders, CHGs, Trained Dais, AWWs for promoting family welfare program.
5. Attend Anganwadi and MCC (Sishukalyani Center) Centers, arrange immunization of the mothers and children, health care of the mothers and children and help AWWs in the implementation of the Supplementary Nutrition Program under ICDS.
6. Collect monthly monitoring report from the AWWs and submit those after compilation to PHN/LHV or HS(F).

V. Miscellaneous

1. Remain in charge of the SC and maintain cleanliness of the same.
2. Attend weekly meeting and submit performance report in conjoin with that of the HA (M).
3. Involve local Dais in FW programme and IUD Campaign.
4. Help HS(F) in training the Indigenous Dais.
5. Take help of her HS(F) and allow her supervision and monitoring, when required.
6. Help HS(F) in conducting School Health Programme.
7. Participate in the organization of Eye Operation Camps, Eye Health Care Camps, Sterilization and Laparoscopy Camps and discharge nursing skill to the patients admitted/operated in the institutions.
8. Detect the physically handicapped from the field and refer those to the nearest health institution.
9. Prepare and maintain all registers, records, maps and charts in her sub-centre and submit the prescribed periodical reports to the HS(F) in time.
10. Maintain field diary for her own performance and exhibit the same for inspection to the HS(F) when called for.
11. Perform any other job as may be assigned to her from time to time by the BMOH or any other Officer authorized by him.

b. Blindness Control Program

National Programme for Control of Blindness (NPCB) was launched in the year 1976 as a 100% centrally sponsored scheme with the goal to reduce the prevalence of blindness from 1.4% to 0.3%. As per Survey in 2001–02, prevalence of blindness is estimated to be 1.1%. Rapid Survey on Avoidable Blindness conducted under NPCB during 2006-07 showed reduction in the prevalence of blindness from 1.1% (2001–02) to 1% (2006-07). Various activities/initiatives undertaken during the Five Year Plans under NPCB are targeted towards achieving the goal of reducing the prevalence of blindness to 0.3% by the year 2020

Main causes of blindness are as follows: - Cataract (62.6%) Refractive Error (19.70%) Corneal Blindness (0.90%), Glaucoma (5.80%), Surgical Complication (1.20%) Posterior Capsular Opacification (0.90%) Posterior Segment Disorder (4.70%), Others (4.19%) Estimated National Prevalence of Childhood Blindness /Low Vision is 0.80 per thousand

Goals and Objectives of NPCB in the XII Plan

1. To reduce the backlog of blindness through identification and treatment of blind at primary, secondary and tertiary levels based on assessment of the overall burden of visual impairment in the country.
2. Develop and strengthen the strategy of NPCB for "Eye Health" and prevention of visual impairment; through provision of comprehensive eye care services and quality service delivery.
3. Strengthening and upgradation of RIOs to become center of excellence in various subspecialties of ophthalmology.
4. Strengthening the existing and developing additional human resources and infrastructure facilities for providing high quality comprehensive Eye Care in all Districts of the country.
5. To enhance community awareness on eye care and lay stress on preventive measures.
6. Increase and expand research for prevention of blindness and visual impairment.
7. To secure participation of voluntary organizations/private practitioners in eye care.

c. Temporary family planning methods

Family planning allows women and couples to determine whether and when to have children. The ability to make these choices is fundamental to healthy families and communities worldwide. Family planning programs should offer a well-balanced mix of contraceptive methods, including those that are short- and long-acting, hormonal and non-hormonal, provider-dependent and client-controlled, and natural and clinical.

1. Natural methods: Abstinence, lactation, withdrawal, and safe period methods.
2. Barrier methods: Condoms with/without spermicide, diaphragm, cervical cap, sponge, vaginal spermicides.
3. Hormonal methods: Oral pills, Injectables, Implants.
4. Others: Intrauterine devices e.g. Cu T.

d. Infertility

Infertility means that couples have been trying to get pregnant with frequent intercourse for at least a year with no success. Female infertility, male infertility or a combination of the two affects millions of couples in the United States. An estimated 10–15% of couples have trouble getting pregnant or getting to a successful delivery. Infertility results from female infertility factors about one-third of the time and male infertility factors about one-third of the time. In the rest, the cause is either unknown or a combination of male and female factors. The cause of female infertility can be difficult to diagnose, but many treatments are available. Treatment options depend on the underlying problem. Treatment isn't always necessary- many infertile couples will go on to conceive a child spontaneously.

Damage to the fallopian tubes (which carry the eggs from the ovaries to the uterus) can prevent contact between the egg and sperm. Pelvic infections, endometriosis, and pelvic surgeries may lead to scar formation and fallopian tube damage. Hormonal causes. Some women have problems with ovulation.

IX. a. What is National Malaria Control Program?, b. Discuss the role of nurse in National Malaria Control Program?

Malaria has been a major cause of poverty and low productivity accounting for about 32.5% of all OPD attendances and 48.8% of under five years admissions in the country (NMCP Annual Report, 2009). The attempt to control malaria in Ghana began in the 1950s. It was aimed at reducing the malaria disease burden till its no longer of public health significance. It was also recognized that malaria cannot be controlled by the health sector alone therefore multiple strategies were being pursued with other health related sectors. In view of this, interventions were put in place to help in the control of the deadly disease. Some of the interventions applied at the time included residual insecticide application against adult mosquitoes, mass chemoprophylaxis with pyrimethamine medicated salt and improvement of drainage system. But malaria continued to be the leading cause of morbidity (illness) in the country.

Mission: To reduce the morbidity and mortality due to malaria and improving the quality of life, thereby contributing to health and alleviation of poverty in the country.

Goals

1. Screening all fever cases suspected for malaria (60% through quality microscopy and 40% by rapid diagnostic test)

2. Treating all *P. falciparum* cases with full course of effective ACT and primaquine and all *P. vivax* cases with 3 days chloroquine and 14 days primaquine.
3. Equipping all health Institutions (PHC level and above), especially in high-risk areas, with microscopy facility and RDT for emergency use and injectable artemisinin derivatives.
4. Strengthening all district and sub-district hospitals in malaria endemic areas as per IPHS with facilities for management of severe malaria cases.

The objectives of this new Malaria Action Program are:
1. Management of serious and complicated malaria cases.
2. Prevention of mortality with particular reference to high risk groups
3. Reduction of morbidity
4. Control of outbreaks and epidemics
5. Reduction of falctparum
6. Incidence and containment resistance malaria
7. Maintenance of low incidence status.
8. The recent resurgence of malaria in many parts of the country necessitated the need to strengthen the health promotion component of the programme.
9. It has been decided to observe Anti Malaria Month before the onset of monsoon ie. month of June every year.

X. a. Define vital statistics, b. Explain briefly the concept and sources of vital statistics. c. Enumerate the uses of vital health statistics.

Vital statistics are statistics on live births, deaths, fetal deaths, marriages and divorces. The most common way of collecting information on these events is through civil registration an administrative system used by governments to record vital events which occur in their populations. Efforts to improve the quality of vital statistics will therefore be closely related to the development of civil registration systems in countries. Vital statistics are, well, vital to public health. Vital statistics include information on births, deaths and a lot of health information generated in between. Before public health officials can know what the needs of a population are and how to address them, they must have data on the prevalence of disease and major health issues. Most national governments by law mandate the collection of vital statistics.

Definition of Vital Statistics

1. Vital statistics are conventionally numerical records of marriage, births, sickness and deaths by which the health and growth of community may be studied.
2. Vital statistics is a part of demography and collective study of mankind. It deals with the data's related to vital events.
3. It is a branch of biometry deals with data and law of human mortality, morbidity and demography.
4. Vital statistics is the numerical description of birth, death, absorption, marriage, divorce, adoption and judicial separation—UNO.

Meaning of Vital Statistics

1. Vital statistics has been used to denote acts systematically collected and compiled in numerical form relating to or derived from records of vital events namely, live birth, death, fetal death, marriage, divorce, adoption, legitimating, recognition, annulment or legal separation.

2. Vital statistics provide a tool for measuring the dynamics of change which continuously occur in population. Vital statistics are derived from legally registrable events without including population data or morbidity statistics.

Purpose of Vital Statistics
1. Community health: To describe the level community health, to diagnose community illness, and to discover solutions to health problems.
2. Administrative purpose: It provides clues for administrative action and to create administrative standards of health activities.
3. Health programmed organization: To determine success or failure of specific health programmed or undertake overall evaluation of public health work.
4. Legislative purpose: To promote health legislation at local, state and national level.
5. Governmental purpose: To develop policies procedures, at state and central level.

Sources of vital statistics: There are four major sources of vital statistics in India, namely (a) the Sample Registration System (SRS), (b) the Civil Registration System (CRS), (c) Indirect estimates from the decennial census and (d) Indirect estimates from the National Family Health Surveys (NFHS). The SRS is the most regular source of demographic statistics in India. It is based on a system of dual recording of births and deaths in fairly representative sample units spread all over the country. The SRS provides annual estimates of (a) population composition, (b) fertility, (c) mortality, and (d) medical attention at the time of birth or death which give some idea about access to medical care. The population composition from SRS coupled with the decennial census counts, enables fairly reliable estimate of population in the intercensal periods. Average time to publication of SRS annual reports is about two years. SRS estimates are generally valid and reliable for the country as a whole and for bigger states with more than 10 million populations. Recently the sample size of SRS has been increased to allow for estimates by natural divisions within the bigger states. Evaluations during 1970s and 1980s showed that completeness of recording of births and deaths by the SRS, was generally good, and errors in recording of events minimal. However, systematic evaluation of the SRS has not been taken up for quite some time. Indirect estimates for 1990s and after suggests that registration completeness has worsened and interstate variations widened. A pluralistic evaluation framework is recommended.

Uses of Vital Statistics
1. To evaluate the impact of various national health programmers.
2. To plan for better future measures of disease control.
3. To elucidate the hereditary nature of disease
4. To plan and evaluate economic and social development.
5. It is a primary tool in research activities.
6. To determine the health status of individual.
7. To compare the health status of one nation with others.

Maternity: Many of the greatest advances in medicine have come as a result of public health interventions rather than individual treatments. The ability to intervene in the health of populations is dependent upon development of appropriate tools for measuring health, illness, and interventions. Only by standardizing communication on such issues as infant mortality can physicians hope to target high-risk populations with effective interventions. Despite the lack of clinical glamour associated with the subject of vital statistics, understanding the common language of public health is vital.

2015
Community Health Nursing

SECTION-I

I. **Give the meaning of the following:**
   a. Cold chain
   b. Infant mortality rate
   c. Demography
   d. Community development.

II. **State whether the following statement are *true* or *false*:**
   a. The road to health card is a important tools for monitoring growth of under five children.
   b. The world tuberculosis day is celebrated on 5th September
   c. In India, there is one primary health center for every 30,000 population
   d. The route of administration of BCG is intramuscular.

III. **Write short notes on any *three* of the following:**
   a. Health organization at district level
   b. Reproductive child health services
   c. Under-five clinic
   d. Preventive and promotive school health services.

IV. a. Define MCH services
    b. Write the objectives of MCH services
    c. Explain the role of community health nurse in MCH services.
    OR
    a. What is occupational health
    b. List the important occupational diseases
    c. Discuss the role of a nurse in industrial health nursing

V. a. Define primary health care
   b. Write the elements of primary health care
   c. Explain the role of a nurse in primary health care.

SECTION-II

VI. **Choose the correct answer and write:**
   a. The state of highest literacy rate in India is: _____
      i. Maharashtra   ii. Tamil Nadu   iii. Kerala
   b. The year of last census done in India: _____
      i. 2010   ii. 2011   iii. 2012

c. The route of administration of measles vaccine is: _____
   i. Subcutaneous   ii. Intradermal   iii. Intramuscular
d. The world AIDS day is celebrated on: _____
   i. 20th august   ii. 1st December   iii. 14th November

VII. State whether the following statement are *true* or *false*
  a. The number of death occurs before 28 days of birth per 1000 live births is termed as under five mortality rate.
  b. The branch of statistics related to biological events and to mathematical facts is called biostatistics
  c. Malaria is transmitted by anopheles mosquito.

VIII. Write short notes on any *three* of the following:
  a. AIDS Control Program
  b. Importance of vital statistics
  c. National methods of family planning
  d. Intrauterine contraceptives.

IX. a. Define community health team
  b. List the members of community health team
  c. Explain the role of male health worker in community health team.
  OR
  a. Define fertility
  b. List the determinants of fertility
  c. Explain the benefits of fertility regulation.

X. a. What is expanded program of immunization
  b. Explain the role of a nurse in Pulse Polio Program.

SECTION-I

I. Give the meaning of the following:

a. Cold chain

The "cold chain" is the name given to a system of people and equipment which ensures that the correct quantity of potent vaccine reaches the women and children who need it from the point of production. The cold chain system is necessary because vaccines are delicate substances that lose potency if they are exposed to temperatures that are too warm or too cold. High levels of immunization coverage are useless if the vaccine that was used is not potent!

The "cold chain" is a system of transporting and storing vaccines within a recommended temperature range of +2 to +8 degrees Celsius (°C). This temperature range has been selected by the World Health Organization (WHO), and adopted by the Australian Technical Advisory Group on Immunization (ATAGI) for the National Immunization Programme (NIP), as a guide to protect vaccines against loss of vaccine potency due to excessive cold or heat1

b. Infant mortality rate

The **infant mortality rate** (IMR) is the number of **deaths** of **infants** under one year old per 1,000 live births. This **rate** is often used as an indicator of the level of health in a country. The **infant mortality rate** of the world is 49.4 according to the United Nations and 42.09 according to the CIA World Fact book.

c. Demography

Demography is derived from two Greek words "demos" meaning the people and graphein" meaning the record. Demography deals with the study of the size, the composition and the distribution of human population at a point of time. Community health nursing and population plays a significant relationship people is the basic unity of community health care.

Definitions of Demography

Demography is as branch of science which studies the human population and their elements. The elements are change in the size of population, structure of population and geographical distribution of population.

Demography is the scientific study of human population, such as changes in population size, the composition of the population and distribution of population in space. It also deals with five "demographic process" namely fertility, mortality, marriage, migration and social mobility.

Sources of Demography

Census: The word census originated from the Latin word censere which means to Assess or to rate. The first census of India was conducted in 1872, hence the census of 1881 is considered as the first systematic census of India. Census 2001 is the 14th census, the 6th census of independent India and the first of 21st century.

Vital registration: It is a process of recording vital events that occur in a population from time to time, the events registered related to births, deaths and marriage. Vital registration helps in planning, implementation and evaluation of community health services/programs.

Institutional records: The records are routinely maintained by various categories of hospitals and health care institutions, operating at various levels, have limited public health relevance.

d. Community development

Community development is a process where **community** members come together to take collective action and generate solutions to common problems.

Community development is a way of strengthening civil society by prioritising the actions of communities, and their perspectives in the development of social, economic and environmental policy. It seeks the empowerment of local communities, taken to mean both geographical communities, communities of interest or identity and communities organizing around specific themes or policy initiatives. It strengthens the capacity of people as active citizens through their community groups, organizations and networks; and the capacity of institutions and agencies (public, private and non-governmental) to work in dialogue with citizens to shape and determine change in their communities. It plays a crucial role in supporting active democratic life by promoting the autonomous voice of disadvantaged and vulnerable communities. It has a set of core values/social principles covering human rights, social inclusion, equality and respect for diversity; and a specific skills and knowledge base. Good community development is action that helps people to recognize and develop their ability and potential and organize themselves to respond to problems and needs which they share. It supports the establishment of strong communities that control and use assets to promote social justice and help improve the quality of community life. It also enables community and public agencies to work together to improve the quality of government.

II. State whether the following statement are *true* or *false*

a. The road to health card is a important tools for monitoring growth of under five children: **TRUE**
b. The world tuberculosis day is celebrated on 5th September: **FALSE**
c. In India there is one primary health center for every 30,000 population: **FALSE**
d. The route of administration of BCG is intramuscular: **FALSE**

III. Write short notes on any *three* of the following:

a. Health organization at district level

Bhore Committee 1946 recommended integrated services at all levels and the setting up of a unified health authority in each district. The principal unit of administration in India is the district under The district health organization is headed by chief medical officer of health (CMOH) who is the director of health service at the district. He is assisted by a number of officer's in-charge of different programs. They are district family welfare officer (DFWO), district malaria officer (DMO), district leprosy officer (DLO), district health officer (DHO), civil surgeon in-charge district hospital.

The health organization at the district level includes:
a. The chief medical officer of the district and his assistant staff
b. The district hospital and the district stores
c. The network of primary health centers and dispensaries.

Functions of District Health Organization
1. Primary health care
2. Secondary and referral health care.
3. Family welfare
4. National health programs.

Bhore Committee 1946 recommended integrated services at all levels and the setting up of a unified health authority in each district. The principal unit of administration in India is the district under a collector. There are 593 (year 2001) districts in India. The districts vary widely in area and population.

Each district has 6 types of administrative areas – sub-divisions, Tehsils (Talukas), community development blocks, municipalities and corporations, villages and panchayats. Most of the districts in India are divided into (two or more sub divisions, each in charge of an assistant collector or subcollector. Each division is again divided into tehsils (taluks) in charge of a tehsildar. A tehsildar usually comprises between 200 to 600 villages.

The district officer is in charge of all health administration and all National health programs are implemented in the district except family welfare program. The district family welfare and maternal and child health officer is in charge of family welfare program. Both of them have control over primary health center

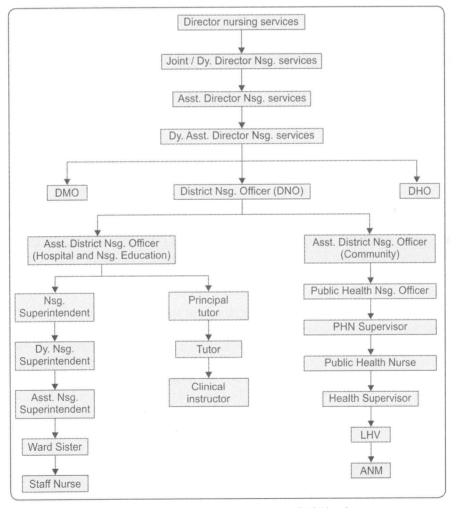

Recommended organizational set-up at district level

The district health organization is headed by chief medical officer of health (CMOH) who is the director of health service at the district. He is assisted by a number of officers in charge of different programs. They are district family welfare officer (DFWO) District Malaria officer (DMO), District Leprosy officer (DLO), District Health officer (DHO), Civil Surgeon in charge district hospital.

The health organization at the district level includes
a. The chief medical officer of the district and his assistant staff
b. The district hospital and the district stores
c. The network of Primary health centers and dispensaries.

Functions of district health organization
1. Primary health care
2. Secondary and referral health care.
3. Family welfare
4. National health programs

b. Reproductive and child health services

Reproductive and child health approach has been defined as "people having the ability to reproduce and regulate their fertility". Women are able to go through pregnancy and child birth safely. The outcome of pregnancies is successful in terms of maternal and Infant Survival and well-being and couples are able to have sexual relations free of fear of pregnancy and of contracting diseases. This concept is in keeping with the evolution of an integrated approach to the programmes aimed at improving the health status of young women and children, namely, National Family Welfare Programme, Universal Immunization Programme. Oral Rehydration Therapy, Child Survival and Safe, Motherhood (CSSM) Programme.

The RCH programme incorporates the components relating to CSSM and includes two addition components, one relating to sexually transmitted diseases (STD) and other relating to reproductive tract infections (RTI). The Universal Immunization Programme (UIP) became a part of CSSM programme in 1992 and RCH programme in 1997. It will continue to provide vaccines for polio, tetanus, DPT, DT, measles and tuberculosis. The cold chain established so far will be maintained and additional items will be provided to new health facilities.

c. Under-five clinic

The under-five's clinic or well baby clinic's combines the concepts of prevention, treatment, health supervision, nutritional surveillance and education into a system of comprehensive health care within the resources available in the country, making use of non professional auxillaries, thus making the service not only economical but also available to a larger proportion of children in the community. Under-five clinics must provide for courteous reception of mother and children, with enthusiasm and zeal on the part of each member of the team.

Aims of Under-five Clinics

Care in illness: The basic philosophy of the "under-five's" clinic to give nurses effective training and responsibility for handling the child healthcare service. The illness care for children will comprise of diagnosis and treatment, X-ray and laboratory services and referral services.

Preventive care: The prevent care give on the bases of immunization, nutritional surveillance, health checkups, oral rehydration, family planning and health education.

Growth monitoring: For under five clinic to weigh the child periodically at monthly intervals during the first year, every 2 months during the second year and every 3 months thereafter up to the age of 5–6 years. The growth curve will help the health worker to detect early onset of growth failure.

Objectives of under-five clinic's
1. The prevention of malnutrition, pertussis, tuberclosis, poliomyelitis, diphtheria, tetanus and measles.
2. The supervision of the health of all children upon the age of five.
3. The education of parents to promote health and family planning.
4. The provision of simple treatment for diarrhea, with or without dehydration, pneumonia, skin conditions and other common disorders.

Role of a nurse in under-fives clinic
1. Treating minor illness
2. Referring the more seriously ill children.
3. Instructing about feeding, nutrition and hygiene.
4. Encouraging child spacing and family planning.
5. Maintaining the children's weight cards, e.g. road to good health cards.
6. Being alert in every in which the effectiveness of the service can be improved.

Physical Facilities for a children's clinic
1. Outside compound: Playground for children waiting to be served including swings slides and sand box are needed. These facilities may be provided by the community volunteer group or by the health committee.
2. Waiting room should include a reception table and the record. The area should include child health posters, display exhibits and play are for the children.
3. Weighing and measuring should be provided in a separate area if possible or it may be part of the waiting room.
4. Isolation area for children with signs and symptoms of illness is essential for every child health clinic.

d. Preventive and promotive school health services

A health promoting school is one that constantly strengthens its capacity as a healthy setting for living, learning and working. A health promoting school:
1. Fosters health and learning with all the measures at its disposal.
2. Engages health and education officials, teachers, teachers' unions, students, parents, health providers and community leaders in efforts to make the school a healthy place.
3. Strives to provide a healthy environment, school health education, and school health services along with school/community projects and outreach, health promotion programs for staff, nutrition and food safety programs, opportunities for physical education and recreation, and programs for counseling, social support and mental health promotion.
4. Implements policies and practices that respect an individual's well being and dignity, provide multiple opportunities for success, and acknowledge good efforts and intentions as well as personal achievements.
5. Strives to improve the health of school personnel, families and community members as well as pupils; and works with community leaders to help them understand how the community contributes to, or undermines, health and education.

IV. a. Define MCH services. b. Write the objectives of MCH services. c. Explain the role of community health nurse in MCH services

Maternal and child health services are directed towards children in order to maintain total well-being of the child within the framework of the family and the community. Every aspect of community health programs in India has marked effects on the health and welfare of expectant mothers and particularly of infants and children. New maternal and child health care (MCH) which now also being described as reproductive and child health (RCH). Reproductive child health can be defined as a state in which "people have the ability to reproduce and regulate their fertility or women have the ability to reproduce and regulate their fertility or women are able to go through pregnancy and childbirth safety."

Objectives of MCH services
1. To give expert advice to the couples to plan their families.
2. To identify "high risk" cases so that can give them special attention.
3. To provide health supervision for antenatal mothers also to foresee complications and prevention.
4. To give skilled assistance at the time of child birth and during puerperium.
5. To supervise trained dais, community health volunteers and community health workers.
6. To impart useful knowledge on desirable health practices which mother should carry out during pregnancy, labor and during puerperium.
7. Encourage the deliveries by trained workers in the safe and clean environment.
8. Prevent communicable and non-communicable diseases.
9. Educate the mother to improve their own and children's health.

Role of nurse in MCH services:
1. **Reduction of maternal, perinatal, health** is an important function of the primary health centres in India. There should be special clinic days and time set apart for this work. The services of specialists should be enlisted as and when necessary. That is, the school health clinic should be linked up with the PHC and higher levels of health care.
2. **Immunizations:** The school offers excellent opportunities for Immunization for children. Immunization by 1990 was part of a global effort coordinated by the World Health Organization. The national immunization schedule is given below.
3. **School sanitation:** The school should be a model of good sanitation. There should be adequate, safe drinking water facilities preferably supplied by a tube well. Urinals and privies should be provided - one urinal for 60 students and one sanitary latrine for 100 students. Arrangements should be separate for boys and girls. Vendors other than those approved by the school health authority should not be allowed inside school premises. A healthful school environment is necessary for the best emotional, social and personal health of the pupils.
4. **Nutritional services:** A child, who is physically weak because of poor nutrition, cannot be expected to take full advantage of schooling. The community health nurse may be required to administer the following nutrition programs: (a) Midday school meal (b) vitamin A prophylaxis program—administration of a large dose (200,000 IU) of vitamin A orally to children every 6 months up to the age of 6 years or so.
5. **First aid:** In every school, a fully equipped First Aid Box should be at hand. The emergencies commonly met with in schools are: (a) accidents (b) Injuries (c) medical emergencies like abdominal pain, epileptic fits, fainting, etc.

6. **Health education:** Health education has an important role to play in the promotion of both individual and community health. Health education in schools should not be reduced merely to teach the children a set of rules of hygiene. Participation of children in community health programmes (e.g., construction of wells, latrines, vaccination campaigns, etc) should be encouraged, whenever possible. The hygiene of skin, hair, teeth and clothing; the importance of exercise, sleep, nutrition and good habits; the need for Immunization, safe water, control of flies and other/insects are some of the topics on which health education may be profitably-Imparted.
7. **School health records:** The health record of each student should be properly maintained. The record should contain
   1. Identifying data—name, date of birth and address
   2. Past health history
   3. Record of findings of physical examination and screening
   4. Record of services provided.

   These records, besides providing Information on the health aspects of school children, also serve as a useful link between the home, school and community.

Or

a. What is occupational health, b. List the important occupational diseases, c. Discuss the role of a nurse in industrial health nursing

Occupational health refers to the identification and control of the risks arising from physical, chemical, and other workplace hazards in order to establish and maintain a safe and healthy working environment. These hazards may include chemical agents and solvents, heavy metals, such as lead and mercury, physical agents, such as loud noise or vibration, and physical hazards, such as electricity or dangerous machinery. The care of healthy people is the principal function of an occupational health service. This is quite unlike the care of sick people in a hospital setting. Doctors and nurses who are accustomed to the background of illness-oriented or curative medicine may not be quite successful in an occupational setting unless they are oriented to work in the care of healthy groups. The aim of occupational health service is to keep the people at work healthy and to prevent them from falling ill. The whole emphasis is on prevention of ill-health and promotion of health.

Definition
1. Occupational Health is the promotion and maintenance of the highest degree of physical, mental and social well-being of workers in all occupations by preventing departures from health, controlling risks and the adaptation of work to people, and people to their jobs (ILO/WHO 1950).
2. Occupational health nursing is the application of nursing practice and public health procedures for the purpose of conversing, promoting and restoring the health of individuals and groups through their places of employment.

Occupational diseases: Diseases that are peculiar to occupational situations, or that are more common in defined occupations as compared to the general population, are known as occupational diseases. Following are the common occupational diseases and their responsible agents:

Agent Category	Agent	Occupational disease(s)
Physical agents	High pressure	Caisson disease
	Low pressure	Pulmonary edema, air embolism
	Electricity	Shock and burns
	Heat	Stroke, exhaustion and cramps
	Cold	Frost bite, trench foot, chilblains
	Light	Nystagmus
	Noise	Deafness, tympanic membrane rupture
	Vibrations	Raynaud's phenomenon
	Radiations	Leukemia, aplastic anemia, cancers
	Gravity, kinetic energy	Accidents
Chemical agents		
	Dusts	Pneumoconiosis
	Acids, alkalis, resins, etc	Dermatitis, chemical burns
	Lead	Plumbism
	Benzene, vinyl chloride	Cancers
Biological agents	B. anthracis	Anthrax
	B. abortus	Brucellosis
	Cl. tetani	Tetanus
	L. icterohemorrhagiea	Leptospirosis

Biological hazards and occupational health: Workers occupied in Agriculture dealing with infected animals and infected animal material like hides and skins are exposed to a host of zoonotic diseases of viral, bacterial protozoal and metazoal origin. Workers engaged in field areas suffer from a variety of environmental infective diseases which may be dust borne, soil borne, water borne or vector borne.

Diseases of environmental origin
1. **Schistosomiasis:** Occupation hazard of agriculture workers who are exposed to contaminated water containing swimming larcae (cercariae) of the parasites of schistosoma species releasing by snails. Man is the principal reservoir of schistosoma mansoni and *S. haematobium* causes painless terminal haematuria, pulmonary hypertension and cor. pulmonale.
2. **Coccidioidomycosis:** the disease initially resembles an acute fibrile illness characterized by chills, cough, and chest pain. Skin lesions of coccidioi domycosis include erythema nodosum and erythema multiformae.
3. **Blastomycosis:** The disease exists in respiratory and cutaneous forms. The respiratory form presents as upper respiratory tract infection characterized by fever, cough and purulent sputum eventually leading to weight loss and chchexia. The cutaneous form of the disease starts as a papulae which appears at the site of the entry.
4. **Histoplasmosis:** It is transmitted by inhalation of air borne spores of *Histoplasma capsulatum* which is a fungus that grows on soil rich in organic matter. It starts as a mild respiratory illness associated with fever, cough chest pain and malaise. The disease eventually results in splenomegaly and lymphadenopathy.
5. **Nocardiosis:** the disease as a localized lesion (mycetoma) at the site of the entry. It spreads by hematogeous route, including the brain and the meninges.

Diseases of zoonotic origin:
1. **Leptospirosis:** the infected animals that serve as reservoirs are cattle, dogs, hogs, rats and mice. The leptospires penetrate skin or mucous membrane of the host who initially develops

fever, chills, headache, and vomiting and malaise. The disease may eventually lead to myalgia, conjunctivitis, meningeal irritation and jaundice which may progress to hemorrhage anemia, renal insufficiency, and hemorrhage in skin and mucous membranes.

2. **Psittacosis:** Psittacosis or parrot fever is a disease of poultry raisers, duck and turkey raisers, poultry dressers, pet shop keepers, pigeon keepers and zoo attendants. Psittacosis is an acute infectious disease characterized by fever, headache, cough, pneumonia and several systemic manifestations.
3. **Q fever:** It is an air-born disease of wild and domestic animals caused by *Coxiella burneti*. Q fever is acute febrile influenza like illness characterized by sudden onsets, chills, sweats, headache, myalgia and weakness. The disease may also lead to pneumonia associated with mild cough, scanty sputum and chest pain.
4. **Anthrax:** caused by *Bacillus antharacis*. It transmitted by contact with infected animals or contaminated animal material and inhalation of infected dust. The clinical features are skin lesion with cellulites (malignant pustule) sever pneumonia (Woolsorter's disease)
5. **Tularemia:** caused by *Pasteurella tularensis*. The disease transmitted by direct contact with infected animals or infected animal materials. Technical features are cutaneous ulcers, lymphadenitis fever, chills and prostration.

Byssinosis: Byssinosis (from 'byssos,' white thread) also called brown lung: (a misnomer as lung in this condition does not turn brown) occurs in cotton, hemp, flax and sisal mills, cottonseed oil mifis, bedding factories and cotton-waste utilization industries. In the textile mills, the hazardous processes are opening the bales, separation of lint from the impurities, and carding; hazard is moderate in spinning, winding and twisting; and least in weaving. About 8% of workers in textile mills develop byssinosis. The clinical features of byssinosis are chest tightness and shortness of breath. Symptoms are worst on the first day of the working week. There are no characteristic radiological features. Byssinosis is prevented through the following measures:
1. Provision of local exhaust ventilation.
2. Use of masks or respirators with filters by the workers at risk.
3. Rotation of workers.
4. Early detection of byssinosis, and provision for the affected workers of alternative employment in dust free areas

Currently occupational environment in the industrialized world is challenging health and safety of man. The risk associated with modern occupation necessitates the adaptation of man to industrial environment on the one hand and his protection from the risks on the other. These risks referred to occupational hazards threaten the physical, mental, social and psychological health of workers. Occupational hazards are classified as physical, chemical and biological.

I. High temperature-occupational exposure: Extremely high temperature is experienced by construction workers, bakers, blacksmiths, chefs and dry cleaners. Workers working under high temperature may suffer from heat cramps, heat exhaustion or heat strokes.
1. **Heat cramps:** Caused when workers lose fluids and electrolytes from their bodies due to excessive sweating. Cramps develop in limbs and abdomen the pain in the lower limbs starts characteristically from calf muscles.
2. **Heat exhaustion:** There is peripheral vasodilatation leading to circulatory collapse. It may be associated with mild manifestations like headache, fatigue and dizziness.
3. **Heat stroke:** Extreme form of heat stresses which results unconsciousness without any prodromal symptoms.

II. Low temperature: Extreme low temperature in outdoor workers in cold northern regions of the world. Disease associates with cold stress are chilblains, trench foot and frostbite.

1. The common complication of mumps includes orchitis and epididymitis results testicular swelling tenderness, scrotal erythema with or without epididymitis. Mumps meningitis occurs in about 10% of mumps victims and affects male patients three to five times more often than female patients. The symptoms include fever, meningeal irritation (nuchal rigidity, headache and irritability, vomiting, drowsiness and a cerebro spinal fluid (CSF) lymphocyte count from 500–2000/mm^3.
2. Less common complications include pancreatitis, transient sensorineural hearing loss, transverse myelitis, arthritis, myocarditis, pericarditis, oophoritis, pancreatitits, diabetes mellitus, arthritis, thyroiditis and nephritis.

Role of nurses in occupational health services

Nurses will have to function within the framework of the above listed functions, which are mostly preventive in nature.

Accordingly the role of nurses will include the following:
1. She will assist the medical officer at examination of employees.
2. She will take an intelligent interest to protect and improve the physical and mental health of all workers.
3. She will attend to daily treatment of minor injuries, and assist the doctor when necessary.
4. She must have good knowledge of first aid.
5. She must be able to identify, assess and advise management on the control of any health hazards affecting employees.
6. She may have to run an immunization clinic, antenatal clinic or school health clinic.
7. She has to conduct health education in all situations.
8. She may undertake home visiting and propagate the ideas of health and family welfare.

The occupational health nurse must have a strong bias towards preventive medicine. One nurse can deal with between 500 and 2000 work people. She should attend refresher in-service training courses from time to time.

Functions of occupational health nurse

1. Assistance in general administration, maintenance and arrangements of health facilities in the plant.
2. Emergency and primary treatment of accidents and illness based on standing orders from physicians.
3. Arranging follow up treatments, where indicated, including health supervision of employees returning to work after illness.
4. Assistance in general preventive health measures in the plant.
5. Health education and counseling for employees.
6. Assistance in supervision of factory hygiene and accident prevention.
7. Advice on specific health questions to management and workers.
8. Maintenance of records and statistics.
9. Cooperation with and referral of workers to general community agencies for help as and when necessary.
10. Participation in a health surveillance program that includes the assessment and recording of the health status of employees.
11. Participation in the environmental control program the aims to work related.
12. Counseling and crisis intervention for those individuals experiencing work related problems and health promotion through specific health education and screening programs.

Specific Areas and Activities of Occupational Health Nurse
1. Shop floor health care—Field health survey practice
2. Occupational medicine—Clinical practice
3. Occupational hygiene—working environment hazards monitoring
4. Health supervision of worker—Surveillari of health.
5. Health education and counseling.
6. Occupational health services—Administration.

V. a. Define primary health care, b. Write the elements of primary health care, c. Explain the role of a nurse in primary health care

Primary health care shifts the emphasis of health care to the people themselves and their needs, reinforcing and strengthening their own capacity to shape their lives. Hospitals and primary health centers then become only one aspect of the system in which health care is provided. As a philosophy, primary health care is based on the overlap of mutuality, social justice and equality. As a strategy, primary health care focuses on individual and community strengths (assets) and opportunities for change (needs); maximizes the involvement of the community; includes all relevant sectors but avoids duplication of services; and uses only health technologies that are accessible, acceptable, affordable and appropriate.

Definition: Primary health care is essential health care made universally accessible to individuals and families in the community, by means acceptable to them, through their full participation and at a cost that the community and country can afford. It forms an integral part both of the country's health system of which it is the nucleus and the overall social and economic development of the community (Alma Ata 1978).

Essential components: Primary health care needs to be delivered close to the people; thus, should rely on maximum use of both lay and professional healthcare practitioners and includes the following eight essential components:
1. Education for the identification and prevention/control of prevailing health challenges
2. Proper food supplies and nutrition; adequate supply of safe water and basic sanitation
3. Maternal and child care, including family planning
4. Immunization against the major infectious diseases
5. Prevention and control of locally endemic diseases
6. Appropriate treatment of common diseases using appropriate technology
7. Promotion of mental, emotional and spiritual health
8. Provision of essential drugs (WHO and UNICEF, 1978).

Characteristics of health care
1. **Relevance:** Health services should be in accordance with health requirements, priorities, and policies.
2. **Comprehensiveness:** It should incorporate the preventive, therapeutic and health promotion services in suitable proportions.
3. **Availability and adequacy:** Health services should be appropriate and proportionate to the population and also, enough to satisfy people's needs.
4. **Feasibility:** For the skilled management of health services, these should be logical, and in accordance to the available resources like, time, labor and the material, etc.
5. **Accessibility:** Services should be available within the geographical and economic limits. These should be within the reach of citizens and should be taking care of their cultural values and realities.

Goals of primary health care:
The ultimate goal of primary health care is better health for all. The WHO has identified five key elements to achieving that goal:
1. Reducing exclusion and social disparities in health (universal coverage reforms).
2. Organizing health services around people's needs and expectations (service delivery reforms).
3. Integrating health into all sectors (public policy reforms).
4. Pursuing collaborative models of policy dialogue (leadership reforms), and
5. Increasing stakeholder participation.

Attributes of primary health care:
1. **Accessibility:** Primary health care permeates uniformly to reach equitably to all segments of population.
2. **Acceptability:** Primary health care achieves acceptability through cultural assimilation of its policies and programs.
3. **Adaptability:** Primary healthcare system is highly flexible and adaptable. It believes in "adaptation" rather than "adaptation".
4. **Affordability:** Primary health care is affordable to consumer as well as providers.
5. **Availability:** Primary health care is always ready to respond to any demand at any time.
6. **Appropriateness:** Primary healthcare system evolves from the socioeconomic conditions, social values and health situation of a community, it is quite appropriate from all angles.
7. **Closeness:** Primary health center is close at hand to people at their door steps.
8. **Continuity:** Primary health service is a continuous service which extends from "womb" to tomb and addresses the changing needs of an individual in all situations of health and disease.
9. **Comprehensiveness:** Primary health care is comprehensive and the curative needs of the community.
10. **Coordinativeness:** Primary health care is dependent on inner – sectoral coordination and community participation.

Role of nurses in primary health care

Recognizing the substantial contribution made to primary health care by the nursing profession, as stated in resolution WHA30.48, a well as the progress made by WHO in increasing the effectiveness o nursing/midwifery personnel in providing primary health care and Member States in making primary health care available to all groups; Further recognizing the valuable contribution made by other health personnel to primary health care in the Western Pacific Region, and the need for better utilization of basic nursing skill in the multidisciplinary approach to primary health care. REQUESTS the Executive Board to consider recommending to the World Health Assembly that a resolution on the role of nursing in primary health care should be adopted, with the following operative, paragraphs:

URGES Member States
1. To promote and encourage greater emphasis on primary health care in nursing education curricula.
2. To take active steps to increase the participation of health personnel from the nursing discipline in planning, management, training and research in relation to the development of health systems through primary health care.

REQUESTS the Director-General:
1. To support Member States in:
    a. Promoting and encouraging greater emphasis on primary health care in nursing education curricula.

b. Taking active steps to increase the participation of health personnel from the nursing discipline in planning, management, training and research in relation to the development of health systems through primary health care.
2. To ensure that the nursing aspect of WHO's cooperation with Member States in relation to primary health care is strengthened.

SECTION-II

VI. Choose the correct answer and write:
a. The state of highest literacy rate in India is: **iii**
   i. Maharashtra, ii. Tamilnadu, iii. Kerala
b. The year of last census done in India: **ii**
   i. 2010, ii. 2011, iii. 2012
c. The route of administration of measles vaccine is: **i**
   i. subcutaneous, ii. Intradermal, iii. Intramuscular
d. The world AIDS day is celebrated on: **ii**
   i. 20th august, ii. 1st December, iii. 14th November

VII. State whether the following statement are *true* or *false*
a. The number of death occurs before 28 days of birth per 1000 live births is termed as under-five mortality rate: **FALSE**
b. The branch of statistics related to biological events and to mathematical facts is called biostatistics**: TRUE**
c. Malaria is transmitted by anopheles mosquito: **TRUE**

VIII. Write short notes on any *three* of the following:

a. Aids control program
National AIDS Control Programme was launched in India in the year 1987. The Ministry of Health and Family Welfare has set up National AIDS Control Organization (NACO) as a separate wing to implement and closely monitor the various components of the program. The aim of the program is to prevent further transmission of HIV, to decrease morbidity and mortality associated with HIV infection and to minimize the socioeconomic impact resulting from HIV infection.

The national strategy has the following components:
1. Establishment of surveillance centers to cover the whole country.
2. Identification of high risk group and their screening.
3. Issuing specific guidelines for management of detected cases and their follow-up.
4. Formulating guidelines for blood bank, blood product manufacturers, blood donors and dialysis units.
5. Information education and communication activities by involving mass media and research for reduction of personal and social impact of the disease.
6. Control of sexually transmitted disease and condom program.

b. Importance of vital statistics

Vital statistics are statistics on live births, deaths, fetal deaths, marriages and divorces. The most common way of collecting information on these events is through civil registration an administrative system used by governments to record vital events which occur in their populations. Efforts to improve the quality of vital statistics will therefore be closely related to the development of civil registration systems in countries. Vital statistics are, well, vital to public health. Vital statistics include information on births, deaths and a lot of health information generated in between. Before public health officials can know what the needs of a population are and how to address them, they must have data on the prevalence of disease and major health issues. Most national governments by law mandate the collection of vital statistics.

Uses of vital statistics
1. To evaluate the impact of various national health programmers.
2. To plan for better future measures of disease control.
3. To elucidate the hereditary nature of disease
4. To plan and evaluate economic and social development.
5. It is a primary tool in research activities.
6. To determine the health status of individual.
7. To compare the health status of one nation with others.

Maternity: Many of the greatest advances in medicine have come as a result of public health interventions rather than individual treatments. The ability to intervene in the health of populations is dependent upon development of appropriate tools for measuring health, illness, and interventions. Only by standardizing communication on such issues as infant mortality can physicians hope to target high-risk populations with effective interventions. Despite the lack of clinical glamour associated with the subject of vital statistics, understanding the common language of public health is vital.

c. Natural methods of family planning

1. **Total sexual abstinence:** It costs nothing except self denial on the part of the couple.
2. **Periodic abstinence:** It is otherwise called as rhythm or calendar method or safe method. It is based on restricting the sex act to the infertile period of the female partner.
3. **Temperature method:** During ovulation naturally the basal body temperature rise of 0.5°C. Based on prediction of the time of ovulation by taking the basal body temperature daily and avoiding sexual intercourse around the time of ovulation.
4. **Billing method:** It relies on the charges in cervical mucus secretion also called mucus method. This method is based on observation of changes in the characteristics of cervical mucus.
5. **Symptothermic method:** This method combines the use of basal body temperature with analysis of cervical mucus changes to make temperature with analysis of cervical mucus changes to make predictions more accurate.
6. **Coitus interruptus:** It is an ancient method that requires the male to withdraw his penis from the vagina immediately before the ejaculation of the semen.
7. **Coitus reservants:** In this method, penetration of the vagina takes placed but there is little or no motion and the man does not ejaculate into the vagina.
8. **Coitus interfemoris:** The erect penis is placed between the thighs of the female.
9. **Lactation amenorrhea method:** It is believed that there is a high probability that the women who is amenorrheal while breastfeeding, will be able to regulate her fertility in first 6 months postpartum even if she introduces supplementation in the baby's feeding.

10. **Barrier method:** Barrier methods of contraception have a long history. The ancient Egyptians used such methods which consisted of honey-coated pessaries. Honey is effective in killing sperms as well as bacteria.

d. Intrauterine contraceptives

Intrauterine device is inserted into the cavity to prevent conception. The device which are placed in the womb. The device may be inert or medicated. The inert device is made up of plastic material only and the medicated devices are fortified with copper, silver or a progestation preparation.

1. **Lippes loop:** It is a double S shaped serpentine device made of polythene impregnated with barium sulfate for radiopacity. Two pieces of nylon (transcervical threads) are attached to the lower end of the loop forming tail, the nylon tail projects into the vagina. Periodic feeling for the tail reassures the user that the loop is in place. The tail also helps in easy removal of the device.
2. **Copper–T:** The copper T is made of plastic but is wrapped with fine copper which enhances its contraceptive effect. Its acceptance is higher than that of the loop. It is T-shaped bioactive contraceptive device made of polyethylene or any other polymer and reinforced with copper metal. The devices are impregnated with barium sulfate for radiopacity and are fitted with two transcervical threads at the tail end. Metallic copper possess a strong antifertility action.

IX. a. Define community health team, b. List the members of community health team, c. Explain the role of male health worker in community health team

The functions of health team members depend upon their status in health team, qualification or the work assigned to them by the team leader. The work of most of the members of the health team is determined either by their post or according to the job chart. Other members of the team (those who are not related directly to health services) fulfill the responsibilities entrusted to them and in achieving the objectives of the health team.

Staffing pattern in PHC
Staffing pattern at PHC: In the new set-up each PHC will have the following staff:

At the PHC level
- Medical Officer   1
- Pharmacist   1
- Nurse mid-wife   1
- Health worker female   1
- Block extension educator   1
- Health Assistant male   1
- Health assistant Female/LHV   1
- VDC   1
- LDC   1
- LAB Technician   1
- Driver subject to availabilty of vehicle   1
- Class   4

Total   **15**

Staff for Community Health Center
Medical Officer   4
Nurse Mid-Wives   7

Dresser	1
Phamalist/Compounder	1
Laboratory technician	1
Radio grapher	1
Ward boys	2
Dhobi	1
Sweepers	3
Mali	1
Chowkidar	1
Aya	1
Poen	1
Total	**25**

The primary health center is the first contact point between the village community and the medical officer. These are established and maintained by the state government under the Minimum Needs Basic Minimum Services Programme. A PHC is manned by a medical officer, health assistant (female and male), and health worker (female)! ANM, Nurse and Midwife, block extension educator, pharmacy, lab technician and is supported by 14 paramedical and other staff. It acts as a referral unit for six subcenters and has 4–6 beds. The activities of PHCs involve curative, preventive, promotive and family welfare services. The number of PHCs functioning in the country is 22,975.

The mere presence of a variety of health professionals is not sufficient to establish team 'work' it is the props division and combination of their operations from which the benefits of divided labour will be derived.

The health team at the primary health center consists of the following health personnel:

SUBCENTER: The staff at each sub center consists of:
1. Health worker (male)
2. Health worker (female)

Voluntary worker (paid Rs 50 per month as honorarium) The male and female health workers are multipurpose workers trained for definite tasks and functions which comprise the following:
1. Treatment of minor illness.
2. Maternal and child health.
3. Family planning.
4. Control of communicable diseases.
5. Immunization.
6. Dais training.
7. Nutrition (distribution of iron and folic acid tablets and vitamin A, etc).
8. Record keeping.
9. Referral services.

It has been proposed that facilities for IUD insertion and simple laboratory investigations like routine examination of urine for albumin and sugar would be established at each subcenter. The female health assistant supervises the work of female health workers.

Male health worker
At subcenter along with female multipurpose health worker, a male multipurpose health worker is also needed. In this direction, union government has started a training program to

convert single purpose workers into multipurpose workers. Under this program, 10th class pass candidates are selected, trained for one year and then appointed at subcenters. This program was started in 47 health and family welfare training centers' and is 100% central sponsored. In order to compensate the deficiency of male multipurpose workers, 28 family welfare training centers and 23 multipurpose workers (male) basic school, are giving training to the male workers (2005).

Job responsibilities of male health worker: Under the Multipurpose Workers Scheme a health assistant male is expected to cover a population of 30,000 (20,000 in tribal and hilly areas) in which there are six subentries, each with one health worker male. The health assistant male will carry out the following functions:

Supervision and Guidance
1. Supervise and guide the health worker male in the delivery of health care services to the community.
2. Strengthen the knowledge and skills of the health worker male.
3. Help the health worker male in improving his skills in working in the community.
4. Help and guide the health worker male in planning and organizing his programme of activities.
5. Visit each health workers male at least once a week on a fixed day to observe and guide him in his day-to-day activities.
6. Assess monthly the progress of work of the health worker male and submit an assessment report to the medical officer of the primary health center.
7. Carry out supervisory home visits in the area of the health worker male.

Teamwork
1. Help the health workers to work as part of the health team.
2. Co-ordinate his activities with those of the health assistant female and other health personnel, including the health guides and dais.
3. Coordinate the health activities in his area with the activities of workers of other departments and agencies, and attend meetings at PHC level.
4. Conduct staff meetings fortnightly with the health workers in coordination with the health assistant female at one of the subcenter by rotation.
5. Attend staff meetings at the primary health center.
6. Assist the medical officer of the primary health center in the organization of the different health services in the area.
7. Participate as a member of the health team in mass camps and campaigns in health programs.
8. Assist the medical officer of the primary health center in conducting training programs for various categories of health personnel.

Supplies and Equipment
1. In collaboration with the health assistant female, check at regular intervals the stores available at the sub center and ensure timely placement of indent for and procuring the supplies and equipment in good time.
2. Check that the drugs at the subcenter are properly stored and that the equipment is well maintained.
3. Ensure that the health worker male maintains his kits in a proper way.
4. Records and Reports scrutinize the maintenance of records by the health
5. Worker male and guide him in their proper maintenance.

OR

a. Define fertility, b. List the determinants of fertility, c. Explain the benefits of fertility regulation

Fertility is the ability to have reproduced and have children. The definition of fertile means that you are able to initiate the act of intercourse, and cause or sustain a pregnancy with a live fetus. There are many different things that can affect fertility. Men need to have enough healthy sperm available, the sperm needs to be able to make the egg to fertilize, and women need to be able to ovulate. When you think about the factors involved, everything has to be just right for optimal fertility. This article will help you understand fertility and reproduction better.

Definition
Fertility refers to the childbearing performance and **fecundity** to the childbearing capacity. Fertility is a voluntary biological process; fecundity is an inherent physiological capacity.

Fertility means the actual bearing of children; fertility varies between individuals depending upon their reproductive behavior.

Determinants of fertility
Age at marriage: If the marriage of a girl coincides with her menarche, i.e. she is married tat 15 years of age, she has a scope for bearing children for the full reproductive span of about 30 years. A delay in the marriage reduces fertility by reducing the reproductive span.

Duration of marriage: A marital life that outlasts the reproductive span of the female spouse has the maximum fertility by reducing the reproductive span.

Spacing of children: Increase in the interpregnancy intervals reduces fertility, the increase may occur naturally as a consequence of exclusive breastfeeding for long periods or artificially by practicing various methods of contraception.

Child survival: People have no faith in the survival of their children because of high infant and child mortality rates in developing countries.

Educational status: Illiterate women are known to be highly fertile. Increase in educational level of women is associated with decrease in their total fertility rate.

Economic stability: Fertility is high in poor income families an higher the income of families, the lower their fertility rate.

Cultural beliefs and practices: It modifies the lifestyle of people and influences their reproductive behavior and fertility outcome.

General determinants of fertility
1. Heredity
2. Health
3. Age
4. Emotional surroundings
5. Ovulation cycle

6. Lactation
7. Pregnancy wastage

The 7 proximate determinants are:
1. Proportion of married women among all women of reproductive age.
2. Contraceptive use and effectiveness.
3. Duration of postpartum infecundability (or postpartum insusceptibility)
4. Induced abortion.
5. Fecundability (including frequency and timing of intercourse)
6. Prevalence of permanent sterility.

Fertility regulation: Natural fertility refers to the absence of parity-specific family planning, meaning that couples are not regulating their fertility based on their current parity. Family planning, on the other hand, is when couples regulate their fertility (e.g. stop having children) after reaching a specific parity.

Principles of fertility regulation
1. Avoid untimely pregnancies
2. Avoid too close pregnancies
3. Avoid unwanted pregnancies
4. Avoid too many pregnancies
5. Avoid risky pregnancies.

Untimely pregnancies: The pregnancies are those that occur the two ends of the reproductive span of women. Women face increased risk of morbidity and mortality if they become pregnant below the age of 20 or above the age of 30.

Too close pregnancies: They undermine the health of mothers. An adequate interpregnancy interval is beneficial for the mother as well as for the two siblings.

Unwanted pregnancies: They are associated with high maternal and infant mortality. Unwanted pregnancies usually end in unsafe with superadded risks.

Too many pregnancies: They impose a continuous drain on the nutritional reserves of women leading to maternal deprivation depletion, reduced maternal competence and low productivity of mothers.

Pregnancy may aggravate coexisting maternal diseases, diabetes, heart diseases, tuberculosis, psychosis, chronic hypertension, chronic cerebral thrombosis and various types of blood disorders.

Benefits of fertility regulation
1. **Benefits of the mother:** Elimination of physical and mental strain, improvement in nutritional status of women and decrease maternal mortality and morbidity.
2. **Benefits to the child:** Baby get adequate birth weight and affectionate family environment, provision for adequate breast feedings ands reduced risk of congenital abnormalities, genetic disorders and vulnerability to infections.
3. **Benefits to the family:** Reasonable degree of health and happiness, economic security progress in health status, nutritional status, economic status, educational status, residential status and overall social status of the family.
4. **Benefits to the community:** Reduced demand for community facilities like housing, education, health care, water supply, communication, waste disposal services, marketing facilities, etc.

5. **Benefits to the country:** Stabilization and economic progress. Increased resource for providing better facilities of education, nutrition, health care, housing and communication. Decrease in the overall morbidity, mortality and fertility statistics of the country.

Approaches to fertility Regulation
1. **Educational approach:** It increases the awareness and importance of fertility regulation and methods available to practice.
2. **Service approach:** Service approach demands continuity of care as provided in antenatal and under five clinics. Service approach implies maintaining contact with acceptors of contraception and also involves follow up cases.
3. **Motivational approach:** Incentives may be offered to the acceptors on individual basis or on community basis. Those who volunteer for vasectomy or tubectomy may be paid compensation for loss of wages besides a cash incentive.
4. **Legal approach:** The most important legal measure is the child marriage Restraint Act that rises the legal age of marriage of boys and girls. Liberalization of Abortion Act is another legal measure to promote fertility control.
5. **Integrated approach:** It includes the elements of all other approaches and addresses all the problems connected with maternal and child health, inclusive of fertility control.

Methods of fertility regulation
Contraception: It is a process of interruption of conception at any stage preceding, accompanying or immediately following copulation. The methods used may be physiological, mechanical, chemical, hormonal or a combination thereof. Contraception may be achieved by using rhythm method, barrier contraceptives, intrauterine devices, hormonal contraceptives or post coital contraceptives.

Termination: It is a process of dislodging the implantation of a fertilized ovum or disallowing the continuation of a n established pregnancy. Termination can be done within a few days of missing a period or much later in pregnancy.

Sterilization: It is a surgical maneuver that arrests the fertility of an individual on permanent basis. It creates a mechanical barrier to the movement of ovum or sperms. It comprises vasectomy in the males and tubectomy in females.

Fertility Trends
Researches: They indicate that the level of fertility in India is beginning to decline. The crude birth rate was about 49 per 1000 population during 1901–11 has declined to about 13.3. per 1000 in 1991 and 25 per 1000 population in 2002. There are considerable interstate variations in fertility trends.

Birth and death rates: They have considerably declined from 27. in 1951 to an estimated 8.1 per 1000 population in 2002. The birth has declined niggardly from 39.9 in 1951 to an estimated 25 per 1000 in 2002. Demographers opine that further rapid decline in India's death rate may not continue in future. The reason is the widespread use of vaccines, antibiotics, insecticides and other lifesaving measures.

Growth rate: The population in India grew at a slow rate. India is now the second populous country in the world, adding 16 million every year to her 1027 million at the time 2001 census. The most recent data indicates a decline in India's population growth rate. Currently the national health goal is to attain a birth rate of 21 and a death rate of 9 per 1000 by 2027. It is a challenging task to India to achieve the goal of health for all.

X. a. What is expanded programme of immunization, b. Explain the role of a nurse in Pulse Polio Programme?

The Expanded Programme on Immunization (EPI) was initiated in India in 1978 with the objective to reduce morbidity and mortality from diphtheria, pertussis, tetanus, and poliomyelitis and childhood tuberculosis by providing immunization services to all eligible children and pregnant women by 1990. Measles vaccine was included when the EPI was accelerated by launching the Universal Immunization Programme (UIP) in 1985–6. Approximately half of all infants now receive complete primary immunization with diphtheria, polio and tetanus (DPT), oral polio vaccine (OPV) and BCG vaccine. Forty-six percent of pregnant women currently receive a second or booster dose of tetanus toxoid (TT). Surveillance reports from selected areas have documented impact through reduction of disease incidence. Although vaccination coverage levels are increasing, continued acceleration is needed to achieve the universal levels targeted for 1990.

Because of the global burden on child morbidity and mortality, last 1976 the **Expanded Programme on Immunization** shortly known as EPI was developed. It primarily focuses on reaching the bright goal of fully immunized child (FIC) and to improve the rate for child protected at birth (CPAB) in the country. **EPI** was established to ensure the access of infant and children (**0–12 months old**) to the recommended vaccines – which in return could prevent the seven common diseases, i.e.: tuberculosis, poliomyelitis, diphtheria, tetanus, pertussis or whooping cough, measles and hepatitis.

According to DOH, the specific goals for the expanded program on immunization are:

Beneficiaries	Age	Vaccine	Dose	Rout	Amount
a. Infants	At birth (for institutional deliveries)	BCG	Single	Intradermal	0.05 mL
		OPV	Zero dose	Oral	2 drops
	At 6 weeks	BCG (if not given at birth)	Single	Intradermal	0.1 mL
		DTP-1	1st	Intramuscular	0.5 mL
		OPV-1	1st	Oral	2 drops
	At 10 weeks	DTP-2	2nd	Intramuscular	0.5 mL
		OPV-2	2nd	Oral	2 drops
	At 14 weels	DTP-3	3rd	Intramuscular	0.5 mL
		OPV-3	3rd	Oral	2 drops
	At 9 months	Measles	Single	Subcutaneous	0.5 mL
b. Children	At 16–24 months	DTP	Booster	Intramuscular	0.5 mL
		OPV	Booster	Oral	2 drops
	At 5–6 years	DT	Single Intramuscular 0.5 mL *second dose of DT should be given after 4 weeks, if not vaccinated previoulsly with DTP		
	At 10–16 years	TT	Single intramuscular 0.5 mL *seocnd dose of TT should be given if not vaccinated previously		
c. Pregnant women	Early in pregnancy	TT-1	1st	Intramuscular	0.5 mL
	One month after	TT-2	2nd	Intramuscular	0.5 mL

1. **To immunize all infants/children against the most common vaccine-preventable diseases:** To make sure that all children in the country are fully immunized child (FIC), the Department of Health utilizes several strategies, such as the reaching every barangay or REB strategy adapted from WHO-UNICEF's reaching every district (RED) strategy, supplemental immunization activity (SIA) to reduce the rate of missed children or drop outs from routine immunization, and also through a strengthened disease surveillance. The routine schedule for immunization is every Wednesday, which is done monthly in every bagangay health stations and quarterly in far flung areas. A child is said to be a Fully Immunized Child if he receives one dose of BCG, 3 doses of OPV, 3 doses of DPT, 3 doses of HBV and one dose of Measles before his first birthday.
2. **To sustain the polio-free status:** As one concept in the eradication of disease initiative is to sustain the country from being polio- free for global certification. The Polio Eradication Project was established last 1992. It has gained high regard in implementing its core advocacy, achieving 92% of its routine coverage and happy to say that the country has maintained to be polio- free since October 2000. Being polio-free is never an assurance for cases, so there is still an ongoing polio mass immunization for children aging 6 weeks up to 59 months old in high risk areas in the country for neonatal tetanus.
3. **To eliminate measles infection:** All children with ages 9 months up to 8 years were given with one dose of measles-rubella (MR) vaccine. They utilized supplemental immunization strategy and rapid coverage assessment (RCA) to make sure that there is no missed child for the campaign. Reports from the RCA tell that in general, 97.6% were vaccinated with MR in all randomly selected barangays.
4. **To eliminate maternal and neonatal tetanus:** Pregnant women are also the target of this program. Tetanus toxoid (TT) is given not only to protect the mother from tetanus during child birth but also to prevent the occurrence of neonatal tetanus. TT (0.5 mL) is given intramuscularly at the deltoid region of the upper arm. The following schedule for injection should be followed to attain the ideal percentage of protection for both the mother and the infant.
5. **To control diphtheria, pertussis, hepatitis b and German measles:** The recent combination of DPT, Hepatitis B and HIB or *Haemophilus influenza* type B is being continuously given to control the rate of cases of these diseases. One disease that is prevented by giving this recent vaccine for children is purulent meningitis which causes acute inflammation of the epiglottis- leading to suffocation in infants and small children.
6. **To prevent extrapulmonary tuberculosis among children:** Part of the ENC or essential newborn care Package is the giving of BCG and hepatitis B at birth in compliance to RA 10152 or the Mandatory Infants and Children Health Immunization Act of 2011. In adherence to eradication of common preventable disease, vaccines should be well taken care and stored accordingly to maintain its potency. Vaccines are very sensitive substances to heat and cold temperatures. It is also a NO-NO for spoilage thus proper handling, transporting and storing should be put into consideration.

Nursing Roles and Responsibilities
1. Maintain a master list of eligible children for immunization.
2. Administer immunization following the protocols in right administration of vaccines (right dose, right route, right schedule and interval, and proper utilization of cold chain).
3. Infuse proper aseptic technique and infection control (one syringe: one child and proper disposal of syringes)
4. Provide health teachings regarding EPI, i.e. scheduled immunization activity to enhance the awareness of community and motivate them to adhere with the campaigns.

5. Conduct visits in the community to assess their needs and to identify cases of EPI diseases.
6. Have an updated record of children who had received immunization and the like and report cases if there is.

Pulse Polio Programme

The Pulse Polio Initiative was started with an objective of achieving 100% coverage under oral polio vaccine. It aimed to immunize children through improved social mobilization, plan mop-up operations in areas where poliovirus has almost disappeared and maintain high level of morale among the public.

1. Maintaining community immunity through high quality National and Sub National polio rounds each year.
2. An extremely high level of vigilance through surveillance across the country for any importation or circulation of poliovirus and VDPV is being maintained. Environmental surveillance (sewage sampling) have been established to detect poliovirus transmission and as a surrogate indicator of the progress as well for any programmatic interventions strategically in Mumbai, Delhi, Patna, Kolkata, Punjab and Gujarat.
3. All States and Union Territories in the country have developed a Rapid Response Team (RRT) to respond to any polio outbreak in the country. An Emergency Preparedness and Response Plan (EPRP) has also been developed by all States indicating steps to be undertaken in case of detection of a polio case.
4. To reduce risk of importation from neighboring countries, international border vaccination is being provided through continuous vaccination teams (CVT) to all eligible children round the clock. These are provided through special booths set up at the international borders that India shares with Pakistan, Bangladesh, Bhutan Nepal and Myanmar.
5. Government of India has issued guidelines for mandatory requirement of polio vaccination to all international travelers before their departure from India to polio affected countries namely: Afghanistan, Nigeria, Pakistan, Ethiopia, Kenya, Somalia, Syria and Cameroon. The mandatory requirement is effective for travelers from March 1, 2014.
6. A rolling emergency stock of OPV is being maintained to respond to detection/importation of wild poliovirus (WPV) or emergence of circulating vaccine derived poliovirus (cVDPV).
7. National Technical Advisory Group on Immunization (NTAGI) has recommended Injectable Polio Vaccine (IPV) introduction as an additional dose along with 3rd dose of DPT in the entire country in the last quarter of 2015 as a part of polio endgame strategy.

2014
Community Health Nursing

SECTION-I

I. Fill in the blanks:
   a. The Indian Red Cross society was established in the year: _____
   b. Under the ICDS scheme, an *Anganwadi* worker covers a population of: _____
   c. BCG vaccination is administered to protect against: _____
   d. The administrative head of the district is a: _____

II. Write whether the following statements are *true* or *false*:
   a. Rural health scheme is based on the principle of placing people's health in people's hands.
   b. Corporations in urban areas have a population of above 2 lakh.
   c. Farmer's lung is caused due to the inhalation of sugarcane dust.
   d. The 12th five year plan commenced in the year 2010.

III. Write short notes on any *four* of the following:
   a. Functions of village health guides.
   b. Occupational hazards of agricultural workers.
   c. Indigenous system of medicine.
   d. Organization of state level health administration.
   e. Recommendations of the Mudaliar committee.

IV. a. Define maternal and child health service.
   b. List the objectives of maternal and child health services.
   c. Explain the role of a nurse in MCH services.

V. a. Define primary health care.
   b. What are the elements of primary health care?
   c. Explain the principles of primary health care.
                    OR
   a. What is the importance of school health services?
   b. Explain the components of school health program.

SECTION-II

VI. Give the meaning of the following:
   a. Life expectancy.
   b. Health team.
   c. Fertility.
   d. Maternal mortality.

VII. Choose the correct answer and write:
   a. The number of females per 1000 males is called—
      (i) Dependency ratio, (ii) Sex ratio, (iii) Family ratio
   b. An outbreak of disease in a community in excess of normal expectation—
      (i) Epidemic, (ii) Sporadic, (iii) Pandemic
   c. Anti-malaria month campaign is observed every year in—
      (i) January, (ii) June, (iii) September

VIII. Write short notes on any *two* of the following:
   a. Criteria for selection and responsibilities of ASHA.
   b. Census.
   c. Functions or responsibilities of female health worker.
   d. Minimum needs program.

IX. a. List any 10 national health programs in India.
   b. Explain the national rural health mission.

X. a. Define vital statistics.
   b. Write the uses of vital statistics.
   c. List the health records used in the primary health centers.

SECTION-I

I. Fill in the blanks
a. The Indian Red Cross Society was established in the year: **1920**
b. Under the ICDS scheme, an *Anganwadi* worker covers a population of: **1000**
c. BCG vaccination is administered to protect against: **Tuberculosis**
d. The administrative head of the district is a: **District Collector**

II. Write whether the following statements are *true* or *false*:
a. Rural health scheme is based on the principle of placing people's health in people's hands: **TRUE.**
b. Corporations in urban areas have a population of above 2 lakh: **TRUE.**
c. Farmer's lung is caused due to the inhalation of sugarcane dust: **FALSE.**
d. The 12th five year plan commenced in the year 2010: **FALSE.**

III. Write short notes on any *four* of the following:

a. Functions of village health guides

The health care at the village level is in the hands of the Village Health Guide, and the Trained Birth Attendant. The Community Health Workers Scheme, 1977, paved the way for the creation of the cadre of Village Health Guides (VHGs) originally called the community health workers. Under the Scheme, one VHG for every 1,000 (500 in the case of tribal and hilly areas) is appointed in all the states except Jammu and Kashmir, Arunachal Pradesh and Kerala. Of the required 4.5 lakh, so far only 3.5 lakh VHGs have been trained and placed in position.

The trainee is selected from the village where she is going to work. She must be acceptable to all sections of the village. She must be a literate (able to read, write and maintain records). She must be willing, after training, to work for 2–3 hours every day. She is then given 3 months training at the PHC. During training, she is paid a stipend of ₹ 200/month. She is trained in the treatment of common minor ailments, including diarrhea and acute respiratory infections, first aid, personal hygiene, environmental sanitation, nutrition, reproductive and child health, family planning and health education. After training, she is awarded a certificate, and given a manual (in which details of what to do and what not to do are given) and a kit containing medicines (both allopathic and indigenous ones).

After training she goes back to the village and works 2–3 hours in treatment and education about nutrition, family planning, sanitation, etc. Rest of the time she engages in her own pursuits. For her work, she is paid an honorarium of ₹ 600/month. Additionally, she is given drugs worth ₹ 600 every year. She works in liaison with the other village health functionaries. She is not answerable to the medical officer of the concerned PHC. She is answerable to the village health committee composed of 5 members chosen by the Panchayat, at least one of whom is a woman and another member of Scheduled castes.

b. Occupational hazards of agricultural workers

The joint committee of ILO/ WHO on occupational health, held in 1950 for the first time gave the following statements about occupational health. The general aims of occupational health should be the promotion and maintenance of highest degree of physical, mental and social well-being of workers in all occupations, the prevention among workers of departures from health caused by their working conditions the protection of workers in their respective employments from risks resulting from factors adverse to health, the placing and maintenance of the workers in an occupational environment adopted to their physiological and psychological needs.

Health Problems due to Industrialization

1. Air pollution.
2. Water pollution.
3. Soil pollution.
4. Shortage of houses.
5. Communicable diseases.
6. Mental health problems.
7. Accidents.
8. Social problems like alcoholism, drug addiction, gambling, prostitution, juvenile delinquency.
9. High morbidity and mortality from certain diseases, e.g. chronic bronchitis and lung cancer.

c. Indigenous system of medicine

Ayurveda: The doctrine of Ayurveda aims to keep structural and functional entities in a functional state of equilibrium, which signifies good health. Any imbalance due to internal and external factor causes disease and restoring equilibrium through various techniques, procedures, regimes, diet and medicine constitute treatment. The philosophy of Ayurveda is based on the theory of Pancha bhootas (five element theory) of which all the objects and living bodies are composed of.

Siddha: Siddha system of medicine emphasize that medical treatment is oriented not merely to disease, but also has to take into account the patient, environment, age, habits, physical condition. Siddha literature is in Tamil and it is largely practiced in Tamil speaking parts of India and abroad.

Unani: Unani system of medicine is based on established knowledge and practices relating to promotion of positive health and prevention of diseases. Although Unani system originated in Greece, passed through many countries, Arabs enriched it with their aptitude and experience and the system was brought to India during Medieval period. Unani system emphasize the use of naturally occurring, most herbal medicines, though it uses ingredients of animal and marine origin.

Homeopathy: Homeopathy is a system of medicine, which believes in a specialized method of treatment of curing diseases by administration of potency drugs, which have been experimentally proved to possess the power of producing similar artificial systems on human beings.

Yoga and Naturopathy: Yoga is a way of life, which has the potential for improvement of social and personal behavior, improvement of physical health by encouraging better circulation of oxygenated blood in the body, restraining sense organs and thereby inducing tranquility and serenity of mind. Naturopathy is also a way of life, with drugless treatment of diseases. The system is based on the ancient practice of application of simple laws of nature. The advocates of naturopathy focus on eating and living habits, adoption of purification measures, use of hydrotherapy, baths, massage, etc.

d. Organization of state level health administration

The state ministry of health is headed by a minister of health and family welfare and a deputy minister of health and family welfare. These are political appointments and they are elected members of legislative assembly. They have political responsibilities towards their constituencies as per their political agenda and responsibilities for administration and management of health and family welfare services in their state.

Responsibilities

1. **As a member of state legislature:** It is his duty to support, and safeguard the total policies of the government because of the collective responsibility of the cabinet.
2. **As a member of ministry:** He brings all the bills pertaining to his department for approval of the legislature.
3. **As political head of the health department:** He acts as executive and administrator.
4. He is a custodian of the interest of the people in general and of his constituency in particular.
5. As a member of government he performs ceremonial duties.

Health Secretariat

Health secretariat is the official organ of the state health ministry. The secretary of the state government, senior officer of the Indian administrative service, is the administrative head and is assisted by additional deputy and under secretaries. The Bhore committee (1946) recommended that Director of health services should also be secretary to the State Government to facilitate administration.

Responsibilities of Secretariat

1. Assisting the minister in policy-making in modifying policies from time to time and in the discharge of his legislative responsibility.
2. Framing draft legislation and rules and regulations.
3. Coordination of policies and programs, supervision and control over their execution and review of results.
4. Budgeting and control of expenditure.
5. Maintaining contact with the government of India and other state governments.
6. Overseeing the smooth and efficient running of administrative machinery and initiating measures designed to develop greater personnel and organizational competence.

State Health Directorate

The state health directorate has a state family welfare bureau headed by the additional director of family welfare also health and family welfare. The state health directorate is the technical wing of state ministry of health and family welfare. He is also responsible for the organization and direction of all health activities. With the advent of family planning as an important program, the designation of director of health services has been changed in some states and is now known as director of health and family welfare. The director of health and family welfare is assisted by a suitable number of deputies and assistants. The deputy and assistant director of health may be of two types—regional and functional. The regional directors inspect all the branches of public health within their jurisdiction, irrespective of their specialty. The functional directors are usually specialists in a particular branch of public health, such as mother and child health, family planning, nutrition, tuberculosis, leprosy, health education, etc.

Responsibilities of the State Health Services

1. Patient care through a network of hospitals and dispensaries.
2. Primary health care through a network of primary health centers and subcenters.
3. Family welfare and population control.

4. National health programs—organization and implementation.
5. Education and training—health manpower development.
6. Information, education and communication.
7. Laboratory services support.

Responsibilities of State Health Directorate
1. Providing curative and preventive services.
2. Promotion of health education.
3. To do studies in depth the health problems and needs in the state and plans schemes to solve them.
4. Collection, tabulation and publication of vital statistics.
5. Provision for control of milk and food sanitation.
6. Promotion of all health programs, such as school health, family planning, occupational health, maternal and child health.
7. Assumes total responsibility for taking all steps in the prevention of any outbreak of communicable diseases especially during festivals and melas.
8. Recruitment of personnel for rural health services.
9. Planning and carrying out surveys in relation to nutrition, health education, etc.
10. Establishing training courses for health personnel and formulating job descriptions.
11. Coordination of all health services with other ministries of state.
12. Establishment and maintenance of central laboratories for preparation of vaccines, etc.

e. Recommendations of the Mudaliar committee

In 1959, the Government of India appointed another committee known as "health survey and planning committee" popularly known Mudaliar committee after the name of its chairman Dr AL Mudaliar. The Mudaliar committee found the quality of services provided by the primary health centers inadequate and advised strengthening of the existing primary health centers before new centers were established.

Important Recommendations
1. Strengthening of the district hospital with specialist services to serve as central base of regional services.
2. Regional organizations in each state between the head quarters organizations in each state between the head quarters organization and the district in change of a regional deputy or assistant directors— each to supervise 2 or 3 district medical and health officers.
3. Each primary health center not to be served more than 40,000 populations.
4. To improve the quality of health care provided by the primary health centers.
5. Integration of medical and health services as recommended by the Bhore committee.
6. Constitution of All India Health Service on the pattern on Indian Administrative Service.

IV. a. Define maternal and child health service
b. List the objectives of maternal and child health services
c. Explain the role of a nurse in MCH services

Maternal and child health services are directed towards and children in order to maintain total well-being of the child within the framework of the family and the community. Every aspect of community health programs in India has marked effects on the health and welfare of expectant mothers and particularly of infants and children. New maternal and child health care (MCH) which now also being described as reproductive and child health (RCH). Reproductive child health can be defined as a state in which "people have the ability to reproduce and regulate their fertility or women have the ability to reproduce and regulate their fertility or women are able to go through pregnancy and childbirth safety."

Objectives of MCH Programs

1. To give expert advice to the couples to plan their families.
2. To identify "high risk" cases, so that can give them special attention.
3. To provide health supervision for antenatal mothers also to foresee complications and prevention.
4. To give skilled assistance at the time of child birth and during puerperium.
5. To supervise trained dais, community health volunteers and community health workers.
6. To impart useful knowledge on desirable health practices which mother should carry out during pregnancy, labor and during puerperium.
7. Encourage the deliveries by trained workers in the safe and clean environment.
8. Prevent communicable and noncommunicable diseases.
9. Educate the mother to improve their own and children's health.

Aims of MCH Services

1. To pay attention on stability in population, safe childhood and health of children.
2. To pay special attention to the health of women, boys, girls, protection from sexually transmitted diseases, antenatal, intranatal, and postnatal mothers.
3. To have safe pregnancies is successful in terms of safe motherhood, safe child and good health.
4. To provide sound reproductive health for men and women and also safe control of their reproduction activities.
5. To have effective control on maternal morbidity and mortality.

Components of Reproductive and Child Health

1. Family planning services
2. Child survival and safe motherhood program (CSSM)
3. Prevention or management of STD.
4. Providing counseling, information and communication services on health.
5. Referral services.
6. Growth monitoring and nutritional education.

Importance of MCH Services

Mother and child are considered as one unit. Mother and child are "special Risk group" or vulnerable group or dependent or weaker group of community.

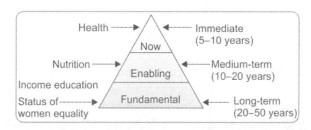

Nurse's Responsibilities in MCH

Responsibilities of community health nurse in maternal health services can be presented under following headings:

Antenatal care

1. Contact: Contacting every pregnant mother in the primary stage of pregnancy.
2. History: Taking history of general health; family environment, social conditions, previous childbirths and present pregnancy.
3. Antenatal examination: Conducting general examination, physical examination and obstetric examination, laboratory examinations, etc.
4. Calculating the expected date of delivery and informing mothers.
5. Conducting antenatal clinics.
6. Identifying high-risk mothers.
7. Providing counseling and health education.
8. Helping mother and other family members in planning the delivery.

Intranatal care

1. Preparing the place for delivery.
2. Arranging necessary equipments and their sterilization.
3. Giving mental support to mother.
4. Preparing mother for delivery.
5. Examining position of fetus, dilation of cervix, and heart of fetus, observing the position of bladder and uterine contractions.
6. Noting general condition of the pregnant mother, process of pains and time of membrane rupture.
7. Ensuring safe delivery, examining umbilical cord and noting abnormalities.
8. If necessary, taking help of doctor or referring patient to a specialist.
9. Taking care of the mother and newborn baby after the delivery.
10. Maintaining through asepsis during delivery.
11. Should be ready to handle complications like bleeding, malpresentation, cord prolapse, etc.
12. Noting the correct time of childbirth.

Postnatal care: The week immediately after the childbirth is called postnatal period. Given below are the duties of community health nurse during this period:

1. Observing the blood pressure, temperature and pulse of mother immediately after the delivery and then during the following period.
2. Collecting information about the general condition of mother, food, sleep, pain and elimination, etc. and, accordingly providing the nursing care.
3. Observing fundus, perineum, lochia, bladder, etc.
4. Protecting the mother from complications like puerperal sepsis, breast inflammation, postpartum hemorrhage, urinary incontinence, urinary retention and thrombophlebitis and providing required treatment.

Neonatal care

1. Observing the respiration of newborn, immediately after birth and if necessary providing resuscitation.

2. Taking care of the umbilical cord and cutting the cord and tying It using proper techniques.
3. Taking notice of abnormalities or congenital defects and informing the relatives.
4. Assessing the physical condition of the newborn by his Apgar score (9 or 10 is ideal score).
5. Cleaning the newborn child (giving bath to the newborn has become less popular. Follow the doctor's order or hospital policy).
6. Taking care of the newborn's skin and eyes.
7. Keeping the newborn child on safe bed and providing breastfeeding to baby at the earliest.
8. Maintaining normal body temperature of the newborn. Give Kangaroo care.
9. Observe the crying, intestinal activity, urination, sleep and feeding pattern of the newborn child and accordingly giving the treatment or nursing care.

Functions related to maternal clinics: In maternal services, community health nurse has to assume the responsibilities of conducting antenatal and postnatal clinics also.

Home visits: Home visits are the backbone of maternal and community health services. In maternal services, home visits can be antenatal. Home visits increase the utility of maternal and child health services, and reduces the mortality and morbidity rate in both the segments.

V. a. Define primary health care.
   b. What are the elements of primary health care?
   c. Explain the principles of primary health care.

Primary health care is essential health care made universally accessible to individuals and families in the community, by means acceptable to them, through their full participation and at a cost that the community and country can afford. It forms an integral part of both the country's health system of which it is the nucleus and the overall social and economic development of the community (Alma-Ata, 1978).

Principles of Primary Health Care
1. **Equitable distribution:** Primary health care services must be shared equally by all people irrespective of their ability to pay (rich, poor, urban or rural).
2. **Community participation:** Primary health care must be a continuing effort to secure meaningful involvement of the community in the planning, implementation and maintenance of health services.
3. **Coverage and accessibility:** Primary health care implies providing health care services to all which are required by them. The care has to be appropriate and adequate in content and in amount to satisfy the essential health needs of the people and has to be provided by methods acceptable to them.
4. **Intersectoral coordination:** Primary health care requires joint efforts of other health related sectors such as agriculture, animal husbandry, food, industry, housing, social welfare, public works, communication and other sectors.
5. **Appropriate health technology**: The technology that is scientific, adaptable to local need and socially acceptable instead of costly methods, equipment and technology.
6. **Human resource:** Health resource is very essential to make full use of all the available resources including the human potential of the entire community.
7. **Referral system:** Referral system would be desirable to develop referring from one level to another with laid down procedures and policies.
8. **Logistics of supply:** The logistic of supply include planning and budgeting for the supplies required procurement or manufacture, storage distribution and control.

9. **The physical facilities:** The physical facilities for primary health care need to be simple and clean. It should have a spacious waiting area with toilet facility.
10. **Control and evaluation:** A process of evaluation has to be built into assess the relevance, progress, efficiency, effectiveness and impact of the services.

Role of community health nurse in PHC: An extent committee on community health nursing was concerned by WHO executive board in July 1974 to recommend way in which nursing could have critical impact on the urgent health problems throughout the world.

The committee made specific recommendations:
1. The development of community health nursing services, responsive to community health needs that would assure primary health care coverage for all.
2. The reformulation of basic and post basic nursing education as to prepare all nurses for community health nursing.
3. The inclusion of nursing in national development plans in a way that would ensure the rational distribution and the appropriate utilization and support of nursing personnel.

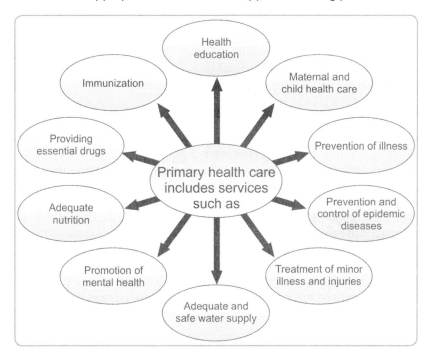

Role of Nurse in PHC
1. Community health nurse work with population, community, family, individual. The focus is multiple or promoting health maintaining a degree of balance toward health.
2. Community health nurse focus on assessment of the impact of the socioeconomical and cultural factors affecting health measures that must constantly be dealt with and take priority in order to make family assume health measures.
3. The community health nurse works with entire spectrum of health and illness conditions from optimal health to minor or severe conditions from acute to chronic illness.
4. The community health nurse works in all kinds of setting, such as home, school, clinic, industry, etc.

5. The community health nurse works in school where primary goal is health education and disease prevention.
6. The community health nurse works in industry is to improve the production and employers' safety.
7. The community health nurse is responsible for assisting patients and families to coordinate health care, which necessitates contact with personnel from health, welfare and other significant community agencies.
8. Community health nurse has responsibilities in education and training of individuals, auxiliaries and others.
9. The community health nurse involves in provision of direct services to patients both preventive and curative at the outpatient, inpatient clinics and community.

OR

a. What is the importance of school health services?

School is defined as an educational institution where groups of pupils pursue defined studies at defined levels, receive instructions from one or more teachers, and frequently interact with other officers and employees, such as principal, various supervisors/instructors, and maintenance staff, etc. usually housed in a single building. School health services referred to need based comprehensive services rendered to pupils, teachers and other personnel in the school to promote and protect their health, control diseases and maintain the health.

Objectives of School Health Programs

1. To increase health awareness in children to a level where they can treat health as a valuable personal family, community and national asset.
2. To educate and guide the school children and prompt them to adopt health giving habits and healthy lifestyle and give up injurious habits practices and urges that can undermine their health.
3. To facilitate early diagnosis and prompt treatment of diseases in school children and arrest their propagation, if communicable.
4. To promote interest of students in individual and community health activities and to use them as "change agents" in various areas of public health significance.
5. To work towards a total personality development of school children in all dimensions physical, mental, social, moral and emotional treating them as a valuable national asset and useful community resources.

Importance/Scope of Community Health Program

1. **Growth and development:** School life is the state of physical and mental growth and intense development of the children.
2. **Socioeconomic development:** One fourth of the India's population is comprized of children between 5–14 years of age. Social and economic development of the nation is possible only through care and development of this group.
3. **Socialization:** School is another social group the child gets after family. They get much experience through this social life. Contribution of school is vital in the socialization of children.
4. **Easy Implementation:** School going children from a specific age group, otherwise called controlled population. They are within the easy reach for the implementation.
5. **Early detection and diagnosis:** Infectious diseases, physical and mental disorders can be detected at early stage in school going children.

6. **Adaptability:** School going children have the ability to quickly adopt and acquire new knowledge therefore school children can be used for giving effective health education to children and to develop healthy habits in them.

b. Explain the components of school health program

The components of school health services include all those aspects which help achieve its aim and objectives. The service need to be comprehensive in nature and include all elements of promotive, preventive, therapeutic and rehabilitative care.
  1. **Health appraisal:** Health appraisal should cover not only the student but also the teacher and other school personnel. Health appraisal consists of periodic medical examination and observation of children by the class teacher.
  2. **Remedial measures and follow up:** Medical examination is not an end in them. They should be followed by appropriate treatment and follow up. Special clinics should be conducted exclusively for school children at primary health centers.
  3. **Prevention of communicable disease:** Protection of all school going children against preventable disease by immunization according to the national immunization schedule.
  4. **Healthful school environment:** The school building site and equipment are part of the environment in which the child grows and develops healthful school environment therefore is necessary for the best emotional, social and personal health of the pupils, e.g. as regards safe drinking water, sanitation accident prevention, food hygiene, etc.
  5. **Nutritional services:** Good nutrition is very essential not only for optimal health. Growth and development of the school child but also for his/her educational achievement. A nutritious mid-day meal for children in the school is considered a practical solution to combat malnutrition in children.
  6. **First aid and emergency:** The school must have an arrangement for providing first aid and emergency care to children who get injured or sick at the school. So all the teachers should receive adequate training during teacher training program or in service training programs to prepare them to carry out this obligation.
  7. **Mental health:** The mental health of the child affects his physical health and the learning process. Juvenile delinquency, maladjustment and drug addiction are becoming problems among school children. They need to plan and organize well balanced curricular, co-curricular and extracurricular activities, so that students are not over burdened and have sufficient relaxation and recreation, etc.
  8. **Dental health:** Dental caries and periodontal disease are the two common dental diseases in India. A school health program should have provision for dental examination, at least once a year.
  9. **Eye health services:** Schools should be responsible for the early detection of refractive errors, treatment of squint and amblyopia and detection and treatment of eye infection, such as trachoma.
  10. **Health education:** Health education is very important for school children. It creates awareness, provides them knowledge regarding health matter, develops motivation and promotes change in health behavior and health attitudes in them. Therefore, health education is considered as one of the crucial and key element of school health services. Health education content areas include personal hygiene, environmental health, nutrition, prevention and control of communicable and non-communicable diseases.
  11. **Education of handicapped children:** The ultimate, so that the child will be able to reach his maximum potential to lead as normal a life as possible to become as independent as possible and to become a production and self supporting member of society.

12. **School health records:** It is essential to maintain complete, accurate and continuous health records of school children. Such health records will be useful for providing need based health care and guidance to children. It will also help evaluate the school health services and assist further development and improvement of health services considered to school children.

SECTION-II

VI. Give the meaning of the following:

a. Life expectancy

Life expectancy is the expected (in the statistical sense) number of years of life remaining at a given age. It is denoted by e_x, which means the average number of subsequent years of life for someone now aged x, according to a particular mortality experience. Because life expectancy is an average, a particular person may well die many years before or many years after their "expected" survival. The term "maximum life span" has a quite different meaning. The "median life span" is also a different concept although fairly similar to life expectancy numerically in most developed countries.

It is important to note that life expectancy is an average value. In many cultures, particularly before modern medicine was widely available, the combination of high infant mortality and deaths in young adulthood from accidents, epidemics, plagues, wars, and childbirth, significantly lowers the overall life expectancy. But for someone who survived past these early hazards, living into their sixties or seventies would not be uncommon. For example, a society with a life expectancy of 40 may have very few people dying at age 40: most will die before 30 years of age or after 55.

b. Health team

The PHCT might therefore be considered to incorporate a much wider range of activities and professional groups, including: The traditional PHCT, for example:
1. Practice manager.
2. Doctors: GP partners, GP assistants and other salaried doctors, GP registrars.
3. Nurses: Practice nurses, nurse practitioners, community nurses; appropriately trained and supported nurses can produce high-quality care and achieve as good health outcomes for patients.
4. Support staff: Receptionists, secretaries, clerical staff.
5. Midwives.
6. Health visitors.

Primary care premises may also be used for selected secondary care services, e.g. hospital consultant clinics, diagnostic imaging, operating services. Allied health professionals may also work closely with the PHCT, e.g. physiotherapy, dietetics, podiatry, pharmacy, counseling.

c. Fertility

Fertility is the natural capability to produce offspring. As a measure, "fertility rate" is the number of offspring born per mating pair, individual or population. Fertility differs from fecundity, which is defined as the potential for reproduction (influenced by gamete production, fertilization and carrying a pregnancy to term) A lack of fertility is infertility while a lack of fecundity would be called sterility. Ability of an individual or couple to reproduce through normal sexual activity. About 90% of healthy, fertile women are able to conceive within one year if they have intercourse regularly without contraception. Normal fertility requires the production of enough healthy sperm by the male and viable eggs by the female, successful passage of the sperm through open ducts from the male testes to the female fallopian tubes, penetration of a healthy egg, and implantation of the fertilized egg in the lining of the uterus.

d. Maternal mortality

According to WHO, a maternal death is defined as "the death of a women who is pregnant (or) within 42 days of the termination of pregnancy irrespective of the duration and site of pregnancy from any cause related to (or) aggravated by the pregnancy (or) its management but not from accidental (or) incidental causes".

Maternal mortality rate (MMR): The MMR is expressed in terms of such maternal deaths per 1, 00,000 live birth. Maternal mortality rate measures the risk of women dying from "puerperal causes" and is defined as

$$MMR = \frac{\text{Total number of female death due to complications of pregnancy, child birth (or) within 42 days of delivery from "puerperal causes" in an area during a given year}}{\text{Total number of live births in the same area and year}} \times 1000$$

In most developed countries, MMR varies from 4% to 40% 100,000 live births. In developing countries, it varies from 100–700 with India having about 460 per 100,000 live birth.

The term reproductive mortality is used currently to include maternal mortality and mortality from use of contraception.

Severity (or) magnitude of the problem: According to WHO estimates, about 50,000 maternal death (about 0.9% of total death) occurred globally during the year 2002, of this deaths about 231,000 occurred in African countries, 17,000 in America, 68,000 Eastern Mediterranean, 3,000 in European, 171,000 in South East Asia and 21,000 in Western Pacific countries.

In India: The shocking scenario reveled when MMR expressed in terms that in developing countries, there has been one maternal death per minute. In India, 148,000 women die every year as a result of pregnancy and child birth which means one maternal death every 4 minutes. It is further estimated that for one maternal death at least 15 more suffer from severe morbidities.

VII. Choose the correct answer and write:

a. The number of females per 1000 males is called: **Sex Ratio**
   (i. Dependency ratio, ii. Sex ratio, iii. Family ratio)
b. An outbreak of disease in a community in excess of normal expectation: **Epidemic**
   (i. Epidemic, ii. Sporadic, iii. Pandemic)
c. Anti-malaria month campaign is observed every year in: **June**
   (i. January, ii. June, iii. September)

VIII. Write short notes on any *two* of the following:

a. Criteria for selection and responsibilities of ASHA

Accredited social health activist (ASHA) is a key link to public health services in villages in India. We conducted a cross-sectional study to determine the proportion of women utilizing services of the ASHA for pregnancy-related conditions. We assessed the knowledge, attitude, practices, hindrances and motivation factors among ASHAs regarding pregnancy-related conditions. We also sought to determine the factors associated with the utilization of ASHAs for pregnancy-related services. One of the key components of the National Rural Health Mission is to provide every village in the country with a trained female community health activist ASHA or Accredited Social Health Activist. Selected from the village itself and accountable to it, the ASHA will be trained to work as an interface between the community and the public health system.

Criteria for selection: One ASHA Sahyogini for each Anganwadi Center.
1. Woman resident of that area, married/widow/divorcee.
2. Age between 21–45 years.
3. ASHA Sahyogini should have effective communication skills, leadership qualities and be able to reach out to the community.
4. ASHA Sahyogini should be literate woman with formal education up to eighth class, In tribal and desert areas the educational qualification may be relaxed if the 8th pass candidate is not available. This is permitted only after the approval of State level Committee.
5. Adequate representation from disadvantaged population groups.

Following are the key components of ASHA:
1. ASHA must primarily be a woman resident of the village married/widowed/divorced, preferably in the age group of 25–45 years.
2. She should be a literate woman with formal education up to class eight. This may be relaxed only if no suitable person with this qualification is available.
3. ASHA will be chosen through a rigorous process of selection involving various community groups, self-help groups, Anganwadi Institutions, the Block Nodal officer District Nodal officer, the village Health Committee and the Gram Sabha. Capacity building of ASHA is being seen as a continuous process. ASHA will have to undergo series of training episodes to acquire the necessary knowledge, skills and confidence for performing her spelled out roles.
4. The ASHAs will receive performance-based incentives for promoting universal immunization, referral and escort services for Reproductive and Child Health (RCH) and other healthcare programs, and construction of household toilets.
5. Empowered with knowledge and a drug-kit to deliver first-contact healthcare, every ASHA is expected to be a fountainhead of community participation in public health programs in her village.
6. ASHA will be the first port of call for any health related demands of deprived sections of the population, especially women and children, who find it difficult to access health services.
7. ASHA will be a health activist in the community who will create awareness on health and its social determinants and mobilize the community towards local health planning and increased utilization and accountability of the existing health services.
8. She would be a promoter of good health practices and will also provide a minimum package of curative care as appropriate and feasible for that level and make timely referrals.
9. ASHA will provide information to the community on determinants of health, such as nutrition, basic sanitation and hygienic practices, healthy living and working conditions, information on existing health services and the need for timely utilization of health and family welfare services.
10. She will counsel women on birth preparedness, importance of safe delivery, breastfeeding and complementary feeding, immunization, contraception and prevention of common infections, including Reproductive Tract Infection/Sexually Transmitted Infections (RTIs/STIs) and care of the young child.
11. ASHA will mobilize the community and facilitate them in accessing health and health related services available at the Anganwadi/sub-center/primary health centers, such as immunization,

antenatal check-up (ANC), postnatal check-up supplementary nutrition, sanitation and other services being provided by the government.
12. She will act as depot older for essential provisions being made available to all habitations like oral rehydration therapy (ORS), iron folic acid (IFA), chloroquine, disposable delivery kits (DDK), oral pills and condoms, etc.
13. At the village level, it is recognized that ASHA cannot function without adequate institutional support. Women's committees (like self-help groups or women's health committees), village health and sanitation Committee of the Gram Panchayat, peripheral health workers especially ANMs and Anganwadi workers, and the trainers of ASHA and in-service periodic training would be a major source of support to ASHA.

b. Census

The word census originated from the Latin word censere which means to assess or to rate. The first census of India was conducted in 1872; hence the census of 1881 is considered as the first systematic census of India. Census 2001 is the 14th census the 6th census of independent India and the first of 21st century.

c. Functions or responsibilities of female health worker

I. A Health Worker (female) is to cover a population of 3000 in tribal areas and 5000 in non-tribal areas.
1. She will make a visit to each family once a fortnight according to fixed calendar of visit. She will carry out the following functions.
2. She will register pregnant women from 3 months of pregnancy onwards.
3. She will maintain a register enumerating all the families.
4. She will maintain a register enumerating all the children 0–5 in her area by systematic house visits.
5. She will maintain up-to-date registers and records as prescribed from time to time.
6. Categories the eligible couple according to the number of children and age of mothers.

II. Care at home
1. She will provide care to pregnant women especially registered mothers throughout the pregnancy.
2. Give advice on nutrition to expectant and nursing mothers and responsible for storage, preparation and distribution of food to the expectant and nursing mothers under supplementary feeding.
3. Distribute iron and folic acid tablets to pregnant and nursing mothers, children and family planning adoptors and vitamin "A" solution to children at twice a year from 6 months to 60 months of age.
4. Immunize pregnant mothers with tetanus toxoid; immunize infants with DPT, Polio and measles as per schedule.
5. Refer cases of abnormal/high-risk pregnancy and cases with medical and gynecological problems at Primary Health Center/Hospital.
6. Conduct deliveries as per the norms prescribed in her area.
7. Supervise deliveries conducted by dais and guide them replenish the stock of basic drugs and dressings to dais.
8. Refer cases of difficult labor and newborn with abnormalities and help them to get institutional care and provide follow-up care to patients referred to or discharged from hospital.
9. Provide at least three post-delivery visits for each delivery cases and render advice regarding feeding of the newborn.

10. Distribute conventional contraceptives to the couples, provide facilities and help perspective adopters in getting family planning services, if necessary, by accompanying or arranging dais to accompany them to hospital.
11. Spread the message of family planning to the couples; motivate them for family planning individually and in groups.
12. Provide follow-up services to family planning adopters, identify side effects, give treatment on the spot for side effects and minor complaints and refer these cases that need attention by physicians to the PHC/hospital.
13. Assess the growth and development of the infant and child by taking birth weight of the newborn and monthly weight of children up to 5 years of age and maintain these in the "Health Cards".
14. Do DPT and Polio and measles immunization to all the newborn infants in her area up to one year of age or till the primary immunizations are completed and assist the Health Supervisors (Female) in the immunization program and in carrying out campaign approach activities. She will administer vitamin "A" concentrate to all the children up to 1 year.
15. She will ensure effective sterilization.
16. She will ensure the cold chain requirement for preservation of vaccine.
17. Provide treatment for minor ailments, provide first aid in case of emergencies and refer cases beyond her competency to PHC or nearest hospital.
18. Notify notifiable diseases, which she comes across during her visits to male multipurpose health worker and to the Medical Officers, and PHC.
19. Record and report births and deaths occurring in her area to the local births and deaths registrar and to her supervisor.
20. Test urine for albumin and sugar and do hemoglobin test during her home visits to the pregnant mothers.
21. Identify the case that requires help for medical termination of pregnancy; provide information on the availability of services and refer them to the nearest approved institutions.

III. Care in clinic
1. Arrange and help medical officer and Health Supervisors (Female) in conducting MCH and Family Planning Clinics at the subcenters.
2. Educate mothers individually and in groups in better family health, including MCH and family planning, nutrition, immunization, hygiene and minor ailments.

IV. Care in the community
1. She will identify women leaders and help the health supervisors (female) and participate in training of women leaders.
2. Set up in women depot holders for Nirodh distribution and help the health supervisors (female) in training them.
3. Participate in women welfare meetings and utilize such gatherings for educating the women in family welfare program.
4. Utilize satisfied customers, village leaders, dais and others for promoting health, nutrition, family welfare programs.
5. She will attend to treatment of minor ailments and render immediate first aid as per the standing instructions issued from time to time.
6. She will arrange for oral rehydration in the case of diarrhea cases.

V. Other duties
1. She will maintain the cleanliness of the labor rooms in wards in subcenters.
2. Attend staff meeting at Primary Health Center.
3. List of dais in her area and involve them in promotion of Safe Delivery and Family Welfare practices.

4. Coordinate her activities with health workers (male) in campaign activities.
5. Help the health supervisors (female) in the training program of dais.

d. Minimum needs program

The **minimum needs program** (MNP) was introduced in the first year of the Fifth Five Year Plan (1974–78), to provide certain basic minimum needs and improve the living standards of people. It aims at "social and economic development of the community, particularly the underprivileged and underserved population"

Principles

Two basic principles are observed during the implementation of MNP:
1. The facilities under MNP are to be first provided in those areas which are at present undeserved so as to remove disparities among different areas.
2. The facilities under MNP should be provided as a package to an area through intersectorial area projects to have a greater impact.

Objectives

Rural health: The objectives to be achieved by the end of the eight five year plan are:
1. One peripheral health center for 30,000 population in plains and 20,000 population in tribal and hilly areas.
2. One subcenter for a population of 5000 people in the plains and for 3000 in tribal and hilly areas.
3. One community health center for a population of 100,000.

The establishment of peripheral health centers, their upgradation also comes under MNP.

Nutrition

1. To extend support of nutrition to 11 million eligible persons.
2. To consolidate midday meal program and link it to health, potable water and sanitation.

The minimum needs program (MNP) was introduced in the country in the first year of the Fifth Five Year Plan (1974–78). The objective of the program is to provide certain basic minimum needs and thereby improve the living standards of the people. It is the expression of the commitment of the government for the social and economic development of the community particularly the underprivileged and underserved population.

The program includes the following components:
1. Rural health.
2. Rural water supply.
3. Rural electrification.
4. Adult education.
5. Nutrition.
6. Environmental improvement of urban slums.
7. Houses for landless laborers.

There are two basic principles which are to be observed in the implementation of MNP:
1. The facilities under MNP are to be first provided to those areas which are at present underserved so as to remove disparities between different areas.

2. The facilities under MNP should be provided as a package to an area through intersectoral area projects, to have a greater impact. In the field of rural health, the objective is to establish: one PHC for 30,000 population in plains and 20,000 population in tribal and hilly area; one subcenter for a population 5,000 people in the plains and for 3000 in tribal and hilly areas, and one community health center (rural hospital) for a population of one lakh or 1 per 5 primary health centers. The establishment of PHCs, subcentres, upgradation of PHCs, and construction of buildings thereof are all included in the State sector of the Minimum Need Programs.

IX. a. List any 10 National Health Programs in India

Program is an organized aggregate of activities directed towards the attainment of defined objectives and targets National health programs, which have been launched by the Central Government for the control eradication of communicable diseases, improvement of environmental sanitation, raising the standard of nutrition, control of population and improving rural health. National health programs should be consistent with national health policies and should contribute towards the achievement of the goals contained therein. Various international agencies like WHO, UNICEF, UNFPA, World bank, as also a number of foreign agencies like SIDA, DANIDA, NORAD and UNAID have been proving technical and material assistance in the implementation of these programs.

1. National Malaria Eradication Program.
2. National Filarial Control Program.
3. National Leprosy Eradication Program.
4. National Tuberculosis Control Program.
5. National Program for Prevention of Visual Impairment and Control of Blindness.
6. National Sexually Transmitted Disease Control.
7. National AIDS Control Program.
8. Diarrheal Disease Control Program.
9. Child Survival and Safe Motherhood Program.
10. Reproductive and Child Health Program.
11. Universal Immunization Program (UIP —1985).
12. National Family Welfare Program.
13. National Water Supply and Sanitation Program.
14. Guinea Worm Eradication Program.

b. Explain the National Rural Health Mission

The National Rural Health Mission launched on the 12th April 2005, seeks to provide effective, efficient and affordable health care to the rural population in eighteen states with weak public health indicators. One of the key components of the mission is to provide every village in the country with a trained female community health activist—The ASHA or the Accredited Social Health Activist. ASHA will be the first port of call for any health related demands to access health services. ASHA will be a health activist in the community who will create awareness on health and its social determinants and mobilize the community towards local health planning and increased utilization and accountability of the existing health services. She would be a promoter of good health practices. She will also provide a minimum package of curative care as appropriate and feasible for that level and make timely referrals.

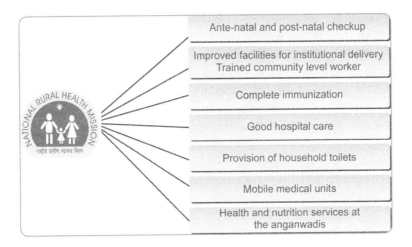

With the sixth year of implementation of National Rural Health Mission (NRHM) in the state the strategies to strengthen the ASHA program year after year has always been a continuous effort. The selection of ASHA in Meghalaya has been such that she has been selected from the village itself and accountable to it. She works on voluntary basis and is actively involved in providing various assistance and help to the community especially with regard to the health services. In the state, the ASHA is also the member secretary of the Village Health and Sanitation Committee (VHSC). At present Meghalaya has 6258 ASHAs in place and have been trained in Module 1–5.

Five Pillars of NRHM

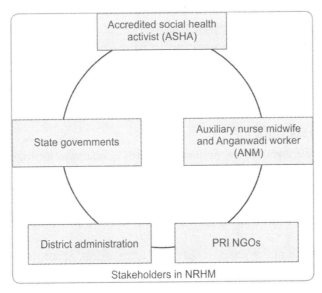

NRHM is organized around five pillars, each of which is made up of a number of overlapping core strategies:

Increasing participation and ownership by the community: Through an increased role for PRIs, the ASHA program, the village health and sanitation committee, increased public participation and NGO participation.

Improved management capacity: Professionalizing management by building up management and public health skills in the existing workforce, supplemented by inculcation of skilled management personnel into the system.

Flexible financing: Provision of united funds to every village health and sanitation committee, to the subcenter, to the PHC, to the CHC including district hospital.

Innovations in human resources development for the health sector: Contractual appointment route to immediately fill gaps as well as ensure local residency, incentive and innovation to find staff to work in hitherto underserved areas and the use of multiskilled and multi-tasking options.

Setting of standards and norms with monitoring: The prescription of the Indian Public Health Standards (IPHS) norms marks one of the most important core strategies of the mission. This has been followed up by a facility survey to identify gaps and funding is directed to close the gaps so identified.

Objectives

1. Reduction in infant mortality rate (IMR) and maternal mortality ratio (MMR).
2. Universal access to public health services, such as women's health, child health, water, sanitation and hygiene, immunization, and nutrition.
3. Prevention and control of communicable and noncommunicable diseases, including locally endemic diseases.
4. Access to integrated comprehensive primary healthcare.
5. Population stabilization, gender and demographic balance.
6. Revitalize local health traditions and mainstream AYUSH.
7. Promotion of healthy lifestyles.

X. a. Define vital statistics.
  b. Write the uses of vital statistics.
  c. List the health records used in the primary health centers.

Vital statistics provide a tool for measuring the dynamics of change which continuously occur in population. Vital statistics are derived from legally registrable events without including population data or morbidity statistics.

Definitions of Vital Statistics

1. Vital statistics are conventionally numerical records of marriage, births, sickness and deaths by which the health and growth of community may be studied.
2. Vital statistics is a part of demography and collective study of mankind. It deals with the data's related to vital events.
3. It is a branch of biometry deals with data and law of human mortality, morbidity and demography.
4. Vital statistics is the numerical description of birth, death, absorption, marriage, divorce, adoption and judicial separation—UNO.

Purpose of Vital Statistics

1. **Community health:** To describe the level of community health, to diagnose community illness, and to discover solutions to health problems.
2. **Administrative purpose:** It provides clues for administrative action and to create administrative standards of health activities.

3. **Health programmed organization:** To determine success or failure of specific health programmed or undertake overall evaluation of public health work.
4. **Legislative purpose:** To promote health legislation at local, state and national level.
5. **Governmental purpose:** To develop policies procedures, at state and central level.

Uses of Vital Statistics

1. To evaluate the impact of various national health programs.
2. To plan for better future measures of disease control.
3. To elucidate the hereditary nature of disease.
4. To plan and evaluate economic and social development.
5. It is a primary tool in research activities.
6. To determine the health status of individual.
7. To compare the health status of one nation with others.

Methods of Obtaining Vital Statistics

1. **Census:** It is a simultaneous recording demographic, social and economic data of individuals. It is an important method of collecting vital statistics. Census is conducted every 10 years.
2. **Registration:** Registration of vital events, e.g. births, deaths. Keep a continuous check on demographic changes. If registration of vital events is complete and accurate, it can serve as a reliable source of health information.
3. **Adhoc survey:** Surveys for evaluating the health status of a population that is community diagnosis of problems of health.

2013
Community Health Nursing

SECTION-I

I. Give the meaning of the following:
   a. Notification of disease.
   b. Immunity.
   c. Maternal mortality rate.
   d. Epidemiology.

II. Fill in the blanks:
   a. World tuberculosis day is on: _____
   b. National health policy was launched in the year: _____
   c. Nursing process is also known as: _____ approach.
   d. _____ is the scientific study of human populations.

III. Write short notes on any *four* of the following:
   a. Bhore Committee Report or recommendations.
   b. RCH program.
   c. Indigenous system of medicine.
   d. Primary health center.
   e. World Health Organization.

IV. a. Define primary health care.
   b. List the function of primary health care.
   c. Write the role of nurse in primary health care.

V. a. Define school health program
   b. Write the components of school health program.
   c. Explain the role of nurse in school health program.

SECTION-II

VI. Choose the correct answer and write:
   a. Time required measuring the Mantoux test:
      (i) 24–48 hours, (ii) 48–72 hours, (iii) 10–24 hours
   b. According to ICDS scheme there is an Anganwadi worker for a population of:
      (i) 500, (ii) 2000, (iii) 1000
   c. Community health is also called:
      (i) Public health, (ii) Community medicine, (iii) All the above

VII. Differentiate between the following:
   a. Balwadi Nutrition Program and Midday Meal Program.
   b. Control and eradication.

VIII. Write short notes on any *two* of the following:
   a. National immunization schedule.
   b. Employees State Insurance Scheme.
   c. Prevention and control of vitamin A deficiency.

IX. a. Define health team.
   b. List the members of health team.
   c. Explain the role of male health worker in health team.

X. a. Define Family Welfare Program.
   b. What are the aims and objectives of Family Welfare Program?
   c. Explain the nurse's role in Family Welfare Program.

OR

   a. What is National Leprosy Eradication Program?
   b. Explain the role of community health nurse in implementation of national health program.

SECTION-I

I. Give the meaning of the following:

a. Notification of disease

A **notifiable disease** is any disease that is required by law to be reported to government authorities. The collation of information allows the authorities to monitor the disease, and provides early warning of possible outbreaks. In the case of livestock diseases, there may also be the legal requirement to destroy the infected livestock upon notification. Many governments have enacted regulations for reporting of both human and animal (generally livestock) diseases. This usually happens during pandemics.

"The purpose of notification is disease control". It is therefore important that we should all notify cases and deaths due to a notifiable condition. This will assist the health authorities to speedily implement measures that will prevent the spread of that disease. Notification of a suspected case of meningococcal disease will allow rapid tracing of close contacts for administration of postexposure chemoprophylaxis to prevent secondary cases. If there are cases of cholera that are notified early, this prevents the spread of the disease and the unnecessary loss of human life. Experts in disease control and epidemiology are often called upon to investigate diseases to determine the cause of the disease (in this case cholera) and put measures to prevent the further spread, e.g. health promotion activities in the communities and in health facilities to improve hygiene practices, water supply and sanitation.

b. Immunity

Immunity is the state of having sufficient biological defences to avoid infection, disease, or other unwanted biological invasion. It is the capability of the body to resist harmful microbes from entering it. Immunity involves both specific and nonspecific components. The nonspecific components act either as barriers or as eliminators of wide range of pathogens irrespective of antigenic specificity. Other components of the immune system adapt themselves to each new disease encountered and are able to generate pathogen-specific immunity.

Innate immunity or nonspecific immunity is the natural resistances with which a person is born. It provides resistances through several physical, chemical and cellular approaches. Microbes first encounter the epithelial layers, physical barriers that line skin and mucous membranes. Subsequent general defences include secreted chemical signals (cytokines), antimicrobial substances, fever, and phagocytic activity associated with the inflammatory responses. The phagocytes express cell surface receptors that can bind and respond to common molecular patterns expressed on the surface of invading microbes. Through these approaches, innate immunity can prevent the colonization, entry and spread of microbes.

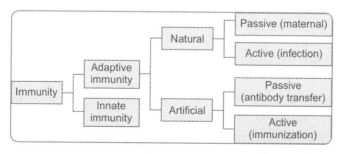

Adaptive immunity is often subdivided into two major types depending on how the immunity was introduced. **Naturally acquired immunity** occurs through contact with a disease causing agent, when the contact was not deliberate, whereas **artificially acquired immunity** develops only through deliberate actions, such as vaccination. Both naturally and artificially acquired immunity can be further subdivided depending on whether immunity is induced in the host or passively transferred from an immune host. **Passive immunity** is acquired through transfer of antibodies or activated T-cells from an immune host, and is short lived—usually lasting only a few months—whereas **active immunity** is induced in the host itself by antigen and lasts much longer, sometimes lifelong. The diagram below summarizes these divisions of immunity.

c. Maternal mortality rate

See question no. VI-d of GNM Paper-3-2014.

d. Epidemiology.

Epidemiology is the study of frequency, distribution and determinants of health related states in human populations. The study is followed by establishing programs to prevent or control health problems. The objective of epidemiology is to determine the effective strategies for the control of diseases. These are based on the elimination, modification and manipulation of the determinants and risk factors of diseases. Epidemiology is a body of knowledge culled through field studies. The aim of these studies is to find out the differences between (a) those persons who have the disease and those who do not, (b) those places where the disease is common and those places where it is rare, and (c) those times when the disease is common and those when it is uncommon.

Epidemiology process is bound to continue in future adding new challenges to the practice of public health. In these circumstances epidemiology is designed to play an increasingly important role in defining the magnitude of the problems, forecasting their long-term consequences and deriving appropriate strategies for their promotion and control. Presently, the use of epidemiology is mainly confined to following areas:

1. **Disease antecedents:** Epidemiology has always stressed the importance of exploring the natural history of disease in their entirely, with special stress on the identification of disease antecedents rather than disease consequents.
2. **Disease correlates:** Epidemiology has revolutionized the concept of etiology and etiogenesis. Epidemiological studies identified a variety of diseases correlate not all of which are casually associated diseases, and some of which behave as risk factors. The risk factors increase the probability of contracting a particular disease.
3. **Disease behavior:** Epidemiological surveillance is applied to disease of international significance. Disease behavior is studied by a process of epidemiological surveillance whereby diseases are kept under constant observation firstly to identify their normal distribution patterns and normal temporal fluctuations, and secondly to detect any deviation in their expected behavior patterns.
4. **Disease and causation:** Epidemiological studies not only establish cause effect association of many noncommunicable diseases, but also estimate the strength of associations in terms of relative and absolute risks. The most notable example is the cause effect associations established by epidemiological studies between smoking and lung cancer and smoking and coronary heart diseases.
5. **Strategy formulation:** Epidemiology plays an important role in strategy formulation for disease control programs and improves program efficiency and effectiveness. Control and

eradication of disease is much more complex than their prevention or treatment. A sound control strategy is one that epidemiologically relevant and operationally feasible.
6. **Program evaluation:** Program performance is evaluated by measuring achievements in various operational areas of the program. Evaluation of public health program is both managerial and epidemiological process.

II. Fill in the blanks

a. World tuberculosis day is on: **March-24.**
b. National health policy was launched in the year: **1983.**
c. Nursing process is also known as: **Systematic Scientific** approach.
d. **Demography** is the scientific study of human population.

III. Write short notes on any *four* of the following:

a. Bhore Committee Report or recommendations

In 1943, the Government of India appointed a committee as the Bhore Committee for the health survey and development committee with Sir, Joseph Bhore as Chairman. Its aim was to survey the existing position regarding the health conditions and health organization in the committee which had among its members some of the pioneers of the health, met regularly for 2 years and submitted its famous report in 1946 which runs into 4 volumes.

Important Recommendations

1. **Nutrition of the people:** They pointed out the main defects of the average Indian diet results from the insufficiency of proteins, mineral salts and vitamins. They also recommend special measures to increase the production of food rich in proteins. Also prevention of food adulteration and improvement of the quality of the food.
2. **Health education:** Bhore Committee suggested that health education to school children on hygiene should begin at the earliest. The doctors, nurses, midwife and in fact every health worker will discharge his or her duties and by educating the persons with whom they deal with regard to prevention of disease and the promotion of positive health.
3. **Physical examination:** Committee stated that there is great dearth of suitable and qualified teachers for imparting instructions in this subject. Also physical training program for the community with emphasis on national games and exercises.
4. **Health services for mothers and children:** At the headquarters of each primary unit and in place where 30 bed hospitals are located the service for mothers and children should be available.
5. **Health services of the school children:** The school teachers who have to carry or certain health duties require careful training and continuous supervision. They have to conduct health education programs. In each primary unit, the male medical officer should take charge of the school health services.
6. **Occupational heath including industrial health:** The Committee recommended that the industrial health organization should form an integral part of the provincial health department and government.
7. **Health services for certain important diseases:** Bhore Committee studied the existing legal and administrative provisions to deal with communicable diseases and suggested certain measures for controlling communicable diseases.

8. **Environmental hygiene:** An essential part of the campaign for promoting public health was to improve man's physical environment. The Committee's main recommendations were improvement in village and town planning.
9. **Vital Statistics:** The Committee recommended administrative organization at the center, organization at provincial head quarters and district organization. Another recommendation is provision of training facilities for statistics.
10. **Professional education:** The main objective of the Committee during his period was the provision of adequate and suitably trained staff to enable the plan of health work effectively.
11. **Drug and medical requisites:** They recommended our universities should undertake research with a view to produce life saving drugs in this country.

b. RCH program

Reproductive child health (RCH) can be defined as a state in which people have the ability to reproduce and regulate their fertility, women are able to go through pregnancy and child birth safely, the outcome of pregnancy is successful in terms of maternal and infant survival and well being, and couples are able to have sexual relations free of the fear of pregnancy and contracting disease.

The origin of the RCH initiative can be justifiably traced from the Alma Ata declaration wherein maternal and child health care including family planning was identified as an important element in the primary health care package. In 1994, the CSSM was replaced by RCH (Reproductive Child health) program in India. RCH incorporates all the elements of the parent CSSM program besides including two more elements namely, the control of sexually transmitted infections (STIs) and the control of reproductive tract infections (RTIs).

RCH program is a joint venture supported by inputs from the Government of India and various donors' agencies, including the World Bank and the European Commission. The program is envisaged to provide need-based, client centered, demand driven high quality, integrated services to the eligible population of young women and children. The program was formally launched on 15th October 1997.

Objectives of RCH

1. The immediate objective is the promotion of maternal and child health to ensure safe method and child survival.
2. The intermediate objective is the reduction of maternal and child morbidity and mortality.
3. The ultimate objective is the attainment of population stabilization through responsible reproductive behavior, expected to emerge in response to reduced risk to child survival.

Organization and Administration

1. **Organizational infrastructure:** The very facts that MCH is service activity of the primary healthcare system makes it an ideal organization for offering RCH services to the community through its nationwide network of community health centers, primary health centers and subcenters.
2. **Consultants:** There is provision for the engagement of consultants for the project period. The appointment of consultants is on contractual basis in keeping with the World Bank procedure. The service of consultants are needed for improving the management, implementation and monitoring RCH program.
3. **Traditional practitioners:** There is a provision for involvement traditional practitioners have to receive an orientation training course to update their knowledge and improve their skills in the areas of RCH activity.

4. **Nongovernmental organizations:** It is felt that NGO's would serve as complementary agency for optimizing the functioning of RCH program. They are better place to try innovative approaches which the conventional government system cannot afford.
5. **Equipment and supplies:** There is provision for supplying equipment kits, surgical kits, delivery kits, IUD kits and MTP kits to help in improving the quality and content of RCH service to the eligible population.

Maternal Health

1. **Obstetric care:** It is provided to all the pregnant women on a longitudinal basis, it starts from early pregnancy and spans over a prenatal, intranatal and postnatal phases.
2. **Infection control:** Observation of cleanliness is the simplest way of avoiding infection. It means clean hands and clean surface. The birth attendant washes her hands thoroughly with soap and water and puts on presterilized gloves before assisting delivery.
3. **Nutrition promotion:** All young women are advised to build up their prepregnancy nutritional reserves. They are instructed to consume foods rich in iron content. Additionally, every pregnant woman is motivated to consume one large Iron folic acid tablet once daily for 100 days, starting from the end of the first trimester of pregnancy.

Child Health

1. **Neonatal care:** It is provided to all the newborns the components of the care being eye care, cord care, recording of birth weight and prevention of cord injury.
2. **Infection control:** Its observation of hygienic precautions during delivery by way of clean attendant hands, clean delivery surface, clean razor blade, clean cord tie and clean cord stump are crucial elements for avoiding infection.
3. **Nutrition promotion:** The mother encouraged to practice exclusive breastfeeding. She is advised to include carotene rich vegetables and fruits in the diet of her children and avail of vitamin A supplements for children available at health facilities.

Reproductive Health

1. **Fertility control:** RCH program has provision for universalizing contraceptive practices and extending sterilization facilities to the eligible couple population.
2. **MTP service:** RCH program provides for legalized MTP service. The facilities are available in all district hospitals, subdivisional hospitals, community health centers and primary health centers that have operation theaters and MTP trained doctors.
3. **Adolescent counseling:** The scheme provides for counseling of adolescents on problems related to sex, and sexuality, including various forms of sexual dysfunction, sexual aberration, sexual abuse, importance, etc.

c. Indigenous system of medicine

Ayurveda: The doctrine of Ayurveda aims to keep structural and functional entities in a functional state of equilibrium, which signifies good health. Any imbalance due to internal and external factor causes disease and restoring equilibrium through various techniques, procedures, regimes, diet and medicine constitute treatment. The philosophy of Ayurveda is based on the theory of *Pancha bhootas* (five element theory) of which all the objects and living bodies are composed of.

Siddha: Siddha System of Medicine emphasize that medical treatment is oriented not merely to disease, but also has to take into account the patient, environment, age, habits, physical condition. Siddha literature is in Tamil, and it is largely practiced in Tamil speaking parts of India and abroad.

Unani: Unani System of Medicine is based on established knowledge and practices relating to promotion of positive health and prevention of diseases. Although Unani system originated in Greece, passed through many countries, Arabs enriched it with their aptitude and experience and the system was brought to India during medieval period. Unani system emphasizes the use of naturally occurring, most herbal medicines, though it uses ingredients of animal and marine origin.

Homeopathy: Homeopathy is a system of medicine, which believes in a specialized method of treatment of curing diseases by administration of potency drugs, which have been experimentally proved to possess the power of producing similar artificial systems on human beings.

Yoga and Naturopathy: Yoga is a way of life, which has the potential for improvement of social and personal behavior, improvement of physical health by encouraging better circulation of oxygenated blood in the body, restraining sense organs and thereby inducing tranquility and serenity of mind. Naturopathy is also a way of life, with drugless treatment of diseases. The system is based on the ancient practice of application of simple laws of nature. The advocates of naturopathy focus on eating and living habits, adoption of purification measures, use of hydrotherapy, baths, massage, etc.

d. Primary health center

Primary health center is essential health care made universally accessible to individuals and families in the community by means acceptable to them, through their full participation and at a cost that the community and country can afford. Primary health centers were started in 1952 as part of community development program in order to provide comprehensive health care to people in rural areas. The community development blocks covering approximately 100 villages and about 80,000 populations. The primary health care consists of a main building and three subcenters.

Primary health center setup: Primary health center is the first contact print between people and doctor. Primary health center is established to cover 30,000 populations in plains and 20,000 populations in hilly/tribal areas. Establishment and maintenance of these centers are done under the minimum basic need program of the State Governments. The work of PHC is looked after by a Medical Officer. There are 4–6 beds for patients and come diagnostic facilities for patients are also available at PHC.

Attributes of PHC

1. **Accessibility:** It denotes reachability of a service, notwithstanding social cultural or geographic barriers.
2. **Acceptability:** It is a measure of community approval. Acceptability achieves through cultural assimilation of its policies and programs.
3. **Adaptability:** It is a measure of flexibility, denoting the ability of a system to permit alterations and modifications.
4. **Affordability:** It signifies the financial and economical dimension of a health care system.
5. **Availability:** Availability is a time function, demanding round the clock presence of a service.
6. **Appropriateness:** It is a measure of relevance in terms of needs and demands of the consumers.
7. **Closeness:** It is measure of proximity between the providers and consumers of a service.
8. **Continuity:** Continuity of a service is a measure of its length of association.

9. **Comprehensiveness:** Comprehensiveness of a service is a measure of its ability to meet the total needs of a community.
10. **Coordinative:** It is a measure of participation, cooperation, coordination and community participation.

e. World Health Organization

The WHO is specified non-political health agency of the United Nations with its head quarters at Geneva. WHO had its origin in April 1945 during the conference held at San Francisco to set up the United Nations. The constitution for WHO was drawn up under the chairmanship of Rene Sand at an international health conference in New York in 1946.

The constitution came into action on April 7, 1948 which is celebrated every year as "**World Health Day**". A world health day theme is chosen each year to focus attention on specific aspect of public health. After an examination of the various methods used by countries throughout the world in producing health care. WHO introduces primary health center concept in 1975.

Objective: The main objective is attainment of health for all people. The current objective is to attain health by all people of the world by the year 2000 AD. The level of health which will permit the people to lead a socially and economically produce life known as "Health for All by 2000 AD".

Functions of WHO

1. WHO is the World's directing and coordinating authority on International health aspect?
2. It provides cooperation with other organizations collaborates with UN and with the other specialized agencies and maintains various degrees of working relationships.
3. In the aspects of health statistics, it concentrates on morbidity and mortality statistics relating to health problems.
4. Regarding environmental health, it advises governments on countries to do the same.
5. It carries out various research studies and also motivates informations.
6. Acts as a world library issuing health literature and informations.
7. Its work extends for prevention and control of specific disease, e.g. global eradication of smallpox, communicable diseases and non-communicable diseases as cancer, cardiovascular diseases, genetic disorders, mental disorders, drug addiction and dental diseases.
8. WHO aimed for the development of comprehensive health services like developing primary health centers for the whole population and development of health man power utilization.

Specific global targets of WHO

1. Every one in every country will have at least ready access to essential health care and to first level referral facilities.
2. Everyone will be actively involved in caring for themselves and their families as far as they can in community action for health.
3. Communities throughout the world will share with governments the responsibility for the health care of their members for the health of their people.
4. All governments will have assumed overall responsibilities to all people.
5. Safe drinking water and sanitation will be available to all people.
6. All people will be adequately nourished.
7. All children will be immunized against the major infectious diseases of childhood.
8. Communicable diseases in the developing countries will be of no greater public health significance in the year 2000 than they are in developed countries in the year 1980.

9. All possible ways will be applied to prevent and control communicable diseases and promote mental health through influencing lifestyle and controlling the physical and psychological environment.
10. Essential drugs will be available to all.

Health contribution to India
1. The control of communicable diseases, such as smallpox, leprosy, cholera, malaria, and tuberculosis.
2. Assists in biomedical research program in India, including research in family planning methods.
3. Education and training of all types of professional and auxiliary health workers. For example, post – certificate BSc Nursing Programs at College of Nursing, Chennai and at Chandigarh were initiated by WHO.
4. Strengthening the public health administration.
5. Improving environmental sanitation.

IV. a. Define primary health care
    b. List the function of primary health care
    c. Write the role of nurse in primary health care

See question no. V of GNM Paper-3-2014.

V. a. Define school health program
    b. Write the components of school health program
    c. Explain the role of nurse in school health program

The second component of a comprehensive School Health Program is health services. The main objective of school health services is to look after the health of children, prevent and control of common diseases, provide first aid in emergency and refer those who need specialized treatment.

Health appraisal: This includes an assessment of the present health and health needs of students as well as teachers. Both health personnel and teachers participate in this activity. Observation, identification and encouragement in the correction of remedial defects are important steps in health appraisal. At the time of the health check-up of children, the parents should preferably be present to give the full history of the child and the present illness if there is any. All possible measures should be taken to promote normal health and development of the child. Health counseling of pupils and parents is also part of health appraisal. School health services assist in the identification and education of scholastically backward or handicapped (physically, mentally and psychologically) or sick children and their follow-up.

Remedial measures: These include curative, corrective and rehabilitative aspects (for example, providing spectacles, hearing aids or orthopedics aids). The doctors, teachers and parents should plan for the follow-up treatment of children after the diagnosis is made.

Provision of first-aid and emergency care: Every school should be equipped with the first-aid amenities. All teachers should be trained in first-aid and kits should be provided according to the strength of the children and the list of the drugs is as advised by the Medical Officer which are very essential for certain emergencies. Promotive and preventive services these include control of communicable diseases, immunization, isolation, and supplementary nutrition. Health education and healthful school living are certainly a part of promotive services. Maintenance of health records is also part of school health services.

Nature of School Health Program

1. School health program is an integral part of community health. It is the phase of community health and family health service that promotes the well-being of the child and his education for healthful living.
2. School health program can be a powerful influence for shaping health behavior. There is a unique opportunity to promote, maintain and improve health and well-being since teachers reach most people early in life where attitudes and values are most readily developed.
3. School health service is a personal health service. It stresses the role of the child as a "change agent for community. A child has greater capacity to observe, learn, experiment and then transfer knowledge to others.
4. School health helps in formation of health habits and practices of healthful living throughout school life, which are very important during the formative period of one's life. Continuous practice and experience will help and individual to lead a healthy life.
5. School health program helps the younger generation become healthy and useful citizens, who will be able to perform their role effectively for the welfare of themselves, their families the community at large and country as a whole.

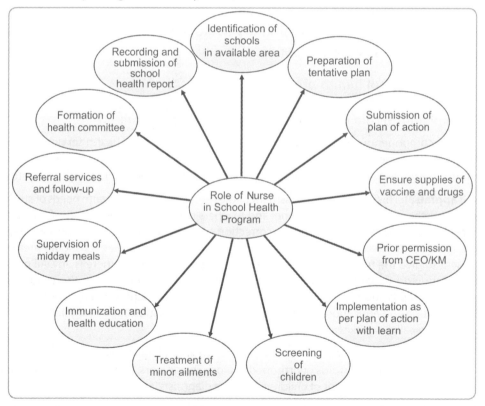

Role of Nurse in School Health Services

1. **Initiation and implementation:** Beginning and implementation of school health service is the responsibility of community health nurse. Before initiating school health services, the nurse should collect complete information about school administration, number of students and teachers, available resources, school environment, facilities of entertainment and sports, etc.

2. **Liaison activities:** The main role of school health nurse is to establish liaison between the school, home and the community. The school health nurse also interacts, involve and coordinate with governmental or non-governmental national or international health agencies.
3. **Coordination:** The school health nurse takes up the responsibility of coordination between doctors, teachers, parent's local leadership, NGOs and voluntary organizations, etc.
4. **Evaluation:** The school health nurse evaluates school health services on the basis of different facts, documents and information. She also provides feed-back on these services on the basis of her knowledge and experience.
5. **Training and guidance:** School health nurse plays an important role in training of teachers about daily check-up, maintaining health records and providing first aid. She contributes effectively in developing healthy habits in children.
6. **Active participation:** In organizing health check-up, providing treatment, immunization programs, nutritional programs, maintaining school health records, good environment at school and providing follow up services.

SECTION-II

VI. Choose the correct answer and write:
a. Time required measuring the Mantoux test: **48–72 hours.**
   (i) 24–48 hours, (ii) 48–72 hours, (iii) 10–24 hours
b. According to ICDS scheme there is an Anganwadi worker for a population of: **1000.**
   (i) 500, (ii) 2000, (iii)1000
c. Community health is also called: **Public health.**
   (i) Public health, (ii) Community medicine, (iii) All the above

VII. Differentiate between the following:

a. Balwadi nutrition program and Midday Meal Program

Balwadi nutrition program is a healthcare and education program launched by the government of India to provide food supplementation at balwadis to children of the age group 3–6 years in rural areas. This program was started in 1970 under the Department of Social Welfare, Government of India. Four national level organizations including the Indian Council of Child Welfare are given grants to implement this program. The food supplement provides 300 calories of energy and 10 g of protein per child per day. Balwadis are being phased out because of the implementation of the integrated child development services program.

Midday meal program has an important role in providing balanced diet to school children. This is an effort taken by Government of India. Since 1960s to provide at least one nutritious meal and diet supplements to children in primary and middle schools. It was first organized in 1957 in Tamil Nadu successfully. In this program, one third of the child's daily requirement can be fulfilled. CARE, UNICEF and many international, governmental voluntary agencies give their contribution in this. The primary objective of midday meal program is to improve the nutritional status of children and imparting nutritional education and to ensure universal primary education.

b. Control and eradication

Control: Although control is a range rather than a level, a particular level of control may be an aim of policy. Because every choice entails consequences, choice of the "optimal" level of control requires economic analysis. *Optimal,* here is defined in relation to the model that gives rise to the result.

Control is local and so needs to be looked at from the local perspective. Because one country's (or region's) control may affect other countries (regions), a global perspective exists as well. The level of control that is optimal for one country (region) may not be optimal from the perspective of the world as a whole. Thus, a need exists to distinguish between, say, a locally optimal level of control and one that is globally optimal. Finally, control requires ongoing intervention. Sustaining a given level of control requires an annual expenditure.

Eradication: Eradication differs from control in that it is global. The term denotes the certified total absence of human cases, the absence of a reservoir for the organism in nature, and absolute containment of any infectious source. Eradication permits control interventions to stop or at least to be curtailed significantly. Finally, eradication is binary. Control levels can vary, but a disease is either certified as eradicated or not. Every disease can be controlled, even if only by using simple measures, such as quarantine. The ultimate achievement of control is eradication. But not every disease that can be controlled can be eradicated. Very few diseases, in fact, are potential candidates for eradication. The criteria for the feasibility for eradication as a preference over control are discussed in the section titled "Economic Considerations."

VIII. Write short notes on any *two* of the following:

a. National Immunization Schedule

Immunization schedule should be planned according to the needs of the community. It should be relevant with existing community health problems. It must be effective, feasible and acceptable by the community. Every country has its own immunization schedule. The WHO, launched global immunization program in 1974, known as Expanded Program on Immunization (EPI) to protect all children of the world against six killer diseases. In India, EPI was launched in January 1978. The EPI is now renamed as Universal Child Immunization, as per declaration sponsored by UNICEF. In India, it is called as Universal Immunization Program (UIP) and was launched in 1985, November, for the universal coverage of immunization to the eligible population.

Beneficiaries	Age	Vaccine	Dose	Route	Amount
(a) Infants	• At Birth (for institutional deliveries)	• BCG • OPV	• Single • Zero dose	Intradermal Oral	0.05 mL 2 drops
	• At 6 weeks	• BCG (it not given at birth) • DTP-1 • OPV-1	• Single 1st 1st	Intradermal Intramuscular Oral	0.1 mL 0.5 mL 2 drops
	• At 10 weeks	• DTP-2 • OPV-2	2nd 2nd	Intramuscular Oral	0.5 mL 2 drops
	• At 14 weeks	• DTP-3 • OPV-3	3rd 3rd	Intramuscular Oral	0.5 mL 2 drops
	• At 9 months	• Measles	Single	Subcutaneous	0.5 mL
(b) Children	• At 16–24 months	• DTP • OPV	Booster Booster	Intramuscular Oral	0.5 mL 2 drops
	At 5–6 years	DTP	Single intramuscular 0.5 mL • second dose of DT should be given after 4 weeks, it not vaccinated previously with DTP		
	At 10–16 yesrs	TT	Single intramuscular 0.5 mL • second dose of DT should be given if not vaccinated previously		
(c) Pregnant women	• Early in pregnancy • One month after	• TT-1 • TT-2	1st 2nd	Intramuscular Intramuscular	0.5 mL 0.5 mL

The Global Alliance for Vaccines and Immunization (GAVI) is worldwide coalition of organization, established in 1999, to reduce disparities in lifesaving vaccine access and increase global immunization coverage. GAVI is collaborative mission of Government, NGOs, UNICEF, WHO and World Bank. The objective of introduction new but under used vaccines in the developing countries, where the diseases like hepatitis-B and *H. influenza* 'B' (Hib) are highly prevalent. National Immunization Schedule as recommended by Government of India for uniform implementation throughout the country was formulated. The schedule contents the age at which the vaccines are best given and the number of doses recommended for each vaccine. The schedule also covers immunization of women during pregnancy against tetanus.

Note:
1. Interval between 2 doses should not be less than one month.
2. Minor cough, colds and mild fever or diarrhea are not a contraindication to vaccination.
3. In some states, hepatitis B vaccine is given as routine immunization.
4. Interruption of the schedule with a delay between doses not interferes with the final immunity achieved. There is no basis for the mistaken belief, that if a second or third dose in an immunization is delayed, the immunization schedule must be started all over again. So, if the child missed a dose, the whole schedule need not be repeated again.

b. Employees State Insurance Scheme

The ESI of 1948 covered all powers using factories other than seasonal factories wherein 20 or more persons were employed. It proved to be a very beneficial step towards social security of factory workers. The Act alleviates economic and physical suffering by providing benefits in cash and kind during sickness, maternity and occupational injury.

Benefits of ESI Act

1. **Medical benefits:** Implying comprehensive medical care including outpatient, inpatient domiciliary investigational and MCH services.
2. **Sickness benefits:** Implying periodical payments to workers during pregnancy and pregnancy related disorders.
3. **Maternity benefits:** Implying periodical payments to workers disabled as a result of an employment injury.
4. **Dependent's benefit:** Implying periodical payments to the dependent of a deceased worker.
5. **Disablement benefit:** Benefit for temporary disablement is paid at the rate about 75% of the wages for the education of disablement. For permanent total disablement, the payment is made at the same rate for the whole life in the form of pension and at a proportional rate in case of permanent partial disablement.
6. **Funeral benefits:** The maximum amount of ₹ 1000 for funeral expenses is given to the eldest surviving member on death of insured worker.
7. **Rehabilitation benefits:** Ensured workers who require artificial limbs are provided with artificial limbs and also the cash allowance equivalent to the sickness benefit rate at the time when they are admitted for provision/replacement of artificial limbs.

ESI—pattern of Financial Support

1. The employer pays 4.75 percentages of total wages.
2. The employee contributes 1.75% of his/her wage.

3. The state government shares 7/8th of the total expenditure on medical care.
4. The ESI corporation shares 7/8th of a total expenditure on medical care.
5. As far the central government is concerned it supports 2/3 of the administrative expenditure.

ESI—Administrative members:
1. Minister of labor—Chairperson.
2. The secretary-ministry of labor—Vice chairperson.
3. Representatives of central government—5 members.
4. Representatives from the states—one from each state.
5. Representatives from union territories—one member from each UT.
6. Representatives of employees—5 members.
7. Representatives of employers—5 members.
8. Representatives of medical profession—2 members.
9. Representatives of parliament—3 members.
10. Director General of the ESI—member.

c. Prevention and control of vitamin A deficiency

Vitamin A occurs only in foods of animal origin. Vitamin A activity is also possessed by carotenoids found in plants. Hence, carotenoids are called provitamin A. Vitamin A is not synthesized in the body and must by supplied by food supplements. One of the best defined role of vitamin A is its requirements for normal vision. Vitamin A is necessary for the health of the epithelial cells.

Vitamin A deficiency is one of the main causes of blindness in India. The signs of vitamin A deficiency are predominantly ocular. They include night blindness, conjunctival xerosis, Bitot's spots corned xerosis and keratomalacia. The term "xerophthalmia" (dry eye) comprises all the ocular manifestations of vitamin A deficiency ranging from night blindness to keratomalacia.

Nonocular features. Increased susceptibility to infections (including diarrheas and urinary tract infections), hyperfollicular keratosis, phrynoderma (toad skin), and bladder calculi are associated with vitamin A deficiency.

Treatment: Vitamin A deficiency is treated with 110 mg of retinol palmitate orally or 55 mg intramuscularly followed by a similar dose 2 days later.

Prevention: Five doses of oral vitamin A concentrate are given. The first dose of 1 lakh IU (3.3 mg) is given to 9–12 months old infants along with the measles immunization. The second dose of 2 lath IU (6.6 mg) is given at 16–18 months of age along with the booster of OPV and DT. The last three doses each of 2 lakh IU are given when the child is aged 2, 2½, and 3 years. People are educated to grow GLVs, tomatoes, carrots, beet, papaya, mangoes, etc., and consume them liberally. Conditioning factors are eliminated with immunization of children against vaccine preventable disease, and improvement in water supply and sanitation.

Following are possible: (a) Fortification of cereal powder and wheat flour, sugar or tea with retinol. (b) Retinol injections to pregnant women to protect the fetus and the future baby.

IX. a. Define health team
   b. List the members of health team
   c. Explain the role of male health worker in health team

The health team consists of a medical officer, health assistant (female and male), and health worker (female)! ANM, nurse and midwife, block extension educator, pharmacy, laboratory technician and is supported by 14 paramedical and other staff. It acts as a referral unit for six sib centers and has

4–6 beds. The activities of PHCs involve curative, preventive, promotive and family welfare services. The number of PHCs functioning in the country is 22,975. The mere presence of a variety of health professionals is not sufficient to establish team 'work', it is the props division and combination of their operations from which the benefits of divided labor will be derived. The health team at the primary health center consists of the following health personnel:

Staffing Pattern at PHC: In the new set-up each PHC will have the following staff.
- Medical officer   1
- Pharmacist   1
- Nurse mid-wife   1
- Health worker female   1
- Block extension education   1
- Health assistant male   1
- Health assistant female/LHV   1
- VDC   1
- LDC   1
- Lab technician   1
- Driver subject to availability of vehicle   1
- Class   4
-           Total   15

Staff for community health center:
- Medical officer   4
- Nurse Mid-wives   7
- Dresser   1
- Pharmacist/compounder   1
- Lab technician   1
- Radiographer   1
- Ward boys   2
- Dhobi   1
- Sweepers   3
- Mali   1
- Chowkidar   1
- Aya   1
- Peon   1
-           Total   25

Role of male health worker in health team

At subcenter along with female multipurpose health worker, a male multipurpose health worker is also needed. In this direction, union government has started a training program to convert single purpose workers into multipurpose workers. Under this program, 10th class pass candidates are selected, trained for one year and then appointed at subcenters. This program was started in 47 health and family welfare training centers and is 100% central sponsored. In order to compensate the deficiency of male multipurpose workers, 28 family welfare training centers and 23 multipurpose workers (male) basic school are giving training to the male workers (2005).

Job responsibilities of male health worker: Under the multipurpose workers scheme a health assistant male is expected to cover a population of 30,000 (20,000 in tribal and hilly areas) in which there are six subentries, each with one health worker male. The health assistant male will carry out the following functions:

Supervision and guidance
1. Supervise and guide the health worker male in the delivery of healthcare services to the community.
2. Strengthen the knowledge and skills of the health worker male.
3. Help the health worker male in improving his skills in working in the community.
4. Help and guide the health worker male in planning and organizing his program of activities.
5. Visit each health workers male at least once a week on a fixed day to observe and guide him in his day-to-day activities.
6. Assess monthly the progress of work of the health worker male and submit an assessment report to the medical officer of the primary health center.
7. Carry out supervisory home visits in the area of the health worker male.

Teamwork
1. Help the health workers to work as part of the health team.
2. Coordinate his activities with those of the health assistant female and other health personnel, including the health guides and dais.
3. Coordinate the health activities in his area with the activities of workers of other departments and agencies, and attend meetings at PHC level.
4. Conduct staff meetings fortnightly with the health workers in coordination with the health assistant female at one of the subcenter by rotation.
5. Attend staff meetings at the primary health center.
6. Assist the medical officer of the primary health center in the organization of the different health services in the area.
7. Participate as a member of the health team in mass camps and campaigns in health programs.
8. Assist the medical officer of the primary health center in conducting training programs for various categories of health personnel.

Supplies and equipment
1. In collaboration with the health assistant female, check at regular intervals the stores available at the sub center and ensure timely placement of indent for and procuring the supplies and equipment in good time.
2. Check that the drugs at the subcenter are properly stored and that the equipment is well maintained.
3. Ensure that the health worker male maintains his kits in a proper way.
4. Records and reports scrutinize the maintenance of records by the health worker male and guide him in their proper maintenance.
5. Review records received from the health worker male, consolidate them and submit report to the medical officer of the primary health center.

X. a. Define family welfare program.
  b. What is the aims and objectives of family welfare program.
  c. Explain the nurse's role in family welfare program.

a. Define Family Welfare Program.

India launched a nationwide family planning program in 1952, making it the first country in the world to do so, though records show that birth control clinics have been functioning in the country since 1930. The first family planning clinic was opened at Poona by Professor RD Karve in 1923.

In **1946**, a health survey and development committee, chaired by Sir Joseph Bhore, advised for deliberate limitation of family size and recommended the provision of integrated preventive, promotive and curative primary healthcare services with high priority for improving nutritional and health status of mother and child.

The early beginnings of the program were modest with the establishment of a few clinics and distribution of educational material training and research. During the Third five year plan (1961–66), family planning was declared as "the very center of planned development".

The emphasis was shifted from the purely "clinic approach" to the more vigorous "extension education approach" for motivating the people for acceptance of the "small necessitated a major structural reorganization of the program, leading to the creation of a separate department of family planning in 1966 in the Ministry of Health.

During the fourth five year plan, the program was made an integral part of MCH activities of PHC's and their subcenters. In 1970, an all India Hospital postpartum program and in 1972 the medical termination of pregnancy (MTP) were introduced. During Fifth five year plan (1975–80), there have been major changes. In April 1976, the country framed its first "National Population Policy".

The National Health Policy has also called for restricting the healthcare delivery system to achieve HFA/2000 AD and family planning has been accorded a central place in health development.

b. What are the aims and objectives of Family Welfare Program?

1. To avoid unwanted births.
2. To bring about wanted births.
3. To regulate the intervals between pregnancies.
4. To control the time at which birth occurs in relation to the age of the parents.
5. To determine the number of children in the family.

Planning Commission Recommendations

1. Widespread education creates necessary social background for the success of family planning program.
2. Integration of family planning with the normal health services.
3. Provision of family planning services, even sterilization through medical and health centers.
4. To develop training program in teaching hospitals and medical college.
5. To stimulate and utilize the voluntary leadership.

c. Explain the nurse's role in Family Welfare Program

The role of the nurse in family welfare will be governed by the policy of the government or the health institution employing them. Policies may vary from those that require nurses to participate in family welfare activities to those that forbid them to do so or that limit their participation to giving advice to high risk mothers eligible because of specific health reasons.

1. **Administrative role:** The community health nurse has to participate and organize family welfare programs at national, regional, and community level as an administrator.
2. **Functional role:** Community health nurse functions include assisting doctor in prenatal, postnatal examination and with various clinical and biological tests. Also helps in family planning and provides opportunity to choose suitable methods of contraception.

3. **Supervisory role:** As a supervisor community health nurses should encourage their staff to participate actively in family welfare program. The community health nurse should organize in service program to other health workers, professionals and auxiliary nursing personnels.
4. **Education role:** As a basis for counseling in family planning, nurses must have sound knowledge of the biology of human reproduction, education for family life, the concept and principles underlying family planning. The community health nurse should play as effective educator for the individual, family, community in family welfare activities.
5. **Role in research:** The community health nurse is a primary member of the multidisciplinary research team. She has to extend directly or indirectly to cooperate, participate and motivate all research activities on family welfare activities.
6. **Evaluation role:** The community health nurse is a primary member of the multidisciplinary research team. She has to extend directly or indirectly to cooperate, participate and motivate all research activities on family welfare activities.

Family Welfare Nurse Activities

1. **Antenatal care:** Registration and provision of antenatal mothers, detection and treatment of anemic pregnant mothers. Timely detection and referral of high-risk pregnant mothers.
2. **Natal care:** As far as possible delivery should take place under the supervision of qualified personnel. Detection and referral of high-risk labor cases. Identification of existing dais and organizing training.
3. **Postnatal care:** Natal resuscitation, growth monitoring and early detection and referral of high-risk newborn babies.
4. **Immunization:** Immunization services against following communicable diseases like polio, diphtheria, whooping cough, and measles, etc.
5. **Contraceptive services:** Community health nurse involves various activities like male or female sterilization, copper-T insertion, oral pill distribution, Nirodh distribution and indigenous traditional methods.
6. **Medical termination of pregnancy (MTP):** The community health nurse assist in MTP along with the medical officer.
7. **Guide:** The community health nurse should guide the female health worker regarding distribution of contraceptives.
8. **Health education:** In health education through various media she could involve community leaders to participate in the programme and through them, she could carry out family planning work.
9. **Follow up activities:** The community health nurse does follow up through home visits, clinical visits and maintaining careful record of follow up, findings and date of supplying device, etc.

OR

a. **What is National Leprosy Eradication Program?**
b. **Explain the role of community health nurse in implementation of national health program**

Leprosy is one of the major health and socioeconomic problems in the country; it is a chronic infectious disease and spreads mainly by dose contracts with infected patients. However, droplet infection is also considered responsible for spread of disease. The average prevalence of disease in 1981 was 5.77 per 1000. Disease carried by *M. leprae* affects mainly the peripheral nerves, partial or total loss of cutaneous sensation in the affected area, presence of thickened nerves and presence of acid fast bacilli in the skin or nasal smears.

The **National Leprosy Control Program**, in operation since 1955, is a centrally aided program to achieve control of leprosy thorough early detection of cases and DDS (dapson) monotheraphy on an ambulatory basis. In 1980 the government of India declared its resolve to "eradicate" leprosy by the year 2000 and constituted a working group to advice accordingly.

In 1983 the Control Program was redesigned as National Leprosy "Eradication" Program with the goal of eradicating the disease by the turn of the country. The aim was to reduce case lead to 1 or less than 1 per 10,000 populations.

Development of Infrastructure NLEP

1. Leprosy control unit or modified leprosy control unit   778
2. Urban leprosy center   907
3. Survey education and treatment center   5744
4. Temporary hospitalization ward   290
5. Reconstructive surgery unit   75
6. Sample survey cum assessment unit   40
7. Mobile leprosy treatment units   350

World Bank Supported Project

The first phase of the World Bank supported NLEP project was completed on 31st March 2000 and it was extended for 6 months to complete the preparation of proposed 2nd phase project. During the 1st phase the case detected was 3.8 million patients and case cure with MDT was 4.4. Million old and new cases. The phase 2nd project of World Bank has been approved for a period of 3 years starting from June 2001.

Tenth Five year Plan for Leprosy Elimination

The tenth five year plan goal is to bring prevalence of leprosy to less than 1 case per 10,000 populations.

Strategies of Xth 5-year-plan:
1. Completing horizontal integration of he program into the general health care system by 2007. The personnel employee under NLEP will be transferred to the states.
2. Skill up gradation and redeployment of the over 30,000 leprosy workers and laboratory technicians get integrated in primary health care institutions for the early detection and management of leprosy patients.
3. Training of existing personnel in primary health care institutions for the early detection and management of leprosy patients.
4. Reconstructive surgery to improve functional status of the individual's methods of leprosy control.

In 1982, WHO regimens of chemotherapy

1. **Multidrug therapy:** The following combinations of drugs for the treatment of multi bacillary cases of leprosy—Rifampcin 600 mg once a month, daspone 100 mg OD and clofazamine 300 mg once a month—the duration of treatment is 2 years.
2. **Aucibacillary terapy:** The recommended drug regimen under PBT Rifampicin 600 mg once a month for 6 months and dapsone 100 mg daily for 6 months—the duration of treatment is 6 months.
3. **Other measure:** Selective isolation, follow up cases protection of children (BCG vaccinations) rehabilitation ad health education.

2012
Community Health Nursing

SECTION-I

I. Fill in the blanks:
   a. Farmer's lung is due to the inhalation of: _____
   b. The 12th five year plan covers the period from: _____
   c. The indicator of the prevalence of contraceptive practice in the community is: _____
   d. The term Siddha implies: _____

II. State whether the following statement are *true* or *false*:
   a. In India, there is one primary health center for every 30,000 population.
   b. The road to health card is important tool for monitoring growth of under five children.
   c. Weight gain during pregnancy in a healthy mother is 6–8 kg.
   d. WHO headquarters is in Geneva.

III. Write short notes on any four of the following:
   a. Role of community health nurse towards care of physically challenged.
   b. Recommendations of high power committee.
   c. National Health Policy-2002.
   d. Eleventh Five Year Plan.
   e. Integrated Child Development Program.

IV. a. What is occupational health?
   b. List important occupational diseases.
   c. Explain the role of a nurse in industrial nursing.

V. a. What are school health services?
   b. Explain the role of a nurse in school health services.

SECTION-II

VI. Choose the correct answer and write:
   a. Anti-leprosy day is celebrated on:
      (i) January 30th, (ii) January 13th, (iii) Janurary 3rd
   b. In India the last census was done in the year:
      (i) 2010, (ii) 2011, (iii) 2000
   c. Number of deaths under 1 year of age per 1000 live birth in a year is term as:
      (i) Infant mortality rate, (ii) Neonatal mortality rate, (iii) Perinatal mortality rate.

VII. Differentiate between the following:
   a. Mortality and morbidity.
   b. Eligible couple and target couple.

VIII. Write short notes on any two of the following:
   a. Health team.
   b. Major health problems in India.
   c. Uses and sources of vital statistics.

IX. a. What is fertility?
   b. Explain in detail the methods of family planning.

X. a. Classify the sexually transmitted diseases.
   b. Write in detail the role of a nurse in control of sexually transmitted diseases.

SECTION-I

I. Fill in the blanks

a. Farmer's lung is due to the inhalation of: **Mouldy Hay or Grain Dust.**
b. The 12th five year plan covers the period from: **2012–2017.**
c. The indicator of the prevalence of contraceptive practice in the community is: **Women empowerment.**
d. The term Siddha implies: **Knowledge of life.**

II. State whether the following statement are *true* or *false*

a. In India, there is one primary health center for every 30,000 population: **TRUE.**
b. The road to health card is important tool for monitoring growth of under five children: **TRUE.**
c. Weight gain during pregnancy in a healthy mother is 6–8 kg: **FALSE.**
d. WHO head quarters is in Geneva: **TRUE.**

III. Write short notes on any *four* of the following:

a. Role of community health nurse towards care of physically challenged

A physical handicap is a physical or mental disability making participation in certain of the usual activities of daily living more difficult according to Noel (2010). There are many types of physical handicaps that people can acquire. They come in all shades, shapes and sizes. Some examples of handicaps can result from a disability such as blindness, deafness or injuries that can lead to paralysis or amputations. Noel (2010) tells us that some physical handicaps are not always a hindrance to someone's everyday lifestyle. This paper analyses this aspect of humanity in six sections. First is a brief discussion on physical handicaps. Second are the causes and characteristics of common physical disabilities. Third is the educational intervention towards physical handicaps while fourth comes a section discussing methods of prevention of these disabilities. Lastly, the paper draws a conclusion that after all, disability is not inability.

People who have a handicap can still have a normal life. They may not be able to do what they would like to do much less do regular activities like others. However, they are capable of being happy and productive. Many face discrimination or get treated as second class citizens or worse seen as a "poor soul." As a result, there were reportedly over 19,000 charges filed in 2008 claiming discrimination from disabled workers. People often mistake being disabled as handicapped and vice versa. Although both refer to someone being at a disadvantage, they are not the same. Noel (2010) is clear in his definition that a disability is the limitations of a function due to injury or illness such as being paralyzed or blind. Examples of someone with a handicap are not having the speed to make a track relay squad or the size and power to make a football team. A person suffering from a physical handicap that severely impairs someone's judgment and ability can become a hazard to themselves as well as others.

b. Recommendations of high power committee

It was observed that nurses are not involved in making policies that govern their status and practice. They are invariably excluded from the government bodies that decide these policies. Most of the decisions concerning nursing care and nurses are made by other people, usually physicians without the benefit of professional input from by nurses. It is possible that this situation is the direct result of lack of appropriate status accorded to the nursing staff. Nearly 97% of nursing staff are in group "C" category and their status are too low.

c. National Health Policy-2002

The National Health Policy-2002 (NHP-2002) has been cleared by the Union Cabinet. This is the second such policy adopted by the Government after a gap of 19 years. The National Health Policy-2002 (NHP) gives prime importance to ensure a more equitable access to health services across the social and geographical expanse of the country. It calls for a strong primary health network in rural India. Emphasis has been given to increase the aggregate public health investment through a substantially increased contribution by the Central Government. Priority has been given to preventive and curative initiatives at the primary health level through increased sectoral share of allocation.

d. Eleventh Five Year Plan (2007–2012)

Goals

1. Accelerate GDP growth from 8% to 10%. Increase agricultural GDP growth rate to 4% per year.
2. Create 70 million new work opportunities and reduce educated unemployment to below 5%.
3. Raise real wage rate of unskilled workers by 20%.
4. Reduce dropout rates of children from elementary school from 52.2% in 2003–04 to 20% by 2011–12. Increase literacy rate for persons of age 7 years or above to 85%.
5. Lower gender gap in literacy to 10 percentage point. Increase the percentage of each cohort going to higher education from the present 10% to 15%.
6. Reduce infant mortality rate to 28 and maternal mortality ratio to 1 per 1000 live births.
7. Reduce total fertility rate to 2.1.
8. Provide clean drinking water for all by 2009. Reduce malnutrition among children between 0 year to 3 years to half its present level. Reduce anemia among women and girls by 50%.
9. Raise the sex ratio for age group 0–6 to 935 by 2011–12 and to 950 by 2016–17.
10. Ensure that at least 33% of the direct and indirect beneficiaries of all government schemes are women and girl children.
11. Ensure all-weather road connection to all habitation with population 1000 and above (500 in hilly and tribal areas) by 2009, and ensure coverage of all significant habitation by 2015.
12. Connect every village by telephone by November 2007 and provide broadband connectivity to all villages by 2012.
13. Increase forest and tree cover by 5 percentage points.
14. Attain WHO standards of air quality in all major cities by 2011–12. Treat all urban waste water by 2011–12 to clean river waters.
15. Increase energy efficiency by 20 percentage points by 2016–17.

e. Integrated Child Development Program

Importance of Child Survival and Safe Motherhood Program (CSSM) Health Services

1. Since the conception the development of fetus (280 days) takes place in the mother's womb and receives all nutrition and oxygen from the mother.
2. Health mother brings forth a healthy child. Healthy mother can avoid premature birth, stillbirth or abortion.
3. Certain habits and diseases conditions of expected mother will affect the child health, i.e. taking drugs, syphilis, German measles.

4. After birth, the child is completely dependent upon the mother for various reasons at least for a year separation of child from mother hinders the growth and development.
5. Child learns many self care tasks from the mother.

Objectives of CSSM

1. Sustaining and strengthening the ongoing universal immunization program (UIP), continuing oral rehydration therapy (ORT) program for children below the age of 5 years, introducing and expanding the program for control of acute respiratory infection for children below 5 years of age.
2. Universalizing the existing prophylaxis scheme for control of blindness due to deficiency of vitamin A for children up to the age of 3 years and prophylaxis scheme against nutritional anemia among pregnant and lactating mothers as well as children up to 5 years of age through administration of iron and folic acid tablets.
3. Improving newborn care and maternal care at the community level.

Components of CSSM

1. Early registration of pregnancy.
2. To provide minimum three antenatal checkups.
3. Universal coverage of all pregnant women with TT immunization.
4. Advice on food, nutrition and rest.
5. Detection of high risk pregnancies and prompt referral.
6. Clean deliveries by trained personnel.
7. Birth spacing.
8. Promotion of institutional deliveries.

Strategies of CSSM

1. Train medical and other health personnel in essential newborn care.
2. Provide basic facilities for care for low birth weight and sick newborns in the first referral units and district hospitals.
3. Create awareness about essential newborn among healthcare providers, pregnant women and mothers of the newborns.
4. Use of low cost effective and locally available equipment for newborn care.
5. Improve maternal care and promote birth spacing.

Goals of CSSM

1. IMR, MMR, and under five mortality rates mentioned in MCH goals.
2. Polio eradication by 2000 AD.
3. Neonatal tetanus elimination by 1995.
4. Measles prevention.

IV. a. What is occupational health?
b. List important occupational diseases
c. Explain the role of a nurse in industrial nursing

Occupational health is the art and science of conserving and promoting the health and efficiency of individuals at their workplace during and throughout the course of their employment.

Objectives of Occupational Health Services

1. To improve human efficiency in his work by applying ergonomics (human engineering).
2. To promote and maintain the highest degree of positive health and welfare of workers in all occupations.
3. To provide a self-occupational environment in order to safeguard the health of the workers and to set up industrial production.
4. To protect from factors adverse to health during their employment.
5. To assist the injured and disabled for rehabilitation.
6. To ensure that physical and psychological demands imposed on workers by their respective job are properly matched with their individual anatomical, physical and psychological needs, capabilities and limitations.
7. To educate workers to promote and maintain their health.
8. To provide care during emergencies.
9. To promote general health and welfare of each worker by providing a good and safe working environment.

Aims: Following are the aims of occupational health:
1. Promotion of physical, mental and social wellbeing of workers and securing their adaptation to work.
2. Maintenance of their physical, mental and social health at the highest possible level.
3. Elimination or at least suppression, of factors in their work environment inimical to the workers' health.
4. Prevention of diseases among them.
5. Modifying their environment to suit their physiological and psychological aptitudes.
6. Raising the level of productivity.

Occupational Diseases: Agent-wise

Diseases that are peculiar to occupational situations, or that are more common in defined occupations as compared to the general population, are known as occupational diseases. Following are the common occupational diseases and their responsible agents:

In India, the following are the occupational disorders in the order of decreasing prevalence:
1. Occupational dermatitis.
2. Industrial accidents.
3. Noise induced disorders.
4. Vibration induced disorders.
5. Ionizing radiation induced disorders.
6. High temperature induced disorders.
7. Dust-induced disorders.
8. Chronic lead poisoning.
9. Stress-induced disorders.

Occupational health nursing: The application of nursing principles in conserving the health of worker in all occupations. It involves prevention recognition and treatment of illness and injury, and requires special skills and knowledge in the fields of health, education and counseling environmental health, rehabilitation and human relations"—American Association of occupational health nurses.

Agent category	Agent	Occupational disease (S)
Physical agents	High pressure	Caisson disease
	Low pressure	Pulmonary edema, air embolism
	Electricity	Shock and burns
	Heat	Stroke, exhaustion and cramps
	Cold	Frostbite, trench foot, chilblains
	Light	Nystagmus
	Noise	Deafness, tympanic membrane rupture
	Vibrations	Raynaud's phenomenon
	Radiations	Raynaud's phenomenon
	Radiations	Leukernia, aplastic anemia, cancers
	Gravity, kinetic energy	Accidents
Chemical agents	Dusts	Pneumoconiosis
	Acids, alkalis, resins, etc.	Dermatitis, chemical burns
	Lead	Plumbism
	Benzene, vinyl chloride	Cancers
Biological agents	*Bacillus anthracis*	Anthrax
	Brucella abortus	Brucellosis
	Clostridium tetani	Tetanus
	Leptospira icterohaemorrhagiae	Leptospirosis

Roles of Occupational Health Nurse

1. Nurse practitioner.
2. Nurse educator.
3. Health administrator/manager.
4. Counselor.

Functions of Occupational Health Nurse

1. Assistance in general administration, maintenance and arrangements of health facilities in the plant.
2. Emergency and primary treatment of accidents and illness based on standing orders from physicians.
3. Arranging follow up treatments, where indicated, including health supervision of employees returning to work after illness.
4. Assistance in general preventive health measures in the plant.
5. Health education and counseling for employees.
6. Assistance in supervision of factory hygiene and accident prevention.
7. Advice on specific health questions to management and workers.
8. Maintenance of records and statistics.
9. Cooperation with and referral of workers to general community agencies for help as and when necessary.
10. Participation in a health surveillance program that includes the assessment and recording of the health status of employees.

11. Participation in the environmental control program the aims to work related.
12. Counseling and crisis intervention for those individuals experiencing work related problems and health promotion through specific health education and screening programs.

V. a. What are school health services? b. Explain the role of a nurse in school health services

See Question no. V of GNM Paper-3-2014

SECTION-II

VI. Choose the correct answer and write:

a. Anti-leprosy day is celebrated on: **January-30th.**
   (i) January 30th, (ii) January 13th, (iii) Janurary 3rd.
b. In India the last census was done in the year: **2011.**
   (i) 2010, (ii) 2011, (iii) 2001
c. Number of deaths under 1 year of age per 1000 live birth in a year is termed as: **Infant mortality rate.**
   (i) Infant mortality rate, (ii) Neonatal mortality rate, (iii) Perinatal mortality rate

VII. Differentiate between the following:

a. Mortality and morbidity

Mortality rate can be distinguished into a crude death rate, which is the total death per year in the world; Perinatal mortality rate (neonatal and fetal deaths per year); Maternal mortality rate (number of deaths of mothers due to childbearing); Infant mortality rate (number of deaths of children less than one years of age); Child mortality rate (number of deaths of children less than 5 years old); Standardized mortality rate (adjusted according to the standard composition in terms of age, gender and other factors); and Age-specific mortality rate (total number of deaths of a particular given age).

Morbidity scores or predicted morbidity are assigned to ill patients with the help of systems, such as the Acute Physiology and Chronic Health Evaluation II (APACHE II), Simplified Acute Physiology Score II and III (SAPS II and III), Glasgow Coma scale, Pediatric Index of Mortality 2 (PIM2), and Sequential Organ Failure Assessment (SOFA). Morbidity scores help decide the kind of treatment or medicine that should be given to the patient. Predicted morbidity describes the morbidity of patients, and is also useful when comparing two sets of patients or different time points in hospitals.

b. Eligible couple and target couple

Eligible couples: A couple of things right now a married couple where the woman of childbearing age is generally believed to be aged 15–45 years. At least 150–180 pairs in 1000, the population of India. These pairs are in need of family planning. About 20% of eligible couples can be found in the 15–24 age group. On average, 2.5 million couples will increase the population every year. The right to register the pair is the basic document for the organization of family planning. Target couples: pairs of long-term goal are used to 2–3 children, living and family planning is largely focused on those pairs. Determination of the duo gradually extended to families with children to develop, or even only married couples to accept the idea of family planning as early as possible. Protection pair: A pair of (PPC) is an indicator of the spread of contraception in the community.

This, as a percentage of eligible couples effectively protected against childbirth is defined by one or other approved methods of family planning, sterilization, or spiral, condoms and birth control pills. Sterilization accounts for more than 60% of couples effectively protected. Efforts to improve availability and access to contraceptive care in India in the seventies and early eighties led to a sharp rise in prices for some protection.

VIII. Write short notes on any *two* of the following:

a. Health team

The PHCT might therefore be considered to incorporate a much wider range of activities and professional groups, including the traditional PHCT, for example:
1. Practice manager.
2. Doctors: GP partners, GP assistants and other salaried doctors, GP registrars.
3. Nurses: practice nurses, nurse practitioners, community nurses; appropriately trained and supported nurses can produce high-quality care and achieve as good health outcomes for patients.
3. Support staff: receptionists, secretaries, clerical staff.
4. Midwives.
5. Health visitors.

Primary care premises may also be used for selected secondary care services, e.g. hospital consultant clinics, diagnostic imaging, operating services. Allied health professionals may also work closely with the PHCT, e.g. physiotherapy, dietetics, podiatry, pharmacy, counseling.

b. Major health problems in India

India is a developing country, it faces variety of problems. After detailed analysis of health situation in the light of the data. The health problems and health needs of the community is identified. These problems are then ranked according to priority or urgency for allocation of resources. The health problems of India may be grouped under the following headings:
1. Communicable disease problems
2. Nutritional problems
3. Environmental sanitation problems
4. Medical care problems
5. Population problems.

1. **Communicable Disease problems:** Communicable diseases continue to be India's major health problem of today. Some of them appear in epidemic form and some are endemic. Communicable disease refers to an illness caused be a specific infective agent, transmitting the infection from a reservoir to susceptible host. This transmission is direct or indirect through an intermediate host, vector or the inanimate environment. The common communicable disease are typhoid, cholera, malaria, diphtheria, whooping cough, tuberculosis, measles, mumps, chickenpox, and leprosy.
2. **Nutritional problems:** The nutritional point of view the Indian society is a dual society, consisting of a small group of well fed and a very large group of undernourished. In India, the people are affected with malnutrition and this is found to be one of the greatest health problems facing our communities today. It is reported that 60–70% of young children today have nutritional deficiencies. The surveys conducted by National Institute of Nutrition at Hyderabad showed that 4 out of 10 homes in rural areas consume diets with low calories.

3. **Environmental problems:** The most difficult problem to tackle in this country is environmental sanitation. The twin problems of environmental sanitation are lack of safe water in many areas of the country and primitive methods of excreta disposal. Besides these, there has been a growing concern about the impact of "New" problems resulting from population explosion, urbanization and industrialization leading to hazards to human health in air, in water and in the food chain.
4. **Medical care problems:** The major medical care problem in India is in equable distribution of available health resources between urban and rural areas and lack of penetration of health services to the social periphery. The existing hospital based, disease oriented health care model has provided health benefits mainly to the urban elite. Approximately 80% of health benefits are concentrated in urban areas. Even in urban areas, there is an uneven distribution of doctors. With large migrations occurring from rural to urban areas, urban health problems have been aggravated and include overcrowding in hospitals, inadequate staffing and scarcity of certain essential drugs and medicines. The rural areas where nearly 80 percent of population lives do not enjoy the benefits of the modern curative and preventive health services.
5. **Population problems:** Population problem is one of the biggest problem facing the country with its inevitable consequences on all aspects of development especially employment education housing, health care, sanitation, and environment

c. Uses and sources of vital statistics

1. Vital statistics has been used to denote acts systematically collected and compiled in numerical form relating to or derived from records of vital events namely, live birth, death, fetal death, marriage, divorce, adoption, legitimating, recognition, annulment or legal separation.
2. Vital statistics provide a tool for measuring the dynamics of change which continuously occur in population. Vital statistics are derived from legally registrable events without including population data or morbidity statistics.

Definitions of Vital Statistics

1. Vital statistics are conventionally numerical records of marriage, births, sickness and deaths by which the health and growth of community may be studied.
2. Vital statistics is a part of demography and collective study of mankind. It deals with the data's related to vital events.
3. It is a branch of biometry deals with data and law of human mortality, morbidity and demography.
4. Vital statistics is the numerical description of birth, death, absorption, marriage, divorce, adoption and judicial separation—UNO.

Purpose of Vital Statistics

1. **Community health:** To describe the level community health, to diagnose community illness, and to discover solutions to health problems.
2. **Administrative purpose:** It provides clues for administrative action and to create administrative standards of health activities.
3. **Health programmed organization:** To determine success or failure of specific health programmed or undertake overall evaluation of public health work.
4. **Legislative purpose:** To promote health legislation at local, state and national level.
5. **Governmental purpose:** To develop policies procedures, at state and central level.

Uses of Vital Statistics

1. To evaluate the impact of various national health programmers.
2. To plan for better future measures of disease control.
3. To elucidate the hereditary nature of disease.
4. To plan and evaluate economic and social development.
5. It is a primary tool in research activities.
6. To determine the health status of individual.
7. To compare the health status of one nation with others.

Methods of Obtaining Vital Statistics

1. **Census:** It is a simultaneous recording demographic, social and economic data of individuals. It is an important method of collecting vital statistics. Census is conducted every 10 years.
2. **Registration**: Registration of vital events (e.g. births, deaths) keep a continuous check on demographic changes. If registration of vital events is complete and accurate, it can serve as a reliable source of health information.
3. **Ad hoc survey:** Surveys for evaluating the health status of a population that is community diagnosis of problems of health and disease. It is information about the distribution of these problems over time and space that provides the functional basis for planning and developing needed services.

IX. a. What is fertility?
b. Explain in detail the methods of family planning

Infertility, inability to conceive or carry a child to delivery. The term is usually limited to situations where the couple has had intercourse regularly for one year without using birth control. The term sterility is restricted to lack of sperm production or inability to ovulate. Approximately, 40% of reported cases of infertility are due to problems in the male; another 40% to problems in the female; the remaining 20% are of unknown cause or due to problems in both the male and female.

Causes: Infertility can be caused by any interruption in the usual process of fertilization, pregnancy, and birth, which includes ejaculation of normal amounts of healthy sperm, passage of the sperm through the cervix and into the fallopian tube of the female, passage of an ovum (egg) down the fallopian tube from an ovary, fertilization in the fallopian tube, implantation of the fertilized egg in a receptive uterus, and the ability to carry the fetus to term. In women, the most common problems are failure to ovulate and blockage of the fallopian tubes. In men, low sperm count is the most common problem.

Underlying problems include disease, such as diabetes or mumps in adult men, hormonal imbalances, endometriosis, pelvic inflammatory disease (often caused by sexually transmitted diseases, e.g. *Chlamydia*), the abuse of alcohol and other drugs, and exposure to workplace hazards or environmental toxins. Uterine irritation or infection that sometimes accompanies IUD use can also reduce fertility. Occasionally, there is a chemical or immunological incompatibility between male and female. Psychological factors are difficult to evaluate because of the stressful nature of infertility itself.

The number of couples seeking treatment for infertility has increased as more of them have postponed childbearing to a later age. In women, fertility begins to decline in the mid-twenties, and continues to decline, more and more sharply, until menopause. Male fertility declines gradually until age 40, then declines more quickly.

Natural Methods of Family Planning

1. **Total sexual abstinence:** It costs nothing except self-denial on the part of the couple.
2. **Periodic abstinence:** Otherwise called as rhythm or calendar method or safe method. It is based on restricting the sex act to the infertile period of the female partner.

3. **Temperature method:** During ovulation naturally the basal body temperature rise of 0.5°C. Based on prediction of the time of ovulation by taking the basal body temperature daily and avoiding sexual intercourse around the time of ovulation.
4. **Billing method:** It relies on the charges in cervical mucus secretion also called mucus method. This method is based on observation of changes in the characteristics of cervical mucus.
5. **Symptothermic method:** This method combines the use of basal body temperature with analysis of cervical mucus changes to make temperature with analysis of cervical mucus changes to make predictions more accurate.
6. **Coitus interruptus:** It is an ancient method that requires the male to withdraw his penis from the vagina immediately before the ejaculation of the semen.
7. **Coitus interfemoris:** The erect penis is placed between the thighs of the female.
8. **Lactation amenorrhea method:** It is believed that there is a high probability that the women who is amenorrheal while breastfeeding, will be able to regulate her fertility in first 6 months postpartum even if she introduces supplementation in the baby's feeding.
9. **Barrier method:** Barrier methods of contraception have a long history. The ancient Egyptians used such methods which consisted of honey-coated pessaries. Honey is effective in killing sperms as well as bacteria.

Chemical Methods of Family Planning

Chemical barriers are usually spermicidal or spermistatic. In addition, they may have some blocking action at the cervix. Sperm thrive best at an alkaline pH of 8.5–9.0. Because the vagina is normally acidic until ovulation.
1. **The foam tablets:** The foam tablets which a woman inserts into her birth canal before having sex produce some foam which provides a productive coating to the whole area.
2. **Cream, jelly and paste:** The spermicidal jelly or cream is similarly applied in the vagina with the help of an applicator. It destroys the male sperm on contact in the vaginal canal itself.
3. **Suppositories and soluble film:** The suppositories and soluble films take time to dissolve in the vaginal fluids. It kills the sperm released from the man's body and thus prevents pregnancy.

Mechanical Barriers of Family Planning

These methods are which prevent meeting of sperms with ovum, the sperms are prevented from entering the cervix by mechanical barriers.
1. **Condom:** The condom or nirodh is an extremely thin rubber sheath used by the man. It has been used since 14th century. The condom is fitted on the erect male organ before intercourse. The air must be expelled from the teat before it is put on. Condom acts be preventing the entry sperms into vagina.
2. **Diaphgram:** It is curved rubber dome enclosed by flexible metal ring that rests in the vagina and covers the cervix. It was invented by a German physician in 1882, also known as "Dutch cap". It is made of soft synthetic rubber or plastic with a stiff but flexible rim around the edges. It is available in different sizes ranging from 5 cm to 10 cm.
3. **Cervical cap:** The use of cervical cap is a variation of the diaphgram. It is smaller than diaphgram and is designed to fit over the neck of the womb. Once the cervical cap is placed, it can remain from the end of one menstruation to just before the start of the next.
4. **Vaginal sponge:** A small polyurethane foam sponge measuring 5 cm x 2.5 cm is saturated with spermicide, nonoxynol-9 and inserted into vagina. It is less effective than the diaphgram. It may be inserted 18 his before intercourse. It is more convenient to use it than some of the other vaginal contraceptives.

Intrauterine Devices: Intrauterine device is inserted into the cavity to prevent conception. The device which is placed in the womb may be inert or medicated. The inert device is made up of plastic material only and the medicated devices are fortified with copper, silver or a progestation preparation.

1. **Lippes loop:** It is a double S-shaped serpentine device made of polythene impregnated with barium sulfate for radiopacity.
   Two pieces of nylon (trans-cervical threads) are attached to the lower end of the loop forming tail, the nylon tail projects into the vagina. Periodic feeling for the tail reassures the user that the loop is in place. The tail also helps in easy removal of the device.
2. **Copper-T:** The copper-T is made of plastic but is wrapped with fine copper which enhances its contraceptive effect. Its acceptance is higher than that of the loop. It is I shaped bioactive contraceptive device made of polyethylene or any other polymer and reinforced with copper metal. The devices are impregnated with barium sulfate for radio opacity and are fitted with two transcervical threads at the tail end. Metallic copper possess a strong antifertility action.

Hormonal contraceptives methods of family planning: Hormonal contraceptives are composed of synthetic gonadal steroids—estrogens and progestogens. Estrogens used are ethinyl estradiol and mestranol. The synthetic progestogens usually used are norethindrone and norgestrel. Hormonal contraceptives are available as pills, injectables, implants an devices.

Oral Pills

1. **Combined pill:** The main action of the combined pill is inhibition of ovulation by blocking the secretion of gonadotropin from pituitary gland. The progestogen also alters the cervical mucosa which prevents the entry of sperms into genital canal. There are two types of pills which are available under the brand name of mala-N and mala-D. Mala-N and Mala-D are available in packet of 28 tablets. The first white tablets are contraceptive pills and the remaining seven pill are iron pills which are brown.
2. **Progesterone only pill:** This pill is also known as minipill. This pill contains only synthetic progesterone in very small quantity. The progesterone thickens the cervical mucus which prevents the entry of sperms into the uterine cavity. Minipills are taken throughout the menstrual cycle.
3. **Once a month pill:** It is a modified combined pill. It contains long-acting estrogen and short-acting progesterone. This pill is not in use because of its poor result and irregularity in menstrual cycle.

Injectable Contraceptives

1. **Progesterone-only injectable:** It contains synthetic progestogen, it prevents ovulation, thickens the cervical mucus which interferes with penetration of sperms into genital canal. DEMPA (Depot-Medroxy- progesterone acetate) available as Noristerat, injectable once in three months and later once in two months (60 days). Another form of injectable is NET-EN (norethisterone enanthate). DEMPA is found to be more successful than NET-EN.
2. **Combined injectable contraceptives:** These contraceptives contain progesterone and estrogen. It prevents ovulation, thickens the cervical mucus which interferes with entry of sperms into the birth canal. The injection is given once in a month. Thorough medical examination must be done by the doctor before prescribing injectable contraceptives.
3. **Subdermal implants:** Subdermal implants are developed by population council of New York. There are two varities, one is nor plant and the latest is Norplant R-2. Norplant R-2 has two small rods; these devices are placed surgically under the skin of the arm by the doctor. After

five years the implant is removed surgically. The actions of these impants are the same as that of injectable contraceptives.

Terminal Methods of Family Planning
1. **Sterilization:** It is the only method which gives permanent protection from contraception. It is safe and a permanent one time means of contraception. Sterilization is a method of the risk of accidental pregnancy. In sterilization either husband or wife can undergo a simple surgical operation, i.e. vasectomy or tubectomy.
2. **Vasectomy:** It is sterilization of male, very simple and minor operation which takes hardly 15–20 minutes. The operation can be done in primary health center under local anesthesia by a trained doctor. A septic technique is to be followed to prevent infection. The operation involves a small cut on both sided of the scrotum, then a small portion of vas deferens on either side of the scrotum, is cut and ligated, folded back and sutured.
3. **Tubectomy:** It is sterilization of females, done by resecting a small part of fallopian tubes and ligated the sected ends. The closing of tubes also be done by using other alternative methods like closing with bands, clips, electrocautery. The operation can be done through abdominal or vaginal approach. The most common abdominal procedures are laparoscopy and minilaparotomy.

X. a. Classify the Sexually transmitted diseases. b. Write in detail the role of a nurse in control of sexually transmitted diseases

Sexually transmissible diseases (STD) are a group of communicable diseases that are transmitted predominantly by sexual contact and caused by a wide range of bacterial, viral, protozoal and fungal agents. The true incidence of STDs is not known because of inadequate reporting and the secrecy that surrounds them. Minimal estimates of yearly incidence of four major bacterial STDs worldwide are (WHO Health for all Series 1981):
1. Gonorrhea.
2. Genital chlamydial infection.
3. Syphilis.
4. Chancroid.

For viral STD, due to the importance of asymptomatic infection, incidence can only be very roughly estimated:
1. Genital herpes 20 million.
2. Genital human papilloma virus infection 30 million.

Trichomoniasis, which is of much less public health importance than the bacterial and viral STD, has an estimated annual incidence of 170 million cases.

Extent of the Problem in India

Sexually transmitted diseases are becoming a major public health problem in India.

Syphilis: Serological surveys continue to be the best source of information on the prevalence of syphilis. The extent of the problem can be gauged from the reports of surveys done in Aurangabad (Maharashtra) and Kerala which showed prevalence of 2.4 and 1.4 respectively (WHO, World Health Report, 1999), which are rather high figures.

Gonorrhea: Accurate information on the morbidity of gonorrhea is lacking, as most cases are not reported. However, the general impression is that gonorrhea is more prevalent than syphilis. An 80% of infected women are reported to be asymptomatic carriers (Park, 2000).

Chancroid: Chancroid or soft sore is reported to be widely prevalent in India.

Chlamydia infections: These are more prevalent in the southern states of India than in the northern states.

Donovanosis: Donovanosis or granuloma inguinale is endemic in Tamil Nadu, Andhra Pradesh, Orissa, Karnataka and Maharashtra. A greater prevalence along the coastal areas has been reported (WHO, World Health Report, 1999). Information about this disease in other states is lacking.

Other STDs: Information about other STDs in India is not readily available as there is no reporting system for these diseases.

Gonorrhea

Gonorrhea is an infectious disease caused by the *Gonococcus, Neisseria gonorrhea*. In the male, the disease is most often an anterior urethritis, whereas in a female, it is a cervicitis.

Pathogenesis
1. *Agent factors*: The causative organisms of gonorrhea are known as *Gonococcus* or *Neisseria gonorrhea*. The gonococci infect mucus secreting epithelial surfaces. They attach to the columnar or transitional epithelium and penetrate through or between the cells to the connective tissue.
2. *Host factors*: Among sexually active individual's incidence rates, are highest in teenagers, non-Whites, the poor, poorly educated, city dwellers and unmarried people who live alone. It is also prevalent in people with multiple partners.
3. *Source of infection*: Human is the only reservoir of this infection. Its organism is present in exudates from mucous membranes of infected person.

Preventive Measures

All those who are conducting delivery, must use chemoprophylactic agents, such as silver nitrate, argyrols, etc.

Control Measures
1. Interview conduct among infected regarding all sexual contacts of 10 days to onset of disease. Also examine serologically for syphilis over a period of several weeks.
2. Keep these patient discharges and dressings separate and either disinfect or burn them. Articles which are contaminated with patient's discharge must be cleaned and disinfected daily before using them for others.
3. Report about the patient to the health authorities.

Nursing Interventions
1. Before treatment determine if the patient has any drug sensitivities. During treatment, watch closely for signs of a drug reaction.
2. Use standard precautions when obtaining specimens for laboratory examination and when caring for the patient. Carefully place all soiled articles in containers and dispose of them according to facility policy.
3. Monitor the patient for complications.
4. Isolate the patient.

5. If the patient has gonococcal arthritis, apply moist heat to ease pain in affected joints. Administer analgesics as ordered.

Syphilis

Management

1. *Antibiotic therapy:* Penicillin administered TM is the treatment of choice. For early syphilis, treatment may consist of a single injection of penicillin C benzathine TM (2.4 million units). Syphilis of more than 1 year duration may respond to penicillin C benzathine TM (2.4 million units 1 week for 3 weeks).
2. Patient who is allergic to penicillin may be successfully treated with tetracycline or erythromycin for 15 days for early syphilis, 30 days for late infections. Tetracycline is contraindicated during pregnancy.

Preventive Measures

1. People of community must be protected from commercialized prostitution and from sexual promiscuity. It is done by enforcing law and social force.
2. Community must get sex education. Adolescents and young adults can have it in the school and colleges. They must know about preparation for marriage and premarital examination and how they contact this disease, etc.
3. Survey of selected groups should be done to find out cases. This group includes industrial workers, contacts of patient, pregnant women, nurses, doctors, etc.
4. Wide publicity and mass education is necessary to prevent people from getting this infection. People must know about personal hygiene.

Control Measures

1. If a pregnant woman has syphilis treats her during pregnancy to prevent her baby from getting congenital syphilis.
2. Interview of patient their contacts, etc. should be carried out by the trained persons to find out the source of infection.
3. Notify about the case to the health authorities.

Nursing Interventions

Follow standard precautions when assessing the patient collecting specimens, and treating lesions. Check for a history of drug sensitivity before administering the first dose of medication. Promote adequate rest and nutrition. Assess the complications of late syphilis; obtain a physical or occupational therapy consultation. Also consult with a social worker to determine homecare needs.

2011

Community Health Nursing

SECTION-I

I. State whether the following statements are *true* or *false*:
   a. There is one PHC for 30,000 populations in tribal and hilly areas.
   b. The family planning associations was found in 1949 with its headquarters at Mumbai.
   c. FAO was established in 1945 with headquarters in Geneva.
   d. The World Health Day theme of 2011 is antimicrobial resistance.

II. Fill in the blanks with suitable answers:
   a. Group on medical education and support man power knows as _____ committee.
   b. Planning prosperity together is the motto of: _____
   c. The fetal point for delivery of ICDS is on: _____
   d. A block contains about: _____ villages.

III. Write short notes on any *four* of the following:
   a. Functions of Directorate General of Health Services.
   b. Care of physically and mentally challenged.
   c. Levels of health care.
   d. Health problems of industrialization.
   e. Primary health center.

IV. a. What are the problems of old age? b. Explain the role of a nurse in geriatric care.

V. a. What is reproductive and child health?
   b. List the aims of reproductive and child health care.
   c. Describe the role of a nurse in reproductive and child health.

SECTION-II

VI. Fill in the blanks:
   a. The kingpin for healthcare delivery at the subcenter level is: _____
   b. The number of live births divided by the mid-year population and multiplied by 1000 is known as: _____
   c. National AIDS Control Program was launched in the year: _____
   d. The pioneer of immunization is: _____

VII. State whether the following are *true* or *false*:
   a. In demography family size means total number of persons in the family.
   b. Census is taken at intervals of 10 years.
   c. For every 5000 rural populations, there are 4 multipurpose health workers.

VIII. a. What is health team?
   b. Explain the role of female health worker in health team.
IX. a. What are the major health problems in India?
   b. Explain the role of a nurse in the National Malaria Control Program.
X. a. Define family planning.
   b. List the scope of family planning services.
   c. Briefly explain the role of a nurse in Family Welfare Program.

SECTION-I

I. State whether the following statements are *true* or *false*:
a. There is one PHC for 30,000 populations in tribal and hilly areas: **TRUE.**
b. The family planning associations was found in 1949 with its headquarters at Mumbai: **FALSE.**
c. FAO was established in 1945 with headquarters in Geneva: **FALSE.**
d. The World Health Day theme of 2011 is antimicrobial resistance: **TRUE.**

II. Fill in the blanks with suitable answers:
a. Group on medical education and support man power knows as **Shrivastav** Committee
b. Planning prosperity together is the motto of: Preventive, curative and promotive care.
c. The fetal point for delivery of ICDS is on: **1975.**
d. A block contains about: **100** villages.

III. Write short notes on any *four* of the following:

a. Functions of Directorate General of Health Services

The Union Ministry of Health and Family Welfare is headed by a cabinet minister, a minister of state, and a deputy health minister. These are political appointments. The union ministry of health and family welfare at the center play a vital role in the governmental efforts to enable the citizen to live a healthier and useful life. Currently, the Union Ministry has the following departments: (i) Department of Health (ii) Department of Family Welfare. The Department of Family Welfare was created in 1966 within the Ministry of Health and Family Welfare for the administrative purpose of the Union Health and Family Welfare minister, which seek the help of health secretariat headed by Secretary. The secretary is assisted by a number of additional, joint, deputy and assistant secretaries and various administrative staff. Department of health deals with planning, coordination, programming, evaluation of medical and public health matters, including drug control and prevention of food adulteration. The department of health functions through the Directorate General of Health Service. Department of Family Welfare is headed by Secretary to the Government of India, Ministry of Health and Family Welfare, who is supported and assisted by a team of two joint secretaries, two chief directors, number of deputy secretaries, deputy commissioners, directors and other technical and administrative officers in hierarchy.

Functions of Central Ministry of Health

Union List
1. International health obligations.
2. Administration of higher central education, technical, vocational and research institutes.
3. Census and publication of statistical data.
4. Interstate quarantine and inter-state migration.
5. Regulation of manufacture and sale of drugs and biological devices.
6. Regulation of labor and safety in mines and oil fields.
7. Regulation of professional bodies.

Concurrent List
1. Prevention of food adulteration.
2. Family planning and population control.
3. Prevention of interstate extension of communicable diseases.
4. Social security and social insurance.
5. Vital statistics and vital registration.
6. Control of drugs and poisons.

b. Care of physically and mentally challenged (handicaped)

Mental retardation is an impaired mental ability. Mental retardation is not primarily a medical problem; moreover, it is an educational, psychological and social problem. Also, it is not a mental illness. Mental retardation is just confined to intellectual retardation; It may influence all aspects of human functioning including speech, language development, hearing and visual functioning as well as muscular coordination. Nowadays, the term mental handicap is more vogue in place of mental retardation.

Definition of mental retardation: According to Persons with Disability Act 1995, "Mental retardation means a condition of arrested or incomplete development of mind of a person which is specially characterized by subnormal intelligence". In other words, we can say that mental retardation or mental handicap is a state of subaverage intellectual function combined with deficits in adaptive behavior (The term idiot, moron, Imbecile are now not used).

Main characteristics of mental retardation: Intelligence should be significantly subaverage. This should have occurred in the developmental period, i.e. up to the age of 18 years. Behavior should be significantly inappropriate.

Management of mentally handicapped
1. Assessing the extent of the problem, informing the reality to relatives/parents.
2. Innovative teaching methodology for providing special education to mentally handicap.
    a. Providing special school or class
    b. Applying more suitable curriculum
    c. A better organized daily teaching routine
    d. Specially trained teachers.
3. Psychotherapeutic intervention as and when needed.
4. Strengthen the family system of mentally handicapped person/child.
5. Taking the help of NGOs, voluntary agencies in the care and management of mentally handicaps along with government measures.
6. Creating a positive attitude in the society towards mentally handicaps.
7. Loving tender care at all levels. Primary, secondary and tertiary.
8. Proper rehabilitation according to individual need, including vocational rehabilitation of the mentally handicaps.

c. Levels of health care

Health care or health facilities have a direct relation to the human being itself. Health facility is the fundamental right of every citizen. Medical services are an integral part of health facilities. Basically, health facilities mean health services. In other words, providing services for prevention, diagnosis, treatment, promotion, rehabilitation and health education are the major constituents of health services. It can be defined as: "Health services are the services provided by health organizations, agencies or their representatives to individuals, families or communities for the promotion, preservation or prevention of health."

Characteristics of Health Care

1. **Relevance:** Health services should be in accordance with health requirements, priorities, and policies.
2. **Comprehensiveness:** It should incorporate the preventive, therapeutic and health promotion services in suitable proportions.
3. **Availability and adequacy:** Health services should be appropriate and proportionate to the population and also, enough to satisfy people's needs.
4. **Feasibility:** For the skilled management of health services, these should be logical, and in accordance to the available resources like, time, labor and the material, etc.
5. **Accessibility:** Services should be available within the geographical and economic limits. These should be within the reach of citizens and should be taking care of their cultural values and realities.

Levels of Health Care

Mainly, health services have three levels. These are the foundation of referral system as well. Here is a short description of these levels:

1. **Primary health care:** At this level, primary contact is established between the individual and the health agencies. Primary health care is very important in diagnosing, solving and treating health problems at grass-roots level. Organizations like health subcenters and primary health centers are very effective in providing primary health services. These health services pay more attention to disease prevention.
2. **Secondary health care:** Some of the complicated problems of health can be faced at this level, and therapeutic services can also be provided. Community health centers and district hospitals provide health services at this level.
3. **Tertiary health care:** Other than providing health services, planning, management, and research work is also executed at this level. Most of the educational and training programs, for the health workers are also conducted at this level. Providing the services of specialists and assisting community at primary and secondary stages is the responsibility of health management at this level. Here, it is worth mentioning that to achieve the goals of community health more attention should be paid to primary level services. Although a lot more is yet to be done in this direction.

d. Health problems of industrialization

Workers occupied in industries dealing with infected animals and infected animal material like hides and skins are exposed to a host of zoonotic diseases of viral, bacterial protozoal and metazoal origin. Workers engaged in field areas suffer from a variety of environmental infective diseases which may be dust borne, soil borne, water borne or vector borne. In India, following are the occupational disorders in the order of decreasing prevalence:

1. Occupational dermatitis.
2. Industrial accidents.
3. Noise induced disorders.
4. Vibration induced disorders.

5. Ionizing radiation induced disorders.
6. High temperature induced disorders.
7. Dust-induced disorders.
8. Chronic lead poisoning.
9. Stress-induced disorders.

Agent category	Agent	Occupational disease (S)
Physical agents	High pressure	Caisson disease
	Low pressure	Pulmonary edema, air embolism
	Electricity	Shock and burns
	Heat	Stroke, exhaustion and cramps
	Cold	Frost bite, trench foot, chilblains
	Light	Nystagmus
	Noise	Deafness, tympanic membrane rupture
	Vibrations	Raynaud's phenomenon
	Radiations	Raynaud's phenomenon
	Radiations	Leukernia, aplastic anemia, cancers
	Gravity, kinetic energy	Accidents
Chemical agents	Dusts	Pneumoconiosis
	Acids, alkalis, resins, etc.	Dermatitis, chemical burns
	Lead	Plumbism
	Benzene, vinyl chloride	Cancers
Biological agents	Bacillus anthracis	Anthrax
	Brucella abortus	Brucellosis
	Clostridium tetani	Tetanus
	Leptospira icterohaemorrhagiae	Leptospirosis

e. Primary health center

Primary health center (**PHC**s), sometimes referred to as **public health center**s, are state-owned rural health care facilities in India. They are essentially single-physician clinics usually with facilities for minor surgeries, too. They are part of the government-funded public health system in India and are the most basic units of this system. Presently there are 23,109 PHCs in India.

Functions of PHC

1. Provision of medical care.
2. Maternal-child health including family planning.
3. Safe water supply and basic sanitation.
4. Prevention and control of locally endemic diseases.
5. Collection and reporting of vital statistics.
6. Education about health.
7. National health programs, as relevant.
8. Referral services.
9. Training of health guides, health workers, local dais and health assistants.
10. Basic laboratory workers.

Apart from the regular medical treatments, PHCs in India have some special focuses.
1. **Infant immunization programs:** Immunization for newborns under the national immunization program is dispensed through the PHCs. This program is fully subsidized.
2. **Antiepidemic programs:** The PHCs act as the primary epidemic diagnostic and control centers for the rural India. Whenever a local epidemic breaks out, the system's doctors are trained for diagnosis. They identify suspected cases and refer for further treatment.
3. **Birth control programs:** Services under the national birth control programs are dispensed through the PHCs. Sterilization surgeries such as vasectomy and tubectomy are done here. These services, too, are fully subsidized.
4. **Pregnancy and related care:** A major focus of the PHC system is medical care for pregnancy and child birth in rural India. This is because people from rural India resist approaching doctors for pregnancy care which increases neonatal death. Hence, pregnancy care is a major focus area for the PHCs.
5. **Emergencies:** All the PHCs store drugs for medical emergencies which could be expected in rural areas. For example, anti-venoms for snake bites, rabies vaccinations, etc.

IV. a. What are the problems of old age? b. Explain the role of a nurse in geriatric care

Geriatric care: This is related to the disease process of old age and it aims at keeping old persons at a state of self dependence as far as possible and to provide facilities to improve their quality of life.

Gerontological nurse: A nurse who has specialization in geriatrics or in the care of old people is called geriatric nurse or gerontological nurse.

Functions of gerontological nurse: The functions of gerontological nurse are mentioned here, on the basis of spelling of the word:

G (Guiding): Giving guidance to people of all ages regarding ageing process.

E (Eliminating): Eliminating agism or considering old age as disease.

R (Respecting): Respecting the rights of old, people.

O (Observing): Observing the facilities provided to old people and improving them.

N (Noticing): Noticing health hazards that may happen in old age and try to reduce them.

T (Teaching): Teaching how to take care of old people, for those who are caring for them (family members, friends, community health worker, voluntary organization, etc.).

O (Opening channels): Opening the channels of developmental activities for the care of the aged.

L (Listening): Listening attentively to the problems of old people and giving due importance to them.

O (Offering): Offering positivism—presenting different possibilities of life.

G (Generating): Generating energy for the participation in the care of aged and researches for new supporting techniques.

I (Implementing): Implementing activities for rehabilitation and readjustment.

C (Coordinating): Coordinating different services related to the care of the aged.

A (Assessing): Assessing the needs and health of the old people.

L (Linking): Linking, contacting services according to need.

N (Nurturing): Preparing future nurses for the care of the aged.

U (Understanding): Understanding every old person as an invaluable asset of the society.

R (Recognizing): Recognizing the moral and religious aspects of old age and giving them recognition.

S (Supporting): Supporting the old people in accepting realities and preparing them mentally for impending death.

E (Education and encouraging): Educating and encouraging old people for self-care.

Responsibilities of Nurse in Aging

The main objective of gerontological nursing is to improve the quality of life of old people. Because of individual variations and the special needs of old age, gerontological nursing is a challenging job. The nurse has to fulfill the following roles in gerontological nursing:
1. Care giver.
2. Health educator.
3. Coordinator of health services.
4. Counselor and guardian (those people who protect the old person or take responsibilities as his guardian, spokesman or responsible person).

The nurse may have to perform different functions in relation to the above roles:
I. **Health assessment:** A nurse should have a detailed examination of the old person and then assess his health. This includes assessment of physical, mental, social and economic resources. In the health assessment of the old person, the following should be included.
   1. Daily activities of living (bathing, excretion, clothing, urinary control, ability to eat, etc.).
   2. Activities related to use of equipment or procedures (Telephone, bank account, food preparation. etc., his ability in these activities).
   3. Health screening: Ability to see and hear, dental problems, blood pressure, examination of breasts and uterus, cancer testing, examination of skin, etc. should be done.
   4. In laboratory tests; blood examination, urine analysis, cholesterol, blood sugar, thyroid, etc. tests should be conducted.
II. **Arranging/promoting good nutrition:** Less financial resources, change in taste, disinterest in food, loss of appetite. trouble of preparing food, non-availability of food stuff, inability to eat, necessity to change food (due to disease), etc. affect the nutrition of old people. Hence, a complete nutritional assessment of the old person should be done and he should be protected from malnutrition and deficiencies by giving balanced and modified diet.
III. **Promoting activity and exercise:** Physical exercises and activity are the basic keys to health in old age. Through this in addition to keeping up physical ability, emotional and mental balance also are maintained. There are many problems in keeping up exercise and activities in old age. Stiffness of joints, arthritis, lack of energy, low blood pressure, lack of motivation or lack of facilities are some of the important ones. In gerontological nursing, it is essential to include exercise, yoga, dhyan, pranayam etc. in their daily activities. Similarly, old people should be encouraged to participate in artistic, cultural, educational or games activities.
IV. **Preventive care of elderly:** In case of the elderly, their physical and mental safety is very important. Gerontological nurse and care givers should pay special attention to the following safety measures:
   1. Protection from unhealthy environment.
   2. Protection from mental tensions.
   3. Special care of personal health.

4. Protection from physical and mental injuries, threats and fatigue.
5. Providing rehabilitation services.

V. **Providing psychological support:** The mental health of old aged person depends upon his mental status in his entire life. Loneliness, neglect, sense of uselessness or being a burden and social inactivity may create imbalance of mind in the old person. The nurse should play an important role in reducing those problems.

V. a. What is reproductive and child health?

Maternal and child health services are directed towards and children in order to maintain total wellbeing of the child within the framework of the family and the community. Every aspect of community health programs in India has marked effects on the health and welfare of expectant mothers and particularly of infants and children.

New maternal and child health care (MCH) which now also being described as reproductive and child health (RCH). Reproductive child health can be defined as a state in which "people have the ability to reproduce and regulate their fertility, women ability to reproduce and regulate their fertility; women are able to go through pregnancy and child birth safety

b. List the aims of reproductive and child health care

Objectives of MCH Programs

1. To give expert advice to the couples to plan their families.
2. To identify "high risk" cases can give them special attention.
3. To provide health supervision for antenatal mothers. Also to foresee complications and prevention.
4. To give skilled assistance at the time of child birth and during puerperium.
5. To supervise trained dais, community health volunteers and community health workers.
6. To impart useful knowledge on desirable health practices which mother should carry out during pregnancy, labor and during puerperium.
7. Encourage the deliveries by trained workers in the safe and clean environment.
8. Prevent communicable and noncommunicable diseases.
9. Educate the mother to improve their own and children's health.

Aims of MCH Services

1. To pay attention on stability in population, safe childhood and health of children.
2. To pay special attention to the health of women, boys, girls, protection from sexually transmitted diseases, antenatal, intranatal, and postnatal mothers.
3. To have safe pregnancies is successful in terms of safe motherhood, safe child and good health.
4. To provide sound reproductive health for men and women and also safe control of their reproduction activities.
5. To have effective control on maternal morbidity and mortality.

c. Describe the role of a nurse in reproductive and child health

Components of Reproductive and Child Health

1. Family planning services.
2. Child survival and safe motherhood program (CSSM).
3. Prevention or management of STD and AIDS.

4. Providing counseling, information and communication services on health.
5. Referral services.
6. Growth monitoring and nutritional education.

Importance of MCH Services

1. Mother and child are considered as one unit.
2. Mother and child are "special Risk group" or vulnerable group or dependent or weaker group of community.
3. Most of the problems of maternal and child health are preventable.
4. Effective maternal and child health protects from infant morbidity and mortality.
5. To maintain the health and wellbeing of pregnant women.
6. To identify risk factors and complications arises during pregnancy.

Major MCH Problems

1. **Nutritional anemia:** Anemia is a condition in which concentration of hemoglobin I the red blood cells is reduced. Hemoglobin is essential for life. It carries oxygen to all parts of the body. Anemia during pregnancy leads to 20% of all maternal deaths, 3 times greater risk of premature delivery and low birth weight babies. Anemia can retard physical and mental development of the child.
2. **Infection:** The common infection causes are urinary tract infection, reproductive tract infection, STD and other common problems. Urinary tract infection causes frequent burning micturition due to *E. coli*, reproductive tract infection/STD caused by bacterial, viral and protozoan, infection occur due to unsafe deliveries and abortion or IVP insertions. Other common problems are toxoplasmosis, rubella; cytomegalovirus and Herpes simplex are common in pregnancy.
3. **Uncontrolled reproduction:** Uncontrolled reproduction has been very well recognized by LBW, severe anemia, abortion, APH, high mortality and perinatal utilization of MCH and family welfare services, MTP sterilization, health education and family welfare counseling.

SECTION-II

VI. Fill in the blanks

a. The kingpin for health care delivery at the subcenter level is: **Panchayat Raj**.
b. The number of live births divided by the mid-year population and multiplied by 1000 is known as: **Early Neonatal Rate**.
c. National AIDS Control Program was launched in the year: **1987**.
d. The pioneer of immunization is: **Edward Jenner**.

VII. State whether the following are *true* or *false*:

a. In demography family size means total number of persons in the family: **TRUE**.
b. Census is taken at intervals of 10 years: **TRUE**.
c. For every 5000 rural populations, there are 4 multipurpose health workers: **FALSE**.

VIII. a. What is health team?

See Question no. IX a of GNM Paper-3-2013

b. Explain the role of female health worker in health team

Community health workers are often responsible for the health of members of the community who may not be cared for by traditional medical institutions. This often includes the uninsured, migrant workers and immigrants. Those served include people of all different ethnicities and cultural backgrounds. Community health workers may be responsible for ensuring that culturally diverse populations and underserved communities receive the proper medical attention. Community health workers may be lay members of the community rather than trained medical personnel and work for pay or as volunteers. Those that work in this field may go by many different titles, including community health adviser, health advocate, community health representative, health promoter or health educator. Community health workers often provide some basic direct services as well, such as first aid and some types of health screening.

IX. a. What are the major health problems in India?

See Question no. VIII-b of GNM Paper-3-2012

b. Explain the role of a nurse in the National Malaria Control Program?

Malaria is a protozoal disease caused by infection with parasites of the genus *Plasmodium* and transmitted to man by certain species of infected female *Anopheles* mosquito.

Pathogenesis

1. **Agent factors:** Malaria caused by *Plasmodium vivax, P. malariae, P. falciparum* and *P. ovale*. As parasites *P. vivax, P. ovale* and *P. malariae* may persist for years in the liver and are responsible for the chronic carrier state. Because blood transfusions and street-drug paraphernalia also can spread malaria, drug –addicts have a higher incidence of the disease.
2. **Host factors:** Malaria affects all ages. Newborn infants have considerable resistance to infection with *P. falciparum*. Males are more frequently exposed to the risk of acquiring malaria than females in India. Malaria is predominantly a rural disease and is closely related to agriculture practices.
3. **Environmental factors:** Malaria is a seasonal disease, in most parts of India; the maximum prevalence is from July to November. Rain in general provides opportunities for the breeding of mosquitoes and may give rise to epidemics of malaria. Burrow pits, garden pools, irrigation channels and engineering projects have led to the breeding of mosquitoes and an increase in malaria. Malaria consequent on human undertaking is called "Man-made malaria".
4. **Mode of transmission:** Malaria is transmitted by the bite of female anopheles mosquitoes. Direct transmissions occur may be induced accidentally by hypodermic intramuscular and intra-injections of blood or plasma. Congenital infection of the newborn from an infected mother may also occur but it is comparatively rare.
5. **Incubation period:** This is the length of time between the infective mosquito bite and the first appearance of clinical signs of which fever is most common. This period is usually not less than 10 days.

Preventive Measures

1. Avoid stagnation of water near the dwelling places and other parts of the city or town or village.
2. Sanitary improvement, such as filling all the pits of depressions, ponds, pools, etc. to eliminate breeding and hiding places of mosquito and larvae.
3. Where residual insecticides are not available then an aerosol preparation or liquid of pyrethrum should be used spray living and sleeping quarters.

4. Until malaria ceases to be in endemic, immediate and yearly application or liquid residual insecticide (e.g. DDT) in suitable dosage and formula on the inside of the walls of houses and surfaces where mosquito habitually rests.

It passes through the punctured skin or makes the skin on its own and finally reaches the system. The dynamics of transmission depends man–mosquito contact.

5. Incubation period—the time interval inoculation of infective larvae and the first appearance of detectable microfilariae (mf) is known as "pre patient period" development of clinical manifestations is known "clinical incubation period". This period most common is 8–16 months.

Antilarval Measures

1. **DDT (dichlorodiphenyl trichloroethane):** It is effectively used in little amount, e.g. 5–10% oily solution used for spraying or 10% used for dusting on larvae.
2. **Gammexane WPD:** It is used in wet breeding places/zones. Gammexane WPD is mixed in 1 gallon water and used. It has non-effect on eggs and pupaes.
3. Paris green or Acetoarsenite of copper, which is mixed with 100 parts of slaked lime, fine road dust, saw dust, sea stone, etc. and the sprayed.

Anti-adult measures: In this method, mosquitoes are killed. Spraying and dusting is done mainly in the houses, building, etc.

1. Protect against bite of mosquitoes by applying repellents. Cover the body with clothes, using mosquito nets and screening houses.
2. Gammexane: Gammexane powder 12 ozs. Mixed with 1 gallon water and sprayed with pressure sprayer.
3. DDT: It is very effective and may be used with kerosene oil, flit, pyrethrum, etc.

Control Measures

1. Isolate patient in screened room or use mosquito net to prevent spread of this diseases.
2. Investigate source of infection, contacts and find out history of previous attack of malaria from the person.
3. Report about the case to the health authorized immediately.
4. Infected places should be disinfected by spraying effective insecticide.
5. As far as possible rigid antimosquito sanitation should be maintained within the mosquitoes fight range of all parts and airports.
6. Survey should be done to know about the number of cases to find out hyperendemic and endemic areas.

Nursing Interventions

1. Assess the patient on admission and daily thereafter for fatigue, fever, orthostatic hypotension, disorientation, myalgia and arthralgia. Enforce bed rest during periods of acute illness.
2. Institute standard precautions. Protect the patient from secondary bacterial infection by following proper hand washing and aseptic techniques. Double bag all contaminated lines and send them to the laundry as an isolation them.
3. When patient gets rigor, give him complete bed rest, enough blankets, hot water bags.
4. During hot stage, watch for rise of temperature, general condition of the patient and record temperature. If it is necessary, give cold compressed ice bag to bring his temperature down.

5. During highest of fever, collect blood sample and prepare the slide and send it for examination.
6. During sweating stage, wipe his body with clean and dry clothes, change his clothes and bed linen. If necessary remove blankets.
7. Given general nursing care: Administer prescribed medications, observe for any complications administer oxygen and blood infusion as per doctor's order.
8. Provide emotional support and reassurance, especially in critical illnesses.
9. Report all cases of malaria to local public health authorities.
10. Encourage frequent coughing and breathing exercises and record amount and color of the sputum.
11. Watch for adverse effects of drug therapy and take measures to relieve them.

X. a. Define family planning, b. List the scope of family planning services, c. Briefly explain the role of a nurse in Family Welfare Program

According to WHO expert committee in 1971 defined and described "Family Planning refers to practices that help individuals and couples to attain certain objectives like, to avoid unwanted births, at which births occur in relation to the ages of the patient and to determine the number of children in the family."

Family planning is the way of thinking and living that it is adopted voluntarily upon the basis of knowledge attitude and responsible decisions by individuals and couples in order to promote the health and welfare of the health and welfare of the family group and thus contribute effectively to the social development of a country.

Objectives of Family Planning (WHO-1971)
1. To avoid unwanted births.
2. To bring about wanted births.
3. To regulate the intervals between pregnancies.
4. To control the time at which birth occurs in relation to the age of the parents.
5. To determine the number of children in the family.

Planning Commission Recommendations
1. Widespread education creates necessary social background for the success of family planning program.
2. Integration of family planning with the normal health services.
3. Provision of family planning services, even sterilization through medical and health centers.
4. To develop training program in teaching hospitals and medical college.
5. To stimulate and utilize the voluntary leadership.

Scope of Family Planning Services: A WHO expert committee (1970) has stated that family planning includes the following services:
1. The proper spacing and limitation of birth.
2. Advice of sterility.
3. Education for parenthood.
4. Sex education.
5. Screening for pathological conditions related to the reproductive system.
6. Genetic counseling.
7. Premarital consultation and examination.
8. Carrying out pregnancy tests.

9. Marriage counseling.
10. The preparation of couple for the arrival of their first child.
11. Providing services for unmarried mothers.
12. Teaching home economics and nutrition.
13. Providing adoption services.

Health Aspects of Family Planning
1. **Women's health:** Maternal mortality and morbidity of women of childbearing age nutritional status (weight changes, hemoglobin level, etc.) preventable complications of pregnancy and abortion.
2. **Fetal health:** Fetal mortality (early and late fetal death).
3. **Infant and child health:** It includes neonatal, infant and preschool mortality, health of the infant at birth (birth weight), and vulnerability to diseases.
4. **The family welfare concept:** It is very comprehensive and is basically related to quality of life. The Family Welfare Program aims at achieving a higher end that is, to improve the quality of life.
5. **Small family norm:** The objective of the Family Welfare Program in India is that people should adopt the "Small family norm to stabilize the country's population at the level of some 1533 million by the year 2050 AD.
6. **Eligible couples:** It refers to a currently married couple wherein the wife is in the reproductive ages of 15 and 45. There will be at least 150–180 couples per 1000 population in India needs family planning services.
7. **Target couples:** It was applied to couples who have had 2–3 living children and family planning was largely directed to such couples.
8. **Couple protection rate (CPR):** It is an indicator of the prevalence of contraceptive practice in the community. National Population Policy was to attain CPR of 42 percent by 1990 and 60% by the year 2000. Couple protection rate is a dominant factor in the reduction of net reproduction rate.

2010
Community Health Nursing

SECTION-I

I. State whether the following are *true* or *false*:
   a. In India, there is one community health center for every 80,000 populations.
   b. The integrated health services was defined by Mukherjee Committee.
   c. About 10% of accidents in industry are said to be due to mechanical causes.
   d. The principle unit of administration in India is the districts.

II. Fill in the blanks with suitable answers:
   a. The most important recommendations of placing health in people's hands was by the: _____
   b. The financial and technical assistance for development of poor countries is provided by: _____
   c. Three-tier structure of local self government in India is known as: _____
   d. The administrative head of a district is: _____

III. Write short notes on any *four* of the following:
   a. Recommendations of Bhore Committee Report.
   b. Child survival and safe motherhood (CSSH) or RCH services.
   c. Voluntary health agencies in India.
   d. Determinants of health.
   e. Epidemiological triad.

IV. a. What is occupational health?
   b. List the important occupational diseases.
   c. Explain the role of a nurse in industrial nursing.

Or

   a. Define health for all by 2000 AD.
   b. List the goals of health for all.
   c. Discuss the role of a nurse in primary health care.

SECTION-II

V. Fill in the blanks with suitable answers:
   a. The cold chain system, all vaccines can be stored for few months at: _____
   b. Objective of Tuberculosis Control Program is to achieve 85% cure rate through: _____
   c. The first step in controlling a communicable disease is: _____
   d. In India, the last census was done in the year: _____

VI. State whether the following are *true* or *false*:
   a. Health survey are used for diagnosing community health problems: _____
   b. Sex ratio is defined as number of males per 1000 females: _____
   c. The concepts of family welfare is basically related to quality of life: _____

VII. a. What are the various national health programs of India?
   b. Explain the universal immunization program.

VIII. a. What is infertility?
   b. Explain in detail the methods of family planning.

IX. a. Define vital statistics.
   b. Explain the sources and uses of health statistics.

SECTION-I

I. State whether the following are *true* or *false*:
a. In India, there is one community health center for every 80,000 populations: **TRUE**.
b. The integrated health services was defined by Mukherjee Committee: **FALSE**.
c. About 10% of accidents in industry are said to be due to mechanical causes: **TRUE**.
d. The principle unit of administration in India is the districts: **TRUE**.

II. Fill in the blanks with suitable answers:
a. The most important recommendations of placing health in people's hands was by the: **Srivastava Committee**.
b. The financial and technical assistance for development of poor countries is provided by: **UNESCO**
c. Three-tier structure of local self government in India is known as: **Panchayat Raj**
d. The administrative head of a district is: **District Collector**

III. Write short notes on any *four* of the following:

a. Recommendations of Bhore Committee Report

In 1943, the Government of India appointed a Committee as the Bhore Committee for the health survey and development committee with Sir, Joseph Bhore as Chairman. Its aim was to survey the existing position regarding the health conditions and health organization in the committee which had among its members some of the pioneers of the health, met regularly for 2 years and submitted its famous report in 1946 which runs into 4 volumes.

Important Recommendations
1. **Nutrition of the people:** They pointed out the main defects of the average Indian diet results from the insufficiency of proteins, mineral salts and vitamins. They also recommend special measures to increase the production of food rich in proteins. Also prevention of food adulteration and improvement of the quality of the food.
2. **Health education:** Bhore Committee suggested that health education to school children on hygiene should begin at the earliest. The doctor, nurse, midwife and in fact every health worker will discharge his or her duties and by educating the persons with whom they deal with regard to prevention of disease and the promotion of positive health.
3. **Physical examination:** Committee stated that there is great dearth of suitable and qualified teachers for imparting instructions in this subject. Also physical training program for the community with emphasis on national games and exercises.
4. **Health services for mothers and children:** At the headquarters of each primary unit and in place where 30 bed hospitals are located the service for mothers and children should be available.
5. **Health services of the school children:** The school teachers who have to carry or certain health duties require careful training and continuous supervision. They have to conduct health education programs. In each primary unit, the male medical officer should take charge of the school health services.
6. **Occupational heath including industrial health:** The committee recommended that the industrial health organization should form an integral part of the provincial health department and government.

7. **Health services for certain important diseases:** Bhore Committee studied the existing legal and administrative provisions to deal with communicable diseases and suggested certain measures for controlling communicable diseases.
8. **Environmental hygiene:** An essential part of the campaign for promoting public health was to improve man's physical environment. The committee's main recommendations were improvement in village and town planning.
9. **Vital Statistics:** The committee recommended administrative organization at the center, organization at provincial head quarters and district organization. Another recommendation is provision of training facilities for statistics.
10. **Professional education:** The main objective of the committee during his period was the provision of adequate and suitably trained staff to enable the plan of health work effectively.
11. **Drug and medical requisites:** They recommended our universities should undertake research with a view to produce life saving drugs in this country.

b. Child survival and safe motherhood (CSSM) or RCH services

Importance of CSSM Health Services

1. Since the conception the development of fetus (280 days) takes place in the mother's womb and receives all nutrition and oxygen from the mother.
2. Healthy mother brings forth a healthy child. Healthy mother can avoid premature birth, stillbirth or abortion.
3. Certain habits and diseases conditions of expected mother will affect the child health, i.e. taking drugs, syphilis, German measles.
4. After birth, the child is completely dependent upon the mother for various reasons at least for a year separation of child from mother hinders the growth and development.
5. Child learns many self care tasks from the mother.

Objectives of CSSM

1. Sustaining and strengthening the ongoing Universal Immunization Program (UIP), continuing oral rehydration therapy (ORT) program for children below the age of 5 years, introducing and expanding the program for control of acute respiratory infection for children below 5 years of age.
2. Universalizing the existing prophylaxis scheme for control of blindness due to deficiency of vitamin A for children up to the age of 3 years and prophylaxis scheme against nutritional anemia among pregnant and lactating mothers as well as children up to 5 years of age through administration of iron and folic acid tablets.
3. Improving newborn care and maternal care at the community level.

Components of CSSM

1. Early registration of pregnancy.
2. To provide minimum three antenatal checkups.
3. Universal coverage of all pregnant women with IT immunization.
4. Advice on food, nutrition and rest.
5. Detection of high risk pregnancies and prompt referral.
6. Clean deliveries by trained personnel.
7. Birth spacing.
8. Promotion of institutional deliveries.

Strategies of CSSM
1. Train medical and other health personnel in essential newborn care.
2. Provide basic facilities for care for low birth weight and sick newborns in the first referral units and district hospitals.
3. Create awareness about essential newborn among health care providers, pregnant women and mothers of the newborns.
4. Use of low cost-effective and locally available equipment for newborn care.
5. Improve maternal care and promote birth spacing.

Goals of CSSM
1. IMR, MMR, and under five mortality rates mentioned in MCH goals.
2. Polio eradication by 2000 AD.
3. Neonatal tetanus elimination by 1995.
4. Measles prevention.

Reproductive and Child Health Program
Reproductive and child health (RCH) can be defined as a state in which "People have the ability to reproduce and regulate their fertility, women are able to go through Pregnancy and childbirth safely, the outcome of pregnancy is successful in terms of maternal and infant survival and wellbeing, and couples are able to have sexual relations free of the fear of pregnancy and contracting disease. The origin of the RCH initiative can be justifiably traced from the Alma Ata declaration wherein maternal and child health care including family planning was identified as an important element in the primary health care package. In 1994, the CSSM was replaced by RCH (Reproductive and Child Health) program in India. RCH incorporates all the elements of the parent CSSM program besides including two more elements namely, the control of sexually transmitted infections (SITs) and the control of reproductive tract infections (RTIs). RCH program is a joint venture supported by inputs for the Government of India and various donors' agencies including the World Bank and the European Commission. The program is envisaged to provide need-based, client centered, demand driven high quality, integrated services to the eligible population of young women and children. The program was formally launched on 15th October, 1997.

Objectives of RCH
1. The immediate objective is the promotion of maternal and child health to ensure safe method and child survival.
2. The intermediate objective is the reduction of maternal and child morbidity and mortality.
3. The ultimate objective is the attainment of population stabilization through responsible reproductive behavior, expected to emerge in response to reduced risk to child survival.

Organization and Administration
1. **Organizational infrastructure:** MCH service activity of the primary health care system makes it an ideal organization for offering RCH services to the community through its nationwide network of community health centers, primary health centers and subcenters.
2. **Consultants:** There is provision for the engagement of consultants for the project period. The appointment of consultants is on contractual basis in keeping with the World Bank procedure.

The service of consultants is needed for improving the management, implementation and monitoring of RCH program.
3. **Traditional practitioners:** There is a provision for involvement traditional practitioners to receive an orientation training course, to update their knowledge and improve their skills in the areas of RCH activity.
4. **Non-governmental organizations:** It is felt that NGOs would serve as complementary agency for optimizing the functioning of RCH program. They are better place to try innovative approaches which the conventional government system cannot afford.
5. **Equipment and supplies:** There is provision for supplying equipment kits, surgical kits, delivery kits, IUD kits and MTP kits to help in improving the quality and content of RCH service to the eligible population.

c. Voluntary health agencies in India

Voluntary health agencies are the private enterprises for social process. Voluntary action is the soul of democracy as this medium secures the active involvement of the people from policy making to implementation of social services. Many organizations at national level are linked with international federation or association. The program of voluntary organizations which is of great and direct relevance to health care administration includes, projects to improve nutritional literacy, provide education and instructional material enhance community development, improve environmental sanitation, child and women welfare, etc.

Functions of Voluntary Health Agencies

1. Creating a sense of responsibility through direct involvement.
2. Channelize human resources.
3. Effective policy formation through interpretation of public opinion.
4. Participation of beneficiaries.
5. Flexibility and experimentation.
6. Initiative and leadership.
7. Supplements the efforts of government.
8. Help in efficient program implementation.
9. Advancing health legislation.

Problems of Voluntary Health Agencies

1. Governmental interference in the activities of voluntary; organizations.
2. Lack of interest among the intellectual elite.
3. Lack of effective collaboration among voluntary agencies themselves.
4. Lack of competence to develop integrated area plan.
5. Poor linkage with the beneficiaries.
6. Absence of sound administrative set-up to deal with social work.

d. Determinants of health

Some of the important health determinants are described here:

Environmental determinants: Environment has the direct impact on the health of individual, family or community. Internal or external and physical, biological and psychosocial components of environment influence the mental, social, spiritual and physical well-being of individuals, Environmental pollution has become a global threat. We must find the ways to reduce and manage the pollution as well as waste. It is worth mentioning that Florence Nightingale had also given importance to environmental factors in the maintenance of the health and care of the sick. Air, water, noise, radiation, housing, waste-management, etc., all affect the health status and quality of life.

Political system: Political system has a great effect on the social climate in which we live. Political influences have the power and authority to regulate much of our surroundings in that, health care is also included. Implementation of any health program cannot be conducted properly without the strong political will. In our country, health is a subject of concurrent list, so there is a need of coordination between the union and state governments in the health-related matters.

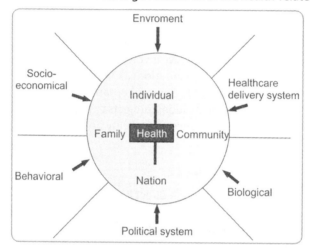

Behavioral determinants: Health is the mirror of a person's lifestyle because faulty and ill habits have the adverse effect on the health of the individual. It is an established fact that culture and ethnic heritage shape much of our lifestyle including the health care.

Socioeconomic determinants: Socioeconomic conditions have the major impact on the health status of any country. Education, economy, occupational opportunities, housing, nutritional level, per capita income, etc. determine the healthcare system and health resources.

Healthcare delivery system determinants: The healthcare delivery system plays a great role in the field of health, This is considered as a disease-oriented system, but in our country which has the second largest population in the world, providing healthcare services at the grass-roots level is a difficult task.

Besides the above-mentioned determinants women's issue, aging population, agriculture, social welfare, rural development, urban improvement, etc. also have a major impact on the health of the nation, its families and individuals.

e. Epidemiological traid

The epidemiology demands a broader concept of disease causation that synthesized the basic factors of agent, host and environment. An individual health is never static and is always in a dynamic equilibrium with his environment. The condition of health is seen as the resultant of various ecologic interactions determines the health status in the human organism.

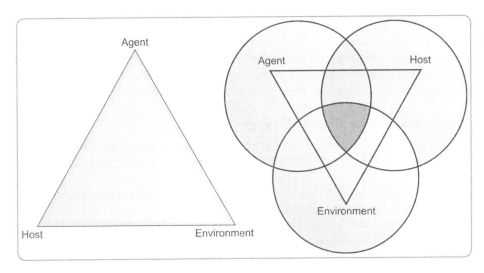

I. **Agent factors:** Disease causing agent in the environment may be classified into the following categories. Inanimate group of agents mainly responsible for noncommunicable disease, such as physical agents, chemical agents, nutritional agents and biological agents.
   a. **Physical agents:** Heat, light, radiation, etc.
   b. **Chemical agents:** Acids, alkalies, metals, etc.
   c. **Nutritional agents:** Lack or excess of nutritional factors.
   Biological agents, the disease caused are always transmissible from one individual to another individual and therefore, they are called "communicable diseases". Some of the communicable diseases are transferable only through another medium like insects, where the agents undergo certain changes in their cycles.
II. **Environmental factors:** Environment is the aggregate of all external conditions and influence affecting the life and development of an organism. It is classified as below:
   a. **Physical environment:** All those inanimate objects like air, water, food, etc.
   b. **Biological environment:** All those animate objects like animals, insects and other humans.
   c. **Socioeconomic environment:** Social and economic factors like housing social group, education, etc.
III. **Host factors:** Age, sex, habits and customs, general and specific defense mechanism genetic makeup and psychobiological characteristics of the host are some of the important factors which determine the outcome of interaction between the agents and host in a suitable environment.

IV. a. What is occupational health?
   b. List the important occupational diseases
   c. Explain the role of a nurse in industrial nursing

The joint committee of ILO/ WHO on occupational health, held in 1950 for the first time gave the following statements about occupational health. The general aims of occupational health should be the promotion and maintenance of highest degree of physical, mental and social wellbeing of workers in all occupations, the prevention among workers of departures from health caused by their working conditions the protection of workers in their respective employments from risks resulting from factors adverse to health, the placing and maintenance of the workers in an occupational environment adopted to their physiological and psychological needs.

Occupational Health Nursing

The application of nursing principles in conserving the health of worker in all occupations. It involves prevention recognition and treatment of illness and injury, and requires special skills and knowledge in the fields of health, education and counseling environmental health, rehabilitation and human relations"—American Association of occupational health nurses.

Objectives of Occupational Health Services

1. To improve human efficiency in his work by applying ergonomics (human engineering).
2. To promote and maintain the highest degree of positive health and welfare of workers in all occupations.
3. To provide a self occupational environment in order to safeguard the health of the workers and to set up industrial production.
4. To protect from factors adverse to health during their employment.
5. To assist the injured and disabled for rehabilitation.
6. To ensure that physical and psychological demands imposed on workers by their respective job are properly matched with their individual anatomical, physical and psychological needs, capabilities and limitations.
7. To educate workers to promote and maintain their health.
8. To provide care during emergencies.
9. To promote general health and welfare of each worker by providing a good and safe working environment.

Health Problems due to Industrialization

1. Air pollution.
2. Water pollution.
3. Soil pollution.
4. Shortage of houses.
5. Communicable diseases.
6. Mental health problems.
7. Accidents.
8. Social problems like alcoholism, drug addiction, gambling, prostitution, juvenile delinquency.
9. High morbidity and mortality from certain diseases, e.g. chronic bronchitis and lung cancer.

Roles of Occupational Health Nurse

1. Nurse practitioner.
2. Nurse educator.
3. Health administrator/manager.
4. Counselor.

Functions of Occupational Health Nurse

1. Assistance in general administration, maintenance and arrangements of health facilities in the plant.
2. Emergency and primary treatment of accidents and illness based on standing orders from physicians.
3. Arranging follow up treatments, where indicated, including health supervision of employees returning to work after illness.

4. Assistance in general preventive health measures in the plant.
5. Health education and counseling for employees.
6. Assistance in supervision of factory hygiene and accident prevention.
7. Advice on specific health questions to management and workers.
8. Maintenance of records and statistics.
9. Cooperation with and referral of workers to general community agencies for help as and when necessary.
10. Participation in a health surveillance program that includes the assessment and recording of the health status of employees.
11. Participation in the environmental control program the aims to work related.

Or

a. Define health for all by 2000 AD
b. List the goals of health for all
c. Discuss the role of a nurse in primary health care

1. The world health assembly in its 30th meeting in 1977 decided the goal of HFA and defined that "Main Social Targets of Governments and WHO" in the coming decades should be the attainment of all citizens of the world by the year 2000 of a level of health that will permit them to lead socially and economically productive life.
2. Attainment of a level of health that will enable every individual to lead a socially and economically productive life.

Goals of Health for All

1. Realization of highest possible of health which includes physical mental and social wellbeing.
2. Attainment of minimum level of health that would enable to the economically productive and participate actively in social life of community in which they live.
3. Removal of obstacles to health, such as unemployment, ignorance, poor living conditions, standards and malnutrition, etc.
4. Healthcare services are within the reach of all in the country.

Strategies for Health for All

The Alma Ata declaration called for global strategy to provide guidelines for member countries to refer. In 1981, the WHO after consultations with member countries developed a global strategy for health for all. The global strategy provides common broad frame work which can be modified and adopted by countries according to their needs.

The global strategy for HFA is based on the following principles:
1. Health is a fundamental human right and a worldwide social goal and an integral part of social and economic development of the communities.
2. People have right and the duty to participate individually and collectively in the planning and implementation of their health care.
3. The existing gross inequality in the health strategies is of common concern of all countries and must be drastically reduced.
4. Government has responsibility for the health of their people.
5. Countries and people must become self-reliant in health matters.
6. Governments and health professionals have the responsibility of providing health information to people.
7. There should be equitable distribution of resources within and among the countries but should be allocated most to those who need most.

8. Primary health care would be the key to the success of HFA and it has to be the integral part of the country's health system.
9. Development and application of appropriate technology according to healthcare system of the nation.
10. Research in the field of biomedical and health services must be conducted and findings should been applied soon.

The national health policy echoes the WHO a call for HFA and the Alma Ata declaration. It had laid down specific goals in respect of various health indicators by different dates such as 1990 and 2000 AD.
1. Reduction of infant mortality from the level of 125 (1978) to below 60.
2. To raise the expectation of life at birth from the level of 52 years to 64.
3. To reduce the crude death rate from the level of 14 per 1000 population to 90.
4. To reduce the crude birthrate from the level of 33 per 1000 population to 21.
5. To achieve a net reproduction rate of one.
6. To provide potable water to the entire rural population.

Millennium Development Goals (MDGs)

September 2000, representatives from 189 countries met at the millennium summit in New York to adopt the United Nations millennium declaration. The goals in the area of development and poverty eradication are now widely referred to as "Millennium Development Goals". Government has set a date of 2015 by which they would meet the MDGs.
1. Eradicate extreme poverty and hunger.
2. Achieve universal primary education.
3. Promote gender equality.
4. Improve maternal health.
5. Combat HIV/AIDS, malaria and other communicable diseases.
6. Ensure environmental sustainability.
7. Global partnership for development.

Health for All through Primary Health Care Strategy

I. Address major health problems of people living in various places.
II. Emphasize on preventive, promotive, curative, and rehabilitative services based on health problems and health needs of people.
III. Including the following services.
   1. Education of people concerning prevailing health problems.
   2. Promotion of nutrition.
   3. Adequate safe water supply and basic sanitation.
   4. Maternal and child health including family planning.
   5. Immunization against major infectious diseases.
   6. Prevention and control of locally endemic diseases.
   7. Appropriate treatment of common ailments and injuries.
   8. The provision of essential drugs.
IV. Take care of the following prerequisites for its successful implementation.
   1. Multisectoral approach.
   2. Community involvement.
   3. Appropriate technology.

Definition of primary health care: Primary health care is essential health care made universally accessible to individuals and families in the community, by means acceptable to them, through their full participation and at a cost that the community and country can afford. It forms an integral part of both the country's health system of which it is the nucleus and the overall social and economic development of the community (Alma Ata 1978).

Role of Nurse in PHC

1. Community health nurse work with population, community, family, individual. The focus is multiple or promoting health maintaining a degree of balance toward health.
2. Community health nurse focus on assessment of the impact of the socioeconomical and cultural factors affecting health measures that must constantly be dealt with and take priority in order to make family assume health measures.
3. The community health nurse works with entire spectrum of health and illness conditions from optimal health to minor or severe conditions from acute to chronic illness.
4. The community health nurse works in all kinds of setting, such as home, school, clinic, industry, etc.
5. The community health nurse works in school where primary goal is health education and disease prevention.
6. The community health nurse works in industry is to improve the production and employers' safety.
7. The community health nurse is responsible for assisting patients and families to coordinate health care, which necessitates contact with personnel from health, welfare and other significant community agencies.
8. Community health nurse has responsibilities in education and training of individuals, auxiliaries and others.
9. The community health nurse involves in provision of direct services to patients both preventive and curative at the out patient, Inpatient clinics and community.

Major Role of CHN in PHC

1. Facilitative role.
2. Developmental role.
3. Supportive role:
    i. Training.
    ii. Management.
    iii. Supervision.
    iv. Program implementation.
    v. Program evaluation.
    vi. Policy making.
    vii. Program planning.
4. Clinical role.

SECTION-II

V. Fill in the blanks with suitable answers

a. The cold chain system, all vaccines can be stored for few months at: **0.4°C.**
b. Objective of Tuberculosis Control Program is to achieve 85% cure rate through: **DOTS**

c. The first step in controlling a communicable disease is: **Vaccination**
d. In India, the last census was done in the year: **2011**.

VI. State whether the following are *true* or *false*:
a. Health survey are used for diagnosing community health problems: **TRUE**
b. Sex ratio is defined as number of males per 1000 females: **TRUE**
c. The concepts of family welfare is basically related to quality of life: **TRUE**

VII. a. What are the various national health programs of India?
b. Explain the Universal Immunization Program

A program is an organized aggregate of activities directed towards the attainment of defined objectives and targets national health programs, which have been launched by the Central Government for the control eradication of communicable diseases, improvement of environmental sanitation, raising the standard of nutrition, control of population and improving rural health. National health programs should be consistent with national health policies and should contribute towards the achievement of the goals contained therein. Various international agencies like WHO, UNICEF, UNFPA, World Bank, and also a number of foreign agencies like SIDA, DANIDA, NORAD and UNAID have been proving technical and material assistance in the implementation of these Programs.

The health problems are listed below:

Eradication Programs
1. National Malaria Eradication Program.
2. National Leprosy Eradication Program.
3. National Guinea Worm Eradication Program.
4. Polio Eradication Program.

Control Programs
1. National Filarial Control Program.
2. National Tuberculosis Control Program.
3. National Goiter Control Program.
4. National Diarrheal Diseases Control Program.
5. Program for Control of Acute Respiratory Infections.
6. Sexually Transmitted Disease Control Program.
7. National AIDS Prevention and Control Program.
8. National Program for Control of Blindness.
9. Anemia Control Program.
10. National Cancer Control Program.

Other Health Programs
1. National Water Supply and Sanitation Program.
2. Universal Immunization Program.
3. National Family Welfare Program.
4. School Health Program.
5. National Program for Maternal and Child Health.

6. Child Survival and Safemotherhood Program.
7. Reproductive Child Health Program.

Universal Immunization Program (UIP-1985): In 1974, WHO launched its "Expanded Program on Immunization"(EPI) against six most common, preventable childhood disease viz diphtheria pertussis (whooping cough) tetanus, polio, tuberculosis and measles. From the beginning of the program, UNICEF has been providing significant support to EPI. The primary healthcare concept as enunciated in the 1978 Alma Ata declaration included immunization as one of the strategies for reaching the goal of "Health for All" by the year 2000. While the WHO's program is called EPI, the UNICEF in 1985 renamed is as "Universal Child Immunization"(UCI).

Program Objectives

1. To reduce morbidity, mortality and disability in children from the six vaccine-preventable diseases to a level where these diseases would cease to be major public health problems.
2. To promote country's self-reliance in the production of vaccines and the delivery of immunization service within the context of comprehensive health care.
3. To eradicate paralytic poliomyelitis before the year 1995, and reduce the incidence of measles by 90% by the year 1995.

Organization and Administration

1. **Organization structure:** UIP is essentially a team activity demanding close cooperation of health functionaries. For operational convenience, it is worthwhile that UIP be integrated with maternal and child health program including reproductive health care. For all these reasons, the primary health care network of the country provides the appropriate infrastructure for the implementation of UIP.
2. **Cold chain system**: The process of preserving the potency of vaccines at low temperature during storage at various levels or during transportation from central stores to state stores and hence to district stores and further onwards to CHC level, PHC level, subcenter level and down to village level is referred to as cold chain.
3. **Logistics and supplies**: The efficiency of the logistic support is therefore dependent upon transport facilities, cold chain arrangements, short period supplies and close and sustainable monitoring operations. The vaccines are kept for as short period of time as possible at the peripheral institutions. Only 1 month's vaccine requirement is permitted in the PHC level and not more than 3 months requirement is maintained at district level.

Program Implementation

I. Immunization schedule
1. **Universal Immunization Program** schedule provides for administering dose of TT to pregnant women, 3 doses of DPT and oral palio vaccine (OPV) and 1 dose each of BCG and measles vaccines to infants and booster does of DT/TT to school children.
2. **Pregnancy:** Immunization of pregnant women with tetanus toxoid stimulates the protection her against puerperal tetanus. It also lends passive immunity to the fetus and protects it against neonatal tetanus.
3. **Infancy:** It is safer to immunize infants against conventional childhood diseases soon after they are 6 weeks old. Accordingly the schedule, recommends DPT and OPV immunization of infants from 6 weeks onwards. BCG vaccination is recommended at birth in institutional deliveries or routinely with any of the DPT/QPV vaccine doses thereafter.

II. Immunization process: Universal immunization program activity was set in two dimensions horizontal and vertical. The horizontal activity is the basic immunization efforts against the six vaccine preventable diseases. The vertical activity is focused on the eradication of poliomyelitis.

VIII. a. What is infertility?
b. Explain in detail the methods of family planning

Infertility, inability to conceive or carry a child to delivery. The term is usually limited to situations where the couple has had intercourse regularly for one year without using birth control. The term *sterility* is restricted to lack of sperm production or inability to ovulate. Approximately, 40% of reported cases of infertility are due to problems in the male; another 40% to problems in the female; the remaining 20% are of unknown cause or due to problems in both the male and female.

Causes: Infertility can be caused by any interruption in the usual process of fertilization, pregnancy, and birth, which includes ejaculation of normal amounts of healthy sperm, passage of the sperm through the cervix and into the fallopian tube of the female, passage of an ovum (egg) down the fallopian tube from an ovary, fertilization in the fallopian tube, implantation of the fertilized egg in a receptive uterus, and the ability to carry the fetus to term. In women, the most common problems are failure to ovulate and blockage of the fallopian tubes. In men, low sperm count is the most common problem.

Underlying problems include disease, such as diabetes or mumps in adult men, hormonal imbalances, endometriosis, pelvic inflammatory disease (often caused by sexually transmitted diseases, e.g. *Chlamydia*), the abuse of alcohol and other drugs, and exposure to workplace hazards or environmental toxins. Uterine irritation or infection that sometimes accompanies IUD use can also reduce fertility. Occasionally, there is a chemical or immunological incompatibility between male and female. Psychological factors are difficult to evaluate because of the stressful nature of infertility itself. The number of couples seeking treatment for infertility has increased as more of them have postponed childbearing to a later age. In women, fertility begins to decline in the mid-twenties, and continues to decline, more and more sharply, until menopause. Male fertility declines gradually until age forty, then declines more quickly.

Natural Methods of Family Planning

1. **Total sexual abstinence:** It costs nothing except self-denial on the part of the couple.
2. **Periodic abstinence:** Otherwise called as rhythm or calendar method or safe method. It is based on restricting the sex act to the infertile period of the female partner.
3. **Temperature method:** During ovulation naturally the basal body temperature rise of 0.5°C. Based on prediction of the time of ovulation by taking the basal body temperature daily and avoiding sexual intercourse around the time of ovulation.
4. **Billing method:** It relies on the charges in cervical mucus secretion also called mucus method. This method is based on observation of changes in the characteristics of cervical mucus.
5. **Symptothermic method:** This method combines the use of basal body temperature with analysis of cervical mucus changes to make temperature with analysis of cervical mucus changes to make predictions more accurate.
6. **Coitus interruptus:** It is an ancient method that requires the male to withdraw his penis from the vagina immediately before the ejaculation of the semen.
7. **Coitus interfemoris:** The erect penis is placed between the thighs of the female.
8. **Lactation amenorrhea method:** It is believed that there is a high probability that the women who is amenorrheal while breastfeeding, will be able to regulate her fertility in first 6 months postpartum even if she introduces supplementation in the baby's feeding.

9. **Barrier method:** Barrier methods of contraception have a long history. The ancient Egyptians used such methods which consisted of honey—coated pessaries. Honey is effective in killing sperms as well as bacteria.

Chemical Methods of Family Planning

Chemical barriers are usually spermicidal or spermistatic. In addition, they may have some blocking action at the cervix. Sperm thrive best at an alkaline pH of 8.5–9.0. Because the vagina is normally acidic until ovulation.
1. **The foam tablets:** The foam tablets which a woman inserts into her birth canal before having sex produce some foam which provides a productive coating to the whole area.
2. **Cream, jelly and paste:** The spermicidal jelly or cream is similarly applied in the vagina with the help of an applicator. It destroys the male sperm on contact in the vaginal canal itself.
3. **Suppositories and soluble film:** The suppositories and soluble films take time to dissolve in the vaginal fluids. It kills the sperm released from the man's body and thus prevents pregnancy.

Mechanical Barriers of Family Planning

These methods are which prevent meeting of sperms with ovum, the sperms are prevented from entering the cervix by mechanical barriers.
1. **Condom:** The condom or nirodh is an extremely thin rubber sheath used by the man. It has been used since 14th century. The condom is fitted on the erect male organ before intercourse. The air must be expelled from the teat before it is put on. Condom acts be preventing the entry sperms into vagina.
2. **Diaphgram:** It is curved rubber dome enclosed by flexible metal ring that rests in the vagina and covers the cervix. It was invented by a German physician in 1882, also known as "Dutch cap". It is made of soft synthetic rubber or plastic with a stiff but flexible rim around the edges. It is available in different sizes ranging from 5–10 cm.
3. **Cervical cap:** The use of cervical cap is a variation of the diaphgram. It is smaller than diaphragm and is designed to fit over the neck of the womb. Once the cervical cap is placed, it can remain from the end of one menstruation to just before the start of the next.
4. **Vaginal sponge:** A small polyurethane foam sponge measuring 5 cm × 2.5 cm is saturated with spermicide, nonoxynol-9 and inserted into vagina. It is less effective than the diaphragm. It may be inserted before intercourse. It is more convenient to use it than some of the other vaginal contraceptives.

Intrauterine Devices

Intrauterine device is inserted into the cavity to prevent conception. The device which is placed in the womb may be inert or medicated. The inert device is made up of plastic material only and the medicated devices are fortified with copper, silver or a progestation preparation.
1. **Lippes loop:** It is a double S-shaped serpentine device made of polythene impregnated with barium sulfate for radiopacity. Two pieces of nylon (transcervical threads) are attached to the lower end of the loop forming tail, the nylon tail projects into the vagina. Periodic feeling for the tail reassures the user that the loop is in place. The tail also helps in easy removal of the device.
2. **Copper-T**: The copper-T is made of plastic but is wrapped with fine copper which enhances its contraceptive effect. Its acceptance is higher than that of the loop. It is I shaped bioactive contraceptive device made of polyethylene or any other polymer and reinforced with copper metal. The devices are impregnated with barium sulfate for radio opacity and are fitted with two transcervical threads at the tail end. Metallic copper possess a strong antifertility action.

Hormonal Contraceptives methods of family planning: Hormonal contraceptives are composed of synthetic gonadal steroids-estrogens and progestogens. Estrogens used are ethinyl estradiol and menstranol. The synthetic progestogens usually used are norethindrone and norgestrel. Hormonal contraceptives are available as pills, injectables, implants an devices.

Oral Pills

1. **Combined pill:** The main action of the combined pill is inhibition of ovulation by blocking the secretion of gonadotropin from pituitary gland. The progestogen also alters the cervical mucosa which prevents the entry of sperms into genital canal. There are two types of pills which are available under the brand name of mala-N and mala-D. Mala-N and Mala-D are available in packet of 28 tablets. The first white tablets are contraceptive pills and the remaining seven pill are iron pills which are brown.
2. **Progesterone only pill:** This pill is also known as minipill. This pill contains only synthetic progesterone in very small quantity. The progesterone thickens the cervical mucus which prevents the entry of sperms into the uterine cavity. Minipills are taken throughout the menstrual cycle.
3. **Once a month pill:** It is a modified combined pill. It contains long-acting estrogen and short-acting progesterone. This pill is not in use because of its poor result and irregularity in menstrual cycle.

Injectable Contraceptives

1. **Progesterone-only injectable:** It contains synthetic progestogen, it prevents ovulation, thickens the cervical mucus which interferes with penetration of sperms into genital canal. DEMPA (Depot-Medroxy, progesterone acetate) available as Noristerat, injectable once in three months and later once in two months (60 days). Another form of injectable is NET-EN (norethisterone anantate). DEMPA is found to be more successful than NET-EN.
2. **Combined injectable contraceptives:** These contraceptives contain progesterone and estrogen. It prevents ovulation, thickens the cervical mucus which interferes with entry of sperms into the birth canal. The injection is given once in a month. Thorough medical examination must be done by the doctor before prescribing injectable contraceptives.
3. **Subdermal implants:** Subdermal Implants are developed by population council of New York. There are two varities, one is nor plant and the latest is Norplant R-2. Norplant R-2 has two small rods; these devices are placed surgically under the skin of the arm by the doctor. After five years, the implant is removed surgically. The actions of these impants are the same as that of injectable contraceptives.

Terminal Methods of Family Planning

1. **Sterilization:** It is the only method which gives permanent protection from contraception. It is safe and a permanent one time means of contraception. Sterilization is a method of the risk of accidental pregnancy. In sterilization, either husband or wife can undergo a simple surgical operation, i.e. vasectomy or tubectomy.
2. **Vasectomy:** It is sterilization of male, very simple and minor operation which takes hardly 15–20 minutes. The operation can be done in primary health center under local anesthesia by a trained doctor. A septic technique is to be followed to prevent infection. The operation involves a small cut on both sided of the scrotum, then a small portion of vas deferens on either side of the scrotum, is cut and ligated, folded back and sutured.
3. **Tubectomy:** It is sterilization of females, done by resecting a small part of fallopian tubes and ligated the sected ends. The closing of tubes also be done by using other alternative

methods like closing with bands, clips, electrocautery. The operation can be done through abdominal or vaginal approach. The most common abdominal procedures are laparoscopy and minilaparotomy.

IX. a. Define vital statistics
b. Explain the sources and uses of vital statistics

Vital statistics provide a tool for measuring the dynamics of change which continuously occur in population. Vital statistics are derived from legally registrable events without including population data or morbidity statistics.

Definitions of Vital Statistics

1. Vital statistics are conventionally numerical records of marriage, births, sickness and deaths by which the health and growth of community may be studied.
2. Vital statistics is a part of demography and collective study of mankind. It deals with the data related to vital events.
3. It is a branch of biometry deals with data and law of human mortality, morbidity and demography.
4. Vital statistics is the numerical description of birth, death, absorption, marriage, divorce, adoption and judicial separation—UNO.

Purpose of Vital Statistics

1. **Community health:** To describe the level of community health, to diagnose community illness, and to discover solutions to health problems.
2. **Administrative purpose:** It provides clues for administrative action and to create administrative standards of health activities.
3. **Health programmed organization:** To determine success or failure of specific health programmed or undertake overall evaluation of public health work.
4. **Legislative purpose:** To promote health legislation at local, state and national level.
5. **Governmental purpose:** To develop policies procedures, at state and central level.

Uses of Vital Statistics

1. To evaluate the impact of various national health programs.
2. To plan for better future measures of disease control.
3. To elucidate the hereditary nature of disease.
4. To plan and evaluate economic and social development.
5. It is a primary tool in research activities.
6. To determine the health status of individual.
7. To compare the health status of one nation with others.

Methods of Obtaining Vital Statistics

1. **Census:** It is a simultaneous recording demographic, social and economic data of individuals. It is an important method of collecting vital statistics. Census is conducted every 10 years.
2. **Registration:** Registration of vital events, e.g. births, deaths. Keep a continuous check on demographic changes. If registration of vital events is complete and accurate, it can serve as a reliable source of health information.
3. **Adhoc survey:** Surveys for evaluating the health status of a population that is community diagnosis of problems of health.